THE
FAMILY
ENCYCLOPEDIA OF
HEALTH

Dr R. Sharma

MB, BCh, LRCP&S[I], MFHom

Dr Rajendra Sharma is former Medical Director of the world-renowned Hale Clinic. He is associated with practices in Europe and the United States, where he blends the culture and medical techniques of East and West. Dr Sharma has studied with specialists in most alternative medical fields. While his particular interest is in working with cancer, HIV/AIDS and other serious and chronic illnesses, Dr Sharma is considered by many to be their family doctor.

THE
FAMILY
ENCYCLOPEDIA OF
HEALTH

A GUIDE TO
INTEGRATED MEDICINE, ENJOYING HEALTH
AND PREVENTING ILLNESS BY COMBINING
COMPLEMENTARY AND ORTHODOX THERAPIES

DR RAJENDRA SHARMA

MB, BCh, LRCP&S[I], MFHom

Thorsons

Thorsons
An Imprint of HarperCollins*Publishers*
77–85 Fulham Palace Road,
Hammersmith, London W6 8JB

The Thorsons website address is:
www.thorsons.com

and *Thorsons*
are trademarks of
HarperCollins*Publishers* Ltd

First published by Element Books Ltd 1998
This updated edition published by Thorsons 2002

1 3 5 7 9 10 8 6 4 2

© Dr Rajendra Sharma 2002

Dr Rajendra Sharma asserts the moral right to
be identified as the author of this work

A catalogue record of this book
is available from the British Library

ISBN 0 00 713766 4

Design by Andrew Sutterby
Illustrated by Michael Courtney, Deborah Maizels,
Anthony Warne, Michael Cole and David Woodroffe
Printed and bound in Great Britain by
The Bath Press, Bath

CONTENTS

Each chapter in Part One deals with health concerns in the following order:

GENERAL,
THE HEAD AND NECK,
THE CHEST,
THE DIGESTIVE SYSTEM,
THE UROGENITAL SYSTEM,
STRUCTURAL MATTERS,
THE SKIN,
THE NERVOUS SYSTEM,
PSYCHOLOGICAL MATTERS.

For easy reference to any specific matter, please refer to the index.

EXTENDED CONTENTS

To
My reasons for being –
Emily, Liam, Madeleine and Bryony

Acknowledgements

Thank you to my late father, Chandra, who was and is the greatest teacher I will ever have and to my mother, Rosemary, for always being there, supporting and believing in me. Thank you to Justin (my loving and much loved brother) and Frankie (and Vivian) for their love and grounding effect.

No Emily, no book. My wife has transcribed and turned this work into a readable form whilst keeping home and children swathed in love. Thank you so much.

Thank you to my friends who encouraged and supported my writing, especially Tibs' mate (Alon) who will, I know, be the literary giant he deserves to be. Thanks also to Ian Fenton who bothered to find me and to Matthew Cory who did all the hard work. Special thanks to Emma Worth for keeping the ball rolling.

Thank you to those who inspired and taught me especially Dr Issac Mathai Nooranal, Dr Harald Gaier, Dr Anthony Soyer and Laurens Holve.

A special thank you to the colleagues I have worked with over the years and from whom I have learned so much – especially the 101 Group of Practitioners and those at Castle Street. Thank you to Fiona Harrold for her support throughout my career. Thanks to my American support especially Dr Woodson Merrell (and, of course, Gaye), Dr Timothy Lynch, Laura Gabbe and Kathy Dunn.

A special thank you to the late Becky and her John as well as Malcolm for keeping me sane.

A very big and special thank you to my team Chan, Mary (and their support team Wendy, Debbie and Jim) for protecting me and to Robin for helping to set it all up. Thank you to those friends who believe in me and help me escape from medicine sometimes, particularly Tina Turner, David Pugh, Kevin and Susie, John Vos, Greg Stuart, Alex Oakes, Richard Berenson and the Arsenal football team!

I am indebted to James and Sheelagh Colton, Dr Stephen Davis, Dr Julian Jessel-Kenyon, Agnes Kernan, Professor D Schweitzer and Annette Wilkinson for providing material for use in this book, and also to the Science Photo Library for permission to use their photographs.

Finally, an apology to those patients who find information or instructions in this book that I failed to give to them in consultations. I have learned a lot in the last three years while preparing this book and if you saw me before the information had come to me, it would not have filtered through to you. Thank you for helping me to learn.

FOREWORD

Medicine, and especially Neurology, has moved forward over the last two decades, driven by technological developments, science, computers and, to a lesser extent, an ever-increasing battery of pharmaceuticals. As a result, medicine has become more and more of a science and less of an art.

As medical students together, Dr Sharma and I were taught the 'art' of medicine with hands-on diagnosis, and a 'common sense' approach to patients as our first line of treatment. I believe, and most medical practitioners would agree, that the art of medicine is waning. Indeed, it has been said that our professional bedside capability and manner has also deteriorated. Whilst I think that many of the technological advances are for the benefit of the patient, the general public are not necessarily in agreement and may actually miss the physical human contact.

Many traditional medical practitioners are sceptical of any treatment that has not been subject to stringent scientific testing. There is a lack of reliable information about the efficacy of alternative treatments, although some intriguing reports have appeared recently, including a study demonstrating the benefit of magnetism on arthritic pain, and another study showing that light exposure to the back of the knees can result in changes in a person's sleep cycle. These results remain to be replicated. With this in mind, an alternative medicine journal, The Scientific Review of Alternative Medicine, was founded in 1997 with the stated purpose of applying 'rational analysis' to alternative treatments.

Alternative medicine has enjoyed a huge upsurge in popularity, forcing traditional medicine to reassess alternative techniques in a critical manner. Interestingly, the American Ivy League schools are at present reassessing their attitude to alternative treatments and at Columbia University a centre for alternative medicine was opened in 1996. Dr Sharma and I have discussed these issues over the years and I have no doubt that he advocates and pursues the scientific study of alternative treatments.

This book will be of use not only to patients and alternative practitioners but also to traditional physicians as many of their patients take a combination of both traditional treatments and alternative ones.

A 1986 study in the United Kingdom showed that there were 13.5 million consultations with alternative practitioners. This number may indeed have grown since in view of the media interest and promotion of these complementary approaches.

Dr Sharma has divided his encyclopedia into various sections based on the age of the patient. He explains that many conditions can occur at any age. I have heard Dr Sharma lecture and found him to be clear, logical and easy to follow. His book follows the same line with well thought-out concepts. It is important to ensure that patients do not spend their time and money on unproved therapies promoted by misguided practitioners. I feel comfortable that Dr Sharma is determined to separate that which is conjecture or anecdotal from that which has some evidence of efficacy and for treatments that are substantiated by proven trials. His book explains things simply and, most importantly, recommends safety above experimentation.

There is an extraordinary amount of interest and information being disseminated by alternative practitioners and the media alike. The former may have vested interests in promoting their own work and may fail to mention other, perhaps more beneficial practices. Media journalists are often interested but are not medically trained and the information they give may sometimes be influenced by a need to increase readership. This encyclopedia shows no such bias and has introduced me to the many alternative medicine concepts that I believe are safe and worthy of recommendation. I believe that this book will act as an invaluable reference guide for physicians, practitioners and families alike in helping to decide what treatments may be beneficial and safe and will steer patients to the most beneficial avenues.

The more that is done to encourage practitioners to gain education and knowledge in both orthodox and alternative practices the better it will be for the health of the individual and society.

Dr Timothy Lynch MB, BSc, MRCP (London),
Consultant Neurologist,
The Mater Misericordiae Hospital,
Dublin, Ireland.

INTRODUCTION

This book has come about because of the need for an easy-reference first-aid book that deals with the problems we are all likely to come across in our lives. The book discusses illnesses such as cancer (one in three people will have to deal with this in their lifetime), AIDS, diabetes and psoriasis, but attention is also paid to options for treatments for conditions that we may all face through our lives.

There is a myriad of books about orthodox, complementary and alternative medical first aid but they are specifically drawn towards one type of treatment, such as homeopathy, herbal treatment or dietetics. An individual requires a veritable library of books to have a reasonable overall knowledge, and selecting the best treatment for a specific problem is not easy. I hope this book will simplify matters.

A UNIFIED APPROACH TO HEALTH

I am the first to admit that to try to encompass a working knowledge of all complementary and orthodox therapies would be beyond all but the most sophisticated computer, but to be aware of the existence and the possibilities that each therapy can offer is both feasible and enjoyable. I have, over the years, come into contact with therapists in most fields of medicine and through discussion and reading about the speciality have learned enough to know when to recommend treatment and which are the appropriate therapies to recommend.

The clinics in which I work have experts in the various fields that I believe have credibility. Such truly holistic practices offer patients a complete understanding of their health and the availability of any treatment necessary to restore their well-being. Using this book will allow the reader to share my experience.

In no way should this book be seen as a replacement for doctors and practitioners. It must be used as a guide to the appropriate courses of treatment. However, it may help not only the reader but also the physician or practitioner whose care the patient is under. Information gleaned from these pages can be presented to your carer for assessment of its use. Do not assume your practitioner knows all the possible treatment routes. All practitioners are constantly learning and should be happy to discuss other therapies apart from their own.

WHAT IS HOLISTIC MEDICINE?

Before the advent of 'modern science' in the West about 150 years ago, medicine and healthcare were based predominantly on trial, error and observation.

Physicians had no more real knowledge than an experienced grandmother. A lack of knowledge concerning viruses and bacteria meant that hygiene was little understood and therefore health was poor and life expectancy was short. As science took hold, the 'art' of medicine became less studied and the birth of modern medicine took us away from some of the gentler skills and techniques that had accrued over centuries.

Thousands of years of traditional knowledge from the Tibetans, Chinese, Ayurvedic (Indian) and other long-established cultures were put aside as the Western world developed. The necessary balance between the modern scientist and the traditional healer was lost and the pendulum swung more towards manufactured drugs and high-technology methods.

Now, however, the pendulum is swinging back and hopefully will settle midway, allowing a balanced attitude towards healing to come to the fore. There is a place for the surgeon's knife and antibiotics alongside the hands of the faith-healer and the brews of the herbalist.

The names 'alternative' and 'fringe' medicine have largely been replaced by 'complementary' medicine. This was an attempt by the practitioners in non-scientific medical art to try to persuade the mighty physician that they were suitable assistants to orthodox medicine. There is no doubt that this attitude was required to create the necessary change, but as we see more and more failures within the modern medical system, the complementary medical practitioner has now suggested a new term – integrated medicine – to try to achieve a level of equal importance with orthodox medicine. It is, in my opinion, as erroneous of an acupuncturist to suggest that he has a higher level of knowledge as it is for a Professor of Surgery to assume an air of superiority.

The term 'holistic' (derived from the Greek *holos*, meaning 'whole') is the closest to the direction in which I believe medicine and healing must go. Unfortunately the term has been associated with quackery and mysticism and thus is not one that an orthodox physician would willingly be labelled.

We all have to learn that there can no longer be any differentiation. The art of healing must draw from all philosophies and all schools of teaching to create a single healthcare system. Divisions will be required because no one individual can retain and use all the available treatment options, but there has to come a time when doctors have as broad a knowledge of the availability of treatments as possible so that they can recommend the most effective and fast-acting repair process to their patients. A GP today should be aware of treatment options such as acupuncture or osteopathy, and a homeopath should be knowledgeable about the potential use of, say, antibiotics. We have, at present, a divisive system that has to change. I hope that this book will help to achieve this.

HEALTH AND HEALING TODAY

The doctors of today, let alone the untrained population, appear to know only a smattering of the simple, non-drug treatments that have much value in treating our common ailments.

In no way do I wish to belittle the work of us Western-trained doctors. More and more patients are, however, becoming disenchanted and alarmed at the advice they receive from their GPs and hospital specialists when seeking advice for general health and non-life-threatening conditions.

CASE HISTORY:

Mrs J B, age 62 years and an active grandmother and homemaker, suffered a stroke three years prior to coming to see me. The stroke had severely affected her speech and the left side of her body had retained less than 10 per cent of its function. Over the three-year period she had regained most of her speech through invaluable speech therapy but, despite physiotherapy, had only managed to regain about 30 per cent of the movement and strength in her left arm. Mrs J B had high blood pressure (until the stroke, when it 'miraculously' reverted to normal) and she had been given, theoretically, adequate blood-pressure control medicine for several years.

After I had examined her I suggested that she try Chinese herbal medicine in conjunction with some osteopathy and acupuncture. Within two months Mrs J B was able to walk more than 200 yards as opposed to the 20 yards that had exhausted her before. Her mood had elevated beyond recognition and she was able to play with and enjoy her grandchildren far more.

When she returned to the GP who had been sympathetic over the previous years, his attitude was not one of surprise and interest: in fact, quite the opposite. He warned Mrs J B about the dangers of herbal medicine and told her that acupuncture was unproved and osteopathy was dangerous.

Apart from the fact that all these statements are untrue, as these therapies had been given by correctly qualified people, the GP managed to frighten Mrs J B and create a negative reaction towards treatments that in two months had done more to help her than three years of the orthodox approach.

This, I think, is typical of the state of healthcare or healing available in the West at the moment. Scientifically trained doctors who have had no teachers to advise them to stay in touch with their instincts, and who have been taught to accept nothing if it does not have a scientific explanation, are losing touch with the principles of healing. This case history is typical of the Western doctor's approach to health and healthcare.

Doctors are trained to memorize facts and stay within specific boundaries or protocols until time and studies prove new techniques and treatments to be safe and effective or until they are shown to be dangerous. This often allows today's orthodox doctor to be completely without responsibility, leaving much to the pharmaceutical industry who are not professional carers (in fact, one might say that they do not care at all) but are money-makers.

The most notorious example of this is the drug thalidomide. Doctors were told that prescribing thalidomide throughout pregnancy was safe, but this proved not to be true. After the damage was done, all the prescribers held up their hands and said 'Do not blame us, not our fault, we did as we were told'. If the doctors had read the facts or even questioned the safety tests, a major disaster might have been averted. This scenario is being repeated constantly. At the time of writing, in the last year alone seven types of contraceptive pill have been shown to be hazardous. In the summer of 1996 a common cardiac drug was scrutinized for safety and failed. In 1995 the efficacy of AZT in the treatment of AIDS was disproved and the year before that, two of the three available measles vaccines were withdrawn. The third vaccine is currently under scrutiny. The list goes on and on.

Of course, the consideration of using any treatment outside the parameters of 'scientifically' proven, and therefore 'safe' (whether or not it has been used for thousands of years), is actively discouraged.

Good health has been defined by the World Health Organization (WHO), and I paraphrase,

The Three Levels of Health

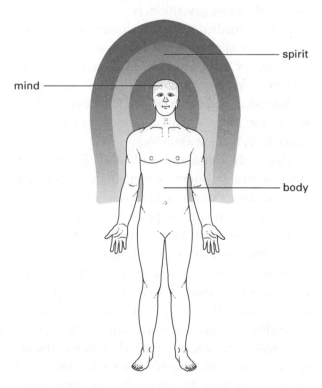

spirit

mind

body

The well-being of an individual depends not only on the health of the mind and body, but also of the spirit, here represented by an aura around the head.

'as a level of health that is not only free from illness but also includes the well-being of an individual in physical, emotional and spiritual terms'. In principle, the WHO is stating that good health requires a level of contentment on the following planes:

- The physical/physiological/biochemical level
- The psychological/conscious level
- The spiritual/subconscious level

For thousands of years physicians, practitioners and healers in many disciplines have worked on the principle that health must be considered at all three levels. We are reaching a time when there is too much knowledge for any one physician to retain. Specialization is a necessity but not only with respect to the physical plane. We need advice on all three levels. We have reached a point where the *life-saving* doctors must work in tandem with the *health-saving* practitioners.

Holistic medicine is about understanding how to deal with all three levels and doing so in simple and effective ways. We all need to have an understanding of the simple processes of health maintenance and repair, with a knowledge of how to use the many disciplines, both orthodox and alternative, that are available.

This body, mind and soul 'stuff' is not some ethereal mumbo-jumbo either. Doctors today are not told about much of the evidence of a strong scientific nature that supports mind/body concepts. The most striking example is that of the psychiatric patient with multiple personalities reported by Drs Braun and Goldman. This patient, not unusual in having multiple personalities, was found to exhibit different diseases depending on who she was at any one time. One personality had diabetes and when this character was in control the patient's sugar levels were very high. As soon as the personality changed, away went the diabetes. Another character developed hives in reaction to certain substances, and these also came and went with this persona.

The hypothesis that living cells contain a vital force is one that is present in many medical philosophies throughout the world. The West has lost sight of this because of an overdependence on science. This is even more strange because the foundations upon which this science is based are very flimsy. Chemistry is founded on physics. Physics has worked itself down to fundamental particles, atoms, electrons, quanta, quarks and so forth, but ask a physicist 'How did it begin?' or 'What is the force holding electrons together or the force that we call gravity?' and there is no definitive answer. We can measure the effects, but the vital force is unknown. If a rock falls to the ground, the vital force is gravity and this is accepted, yet if a tumour disappears by the influence of the vital force of a healer, it is unacceptable.

STAYING HEALTHY

It is much easier to keep someone healthy than to get them better. The bulk of this book is concerned with repair, but ideally one hopes that the reader will not have recourse to look at these sections. The best way to avoid this is to maintain a healthy lifestyle, and the following tips may give some guidance on how to do so.

The 24 hours in a day should be divided into the following:

Sleep	8hrs
Enjoyable, productive work	8hrs
Exercise	40min–1hr
Meditation	1–2hrs
Basic hygiene	$1/2$–1hr
Preparing and eating food	$1^1/2$–2hrs
Having fun	The rest of the time

Of course, all these time suggestions are variable: 10 minutes of exercise is better than none, and the same could be said for meditation.

Sleep should not be cut out for the benefit of any of the other time allocations because sleep is essential for repair and well-being.

A Healthy Day

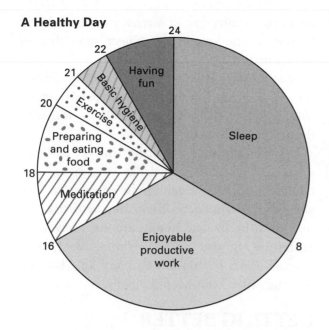

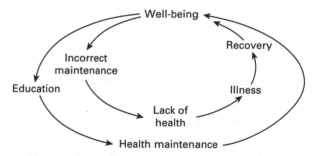

ACTIVITY	0	1	2	3	4	5
• Basic hygiene						
• Doing something creative						
• Eating						
• Exercise						
• Fun						
• Prayer or meditation						
• Sex						
• Sleep						
• Socializing						
• Work						

Wherever possible, work should be enjoyable and serious consideration given to changing employment that is not so.

Exercise and meditation are discussed in their own sections in this book but must make up a part of every day. Eating and the preparation of food is discussed in chapter 7 on nutrition.

Basic hygiene is very often overlooked in the West but is integrated into the social and religious philosophies of Eastern and Middle Eastern cultures. A Hindu, for example, would not consider eating before ablutions. All parts of the body should be considered, starting with a cleansing of the skin and hair, emptying of bowel and bladder and the cleaning of our VIPs (very important places!), which include the oral cavity, genitals, ears, nostrils and anus. Special attention should be paid to the feet, which are often neglected until a problem sets in.

In an attempt to make life simple, I suggest to my patients that they draw themselves the following chart.

I suggest that each day individuals give themselves marks out of five for each of these subjects, aiming to score over 40 points and ensuring at least 3 points in each category.

If sex is not available, score another five points with some other enjoyable activity!

ILLNESS, DISEASE AND HEALTH

Principally, there is a big difference between being ill and lacking health.

Being Well and Staying Well

When we lose control or if we are poorly educated about how to maintain our health, then unhealthy living will lead to a lack of health, which is quite distinct from illness. A lack of health can be corrected merely by re-education and rearrangement of our lifestyles, whereas illness generally requires intervention or treatment. A broad example would be that of a smoker. Inhaling 20 cigarettes a day will initially lead to an increase in the likelihood of coughs, colds, sinusitis, sore throats, which may indicate a lack of health and can be corrected by not smoking. If these early warning signs are ignored then the destruction of lung tissue is inevitable and conditions such as chronic bronchitis, emphysema and cancer may, and usually do, set in. This is illness and requires intervention rather than simply refraining from smoking.

Being well and staying well is a matter of correct education. If we know what we are doing and how to encourage those around us to do the same, then staying well is not that difficult. Persuading those close to us may be relatively easy but, when dealing with large corporations, government and industries, keeping ourselves from pollutants and toxins is, unfortunately, much harder to do. This book will do its best to help you avoid some of the poisons that are fed into our food and atmosphere.

The human being responds to ill-health in three ways.

- **Elimination:** a process that throws things out of the body. Mucus production during a cold, vomiting or diarrhoea, sweating and persistent urination are all elimination reactions.
- **Reaction:** when the body produces symptoms that do not seem to be throwing anything out. Skin rashes such as eczema, asthma, abdominal colic or cramps are a few examples.
- **Retention:** when the body holds on to problems by forming lumps and bumps or stones in the gallbladder or kidney.

Good health is about a balance of all three, although individuals tend towards one type more than another.

It is not more healthy or better to exhibit any one of these three response types because different conditions will be more dangerous in different response groups. A retentive type of person is more likely to be able to deal with problems that stay in the body and will handle cancer cells more effectively than, say, an eliminator who is more geared to throwing things out. Furthermore, food poisoning or a condition such as cholera, which encourages fluid loss through vomiting and diarrhoea, may be far more devastating to a body that habitually throws things out than to one that is geared to holding things in. In contrast, an infection in a retentive type is liable to stay in the system for longer than that of an eliminator.

Reactions are usually warnings and the initiation of a repair process either depends on an elimination or the body being able to deal with the problem internally.

Individuals should establish their type and tendency and use this knowledge to enhance any treatment choices. Establishing your body type will also relieve anxiety. If you are a retentive sort then most lumps and bumps are not likely to be cancerous. If you are an eliminative type a stomach upset should not last very long because the 'bug' will be thrown out rapidly.

GETTING BETTER

This book is about healing, which in turn is about getting better. The body responds to not being well by producing symptoms that fall into one of three categories.

- Warning Symptoms.
- Repair Processes.
- Loss of Control.

The first two categories are the body healing itself and the third is when the body is failing to do so.

The important factor in helping to heal is being able to differentiate between the three categories of symptoms.

WARNING SYMPTOMS

The body may create certain symptoms to advise the patient that a particular action is liable to lead to problems. A good example is the following case history.

CASE HISTORY:
Mr N F, age 38 years, had been advised that he had a stomach ulcer. On close questioning it

became clear that his upper abdominal pain was made worse by drinking coffee. If he did not drink coffee he did not have the pain. Interestingly, on further questioning it became clear that Mr N F was very sensitive to caffeine, which would keep him awake for up to 4 hours if he drank it after his evening meal.

In this simple example Mr N F was being warned by his stomach that the continual use of caffeine was overstimulating his system, which would lead to more serious complications in the future. Most pain is a warning and if the warning is heeded the problems should be healed.

REPAIR PROCESSES

Quite often symptoms are created to repair the body. A cut that hurts, falls into the warning category, telling the individual to protect that area of damaged skin. However, the pain is also sending information to the nervous system, which in turn sends information back, opening up blood vessels and attracting more white blood cells, scar tissue-forming cells and nutrients necessary for repair to rush into the damaged area. In this example the pain is not only warning but also encouraging repair. Taking a painkiller, therefore, cannot only allow further damage to occur, because we become less conscious of the damage, but also interfere with the reflex repair process.

Healing response

One problem with any self-help text associated with alternative medicine is the concept of the healing response. Orthodox medicine is very much geared towards removing unpleasant symptoms, regardless of the effect on the underlying disease. Holistic medicine is about curing the

problem, thereby alleviating the symptoms from a deeper, non-superficial aspect. Many treatments in the complementary medical field will trigger reactions that may be initially unpleasant or worsen the symptoms that the treatment is supposedly curing. It is vital to have an understanding of this and I believe that the case history below illustrates the matter clearly.

CASE HISTORY:

Mrs J D, age 22 years, came to see me with a history of persisting and recurrent 'cold' symptoms. She was very precise about her symptoms and discussed with me at our first meeting the fact that she would sneeze between 10 and 20 times per hour, have a fever that never raised itself above 98°F (38°C) and was able to take warm fluids through her sore throat, but when her symptoms were at a peak she was unable to swallow solids. She was in my consulting room at the zenith of her current cold and told me that the problem would take another week of slow improvement before it disappeared but that she would probably be ill again within the month.

I took her medical history, performed a full examination and initiated the appropriate treatment. I neglected to advise Mrs J D on the principles of the healing reaction and three days later I found her back in my consulting room: 'I don't know what you gave me doctor but I am now sneezing over 30 times an hour, my temperature reached 100°F (39°C) and I am now unable to swallow even fluids.'

I explained that all her symptoms had worsened because the virus was being thrown out quicker by the sneezing, the inflammation in her throat was due to more blood in the area, bringing with it more white blood cells to kill the virus, and that *she* can live at 100°F (39°C) but many viruses cannot! Such healing responses should, therefore, shorten the time of the illness. I explained that her immune system was now fighting a stronger battle and that this indicated that the treatment was working. Mrs J D did improve over the next 24 hours and has since suffered only two 'colds' each year during the last five years.

The Five Reactions of Healing

There are five reactions worth noting as part of the repair process. These are particularly relevant for anybody going through a homeopathic treatment course but also stand in good stead for any naturopathic healing process.

• As mentioned above, symptoms may get worse before they get better.
• Despite symptoms getting worse, an individual will feel better on a psychological level before the physical symptoms resolve. This is an extremely important factor in the healing process whilst waiting for physical effects to take place.
• Problems often leave the body in a downward motion: for instance, a headache may become a backache; an upset stomach may eliminate as diarrhoea; a rash on the chest may leave via the feet.
• Problems will resolve from inside, outwards: internal illness may expel itself as a rash as in the case of measles or chickenpox; food poisoning may cause vomiting; toxins may come out through the hair or nails.
• An illness may regress through symptoms previously suffered. This is described as 'present conditions go to past conditions'. In an acute disease such as pneumonia the patient rarely wakes up with pneumonia but goes through cold symptoms, flu-like symptoms, a mild chest infection to pneumonia; conversely, a patient with pneumonia rarely wakes up

suddenly feeling wonderful but goes through symptoms of a mild chest infection, flu symptoms, a cold and then feeling well again. Chronic conditions may do the same, even though there may be no direct or obvious connection. For example, someone, aged 30 years, with rheumatoid arthritis may find that the condition improves and at the same time they have a rash that reminds them of a problem they had when they were 15 years old. Very often that rash was suppressed, the condition went deeper and is now being resolved. This scenario may occur many years into the future.

It is important to understand these facts because reporting to the complementary medical practitioner can be made more accurate by including any symptoms within these parameters and will also allow the individual to feel confident despite a slow improvement.

LOSS OF CONTROL

When the body loses control of its symptoms then the situation demands medical intervention. A cancer can grow unnoticed in a major organ, showing no signs or symptoms until it is too late to be treated. Other silent conditions, such as AIDS and diabetes, may not present until the disease process is very far gone. It is a sign of ill-health to have a disease process and show no symptoms, which is ironic because a bad cold will bring the patient to a practice complaining that they are 'ill' or at 'death's door' when in fact their variety of symptoms is repairing them. Conversely, someone attending for a check-up who feels fine and 'full of the joys of spring' may be discovered to be ravaged by cancer or slowly damaging their arteries with arteriosclerosis.

ABOUT THIS BOOK

This book has arisen from my experience of helping individuals search for guidance towards optimum healthcare techniques. Until the time comes when all practitioners of medicine are encouraged to broaden their outlook, this book will enable people to understand the available techniques, both modern and traditional, to be well.

The speed with which medical treatments, both orthodox and complementary, are being thrown out to the eager public suggests that by the time you have read this sentence, new ideas and concepts for treatment will have manifested themselves. The subject is so large that I may not have included all possible treatment avenues despite my extensive research. I invite any practitioners or individuals who have had success with treatments not mentioned in this edition to have no hesitation in writing to me with references so that I can continue to update this book in the future.

This book is indexed to allow easy access to any particular condition. Each subject has a brief explanation from both an orthodox and an Eastern medical perspective, where appropriate, and the most effective treatments are mentioned. I have chosen only to list those medicines and therapies that are easily available, and where I make reference to a particular need to see a practitioner or doctor this is because many other treatments are available but may be difficult to obtain or require skilled judgement in prescribing.

I hope that this book will enable individuals to look after themselves and find safe treatments swiftly, by helping them to choose the best option rather than experimenting until the right formula is found. I also believe that this book may be an invaluable companion for general practitioners (GPs), hospital specialists and complementary/alternative practitioners whose training, I am sure they will agree, does not necessarily illustrate the available options from specialities other than their own.

The purpose of this book is to provide a first-aid reference and a mini-encyclopedia for both the initiated and for newcomers to complementary medicine. It would not be possible to cover all health matters in one single volume, and nor is it necessary. There are many books that can provide in-depth details of specific health problems.

I give many recommendations for all the common ailments that we may come across in our personal or family lives. It would take another book of this size to give all the references. One resource centre told me that they have over 40,000 references for papers and trials on complementary medicine. Where I have given advice, be assured that it is from personal experience or from other reputable sources. I have also not given all the reasons why certain compounds may work on a particular condition. Whilst fascinating, this is not the reason for this book, which should act as a reference for home medicine and suggest suitable treatment courses, both orthodox and alternative, and give an understanding of what practitioners are doing and why.

USING THIS BOOK

This encyclopedia follows a format in which ailments that occur *commonly* at particular times of life are discussed. For instance, I write about the best nutrition for pregnancy in the section about pregnancy and childbirth. However, some conditions span many age groups. Eczema can occur at any stage of life but is initially discussed in the section on childhood since this is when eczema most commonly presents itself to a physician. After the discussion of any particular condition, I suggest under the heading RECOMMENDATION(S) the appropriate actions which may be taken.

RECOMMENDATION

- *Check in the index at the back of the book for any specific complaint when using this book as a reference. You may be directed to a different age group but the treatment will be the same for your own.*

COMPLEMENTARY MEDICINE

The complementary medical advice given for any condition is at best curative and at worst ineffectual. Specific treatments may have effects that are unpleasant and 'healing responses' (*see* **Getting Better**) may occur as the body repairs. Certain illnesses such as meningitis can develop rapidly and must be treated by doctors. *Do not ignore the advice in the text if it supports orthodox treatment.*

> RECOMMENDATION
>
> * *For any condition where self-help is initiated, discuss the matter with a professional if improvement is not apparent within 24hr, or sooner if the condition worsens. If in any doubt, consult a professional practitioner immediately.*

REMEDIES

When homeopathic remedies are mentioned, be aware that the list may not include the best remedy for you. Homeopathy is best prescribed by looking at the totality of symptoms, both pleasant and unpleasant, in an individual. The typical modern approach of selecting *one* remedy for *one* symptom is incorrect and most often unsuccessful. It is unlikely that any negative reaction will occur by using an incorrect remedy. Probably nothing will happen at all. Using a recommended remedy is therefore safe.

> RECOMMENDATION
>
> * *Most medication and therapies mentioned are general but when homeopathic remedies are listed please be aware that correct selection depends on a specific symptom picture and reference to a homeopathic manual is highly recommended.*

DOSAGES

When no specific dosage is given for a homeopathic remedy assume that it should be taken as either four pills (round), two tablets (disc shaped) or four drops every two waking hours until improvement is seen, then should be reduced to every four hours. Stop the remedy 24 hours after the condition has gone.

When I recommend a herbal extract you will see the amounts and dosages. If I recommend a therapy, the length of treatment will be decided by the patient's response and the therapist.

FURTHER INFORMATION

Any questions or omissions, corrections or criticisms (constructive only please) should be directed to the attention of :

Dr Sharma
Medical Director
The 101 Group
87 North Road
Parkstone
Dorset
BH14 0LT.

YOUR MEDICINE CABINET

This book covers the most common conditions and describes treatments that are either easily or readily obtainable. Where feasible, treatment recommendations are given that include the amounts and potencies that should be taken. However, certain recommendations include nutrients, vitamins, minerals that are obtainable from food, and these foods have not been listed. I also frequently mention the need to refer to 'Your preferred Homeopathic Manual'. There are many good books but I take the liberty of mentioning those that I think should sit next to the medicine cabinet and I list these at the foot of the following page.

THE MEDICAL KIT

There is a benefit in having certain naturopathic and homeopathic remedies easily at hand in the house. The following is my recommendation for the contents of a first-aid cabinet. Most of these should be available in good health shops and chemists, but if not they are available through mail order from: *Best of Both Worlds Health Care, 87 North Road, Parkstone, Poole, Dorset BH14 0LT, UK.*

Lotions
Arnica Fluid Extract
Calendula Fluid Extract
Hypericum Fluid Extract
Euphrasia Fluid Extract

Creams
Arnica Cream
Calendula Cream
Any cream containing both of the above

Essential oils
Clove oil
Lavender oil
Mullein oil
Olbas oil
Peppermint oil

Homeopathic remedies
The following should be kept at potencies of 6 and 30:

Aconite
Agaricus muscarius
Agnus castus
Allium cepa
Argentum nitricum
Arnica
Arsenicum album
Baptisia
Baryta carbonica
Belladonna
Bellis perennis
Berberis
Bryonia
Calcarea carbonica
Calcarea phosphorica
Calendula
Cantharis
Carbo vegetalis
Caulophyllum

Causticum
Chamomilla
Chelidonium
China arsenicum
Cimicifuga
Coffea
Drosera
Euphrasia
Ferrum phosphoricum
Gelsemium
Hepar sulphuris
Hypericum
Ignatia
Ipecacuanha
Kali bichromicum
Kali bromatum
Kali carbonicum
Lachesis
Lycopodium
Magnesia carbonica
Magnesia phosphorica
Mercurius corrosivus
Mercurius solubilis

Natrum carbonicum
Natrum muriaticum
Natrum sulphuricum
Nitricum acidum
Nux vomica
Pertussin
Phosphorus
Phytolacca
Pothos foetidus
Pulsatilla
Rhus toxicodendron
Ruta graveolens
Secale cornutum
Sepia
Silica
Spongia
Staphysagria
Streptococcus
Sulphur
Thuja
Urtica urens
Veratrum album

- **The Family Guide to Homeopathy,** Dr Andrew Lockie, *Hamish Hamilton Ltd, London, 1992.*
- **The Vitamin Bible,** Earl Mindell, *Warner Books.*
- **The Encyclopedia of Pregnancy and Birth,** Janet Balaskas and Yehudi Gordon, *Little Brown & Co.*
- **Toddler Taming,** Dr Christopher Green, *Vermilion, London, 1992.*

For those interested in more complex homeopathy or for practitioners of homeopathy, the following are a must:

- *The Encyclopedic Dictionary of Homeopathy,* by Harald Gaier – published initially by Harper Collins and republished by Michael O'Mara, UK and by Avery, New York, USA.
- *The Homeopathic Materia Medica,* with repertory by William Boericke MD, is a must for those who intend to use homeopathy accurately.

INVESTIGATIONS

In the text there are indications of suitable investigations or tests that should be available through your doctor, practitioner, hospital or health clinic. If not, then you may contact: *The 101 Group, 87 North Road, Parkstone, Poole, Dorset BH14 0LT, UK.*

Practitioners may liaise with a sympathetic GP or may contact the 101 Group to request tests.

A list of addresses where further information may be sought is placed at the end of this book.

PART ONE

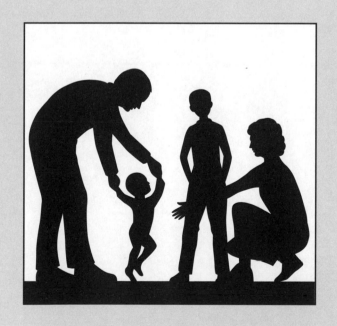

SEX, FERTILITY AND CONCEPTION

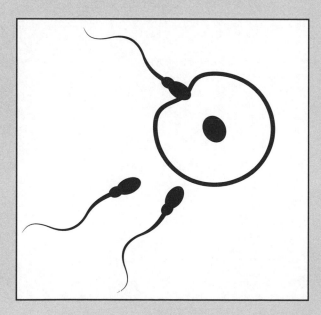

CHAPTER 1

SEX, FERTILITY AND CONCEPTION

'Children are Nature's longing for itself'

So wrote Kahlil Gibran in his magnificent work *The Prophet*. Nature wants us to conceive. However, nature does not want unhealthy or weak genes and will therefore go to great lengths to weed out all but those that are the strongest and most likely to survive.

One Eastern philosophy believes that the spirit of a child will select its parents. If this is the case then the physically healthier and psychologically more secure the parents, the more likely the infant spirits will be to vie for these parents and, through natural selection, the most healthy and psychologically adjusted child will develop from the parents' union. From a more grounded and less ethereal point of view, the healthier the parents, the more psychologically ready and the more spiritually secure the couple are, then clearly the chances of the child being born healthy must increase.

CHOOSING A PARTNER

There are two extremes in choosing a partner. The Eastern philosophy of arranged marriages lies at one end and the romantic notion of falling in love lies at the other. At the first end is the conscious appraisal by elders of two youngsters' attributes and what they would bring to a partnership or to the respective families. At the other end is the emotionally charged, 'love is blind' method. As in most matters, the balance probably lies in-between.

I am not seeking to change religious or ethical inclinations but feel strongly that choosing a partner is such an important decision that neither should it be left solely to others nor left entirely to the vagaries of our emotional states.

On the following pages are a list of questions that should be answered by a prospective couple at some stage through their decision to have a baby. If you wish you may photocopy these pages and send them to *The Right Match, 87 North Road, Parkstone, Poole, Dorset BH14 0LT, UK*, where a relationship counsellor will assess the answers and advise you on areas that may prove problematic.

THE MISCONCEPTIONS OF CONCEPTION

The reasons why we have sex are manifold. The sensory pleasures that are derived from interacting in a sexual way with another human being give both pleasure and comfort. Most people enjoy sex and those who do not, often instead use sex to derive respect, security or to derive some other gain. When all is said and done, however, the one-, two- and three-play that leads up to foreplay and sex are all social distortions of our necessity to create the next generation of our species.

The large majority of women will, at some time in their lives, consider whether they wish to become pregnant. If they did not, we would not be here. The decision is reached when the correct physical age is attained and it is decided that it is time psychologically and spiritually to be a parent.

There are over 750,000 births per year in the UK and five times that number in the USA. It is estimated, however, that as many as two out of every five pregnancies fail to reach maturation (be delivered). This means that there are possibly 2.5 million conceptions in the UK and 12.5 million in the USA each year. Most are not even noticed. The fertilized egg fails to implant in the womb or fails to survive for reasons such as faulty genes in either the sperm or in the egg, or because of problems with the health of the mother. The fertilized egg is then shed imperceptibly, usually at the next period. Problems of conception, however, are not only due to failure once an egg has been fertilized. Many couples failing to conceive do so because the male and female sex cells do not even meet. Problems either with the production of the egg from the ovary or inadequate amounts of sperm or non-viable sperm can also cause infertility.

A minority of the 10 million women in the UK and 50 million in the USA who could conceive at any particular time may have problems in doing so, but what advice and treatment is currently available to those who are unsuccessful?

Approximately 30,000 women, either alone or with their partner, attend clinics or specialists each year in the UK because they have not been able to conceive. Again, an assumption can be drawn that only one-third of those having trouble becoming pregnant actually present themselves to a practitioner. In any particular year, therefore, it can be estimated that 90,000 women in the UK are failing to conceive.

Earlier this decade the orthodox medical establishment stated that only 15 per cent of infertile females respond favourably to orthodox treatment. This figure has probably doubled due to scientific advances. It was also established that various alternative methods gave much the same response. Holistic medicine, effectively being the use of both orthodox and alternative treatments, may, arguably, double the chances of a couple having a child.

The problem of infertility, as with any health matter, should be studied and treated at the three levels of well-being: body, mind and spirit. The actual causes of infertility can be divided into problems arising from the male or the female, but many factors are shared.

CONTRACEPTION

This is the voluntary and temporary prevention of pregnancy and it is generally governed by social, economic, medical or personal reasons. Both as a father and a professional, I rarely find men who think it is the right time to have children, but this may be due to the current Western trend that so ardently promotes convenience. At some point, most women seem to consider pregnancy and motherhood, and they appear to have a better instinct about deciding when the time is right.

Contraception is a rare commodity when looked at worldwide and those who have access to it may underestimate the privilege. Measures ranging from the draconian one-child-per-family rule in parts of China to the disease-spreading use of anal intercourse in parts of Africa are very much part of these cultures. However, the choice of the right form of contraception can still be a problem. Contraception may be divided into the following categories:

Natural

This includes abstinence, the withdrawal method (coitus interruptus) and the rhythm method. Abstinence is, of course, 100 per cent effective! This not being everybody's cup of tea makes withdrawal a popular method, but it is extremely unreliable and fails very frequently.

Sperm can exist quite conformably at the tip of the penis, along the urethra or under the foreskin in the uncircumcised. Sperm may live for up to three days under the right circumstances after emission, so conception may occur from the first penetration. It is also important to note that ejaculation can occur well before orgasm and frequently the first ejaculate happens before a climax.

The rhythm method is safer but is only around 75 per cent secure. Statistically, this means that one in four acts of intercourse using 'safe' times may cause a pregnancy. Part of the problem is the unreliability of our calculations; also, it is thought that intercourse itself may trigger female ovulation. Read the section below, 'Getting the Timing Right', and reverse the logic to avoid conceiving.

Mechanical (barrier methods)

Condoms (sheaths)

These vary in success from 93–97 per cent and usually fail from improper application or from being put on after initial penetration has already occurred. They may break but this is rare.

Cervical Caps (diaphragms)

Most of these are used in conjunction with spermicidal gels, creams or suppositories, all of which should be used for only a short space of time before changing to another one so that local sensitivity does not develop.

It is not advisable to use these chemical barriers without a mechanical one as statistics show an increased risk of conception. The Honey Cap has become a popular natural device. It is so called because it was originally stored and cleansed in honey although modern devices are now impregnated with honey. This acts as a natural barrier and has an antiseptic quality. Many patients in my practice use this method successfully (although I am aware of failures), but the orthodox establishment feels that there is insufficient statistical evidence to support its use and consider it as effective as an ordinary diaphragm without the spermicidal preparations.

Intrauterine devices

This method is discussed in the Adult section of this book (*see* page 435).

Chemical

The use of the oral contraceptive pill (OCP) has grown rapidly since the early 1960s despite concerns about potential side effects and dangers. The OCP tricks the body into believing that it is pregnant by introducing artificial oestrogen and/or progesterone, thereby inducing the command centre (the pituitary gland) not to produce the usual stimulatory hormones. The arguments for and against the use of the OCP are diverse and controversial. There is no doubt that the pill confers a variety of side effects – some mild, others fatal –

including cancer and blood clots. However, one has to balance these misfortunes against social and economic difficulties, as well as the actual dangers of unwanted pregnancies. Termination (abortion), a frequent and commonly abused form of contraception, carries far greater statistical risks.

It has been possible to obtain a progestogen (artificial progesterone) implant that is placed by a doctor under the skin and this provides a slow, steady release of the drug. Considerable controversy arose and, amidst allegations of this process causing considerable suffering, the company responsible have withdrawn the product. This is clearly not something to be recommended at this stage of its development.

RECOMMENDATIONS

General Advice

- *Choice must be made on an individual basis with the advice of a GP or health practitioner with suitable knowledge.*
- *If an application is made of any product, it should be varied with others, or used sporadically to avoid sensitization.*
- *The Honey Cap must be fitted by a doctor and, until proper studies have been carried out, used only by those for whom a pregnancy would not be totally unacceptable or by those who cannot tolerate spermicides.*
- *Decisions concerning the OCP should only be made once a full family history, risk profile and health examination are undertaken, and the user is fully aware of the possible side effects and risks.*
- *Certain types of coil are now impregnated with hormones that are released over a period of time that effectively stops the normal cycle, thereby giving a secondary contraceptive effect. This should be viewed in the same way as the OCP.*

GETTING THE TIMING RIGHT

The average menstrual cycle is 28 days. There is, of course, much variation and some females can have a cycle as long as 40 days whilst others may

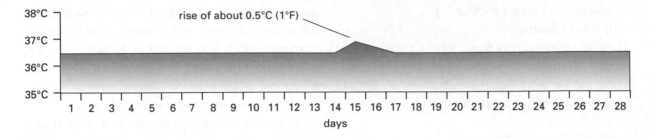

A woman's temperature rise when an egg is ready for fertilization.

have periods every three weeks. As a rule, the egg is ready for fertilization approximately 14 days before the next period is due. For women with a regular cycle this can be calculated quite simply but for others, tests on the urine or the vaginal secretions can accurately suggest the time to get their partner into bed. Kits for such tests can be obtained from a high street chemist. Another common method is to measure the half-degree rise in body temperature, which can be used with some confidence towards its accuracy. Simply measure and record your temperature every morning by placing a thermometer under your tongue. Put the result on a large-scale chart and watch out for a half-degree rise (*see the example above*).

Couples must remember that not every period and not every month necessarily means the eviction of an egg from the ovary and they should not be distressed if the tests show negative during some months.

PHYSICAL PREPARATION FOR CONCEPTION

The Eastern philosophies of medicine all categorically state that the use of drugs, alcohol and tobacco, or any compound that effects the nervous system, will alter the levels of energy through the meridians or energy channels and, if not directly affecting the conception, will affect the pregnancy. Toxins specifically decrease the body's kidney Qi or Chi – pronounced 'chee' – which is thought to be the body's energy store and the main supplier of energy at times of conception and pregnancy. Each individual may have particular likes and dislikes, intolerances or even allergies that should be excluded prior to conceiving (*see* **Chinese and Oriental medicine**).

Successful conception relies upon a healthy sperm meeting a healthy egg. The nutritional status of both partners is paramount. The number of known toxins to both sperm and eggs is limited, namely: tobacco, alcohol and drugs (recreational or prescribed, including the contraceptive pill).

Tobacco

Tobacco is a known teratogen (capable of altering cell structure). Many studies have shown that infants of mothers who smoke are often preterm deliveries and underweight. There is no exception and no quantity that is safe. If you smoke, your baby will be affected to some extent and this effect may take place at any stage during conception and pregnancy. An intended father who smokes may actually cause more birth defects than a smoking mother-to-be by damaging the sperm before it leaves him. The motility (movement) of the sperm is also adversely affected.

> **RECOMMENDATION**
>
> **General Advice**
> * *Women should not smoke for at least one cycle before attempting conception and men should abstain for at least ten days.*

NAME (please print) ....

ADDRESS...

....

GENERAL

	0	1	2	3	4	5

- I am satisfied with the ways we resolve our differences.
- I am confident about our physical and mental health.
- I agree with my partner on our involvement in running our home.
- I agree with my partner's goals and plans.
- I wish to be with my partner and I am not being forced.
- I never have doubts that we are right for each other.
- I share similar interests with my partner.
- I am happy to talk with my partner.
- I am happy with what my partner expects of me.
- I am confident with the compatibility of our education and intelligence.
- I find it easy to express my feelings to my partner.
- I would worry if I thought that we would not be together.
- I feel that we have the same ideas about lifestyle.
- I agree with my partner on how to decorate and furnish our home.
- Our jobs are not interfering with our relationship.
- There are no objections to our being together.
- I understand the circumstances that could end our relationship.
- We agree on when and whether to get married.

HABITS AND HOBBIES

	0	1	2	3	4	5

- My partner does not place too much emphasis on neatness.
- My partner does not worry me about his/her use of alcohol/tobacco/drugs.
- My partner is not too busy for us to do enough things together.
- I am not uncomfortable on occasions with my partner's behaviour.
- My partner does not need more outside activities.
- Our leisure activities are compatible.

FAMILY/FRIENDS

	0	1	2	3	4	5

- My partner's spiritual beliefs are acceptable to me.
- My partner's spiritual beliefs are acceptable to my family.
- Our families have similar cultural/social/economic/ethnic values.
- We share attitudes about values.

	0	1	2	3	4	5

- We share attitudes on children and the attitudes we would like them to have.
- I like my partner's friends.
- I am happy for my partner to spend time with his/her own friends.
- I am happy to spend time with my partner's friends.
- I do *not* worry that either of our families will cause friction between us.
- We have the same feelings about pregnancy, childbirth and adoption.
- We agree on our roles as parents in raising children, if we have them.
- I believe that my partner will make a good parent if we have children.
- We agree on whether to talk about our problems with close friends.
- I believe that we should talk about our problems with each other.
- We agree on whether to talk about our problems with our families.
- My partner is not too dependent on his/her family.
- My partner's family is not too dependent on him/her.
- My family agrees with my choice of partner.
- My partner's family likes me.
- I am comfortable when I am with my partner's family.
- We agree on whether to have children.
- I do *not* worry that my own childhood will badly affect my relationship with our children, if we have any.

PERSONAL

	0	1	2	3	4	5

- My partner is not depressed and does not have major mood swings.
- My partner is very unlikely to hurt my feelings.
- My partner and I have a similar sense of humour.
- My partner is a good companion.
- My partner expresses feelings well.
- My partner does not have a problem with his/her temper.
- I have no doubt my partner has made the right choice in me.
- I have no doubt that I have made the right choice in my partner.
- My partner does not have prejudices that upset me.
- Most of the time I am satisfied with life.
- I find that I feel comfortable with my partner most of the time.
- I try very hard to avoid disagreements with my partner.
- My partner tries very hard to avoid disagreements with me.
- I always feel safe with my partner.
- My partner handles personal problems well.
- My partner is not too possessive.
- I do not get annoyed with any of my partner's mannerisms.

	0	1	2	3	4	5

- I am never embarrassed by my partner's behaviour.
- My partner is not stubborn.
- My partner is there for me when I am down.
- I am comfortable with my partner's moods.
- My partner is a good listener.
- We are able, when necessary, to talk over problems when we disagree.
- My partner is not too aggressive.

SEXUAL COMPATIBILITY

	0	1	2	3	4	5

- I feel good about my sexuality.
- I feel good about my partner's sexuality.
- We agree on the process of lovemaking and intercourse.
- I like the way I look.
- I do not think that sex is the way to sort out our problems.
- I am not embarrassed by sexual contact with my partner.
- I am happy with how sex is initiated.
- I am not worried about being unable to satisfy my partner sexually.
- I am not worried about being unsatisfied by my partner sexually.
- I can trust my partner with members of the opposite sex.
- I am happy in the way we show affection for each other.
- I am not worried that I might be sexually impotent or frigid.
- I am not worried that my partner might be sexually impotent or frigid.
- I understand that if I were unfaithful it could ruin our relationship.
- At times I need my personal space and my partner gives it to me.
- I can discuss sex with my partner.
- My partner and I have the same views on premarital sex.
- The method or absence of birth control is not a problem between us.
- At times, if my partner does not want sex or to be touched, it is all right with me.

RECOMMENDATION

Where the couple have differing or opposing views, the points should be discussed amongst themselves or their friends and family. If resolution is not forthcoming then I strongly advise a session with a relationships counsellor or, in the case of religious disagreements, a suitable spiritual advisor.

Alcohol

I co-published a study in 1984 concerning the Foetal Alcohol Syndrome, which suggested that this potentially lethal and devastating effect by alcohol on foetuses is often underdiagnosed and may be caused by a small amount of alcohol. Throughout this book I will touch upon the dangers and joys of alcohol and principally will not support abstinence. When aiming to conceive and through the early part of pregnancy, however, I am a strong advocate of abstinence. In the male partner alcohol adversely affects the motility of the sperm.

RECOMMENDATION

General Advice
• *Do not drink alcohol for at least ten days before attempting conception.*

Drugs

Drugs are harmful in any case but more so in pregnancy. There are very few orthodox, doctor-prescribed drugs that have been shown to have any level of safety during pregnancy. Very little evidence is available on the effects of drugs during conception but we do know a lot about the dangers of drugs during early pregnancy.

Studies on recreational drugs have clearly stated that they are dangerous. They can alter the genetic material and affect the mother's ability to nourish the child. Drugs also adversely affect the motility of sperm.

RECOMMENDATION

General Advice
• *Do not use a drug, unless absolutely essential, for at least one month before attempting conception.*

Detoxification prior to conception

Once the ovulation cycle and the days when fertility is at a premium have been determined, I recommend a detoxification diet.

RECOMMENDATION

Nutritional
• *See the* **Detox** *(3-day) and* **Semi-fast** *(7-day)* **diets** *in chapter 7. These should be considered at least one week before the period is expected and continued until ten days before the next period is due. The Hay diet (see chapter 7) can be followed in-between attempts to conceive so that the body remains predominantly alkaline- and toxin-free.*

Nutrition pre-pregnancy

The basic rules of general well-being with regards to nutrition hold true for pre-conception. Please review the chapter on nutrition paying particular attention to foods containing folic acid. Foods containing iron should be increased to reach the 30mgs per day recommended level for pregnant women. Try to maintain five portions of fruit and vegetables daily and generally go with your cravings and intuition.

RECOMMENDATIONS

Nutritional
• *Foods containing folic acid include dark green leafy vegetables, carrots, egg yolk, avocados, beans and rye. Many breakfast cereals are now fortified with folic acid but as they have been separated from their natural source, a high absorption level is not guaranteed.*
• *Iron can be increased by eating more red meat and, in particular, kidneys, but for the vegetarian dried peaches, egg yolks, nuts, beans, asparagus and oatmeal are all good sources.*

Psychological Preparedness

Hang out with parents! Very few men are ever particularly ready for fatherhood and most women, especially if they do not have younger brothers or sisters, are surprised at the increase in responsibility, lack of sleep, relationship changes and shifts in behaviour patterns that occur with pregnancy and motherhood.

Try setting your alarm clock to go off every three hours for a week. Walk out of the most exciting parts of your favourite television programmes, spend some time turning down invitations to events and dinner parties, stop all your 'bad' habits such as drinking and smoking, and bring into discussion all the main points of contention between you and your partner! The rewards of your baby's smile, gurgle and undying affection will override all the negative aspects, but if you still do not feel comfortable you may benefit from chatting to young parents or even talking with a psychologist to map things out.

Vitamins and supplements

Principally, a good diet should provide individuals with all the vitamins and supplements they need. There is no specific advice for males other than healthy eating, unless a couple are not conceiving. Women, on the other hand, should add some supplements to their diet for at least one month prior to conception.

RECOMMENDATIONS

Nutritional

- *Visit a nutritionist to establish a clear-cut dietetic regime to follow after the Detox and Semi-fast diets recommended above.*

Supplemental

- *Folic acid (400mg daily) has been shown to reduce the number of neural tube defects (problems with the formation of the spinal column).*
- *A natural multivitamin and mineral complex should be used to avoid any problems that we may not yet be aware of due to deficiencies of the trace elements.*

Homeopathic

- *Visit a homeopath to establish a constitutional pattern (see **Homeopathy**).*

Orthodox

- *Visit a GP for a thorough orthodox check-up.*

THE ENERGY OF CONCEPTION

The vessel of conception and the governing vessel, according to the Chinese, is a term for an energy flow that passes through or over the pituitary and thyroid glands, the pancreas and the uterus. I discuss this vessel in more detail later (*see* **Vessel of conception**). If a woman who is intending to become pregnant has a mother who has had problems with the thyroid, diabetes or the uterus, then she should see a Tibetan or Chinese practitioner for acupuncture, with or without herbal treatments. A weakness in any of these organs may represent a weakness in this midline energy flow, and this may mean that the intended mother has a weakness and a predisposition to developing diabetes or hypothyroidism during a pregnancy.

SEXUAL POSITION AND TECHNIQUE

Physically speaking, the art of lovemaking is important in a successful conception. The male orgasm indicates a successful ejaculation and an improper technique can lead to faulty 'firing'. The woman's orgasm is associated with an increased flow of blood to the genital tract prior to orgasm, which ensures that everything is primed prior to reception of the sperm. The orgasm causes the blood to disperse, which decongests the area and allows the sperm to travel more easily. It is therefore preferable, when trying to conceive, to time a mutual orgasm.

Mutual orgasms are not a prerequisite to successful conception but they are liable to help. Orgasms are moments of physical, psychological and spiritual bliss, so if both partners can share this at a time when a new life is being created then it is a better start from a spiritual, energetic point of view.

On a more practical note, the position of intercourse may be of vital importance. Human beings

UTERUS – Normal and Retroverted

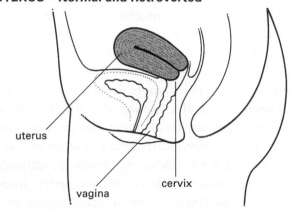
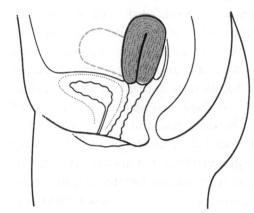

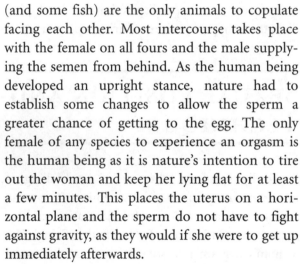

uterus

vagina

cervix

A uterus tilted in the normal position.

The almost vertical position of a retroverted uterus.

(and some fish) are the only animals to copulate facing each other. Most intercourse takes place with the female on all fours and the male supplying the semen from behind. As the human being developed an upright stance, nature had to establish some changes to allow the sperm a greater chance of getting to the egg. The only female of any species to experience an orgasm is the human being as it is nature's intention to tire out the woman and keep her lying flat for at least a few minutes. This places the uterus on a horizontal plane and the sperm do not have to fight against gravity, as they would if she were to get up immediately afterwards.

There is a surprisingly common condition called a retroverted uterus. In this condition the body of the uterus tips or is held backwards towards the spine. The cervix, the opening to the uterus, automatically pushes forward and can push into the front wall of the vagina. During intercourse the semen is fired from the penis at speeds of up to 80mph. If this hits the cervix directly, the sperm obtain quite a head start on their travel from the opening of the cervix to the egg. If the uterus is retroverted and the cervix is pushed forward, then the sperm can be fired into the posterior fornix and then have to swim around, find the cervix and travel a much further distance. Amazingly, during female orgasm, the cervix 'dips' into the pool of semen to help the sperm on their

journey, but even so the sperm are disadvantaged.

The uterus can also have a tendency to tip to the right, to the left or forward, and in each case can cause the cervix to be pushed against any of the sides of the vaginal wall. A basic examination by a qualified doctor can clearly illustrate the position of the cervix. If the cervix is pushing into one of the sides of the vagina, then the woman should take up a position during intercourse that moves the uterus through the pull of gravity, thus moving the cervix away from the vaginal wall.

CASE HISTORY

Mrs J O came to see my late father over 15 years ago. She was from the Cameroon and had undergone tests for infertility there, in Switzerland and in London, all to no avail. She came to see a complementary practitioner as a last resort and was very surprised when my father, after a full examination, gave her a basic homeopathic remedy and told her to lie on her right-hand side whenever she and her husband were trying to conceive. I now look after her and her family of four children, all conceived at times when she was lying on her right-hand side.

For the reasons I have described above, a long penis can find itself passing the cervix and ejaculating into the top of the vagina. At times of attempted fertilization it is wiser to try to keep only two or three inches in the vagina in an attempt to ejaculate onto the cervical opening.

FAILURE TO CONCEIVE

Between 10 and 15 per cent of couples are defined as infertile by having been unable to become pregnant after unprotected sexual intercourse undertaken at the most fertile time over the course of a year. Of these, 35 per cent of cases are caused by female problems and a similar figure is created by male problems; 20 per cent occur because of a combination of the two and 10 per cent remain unexplained. These figures need to be taken into consideration before extensive investigations are mapped out on the female partner since tests and examinations on males are much easier.

One of the most rewarding areas of medicine must be helping a couple to become pregnant who have previously failed to conceive. The majority of those who wish to conceive do so, but for a small percentage conception continues to prove difficult if not impossible. There are many potential causes and each needs to be addressed and suitable treatment applied.

INFERTILITY AND MEN

The following advice is really relevant only after a year of unprotected and well-timed intercourse has been attempted, although the concepts hold true at any time.

Initial testing is undertaken to illustrate inadequate function or amounts of sperm. Male ejaculate (semen) contains spermatozoa (sperm) produced in the testes and they live in and feed from seminal fluid made in the prostate. This fluid contains fructose, a sugar that provides nutrition to the swimming sperm, further nutrients and a small quantity of defence chemicals known as immunoglobulins. Diseases or injury to the testes, the tubes (vas efferens, vas deferens and

Genitals – Male

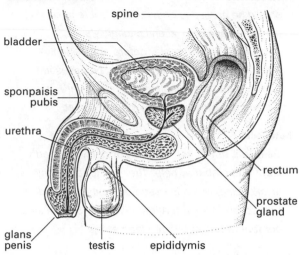

spermatic cord), the prostate, the urethra or penis can all cause a fault in the production of the sperm or its delivery. (Rarely, tumours and hormonal problems can be underlying causes.)

The testes are kept outside of the body, thus allowing them to be maintained at a degree lower in temperature than the rest of the body. It has been shown that the advent of disposable nappies impairs normal testicular cooling mechanisms and may be a cause of infertility in later years.

The first line of treatment in the case of any infertile couple is to check the male out and assure that his sperm count is good. The tests are non-invasive and fast to perform. The male provides a semen sample and a blood test may be taken to check the hormonal situation if the sperm count or motility is low. If something is wrong, the following can be of help.

RECOMMENDATIONS

General Advice

- *Provide a sperm sample after three days if not ejaculating.*
- *Ensure that loose boxer shorts and trousers that are not tight-fitting are worn.*
- *Stress reduction (see **Stress**). Adrenaline reduces sperm production.*

- Reflexology can be of benefit. Gentle pressure should be applied to areas on the feet representing the testes and adrenal and pituitary glands.
- Allow for lengthy foreplay before ejaculation.
- Infertility beyond one year should be assessed and treated by a complementary medical practitioner with knowledge of the subject.

Nutritional

- Believe it or not, half a dozen oysters, lean red meat and crab may help. They all contain a high level of zinc, which is essential for motility and production of sperm. Alternatively, try 5mg of zinc per foot of height before sleep at night.

Supplemental

- Korean, Chinese or Tibetan ginseng (2g twice a day).
- The following may be taken daily with food, in divided doses per foot of height: beta-carotene (3000iu), vitamin C (1g) and vitamin E (100iu).

Orthodox

- Intra-cytoplasmic Sperm Injection (ICSI) selects the most active sperm and directly injects it into the egg. This technique has increased the number of successful pregnancies considerably in the last 20 years.

Assuming that all is well with the male then the investigations turn to the female.

INFERTILITY AND WOMEN

As with men, do not feel a need to concern yourself until conception has not occurred for a year of unprotected and well-timed intercourse. If you are trying to conceive after the age of 38 years, then seek advice after six months.

Women have much the same potential difficulty in producing viable eggs as men do in creating sperm. Girls are born with a finite number of eggs in each ovary. These lie dormant as the ovary and the rest of the female matures. Around the time of the menarche (the starting of the periods), the chemical changes that occur with young girls at that age cause eggs to mature and ripen.

Genitals – Female

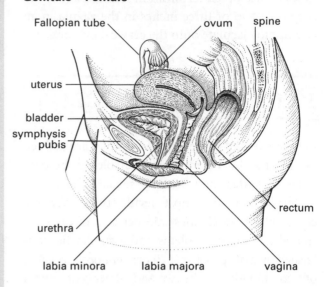

Due to a particular chemical 'cut-out' method, usually only one egg matures each month from either ovary and is released into the opening of the Fallopian tube. Many reasons can account for failure of an egg to ripen: nutritional factors, infections, stress and unhappiness, hormonal imbalances and ovarian pathology.

Practical matters can be a hazard too. Once the egg has passed into the Fallopian tube it has to travel the equivalent of a human being walking from London to Munich. The egg is assisted by peristaltic waves pushing the packet of female genes towards the uterus. Most fertilization occurs in the outer one-third of the Fallopian tube, requiring the more motile sperm to travel a far greater distance. As one can clearly see, there is much scope for structural problems causing a barrier between the two gametes. Previous infections can scar up the Fallopian tubes and difficulties such as endometriosis (misplacement of uterine tissue around the Fallopian tubes onto the ovaries or in the abdominal cavity) can all bar the movement of the microscopic egg and sperm.

CHROMOSOMAL ABNORMALITIES

All our cells contain protein structures (DNA) that carry the memory of our inheritance. These

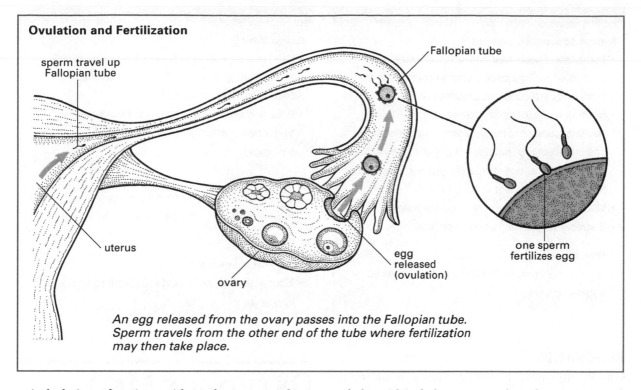

Ovulation and Fertilization

sperm travel up Fallopian tube

Fallopian tube

uterus

egg released (ovulation)

ovary

one sperm fertilizes egg

An egg released from the ovary passes into the Fallopian tube. Sperm travels from the other end of the tube where fertilization may then take place.

spiral chains of amino acids make up our chromosomes, found in the nucleus of most of our cells. There are 46 chromosomes in our cells – the sperm and the egg carrying 23 each. When these join together a full compliment is formed and the fertilized egg can then develop into a foetus. (The gender of a baby is determined by the chromosomes in a sperm. A sperm may carry an X or a Y chromosome. Two X chromosomes become a girl and an X and a Y create a boy).

Problems with chromosomes or the division of the chromosomes while developing into the egg or the sperm (for example 22 or 24 chromosomes being present instead of the normal 23) generally leads to a failure in conception. The best-known chromosomal abnormality is Down's syndrome (*see* **Down's syndrome**) and it is by far the most common of the chromosomal abnormalities that actually survive to become a pregnancy.

HORMONAL MATTERS

Once the basic health of the couple has been checked, the physician may move on to more specific tests. In women, problems such as diabetes

and thyroid imbalances can alter the picture and generally a complete blood screen is performed to check hormone levels. If nothing is found to be wrong, then blood tests are taken at particular times of the cycle to get an idea of the hormonal pattern. The hormones checked are:

- oestrogen and progesterone
- follicle-stimulating hormone
- luteinizing hormone
- prolactin

Oestrogen and progesterone are necessary for the preparation of the uterus to allow the fertilized egg to implant. Follicle-stimulating hormone (FSH) causes an egg within the ovarian tissue to mature and ripen, and the luteinizing hormone causes the shell of the ovary to open and allow the egg to be released into the Fallopian tube. Prolactin is formed to prepare the breasts for lactation; an excess of prolactin, usually due to a non-cancerous tumour in the pituitary gland, can prevent pregnancy, which is why lactation and breast-feeding may prevent pregnancy.

BLOCKAGES

One of the more common causes of infertility is a blockage in the Fallopian tubes, so the specialist's first step is usually to perform a laparoscopy. This is an operation that usually requires a general anaesthetic. A small incision is made underneath the navel and a thin flexible scope is passed through, enabling the surgeon to have a look at the ovaries, Fallopian tubes and surrounding structures. A dye is passed through the cervix and the flow is watched from the two open ends of the Fallopian tube. This is called a hysterosalpingogram. The discovery of a blockage can be cured by operation, as can polycystic ovaries: a condition that can run in families, where the ovaries have multiple fluid-filled cysts that act as a blockage as well as sometimes being associated with hormonal imbalance.

Ideally, before this invasive stage is reached I would recommend that alternatives are assessed. Without the tests one cannot be certain of the diagnosis of a blockage, although a history of infection may point to this. Good pulse-readers claim to be able to diagnose a blockage, as can Kerlian photography (see relevant sections).

ORTHODOX METHODS FOR INFERTILITY

One should always allow a few months for the results of any technique to be conclusive but if the couple remain infertile then one should resort to the orthodox methods with some increased success because all holistic techniques automatically improve the general health of the individual and the area to be treated by drugs or surgery.

Any structural difficulties such as scarred tubes or blockages can sometimes be dealt with operatively. As our scientific techniques become more elaborate, so do our techniques for unblocking the microscopic lumens of the Fallopian tubes. Hormonal imbalances can be corrected chemically and fertility drugs such as clomiphene can be administered, usually with side effects but with some success. Most women react unpleasantly to these drugs and I view them as a last resort rather than first line. In any case, complementary methods can be beneficial in reducing the unwanted side effects.

ARTIFICIAL INSEMINATION

Once initial treatments have failed and the specialist feels that the individual is suitable for artificial techniques, then the 'test-tube baby' concepts come into play. The tried and tested technique of *in-vitro* fertilization (IVF) is one option. This technique requires the removal of mature eggs from the female's ovaries through a specialized laparoscopic procedure after drug inducement of the ovary to produce eggs. The mature eggs are then fertilized under laboratory conditions by the father's or donor's sperm. The fertilized eggs are then replaced in the uterus and hopefully nature takes its course. The uterus is prepared to receive the implant through a programme of administering hormones.

Another successful method is called gamete intra-fallopian transfer (GIFT), which once again entails the removal of an egg from the ovary; the egg is then placed back into the Fallopian tube with an amount of donor sperm. If fertilization occurs, the fertilized egg is then moved down the Fallopian tube naturally into the uterus for implantation.

'Artificial insemination, homologous' (AIH) is a technique initiated by the collection of a number of samples of the partner's semen. This is then concentrated, pooled and placed at the cervical opening, thus shortening the distance that the sperm has to travel. This technique is useful for couples where the male partner has a poor sperm quality or low count. However, AIH is often unsuccessful despite repeated attempts, mainly because there may be other factors involved such as poor motility influencing the sperm efficacy. On the other hand, donor artificial insemination (AID) is about 70 per cent successful even though

several inseminations may be required. AID has raised emotional and ethical questions and so the anonymity of the donor is essential. Donor sperm may often be mixed to block possible legal issues.

The success of these techniques varies greatly from one clinic to the next. There is a 15–20 per cent fertilization rate and one in seven pregnancies that result from artificial fertilization end with a live birth. I feel sure these figures will improve as the techniques get better.

There are always risks with any procedure and the most debilitating (and potentially fatal) is a condition known as ovarian hyperstimulation. This occurs because of the influence of the drugs that stimulate egg production, which causes swelling of the abdomen and vulva, abdominal pain and, a serious sign, vomiting.

THE PSYCHOLOGY OF CONCEPTION

When deciding to have a baby, there are many psychological factors which should be faced and dealt with. For either the male or the female to make a decision to have a baby and a family is a true 'coming of age'. We are stepping away from being the child of our parents to being the parents of a child. We all have to deal with increased responsibility, a loss of freedom, a loss of choice and financial constraints. We also have to face a lifetime of commitment, not only to the child but also to our partner.

Follicle-stimulating hormone (FSH) and luteinizing hormone (LH), which control the ovulation cycle, are produced by a small walnut-sized gland next to the brain, the pituitary gland, so it is perhaps anatomically acceptable that the emotion centres surrounding this gland feed into it chemicals that can block the production or release of FSH

and LH. Long-term unhappiness such as that produced by an unhappy relationship or marriage can put persistent pressure on this gland and hamper its normal production. Stress in males, similarly, can also cause problems. So the simple experience of being happy with your partner can chemically affect your chances of becoming pregnant.

Whilst one is going through all the trials of conceiving, one must not forget that at the end of the day no one is really sure what makes the whole event happen. What is the vital force that gives life to any particular cell? Hindus believe that spirits choose their parents or more scientifically, that a life force enters a fertilized egg. I often see couples where one or both are so full of anger or misery that I find myself asking if I would really want these two as my parents. It is important, I feel, when inviting a spirit into a family unit that the environment is conducive. I always encourage peace and harmony in any infertile situation. Too many marriages and families break up because the parents were not suited, and how many relationships struggle on with the idea that the baby will make things 'right'? It is vitally important for all involved to be content and happy. Choosing and being with the right partner is discussed at the beginning of this chapter, and

THE VESSEL OF CONCEPTION

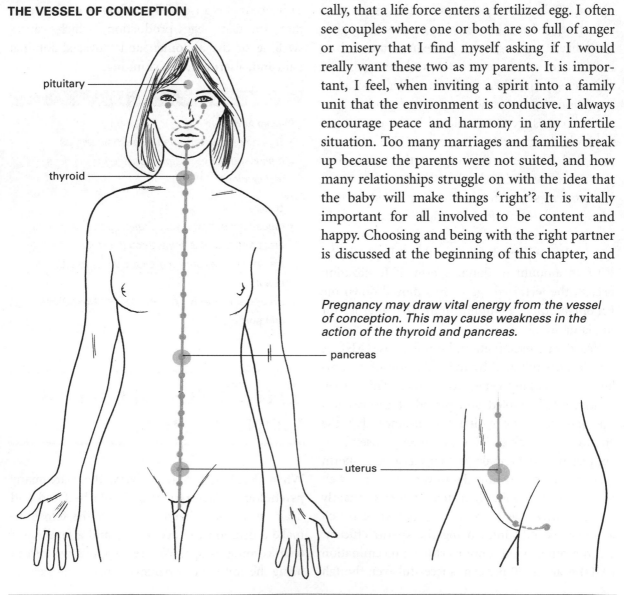

Pregnancy may draw vital energy from the vessel of conception. This may cause weakness in the action of the thyroid and pancreas.

elsewhere, but my experience makes me believe that being with the right or best partner alters conception problems favourably.

THE VESSEL OF CONCEPTION

All philosophies of medicine that include an energy flow through the bodily system describe a mid-line channel or meridian. The Chinese call this the 'vessel of conception', amongst other terms. It is so called because of the establishment, over thousands of years, of an energy flow from the pituitary gland (the hormonal controller of the female cycle) to the uterus. This energy line travels through or over the thyroid gland and the pancreatic gland. It is interesting, is it not, that pregnancy can induce both diabetes and hypothyroidism with no accepted scientific reasoning? This line then travels through the uterus (the testes in the male) to complete this energy channel.

My view is that a pregnancy draws energy into the uterus, thereby diminishing the vital force necessary for the correct maintenance of health within the thyroid and the pancreas. I believe that the vessel of conception receives energy from those close to us. Parents, in particular, pass energy from their vessel of conception to their offspring, and energy is also received from lovers and best friends.

A weakness in the relationship between any of our close contacts, partners and parents will lead to a weak vessel of conception. Energy is passed from both father and mother to their offspring and if the vessel of conception is not initially well supplied or refuelled along the way, then each pregnancy will drain the parents' meridian, leading to problems with subsequent children.

It is essential to have a strong relationship with the partner when conception is considered and the connection between the intended parent and their parents should be strong and positive.

SPIRITUAL MATTERS

Eastern philosophies are much more spiritual in their consideration of pregnancy and use many techniques, including acupuncture, to relieve energy blocks, which in turn interfere with fertility. The West, through its dependence upon science, has lost touch to a great extent with the spiritual aspect of conception. Religions consider a birth 'a blessing' but little, if any, forethought goes into the preparation of starting a new life. Eastern medical philosophies differ substantially.

Mr J G Bennet, a philosopher and student of Gurdjieff, discussed the existence of spiritual genetics. He defined this as an energy that exists on an, as yet, immeasurable plane that travels with individuals and at the time of conception this energy is passed, along with the physical genetic material, into the embryo. Whether this occurs at the moment of conception or at some stage during the pregnancy is open to debate, whether it is the same thing as 'vital force' or the spark of life or whether it is a state of consciousness that may enter the foetus at a later stage are all philosophical points. It is wise, however, to ensure that, when conceiving, both partners:

- are in a non-altered (alcohol and drug-free) state,
- want a child,
- love each other.

These are the three emotional components that traditional Eastern philosophies believe the human spirit can offer and to this you may add the contribution of whichever religion you may follow.

RECOMMENDATIONS

General Advice

- *Sit with your religious advisor and talk.*
- *Those of us who do not have such a teacher should find an Ayurvedic- or Tibetan-trained practitioner to draw on the medically associated aspects of correct spiritual preparedness.*

ASTROLOGY

Lastly, but only because of the scant evidence of accuracy, why not look at astrological patterns? If the Sun and Moon can shift huge bodies of water several miles, as the tides all over the world testify, why should not the small influences of Pluto and Jupiter cause changes in the microscopic amounts of fluid in the egg and sperm?

It is worth checking out whether you and your partner's astrological charts are compatible and when the best time for a child's birth would be. It is an interesting point that the time between conception and delivery is the same time it takes for the planets to reverse their aspects in the heavens. Perhaps charts should be drawn up at the time of conception rather than delivery. Might this rule out the inaccuracies that can occur?

CHAPTER 2
PREGNANCY AND CHILDBIRTH

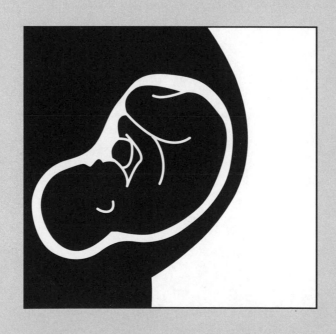

CHAPTER 2

PREGNANCY AND CHILDBIRTH

PREGNANCY

Pregnancy is not a disease process that requires medical intervention. Three out of every five of pregnancies in the world will be managed by unqualified personnel, friends and relatives, common sense and nature.

In the West, due to a lack of nutritional understanding, toxins being knowingly or unwittingly introduced into the body and poor physical preparedness, pregnancies can be uncomfortable and problematic although are safe in comparison to other countries. Problems in these other countries occur mainly due to malnutrition, poor sanitation and negligible emergency services, although pregnancies are generally treated in a more natural manner. As usual, neither the highly-developed countries nor the poorest nations have an ideal situation. The most comfortable and successful pregnancies will have a blend of the best from both. There is a need to mix the high technology of modern science with the intuition and experience of traditional medicines.

DISCOVERING A PREGNANCY

Provided that you are trying, expecting or happy to become pregnant, the revelation is a time of mixed emotions and feelings. The joys of having conceived are tempered with the anxieties of something going wrong. In a first-time pregnancy the fear of the unknown is tempered with the spirit of adventure. The physical symptoms of early pregnancy usually mingle with a profound sensation of well-being. But not always!

Most couples discover that they are pregnant when an expected period is missed. A woman may or may not feel:

- nausea
- mood changes
- aches and pains
- swollen feet and hands

Nausea

At some point in the day nausea is caused by reaction to human chorionic gonadotrophin (HCG), a chemical essential for the survival of the fertilized egg. A Swedish study postulated that mothers with hyperemesis gravidarum (severe vomiting during pregnancy) are more likely to give birth to girls than to boys.

> RECOMMENDATIONS
>
> **General Advice**
> - *Acupressure (see **Nausea**).*
> - *Failing the above, both acupuncture and reflexology can be curative.*
>
> **Nutritional**
> - *Avoid low blood sugar: eat small healthy snacks at regular intervals (see **Hypoglycaemia**).*
> - *A crushed stick of fresh cardamom in yoghurt.*
>
> **Supplemental**
> - *Selenium 20mg per foot of height taken daily with a general multi-mineral supplement.*
> - *Vitamin B6 5mg per foot of height three times daily.*
>
> **Homeopathic**
> - *Homeopathic remedies Ipecacuanha 6, Nux vomica 6 or Cocculus indicus 6 taken every 15 minutes.*
>
> **Herbal/natural extracts**
> - *Ginger: as biscuits (two or three eaten before rising from bed in the morning); as tea (quarter-inch thick, chopped fresh in hot water); as juice (quarter-inch slice with apple, liquidated).*

- *Place a drop of peppermint oil on a sugar cube and suck slowly. You cannot use this if you are using a homeopathic remedy because mint of any sort will inhibit the action of the remedy.*

Mood changes

Mood changes can be either positive or negative. Do not fight the elation! Negative moods may be alleviated by talking, so do so with friends, relatives and even your partner!

RECOMMENDATIONS

General Advice
- *Massage works wonders.*
- *Practise or learn a suitable meditative technique. Self-hypnosis is useful before, after or at delivery.*

Nutritional
- *Keep your blood sugar levels up with healthy snacks.*

Supplemental
- *Depression or anger may respond to D, L-phenylalanine (100mg per foot of height three times a day).*

Homeopathic
- *If depressed, tearful, fearful or angry, use a carefully selected remedy, ideally chosen by a homeopath. Remedies are best given at high potency and many are not recommended during pregnancy.*

Herbal/natural extracts
- *A drop of rose oil on your collar.*
- *Sesame oil rubbed into the feet for five minutes before washing it off.*

Aches and pains

Aches and pains are caused by hormonal effects on ligaments, even this early on in the pregnancy.

RECOMMENDATIONS

General Advice
- *Massage – especially Shiatsu.*

- *Polarity therapy is good at all stages of pregnancy.*
- *Yoga. The earlier in pregnancy that yoga is learned and practised, the better.*

Supplemental
- *Vitamin B_6 (50mg daily) and copper (2mg daily) for up to five days.*

Homeopathic
- *Arnica 6 or Magnesia phosphorica 6 four times a day for up to five days.*

Herbal/natural extracts
- *Comfortably hot baths with chamomile, lavender or rosemary essential oils.*

Swollen feet and hands

Swollen feet and hands are a side effect of the hormones of pregnancy but may be helpful because of a diluting down of the chemical effects on the body tissues. Diuretic treatments should be avoided. If the male partner is experiencing 'sympathetic pregnancy', he may find the following recommendations useful as well. These are all normal and can be alleviated.

RECOMMENDATIONS

General Advice
- *Place swollen hands or feet in hot and cold water alternately.*
- *Lymphatic drainage massage is tremendous.*

Nutritional
- *Increase your protein intake at each meal.*

Homeopathic
- *Natrum muriaticum 6 can be used four times a day for three days.*

SYMPATHETIC PREGNANCY

Male partners often experience similar symptoms to pregnant women. These are known as symptoms of sympathetic pregnancy. The male partner may find all the previous recommendations useful. Why this phenomenon occurs is uncertain and may be purely psychological but possibly pheromonally (inhaled chemical) induced.

PREGNANCY TESTS

Today pregnancy tests are 98 per cent accurate. Two tests having the same result is usually conclusive. The options are:

- home testing
- a test by your local chemist or pharmacy
- a test by your GP or Pregnancy Advisory Clinic.

Your GP will do the test for free, otherwise the tests range from £5 to £15 and they are all equally accurate. A drop of urine is placed on a small pad or a small sample of urine is shaken with a chemical that measures the presence of human chorionic gonadotrophin (HCG). A colour change or the appearance of a line indicates a positive pregnancy test.

A pregnancy test can be carried out as soon as two weeks after fertilization is thought to have occurred. The earlier the test, the greater the chance of a 'false' negative or positive result and it is probably best to wait for two weeks after a missed period.

Home-testing for pregnancy

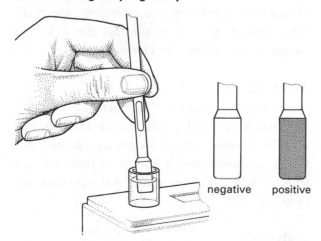

negative   positive

There are many different home-testing kits and they mostly work on the same principle – a particular colour or line indicating the presence of Human Chorionic Gonadotrophin (HCG).

ESTIMATING THE EXPECTED BIRTH DATE

The estimation of a delivery date is always a 'best guess' and not an exact science. Assessing the delivery date is considered in the West to be a mathematical problem. The simplest technique is to add seven days to the first day of your last period and take off three months. For example, if the first day of the last period was 14 July, add seven days to make 21 July and subtract three months. The delivery date is 21 April. You will then be told that the delivery could occur anywhere around that date.

The moon is considered to be very influential in the female hormonal cycle, especially with regard to childbirth. It is worth assessing the stage of the moon around the expected time of conception. If you conceived on a full moon then delivery is more likely to be around the full moon. Conversely, a new moon conception will support a new moon delivery.

CHOOSING YOUR MEDICAL SUPPORT

Pregnancy and childbirth is one of your most exciting and rewarding life experiences. As with any event, it is usually better if it is shared. The choice of your medical advisors is important because they will be sharing this marvellous time with you. If you do not get on with them, much of the enjoyment can be spoiled in much the same way that a prime fillet can be ruined at a shared meal with an ardent vegetarian!

It is essential to visit your maternity unit and meet as many of the midwives as possible. Any one of them could be on duty when you deliver. The obstetrician is, hopefully, not going to be particularly involved unless things go awry, but it helps to get on with the specialist, although not to the same degree as with the midwives.

Ensure that your views concerning position of delivery, water birth and pain relief are shared with the midwives, otherwise friction and doubts can manifest.

To a lesser extent partners should be happy with the team because they too will be part of the event. There are good and bad in all professions and it is very hard for patients or, for that matter, GPs to be able to isolate the jokers in the pack. A conversation with your GP or complementary medical practitioners will probably make the selection process a lot easier.

CHOOSING YOUR HOSPITAL

Ideally each maternity unit would have a blend of the best in orthodox technology with the comforts of your own bedroom. The unit would be staffed by experienced medical personnel with the personal touch of your closest friend and relative. An emergency unit would be next to the birthing unit and your God would be in the waiting room in case anything went wrong. This is not the case and until it is we have to adjust the situation to our best advantage. I am not a great believer in the safety of home births, certainly not for a first pregnancy and delivery. For latter pregnancies when no complications have arisen before and the home midwife and GP are very experienced and emergency facilities are close by, then perhaps the risk is negligible.

I prefer to look upon childbirth as an unusual part of life and not a household activity. In contradiction to this last statement, I feel that if the local hospital facilities are not 'homely' enough then a home delivery may be preferable as long as easy access to the emergency facilities is available. As will be mentioned many times throughout this book, each case should be judged upon its individual merits.

The place of delivery should preferably be in a room with a comfortable atmosphere for the parents. A bed at the correct height which allows Mum to place her feet on the floor and keep her backside on the edge is needed, and also a large tub or bath that can allow her and her birthing partner to relax comfortably with clear access from the sides for the midwives. Full medical facilities should be available within moments in case anything goes wrong.

Such hospitals are few and far between, although their numbers are increasing dramatically.

Access to such units is becoming increasingly available in big cities but still remains out of reach for those in rural areas.

CHOOSING AND USING A COMPLEMENTARY MEDICAL CLINIC

In an ideal situation your GP and your obstetric team will have a liaison with a complementary medical clinic or practitioners. If this is the case, then you simply follow the guidelines set down by your now complete team.

Unfortunately it is rare to find a unit that has all the available options from a complementary point of view. The choice of a clinic is best made by asking friends who have had dealings with clinics in your local area or practitioners within striking distance of your home or place of work. The complementary clinic should have at its disposal the following therapists, practitioners and techniques.

Acupuncturist

Acupuncture can be most beneficial for morning sickness, aches and pains, mood changes and other symptoms during pregnancy. In the right hands, acupuncture can also be of benefit at the time of delivery by speeding up the process and reducing pain.

Bodywork

Bodywork should be an integral part of pregnancy. Any massage technique is liable to be relieving, especially for the inevitable backaches

MORNING SICKNESS – Acupuncture Points

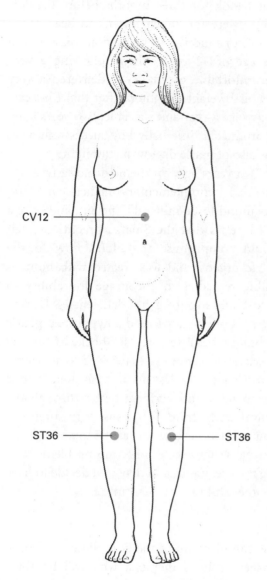

CV12

ST36 — — ST36

Acupressure or acupuncture treatment at Conception Vessel meridian point 12 (CV12) and Stomach meridian point 36 (ST36) may help alleviate morning sickness.

associated with carrying extra weight. Muscles which go into spasm can be relieved through massage. Shiatsu massage is even more beneficial, since it uses acupressure points and meridian stretches as well as muscular pressure. It is useful for the mother-to-be's partner to learn some basic pressure points as these can be useful at the time of delivery.

General Advice

- *A local masseur or one who can visit your home should be found and a weekly massage from three months onwards is ideal. It helps to keep the muscles supple and also creates an amount of endorphin release that is mentally soothing to both the mother and the baby. Partners should be taught some basic massage techniques for use on a daily basis.*
- *Shiatsu massage is of great benefit. Not only is it soothing but it can be useful by teaching the partner specific acupressure points that may help delivery. There are certain Shiatsu techniques and pressure points that should not be used during pregnancy but be assured that any registered and qualified Shiatsu practitioner will know the places to avoid.*
- *Other techniques of bodywork, such as polarity, osteopathy and chiropractic can all be used if aches and pains come to the fore.*

Homeopathy

There has been much anecdotal evidence over the last 150 years to support the use of homeopathy both in the treatment of problems in pregnancy and in aiding the delivery of the baby. Because of the unknown constitution of the foetus/baby, I only recommend the use of this form of medicine under the guidance of a practitioner but, having said that, there is no evidence whatsoever to suggest any dangers to mother or baby with the use of homeopathy. There are many remedies that can encourage the contraction of the uterus, amongst them Caulophyllum, and Secale cornutum. These may be taken at potency 30 as soon as contractions start. Secale cornutum may also be used after the delivery of the baby to encourage the third stage of labour. There are many remedies that can be used for problems associated with pregnancy such as backaches, nausea, discharges and painful breasts. Having a homeopath as part of the 'team' is an extremely useful idea.

Hypnotherapy

An excellent study was concluded in the 1980s and published in the *Journal of Obstetrics and Gynaecology*. It showed that hypnotherapy can reduce the length of labour by as much as one-third and the need for analgesia by up to 50 per cent.

Different hypnotherapists use different techniques but my recommendation is a course of self-hypnotherapy taught two or three months before delivery to help the sleep pattern, which is often disturbed by the discomfort of late pregnancy and the delivery itself.

Nutritionist

The importance of correct nutrition has been discussed in the section **Physical Preparation for Conception** (*see* **Nutrition in pregnancy**).

Psychotherapist or counsellor – *see* **Psychology of conception** *and* **Vessel of conception**.

Yoga or polarity – *see* **Exercise in pregnancy**.

All the above may not necessarily be required but access to them all is preferable just in case. All the above techniques have specific uses at times during normal and complicated pregnancies.

CASE HISTORY:

Mrs E B, age 38 years: 'My first attempts at becoming pregnant were half-hearted and started at the age of 24 years. After several months of not conceiving I visited my GP and was told not to worry until I had not conceived for over a year. When that time came I went back and was promptly pushed through the orthodox system and both my husband and I ended up having a variety of tests, culminating in a laparoscopy under general anaesthetic six months later. At no stage was I advised on my diet, possible nutritional deficiencies or the use of alternative medicines, although I was offered a heavy drug regime that I took for three months before the side effects were too much for me to bear. I was unable to conceive for no obvious reason until the age of 32 years when, following a very uncomfortable pregnancy, I delivered a very low birthweight daughter. After that I miscarried twice a year and was able, two years later, to produce a little baby boy successfully who was also of markedly low birthweight.

Two years ago, on the advice of a friend, I attended a complementary medical clinic and was found to be mineral deficient, and have a tilted pelvis that the Shiatsu practitioner felt would compromise the blood flow to the pelvic organs, and was treated with homeopathic remedies to encourage my ability to absorb and avoid further deficiencies. During the next pregnancy I used a hypnotherapeutic technique because I was so shocked from my previous adventures. I received counselling and a couple of lessons in yoga that helped me to relax and perform better through the delivery. My third baby was born after five hours of labour and was at the top end of the normal weight scale. I had no problems during the pregnancy and may well decide to have another child in the near future.'

Most complementary medical clinics will have a manager or head therapist who will be able to discuss your particular requirements. Your own physician may have some insight and the next few pages will cover a lot of the ground.

INVESTIGATIONS

Your GP or hospital will run routine urinalysis and blood pressure checks and at later stages of the pregnancy will check your haemoglobin levels for anaemia.

I encourage my patients to have their haemoglobin checked early on in the pregnancy and if there is any drop in the level then this should be

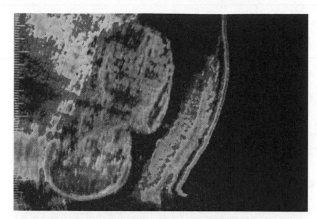

Foetal ultrasound scan.

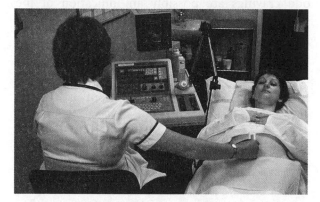

Ultrasound scanning.

compensated for. The orthodox approach is to maintain the haemoglobin level within 'normal limits' and supplemental iron may not be administered until the level drops below 10mmol/l. Each person is an individual and if your haemoglobin starts at 14mmol/l then that is where it should stay. All patients should have a routine antibody screen for:

- Rubella.
- Toxoplasmosis (especially for anyone with a household containing cats).
- A hair analysis or other test for deficiencies (*see* **Bioresonance** and **Hair analysis**). Minor mineral and vitamin deficiencies can be quite devastating to a healthy pregnancy.

Ultrasound scans are not completely safe. Research in the early 1990s suggested that more than eleven ultrasound scans in a pregnancy can lead to a low birthweight baby. For some reason the ultrasound waves inhibit growth. The orthodox world considers that up to ten scans is therefore safe. My experience and common sense do not agree. I feel that the benefits of ultrasound in being able to diagnose problems is enormous but try to confine ultrasounds to a maximum of three per pregnancy unless problems exist. A scan at around 11–16 weeks to confirm a viable foetus, around 20–24 weeks for defects and around 30–34 weeks to check for correct growth is ample investigation.

OTHER ORTHODOX INVESTIGATIONS
Amniocentesis

Amniocentesis (the insertion of a needle and withdrawing of the fluid surrounding the foetus) has its place but not in routine pregnancy care. Much information can be gleaned from analysis of the fluid, including a diagnosis of Down's syndrome and other chromosomal abnormalities.

Amniocentesis

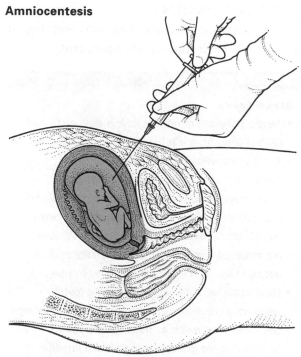

Amniotic fluid, extracted by syringe through the abdomen, is used to diagnose for genetic abnormalities.

There is now, however, a blood test that is becoming more available and accurate, although not as accurate as the amniocentesis. Amniocentesis carries a 2 per cent complication rate (1 in 50 such investigations may cause a problem), whereas the blood test is harmless.

RECOMMENDATIONS

Orthodox

- *Discuss any suggestion of this procedure with more than one obstetrician and ensure that there is a need for such a process. Would you have a termination (an abortion) if something were wrong?*
- *Chorionic villus sampling (CVS). The chorionic villi are on the foetal side of the placenta. The cells are therefore derived from the genetic components of the foetus, and a biopsy or sample of this tissue can be extracted to test for congenital or hereditary defects. The complications and problems are the same as for amniocentesis.*

THE ENVIRONMENT

Please follow these recommendations with regard to the home environment when pregnant.

RECOMMENDATIONS

General Advice

- *Never, pregnant or not, sit nearer than eight feet (2.2m) away from a television.*
- *Avoid VDUs (visual display units). There is evidence that they increase the chances of miscarriage. If you have to use one or are near any, avoid the back or sides. Do not sit at one for more than 20min without a 20-min break, avoid old machines, obtain low-radiation units and do not trust the 'screens': they are next to useless.*
- *Loud music will detrimentally affect the foetus. Apparently, classical music is good, especially Mozart!*
- *Get outside as much as possible and walk barefoot on the grass where safe and possible. If you are a town dweller, make a point of going to the country as often as you can.*

NUTRITION IN PREGNANCY

Once you have established that you are pregnant, the first and possibly the most important thing to do is to ensure that your diet is adequate and that you are supplemented correctly. A well-balanced diet will probably not need any extra nutrition but for those under pressure, with any form of illness, or who are regularly missing meals, or are subjected to fast food or inadequate nutrition, then supplements should be utilized.

There is no set diet for pregnancy and intuition is extremely important. The stories of odd cravings are possibly an indication of the body's requirements. The not-so-unusual cravings for charcoal or chalky substances are suspected to be due to the body's increased requirements for calcium and other minerals. The brain is good at knowing that it needs something but it does not always get it right.

RECOMMENDATIONS

Supplemental

Many of the requirements have been discussed earlier, in chapter 1, and the nutritional requirements throughout your planning to conceive should continue during pregnancy, specifically:

- *Folic acid (400µg) can be taken daily, although the requirement is most important whilst trying to conceive.*
- *Fish oils (omega 3) 500mg daily.*

Most other recommendations are not categorically proven. I think it best, however, to err on the side of caution and anyone who is not well-versed in eating a specifically well-balanced diet should take supplements to allow for the increased demands by the baby and the mother's metabolism, therefore:

- *Multivitamins – most obstetricians and GPs who disagree with additional supplementation do so on the grounds that it is an unnecessary expense, and not because taking extra* supplements could harm the mother or baby. Having said that, an excess of anything may, of course, be harmful, as recently suggested by the vitamin A scare from pregnant women eating too much liver.

- A trace element and mineral compound specifically to cover zinc, manganese and copper.

Nutritional

- Remember to go with your instincts but only if your cravings are for healthy food. If you are yearning for foods that you know are not necessarily healthy, such as chips, specific flavours of crisps and processed foods, then examine the food groups (see **Hay diet**) and select out healthy items from that food group, eat some and see if the unhealthy craving diminishes.
- It is not advisable to change your diet dramatically. Being vegetarian or eating more meat is neither beneficial nor necessary. Aim at a balance.
- Specific foods that you should add to your diet include occasional meals rich in soya or tofu, half-raw/half-cooked vegetables at some time during the day, seaweed every now and then, and ginger.
- Avoid nuts, hazelnuts and oats because they may contain alpha-toxins or promote their production, which can cause foetal damage.

Herbal/natural extracts

- A tablespoon of honey should be eaten per day.

Avoid extra vitamin A

In direct opposition to the need for supplementing the diet with folic acid to avoid birth defects, it is important not to take an excess of vitamin A for exactly the same reasons. Vitamin A content in food does not cause a problem, although eating an excess of liver or carrots may be harmful. It has been shown that more than 10,000iu of vitamin A can increase the risks of developmental problems and should not be taken.

EXERCISE IN PREGNANCY

It is extremely important to maintain a level of fitness and suppleness during pregnancy. A pregnant woman will be carrying extra weight, which will put pressure on joints, ligaments and muscles. The fitter and stronger the muscular framework, the easier the extra weight is dealt with.

RECOMMENDATIONS

General Advice

- Stretching is extremely important and will allow for a much easier delivery.
- Do not commence a heavy exercise programme because you find yourself pregnant. If you are already active then there is no reason why you should stop unless your exercise is a contact sport such as soccer or rugby (many women now play these sports!) or a sport that results in jolting the body. Games such as squash where one places one's feet down heavily and bounces off walls, and activities such as jogging where the downward force on the lower abdomen and pelvis is quite marked, are best avoided.
- Preferably use aerobic exercise such as walking and especially swimming. Dancing is an excellent exercise but avoid your local rave! Many ancient cultures have incorporated dance techniques into the pregnancy period and intuitively moving your body to your favourite piece of music will not only have a beneficial effect on your structure but also be soothing to the baby.

Nothing more needs to be done but:

- I highly recommend learning some basic Alexander Techniques to ensure correct posture. Polarity is equally effective.
- Yoga is, in my opinion, the best form of exercise in pregnancy. Yoga incorporates deep breathing and relaxation techniques, stretching and muscular strengthening along with postural exercises. Certain yoga techniques should not be

Yoga Exercises in Pregnancy

Yoga techniques for relaxation as well as stretching and muscular strengthening are the best form of exercise in pregnancy.

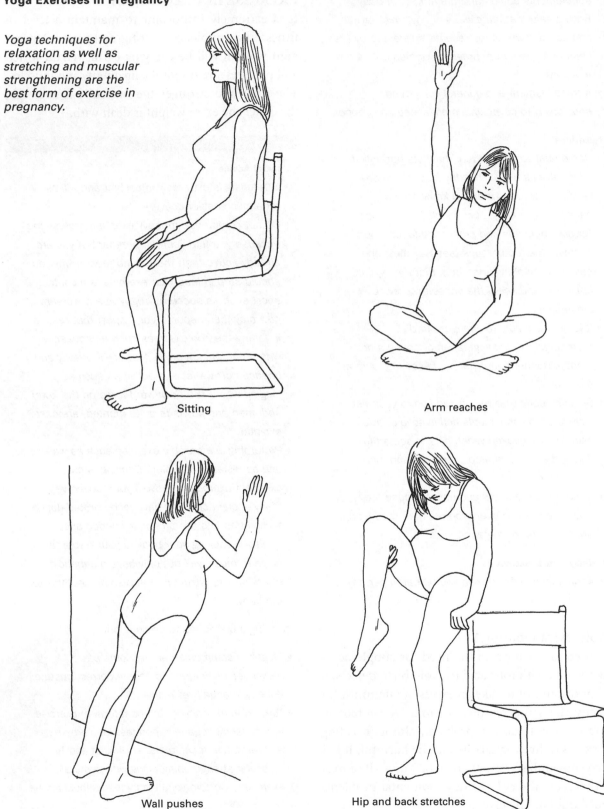

Sitting

Arm reaches

Wall pushes

Hip and back stretches

used during pregnancy and it is best to have a private session or two with a yoga teacher to ensure that you are practising the best techniques.

PSYCHOLOGICAL ASPECTS

Pregnancy should be a time of great joy but almost invariably at some stage during the puerperal (the time you are pregnant) period feelings ranging from ambivalence and indifference, through depression, to anger and anxiety are all commonplace.

Often it is not suitable to use your partner, however close you may be as a couple, for expressing these emotions, but express these emotions you must. Feeling guilty about a state of mind is almost as detrimental to health as the negative emotion itself. Partners, however, are undergoing their own 'crises' and are caught between giving you the best advice and the advice that they think you want to hear. It is an unfair situation to be put in and quite often beyond the intuitive expertise that partners can have.

It is better to face your dilemmas with a 'professional friend' and bring your conclusions to the attention of your partner. Do not hide your feelings from those close to you but do not expect them to have answers. Counsellors are available through any obstetric unit, general practice, complementary clinic or recommendation by friends. It is best to deal with a woman psychotherapist who has been through pregnancy because you will have both the professional and the personal opinion.

Do not be ashamed to ask for support – pregnancy is a time of great change and the psychological help of the extended family is fast dwindling here in the West. It can only be beneficial to be nurtured.

RECOMMENDATIONS

General Advice
• *See a counsellor.*

Herbal/natural extracts
• *Drink strong chamomile tea. This is a great psychological relaxant and can make problems far easier to solve.*
• *Specific essential oils, such as rosemary, chamomile and lavender, can be used as massage oil, in the bath or on the collar.*
• *Homeopathic remedies worth looking up in your preferred homeopathic manual are: Aconitum if fear is the main component; Aurum Metallicum if sad and despairing; Ignatia if your sense of freedom is lost and your sense of responsibility too great; Pulsatilla if your mood is very tearful, although this remedy should not be taken for longer than three days because it may encourage contractions. Other remedies can be of great benefit and your homeopath would be best suited to choose the correct one. All may be taken at potency 30.*
• *The Bach flower remedies are marvellous and a specific book should be reviewed or a therapist's opinion sought to establish the best choice.*

COMMON PROBLEMS ARISING DURING PREGNANCY

Pregnancy is a natural process and not one that requires medication as a rule. Some conditions can arise, however, that may need treating.

ANAEMIA OF PREGNANCY

Anaemia is the medical term given to a range of conditions that are all associated with a lack of the oxygen-carrying compound haemoglobin found in the red blood cells. Assessment of normal levels of haemoglobin vary from laboratory to laboratory around the world but principally the amount we carry in our bloodstreams is 11.5–17mmol/l.

Anaemia is not uncommon in pregnancy due to the baby using up the mother's supply of iron or folic acid. The symptoms of anaemia range from tiredness, lethargy, shortness of breath and irritability to palpitations and fainting. The signs are a pale skin, a pallor under the fingernails and sometimes tingling in the hands and feet. The only way to be certain that anaemia is the cause is by having a blood test which shows your haemoglobin level to be low.

RECOMMENDATIONS

General Advice

- *The orthodox world considers a person to be anaemic only if their haemoglobin level drops below the 'normal' levels. I believe it to be more relevant to have your haemoglobin level checked at an early stage of pregnancy and if your level drops from that figure and any of the aforementioned symptoms are present then consider yourself in need of treatment.*
- *If symptoms persist, acupuncture and especially moxibustion can be administered by a healthcare practitioner who will advise you further.*

Nutritional

- *Increase your input of green-leaf vegetables, especially spinach, and enjoy a little more lamb. Molasses should be used instead of sugar.*

Supplemental

- *Using blood tests, establish the cause of an anaemia. Most often it is due to lack of iron, folic acid or vitamin B_{12} but it may be an amino acid or other vitamin. Once established, replenish with natural food supplements and seek advice from a complementary medical practitioner concerning the correct amount to take.*

Homeopathic

- *The homeopathic remedy Ferrum phosphoricum 30 should be taken twice a day for 10 days.*

Herbal/natural extracts

- *Strawberry tea with half a teaspoon of thyme per mug may taste a bit earthy but helps if taken three times a day.*

BLEEDING IN PREGNANCY

Bleeding from the vagina during pregnancy requires immediate discussion with your GP or obstetric team. Bleeding before the 28th week is classified as a threatened miscarriage and after that week is called an antepartum haemorrhage.

Very often a small bleed lasting a short time is nothing to worry about and is probably due to a burst vein or changes to the vagina or cervix due to the new hormone levels.

RECOMMENDATION

General Advice

- *I do not recommend any home care although treatments from a homeopath or a herbalist can be used to great effect, but only after a doctor has been consulted.*

BREAST PROBLEMS

Many changes will occur to the breasts in response to the hormonal changes of pregnancy. They will feel more sensitive, heavier and more tender, almost to the point of being painful.

The area around the nipples – the areola – may produce little bumps called Montgomery's tubercules, which produce the necessary secretions to help the nipples prepare for breast-feeding. The areola may darken and the nipple may enlarge out of proportion to the rest of the breast. This is all normal and requires no treatment.

RECOMMENDATIONS

General Advice

- *Milk ducts may become blocked and hard, painful swellings may arise within the breast tissue. Apply alternate hot and cold compresses and gently massage the lump in the direction of the nipple. The lump may become slightly red but if it becomes deeply red or inflamed or streaks of red appear, move on to the next recommendation.*
- *Ensure that correct-fitting cotton bras are obtained. Spend as much time as possible with the breasts exposed to air and sunlight.*
- *Comfortably hot baths can be very relieving for painful breasts.*

Homeopathic

- *If the breast lump becomes red or inflamed use Belladonna 6 every 15min for three doses and then every 2hr until the matter settles. If it does not settle after 24hr, talk to a healthcare practitioner but avoid antibiotics as a first-line treatment.*

CONSTIPATION

Constipation occurs for several reasons: the direct effect of the hormones on the bowel musculature, the body naturally slowing down the transit time (the time taken for food to travel from the stomach to the rectum) to allow more digestive process and absorption; reduced activity, dehydration and the taking of iron supplements.

Common sense approaches such as drinking more water and maintaining activity levels are essential. If the problem continues, the following recommendations can help.

RECOMMENDATIONS

General Advice

- *Massage in general but abdominal massage in particular can be very relieving.*
- *Drink at least three pints of water per day.*
- *Laxatives are not an option. If constipation continues despite the measures mentioned above, bring the problem to the attention of a complementary health professional.*
- *Also see section on constipation.*

Nutritional

- *Reduce dairy products, meat and eggs. Increase your fibre intake (see chapter 7) and ensure that you are taking multivitamins because deficiencies in several vitamins can worsen the problem.*
- *Four ounces of yoghurt, two teaspoonfuls of olive oil and a clove of garlic, mixed and eaten with wholegrain pitta bread.*
- *A mildly spicy vegetable dish (Indian, Thai, etc).*
- *Molasses instead of other sweeteners is a help or it can be taken as 2 dessertspoonfuls before bed.*

Supplemental

- *Lactobacillus acidophilus – two million bacteria with each meal will encourage the bowel flora to break down the faeces.*
- *Pure liquorice comes as a soft bar and is distinct from the children's sweetened rubbery liquorice; 10–20g eaten before bedtime will help.*

CRAMPS

RECOMMENDATIONS

General Advice

- *Increase water input.*
- *Massage, Shiatsu and yoga techniques will all relieve cramping.*

Supplemental

- *Calcium (500mg daily), copper (2mg daily), zinc (15mg at night) and magnesium (400mg daily) should all be taken for up to one week. If the problem persists, speak to your health professional.*

Herbal/natural extracts

- *Drink strong chamomile tea.*

DIABETES IN PREGNANCY

Diabetes mellitus is caused by an insufficiency of naturally occurring insulin from the pancreas. It causes a rise in the sugar level in the blood, which is detrimental to most organs and systems in the body.

Diabetes, like thyroid problems, can occur during pregnancy despite not being a problem in the same person when they are not pregnant. The Chinese have a meridian or energy line that travels from the top of the head down the mid-line of the body. This meridian is called the vessel of conception, or the directing vessel, and is of paramount importance in the reproductive systems of both men and women. The orthodox world considers problems in the pancreas or the thyroid to be due to chemical overdemand but all

Eastern medical philosophies have an energy line such as the vessel of conception, which connects the pituitary gland (control of the cycle), the thyroid gland, the pancreatic gland and the uterus (*see* **Vessel of conception**).

Weakness in this energy channel is brought on by poor health throughout the system but also by a lack of energy received from the relationship of the pregnant woman with her partner and her parents.

General Advice

- *Because of the association of diabetes with the vessel of conception, see a Chinese or Tibetan practitioner for acupuncture and possible herbal treatment.*

Nutritional

- *Discuss diabetes situation with a nutritionist to adjust the diet correctly.*

Herbal/natural extracts

- *Once a nutritionist has adjusted your diet, you may use dandelion (Taraxacum) fluid extract (five drops in water) 10mins before each meal.*

HYPOTHYROIDISM

Hypothyroidism occurs infrequently in pregnancy. The orthodox world has some belief that this is caused by an excessive demand or by some suppression of the thyroid gland by chemicals produced by the baby or by the mother herself. The Eastern philosophies consider that the energy is being pulled down into the uterus, leaving less for the organs associated with the vessel of conception (*see* **Vessel of conception**).

Any symptoms of hypothyroidism, especially excessive tiredness, feeling cold, dulled concentration and excessive water retention, should all arouse suspicion. Most pregnant women like to sleep more but an excessive sleep requirement in association with tiredness regardless of the rest received should also arouse suspicion.

General Advice

- *Please obtain the opinion of your GP and complementary medical practitioner.*
- *Please follow the advice and recommendations given in the section in this book on hypothyroidism.*

MISCARRIAGE

Sadly, some pregnancies do not reach a satisfactory conclusion. One Eastern philosophy believes that a pregnancy that ends in a miscarriage is a tremendous blessing for the parents, who had vested upon them a spirit requiring a very short incarnation that is usually associated with an Advanced Soul. However, this information does not take away the devastating sadness of the loss of a baby. If a miscarriage takes place, please follow the recommendations below.

Recurrent Miscarriage

Repetitive miscarriages are rare. (This is despite the theory that one in three pregnancies fail – a perception that comes from poor recognition of a pregnancy.) Recurrence is frequently a genetic problem and other factors such as environmental toxins or poor health need to be assessed by a specialist in alternative medicine rather than attempting self-help.

General Advice

- *To try to help avoid a miscarriage once it is suspected to be likely, contact your complementary medical practitioner for a reference to someone in the alternative medical field who has some knowledge of this subject. That person or your own practitioner may be able to help but your home medical kit is unlikely to be enough.*
- *Visit a counsellor, however well you feel that you are dealing with the event.*

- The sudden change in hormonal structure is best dealt with by a health professional. Please see your complementary practitioner.

Homeopathic

- If a miscarriage has occurred and bleeding continues, use the homeopathic remedy Phosphorus 6 or Secale cornutum 6 (four pills every hour) until the bleeding and discharge stops. Once this has occurred, take Arnica 200 (one dose twice a day for five days).
- The male partner should take Arnica 200 (one dose twice a day for five days) and would also benefit from a counselling session.

PRE-TERM DELIVERY

An uncommon problem is the development of major contractions before the 40 weeks gestation period has arrived. Few physicians or midwives are concerned if delivery occurs in the 39th week and little intervention is brought into play after the 37th week. Attempts to delay the onset of labour are usually considered at 36 weeks, taking in to account factors such as the size of the baby and of the mother's pelvis, as well as the general well-being of the mother and baby.

Orthodox drugs can be used to relax uterine muscle, but most inhibition is geared towards preventing delivery for long enough for the mother and baby to be transferred to a hospital unit.

As little is known why premature delivery takes place (unless there is an obvious lack of health in the mother), there are no preventative measures to take unless the problem has occurred before. There seems to be an increased chance of premature delivery in those who have experienced this in a previous pregnancy. Poor nutrition and overall poor health are a cause of premature labour. There is also a possible link to smoking. Cervical incompetence (a weak cervix), twin pregnancies, trauma to the abdomen and raised blood pressure (pre-eclampsia) can all predispose to pre-term delivery.

Some Eastern philosophies believe that labour commences because of a build-up of energy that reaches a threshold nine moon phases after conception. Pre-term labour is viewed as a premature build-up of this energy due to a block in the flow of energy from the lower energy centres (chakras). Suppressing emotions, not expressing feelings and giving in to sensual desires (sex, drugs, etc) are all effective methods of keeping energy in the lower areas. Too much energy in and around the lower chakras may cause the uterus to contract too soon.

RECOMMENDATIONS

General Advice

- Lie down. Statistics suggest that this will not make a big difference to the outcome but it may slow down the progress sufficiently in order to allow transfer to hospital.
- If a recurrent problem, learn a meditation technique and consider employing yoga early on in the pregnancy. Use the techniques if a problem is suspected.
- If you have psychological blocks, suppressed feelings or are unable to express your anxieties, visit a counsellor.

Nutritional

- Please see nutritional advice in the pregnancy and pre-conception sections.

Supplemental

- Omega 3 essential fatty acids, 500mg per foot of height in divided doses each day taken from around 20 weeks of pregnancy. In women with a history of pre-term delivery, this cuts the risk of recurrence from about 33 per cent to 21 per cent.

Homeopathic

- Women with a tendency to abort before the third month should consider taking Cimicifuga, Sabadilla or Secale cornutum potency 30, twice a day for the first three months.

- *A tendency to abort after this may be prevented by the remedies Caulophyllum, Helonius or Sepia. It is not advisable to take a remedy persistently so start three weeks prior to the previous time of delivery using potency 30 twice a day.*
- *Care under a qualified homeopath is recommended.*

Herbal/natural extracts

- *I would recommend the use of orthodox drugs as their risk to pregnancy is better established although a medically qualified herbalist could administer herbs.*
- *The daily use of chamomile tea as a relaxant can be considered a safe option.*

Orthodox

- *Uterine muscle relaxants such as beta 2-adrenoceptor stimulants and oxytocin receptor antagonists both inhibit uterine contraction. These must be administered by a doctor.*
- *Pain relief should be accepted if required with no anxiety about damage to the baby.*
- *Given a choice, try to deliver the baby with the foetal membranes ('waters') intact as this gives protection to the baby's soft skull.*

PRE-ECLAMPSIA AND ECLAMPSIA

Pre-eclampsia refers to a rising blood pressure and the presence of protein in the mother's urine. These two parameters are constantly checked because the development of eclampsia can be extremely dangerous. Eclampsia is characterized by convulsions due to the effects of swelling in the brain.

A study of women at high risk of developing pre-eclampsia found that those who took high doses of vitamin C and vitamin E were 76 per cent less likely to suffer from the condition than those who only took a placebo. The obvious conclusion, although not yet proven, is that vitamins C and E, taken through pregnancy, may reduce the chance of this condition. One has to be wary of the use of high doses of vitamin E since this may induce bleeding, thereby jeopardizing the placenta as well as prolonging bleeding after delivery. Vitamin C is also under investigation regarding altering DNA if it is taken in high doses – so stay below 2000mgs daily.

Lead poisoning, and deficiencies in magnesium and zinc may be associated with narrowing of the placental blood vessels and this encourages the mother to raise her blood pressure. Essential fatty acid deficiency and low protein diets have also been linked to pre-eclampsia.

RECOMMENDATIONS

General Advice

- *A pre-eclamptic condition must be monitored by a gynaecologist and a GP.*
- *A naturopathic physician should be consulted and homeopathy, herbal medicine, acupuncture and meditation/relaxation treatments can be effective, reducing the risk of hospitalization. Delivery is usually by Caesarean section if the pre-eclamptic condition is not controlled.*
- *Undergo hair, sweat and blood tests for lead poisoning and mineral deficiencies.*

Nutritional

- *Increase protein intake and eat a variety of vegetables to avoid deficiency.*

Supplemental

- *Vitamin C 200mg per foot of height and vitamin E 50iu per foot of height could be taken as part of a routine supplemental intake. If a previous pregnancy has induced pre-eclampsia or eclampsia, then consider discussing the matter with a medically qualified naturopathic physician or with your obstetrician.*

DIZZY SPELLS AND FAINTING

Dizziness and fainting are usually due to lowered blood sugar levels, nutritional deficiencies and just plain exhaustion. If the following recommendations do not help with dizziness within a few days or if you have more than one faint, bring yourself along to your health practitioner and advise your GP that you are doing so.

General Advice
- *Ensure that clothes are not too tight around the waist.*

Nutritional
- *Eat small snacks in-between meals if dizzy spells or a single faint should occur (see **Hypoglycaemia diet**).*
- *Consult a nutritionist to establish correct dietetics.*

Homeopathic
- *Use the homeopathic remedy Aconite 6 (four pills every 15min). If the fainting or dizziness is associated with a flush use Belladonna 6 and if the dizziness is noticeable when rising from bed or a chair take Bryonia 30, one dose three times a day for five days.*

NAUSEA AND HYPEREMESIS GRAVIDARUM

Hyperemesis gravidarum is the Latin terminology for severe nausea of pregnancy. The most effective treatments that I have come across are mentioned at the start of this chapter under the heading 'Discovering a Pregnancy', but if they do not work consider the following.

General Advice
- *Regular visits to an acupuncturist to obtain a suitable acupressure technique.*

Orthodox
- *Severe nausea and vomiting can lead to malnutrition and may need to be controlled by orthodox drugs via your GP.*

POLYHYDRAMNIOS

Polyhydramnios is the presence of too much amniotic fluid and can be associated with twins or diabetes. Symptoms are abdominal pressure and distension, in association with a tense and larger-than-expected abdomen.

General Advice
- *I have not seen alternative techniques correct this situation, although bed rest and massage can be relieving.*

Herbal/natural extracts
- *Do not be tempted to use herbal treatments because anything that can affect the production of amniotic fluid is liable to affect the foetus.*

Orthodox
- *A gynaecologist can drain excess fluid under ultrasound guidance, which is a comparatively safe and effective procedure.*

SWELLING AND OEDEMA

This has been discussed earlier in the chapter but if the recommendations do not ease the problem, then visit your health practitioner for their expert advice. *See* **Polyhydramnios** *and* **Swollen feet and hands**.

URINARY TRACT PROBLEMS
Infections

During the pregnancy urine tests will be performed. Whilst looking for sugar to show diabetes, the urine will also be checked for the presence of protein or nitrites. Evidence of either of these

Urine Analysis

pH	7.0
Protein	+ (0.30g/L)
Glucose	Negative
Ketone	Negative
Blood	+

Microscopy

WBCs	>100/HPF
RBCs	Not seen
Casts	Not seen
Epithelial cells	+
Crystals	Not seen
Organisms	++
Culture	No bacterial growth

Example of the results of urine analysis showing the chemistry and biology of the urine sample.

leads to a suspicion of a urinary tract infection and the orthodox world is divided as to whether to treat this finding with antibiotics or not. One must not allow a bladder infection to travel into the kidneys, which can lead to spontaneous abortion. On the other hand, one does not want to give antibiotics, which can affect the normal bowel bacteria and lead to absorption problems.

RECOMMENDATIONS

General Advice

- *Any discomfort in the bladder or in the lower back (the kidney area) must be brought to the attention of your health practitioner.*
- *Apply reflexology to the bladder and kidney points on your feet (see **Reflexology**).*
- *Drink one glass (6–8oz) of water or herbal tea every hour and put half a teaspoonful of sodium bicarbonate (baking soda) into every other glass (maximum of 4 pints of water per day).*

Homeopathic

- *Depending on the symptoms, the following homeopathic remedies should be reviewed: Cantharis, Pulsatilla, Equisetum, Staphysagria, Phosphorus and Mercurius.*

Herbal/natural extracts

- *In the early stages of a mild discomfort you may use cranberry tablets or powder, as directed by a practitioner or pharmacist. There is no standard strength for cranberry preparations. Do not use the sweetened cranberry juices. The sugar content will encourage bacterial growth.*
- *Juniper or Berberis vulgaris fluid extracts (ten drops four times a day in water) may be curative.*
- *Add 20 drops of eucalyptus and sandalwood essential oils to a hot bath.*

Orthodox

- *If proteins or nitrites are found in the urine sample, insist that the sample be sent to a laboratory for culture and sensitivity. This means that any bacteria will be grown and tested against antibiotics so that a correct drug is given if the need arises.*

Frequency and urgency

The need to pass urine and having difficulty in holding a full bladder are symptoms that can occur very early in pregnancy but will definitely occur as the pressure on the bladder increases with the growth of the baby.

RECOMMENDATIONS

General Advice

- *Yoga and pelvic floor exercises are essential.*
- *Try not to drink a lot within 2hr of going to bed.*
- *Acupuncture, craniosacral therapy and osteopathy can all make an appreciable difference.*

Homeopathic

- *Two less well-known remedies, Chimaphila umbellata 6 and Linaria 6, can be taken at a dosage of four pills every 4hr but if you find no relief after five days, stop.*

Vaginal discharges

Vaginal discharges are common, usually due to the hormonal changes affecting the cells lining the walls of the vagina. Any bloody or brown (stale blood) discharges should be discussed with a GP or gynaecologist but other minor discharges should be left alone and assumed to be normal.

If the discharge is irritating, copious, coloured or bad smelling then a simple douche technique as described below is acceptable. It may well be a thrush infection so *please see* the section in chapter 4 that deals with this problem.

Concern is sometimes expressed about cleaning the vagina when pregnant because this may introduce infection. To an extent this is true, but since intercourse is permissible with the resultant introduction of another person's bacteria and body fluids, I do not see why the following antiseptic technique is not perfectly safe.

General Advice

• *Obtain a 20ml or 50ml syringe, leave it in recently boiled water for 5min. Mix one tablespoon of live yoghurt with a large mug of boiled water cooled to a warm temperature and pull the milky solution into the syringe. Insert the syringe no more than two inches into the vagina and gently depress the plunger. Thoroughly flush the vaginal vault and perform this each morning for seven days. The procedure should be repeated at night using a tablespoon of cider vinegar in a large mug of warm water.*

Homeopathic

• *The following homeopathic remedies may be helpful: Hydrastis 6 if the discharge is thick and tenacious; Mercurius 6 if greenish yellow, smarting, with some swelling and worse at night; and Stannum metallicum 6 for a white mucusy, profuse discharge, especially if the back aches. As always, refer to a good homeopathic text for a more accurate prescription.*

SKIN PROBLEMS

Skin changes occur in all pregnancies, usually for the better. Sufferers of eczema and psoriasis frequently find that their condition improves, which is good news because the drugs used in psoriasis and the steroid creams used in eczema should be stopped if possible. If you are under any treatment for psoriasis that involves taking oral medication this should be stopped several months before pregnancy is planned (*see* chapter 1).

Stretch marks

The stretching of the skin can lead to shiny streaks over the breasts and abdomen.

RECOMMENDATION

Supplemental

• *Apply a high-dose vitamin E cream or mix vitamin E (1,000iu emptied from capsules) into a tablespoonful of olive oil and massage in twice a day.*

Itching skin

All too frequently at some point during a pregnancy itching skin will become a problem. The cause is uncertain, although there are two possibilities: altered hormone levels and a histamine release in the skin due to the waste products produced by the baby.

RECOMMENDATIONS

General Advice

• *Change your soaps, bath products and washing powder to unmedicated hypoallergenic products. Make sure you only wear natural material such as cotton or wool, avoiding synthetics.*
• *Calamine lotion can be used if the above compounds do not work.*

Supplemental

• *Use Evening Primrose Oil 1g three times a day for five days. Liquorice extracts can be remarkably soothing when applied to the skin.*

Herbal/natural extracts

• *Add chamomile extracts, coconut or almond oil to your baths. Chamomile extracts are very often successful.*
• *Borage oil can be applied either directly or through the bath.*

CHILDBIRTH AND AFTER

The most important aspect of the Eastern philosophy of medicine is the concept of the balance of energy flowing through and contained in the body. The Chinese refer to Yin and Yang as being opposite yet complementary factors. Here are some examples of Yin and Yang.

YIN	YANG
Inferior	Superior
Front (abdomen)	Back

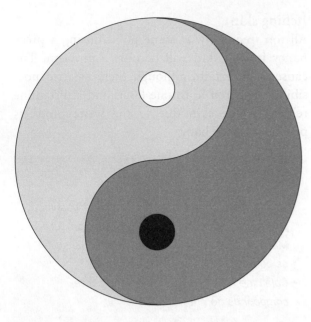

Yin/Yang circle depicting the dynamic relationship between Yin and Yang.

Interior organs	Exterior organs (skin)
Structure	Function
Water	Fire
Quiet	Noise
Wet	Dry
Slow	Rapid
Storage	Distribution
Curled up	Stretched out

From these examples you can see that the process of development in the womb is predominantly influenced by Yin. Life, however, is one of balance and leading up to the delivery the balance is redressed by the more Yang-dominated energy of delivery.

It is best, therefore, to support the promotion of Yang as we move towards the latter part of pregnancy because a deficiency may create the problems that can be associated with delivery.

ONE MONTH BEFORE LABOUR

One month before labour there is going to be a strong desire to get all this hoo-ha over! In some US clinics, weights are attached to the husband's abdomen and chest and they are asked to wander around like that for a short time. We men are not aware of the strain and effort that goes into the later stages of pregnancy. A pregnant mother will be fed up with the restrictions but, hopefully, will have enjoyed the health that is usually associated with pregnancy.

It is around this time that thoughts turn to the preparation for delivery. A lot of intervention is not needed, of course, but certain preparations can be made to try to reduce any delays with the delivery.

RECOMMENDATIONS

General Advice
- *Regular practice of the pain-relieving techniques taught through hypnotherapy earlier in the pregnancy should be practised.*
- *Ensure that, by now, your partner has a grasp of the Shiatsu pressure points; if not, pack him off to the practitioner to learn.*
- *Daily yoga, however uncomfortable it may be, should be continued to ensure good muscular tone.*
- *Ensure relaxation, breathing techniques or meditation is continued to engender a sense of calm leading up to the event.*
- *Contact your preferred complementary medical practitioner and glean any advice.*

Homeopathic
- *Ten days prior to the expected delivery date take the homeopathic remedy Caulophyllum 30 for seven days before bed, and for the last three days before the delivery date use Caulophyllum 200 before bed. This higher potency can be used for up to one week if the delivery date is passed.*

ALTERNATIVE TECHNIQUES FOR INDUCEMENT OF LABOUR

There is rarely a good reason to induce a delivery but if there is no sign of labour two weeks after the expected date (remember that the date calculated from the last period and the day suggested by the scans during pregnancy may differ due to the length of the mother's monthly cycle) then pressure may be applied by the midwives and consultant. The reasons are simple and sound: the baby may grow to a size that may make it difficult to fit through the pelvic rim; and the placenta may be unable to sustain the baby's nutritional and oxygen requirements.

Provided that the obstetrician and the ultrasound scans agree that the baby is of correct size, then alternative techniques for induction of labour can be employed ten days after the expected delivery date.

Shiatsu Points for Inducing Labour

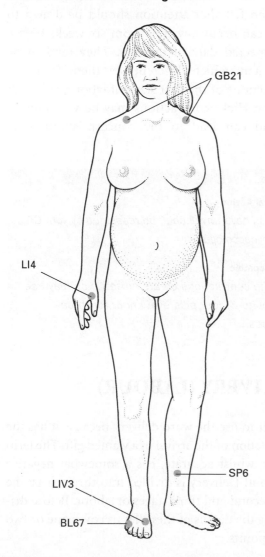

RECOMMENDATIONS

General Advice

• *Acupuncture or specific acupressure (Shiatsu) points can be activated. These are illustrated in the diagram opposite, along with the areas that should not be massaged under normal circumstances at any stage during pregnancy. The specific points are:*

GB21 (gallbladder 21) – on the highest point of the shoulder where a perpendicular line drawn from the nipple crosses the top of the shoulder;

LI4 (large intestine 4) – in the centre of the flesh before the first and second metacarpal bones (in the hand);

LIV3 (liver 3) – in the depression up the foot from the big toe and the second toe.

BL67 (bladder 67) – on the lateral side of the small toe at the base of the toe nail;

SP6 (spleen 6) – three thumb-widths above the tip of the inner ankle bone and backwards to the edge of the bone;

• *Reflexology can be utilized on the uterine and pituitary points on the feet.*
• *A brisk walk.*
• *Sexual intercourse.*

Homeopathic

• *The homeopathic remedy Secale cornutum 30, four pills every 3hr.*

Herbal/natural extracts

• *Fluid extracts of Pulsatilla or, if available, Caulophyllum can be taken, ten drops in water every three hours.*
• *Raspberry leaf tea, one teabag in a mug four times a day.*

Nutrition

There is no need to alter the diet, particularly if all has gone well through the first eight months of a pregnancy. Always consider your intuition and cravings as being the best guidelines. You may encourage Yang energy building up towards the expected delivery date by adding the following foods into the diet. They should not be taken in excess nor too early in the pregnancy because, as explained above, the uterine environment is predominantly Yin and excess Yang may cause problems. The foods to increase are:

- lamb
- lobster and shrimps
- basil, dill, sage, cinnamon, thyme, clove, nutmeg, garlic, ginger and fennel.

Exercise

RECOMMENDATIONS

General Advice
- *Ensure that stretching exercises are practised regularly throughout the day. The act of squatting with your knees as far apart as possible and the back supported by your partner or a wall is excellent.*
- *Practise holding certain positions that you may choose at the delivery and hold these postures for as long as you can.*
- *Walk and swim: 15min of swimming and 40min of walking (provided that your back is all right) is a sensible plan.*

Medication

It is not necessary to consider the use of medication for, or leading up to, delivery. However, certain treatment protocols can be used if mild problems or symptoms are arising. These should be dealt with according to the symptoms and in consultation with your health practitioner.

RECOMMENDATIONS

Homeopathic
- *See earlier in this section for the use of Caulophyllum.*

Herbal/natural extracts
- *Pulsatilla fluid extract – 1 teaspoonful in water four times a day, starting the day before delivery is expected.*
- *Apply a combination cream of Arnica, Calendula and Urtica to the outer aspects of the vagina, the perineum and around the anus. Do so three or four times a day to prepare the area for the stretching that it will undergo. Arnica or Calendula creams will suffice, as will olive oil, if the combination is not readily available.*

BRAXTON HICKS

These contractions, named after the gynaecologist who felt that attention should be drawn to them, can occur any time from six weeks before the expected date of delivery. They tend to be infrequent, which differentiates them from the contractions of the first stage of labour, although Braxton Hicks contractions may be very powerful and can lead to the concern about early labour.

RECOMMENDATIONS

General Advice
- *If you have any doubts, be reassured by your GP or gynaecologist.*

Homeopathic
- *If the contractions create anxiety, you may use Aconite 6, four pills every hour for three doses.*

DELIVERY (LABOUR)

I prefer to use the word delivery because it has the connotation of the arrival of a wanted gift. The term labour, whilst accurate, has a somewhat negative ring to it! Delivery is divided into three parts: the first, second and third stages of labour. Before discussing the details of these, let us cover one or two other points.

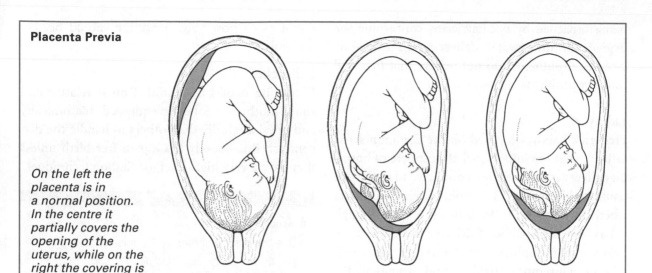

Placenta Previa

On the left the placenta is in a normal position. In the centre it partially covers the opening of the uterus, while on the right the covering is complete.

normal position   partial   complete

At the onset

When delivery seems imminent – by the 'show', the breaking of the waters or by frequent contractions – the following can be recommended.

RECOMMENDATIONS

General Advice
- *Walk about. The Yang energy is encouraged by movement.*
- *Sleep as much as you can, especially in the breaks between contractions.*
- *Cry if you wish and be open to demanding love and support at a notoriously insecure time.*

Nutritional
- *Increase the glucose levels in preparation for expending energy by eating light meals, preferably of complex carbohydrates (whole grain bread, brown rice, honey).*

Placenta previa

Placenta previa is the medical term for the positioning of the placenta within the uterus in such a way that it covers the opening from the uterus through the cervix into the vagina.

A full placenta previa has never been corrected by a complementary medical technique in my experience, although many times I have seen a partial placenta previa 'move' after therapies. It should be mentioned that this may occur in any case as the uterus enlarges.

RECOMMENDATIONS

General Advice
- *Osteopathy in combination with Tibetan or Chinese acupuncture and herbal treatments has most often proved successful.*

Orthodox
- *Do not allow an excess of ultrasound investigation to be performed. Once a scan has identified a placenta previa, do not have repeated tests; have a rescan one month before delivery and if things have not changed then consider orthodox management (see **Ultrasound**).*

Water birth

The use of water has been much publicized. A recent appraisal of the popularity of delivering in water has suggested that many mothers prefer to be in water for the first part of labour but over 50 per cent choose to deliver out of the pool.

There is no advantage or disadvantage to delivering under water, although some questions are being broached by paediatricians concerning the hygiene of underwater deliveries. In a healthy clean environment I do not believe that they will find any problems.

Laboyer

Frederick Laboyer focused on the common sense attitude that the impersonal atmosphere of hospital delivery rooms was not conducive to healthy or comfortable delivery. This point of view has flourished since the early 1970s in the West, although it has been a principle of delivery throughout the Eastern philosophies for thousands of years. Choose your music, lighting and aromas in the delivery suite or room.

DELIVERY – FIRST STAGE OF LABOUR

The first stage of labour includes the 'ripening' (softening) of the cervix and the first 4cm of dilation. At this time a 'show' may occur, which is the exiting of the mucus plug that has been a major protective factor in the cervical 'os' or opening. The 'waters' (the protective amniotic fluid sack) may break before the first stage of labour or in the early part. This natural lubrication is an important indication of delivery and excessive drying of the fluids should be avoided. Contractions should be occurring at 10–20-minute intervals and lasting up to 30 seconds.

Dilation from 4cm to 10cm can take a matter of minutes or several hours. The recommendations below can help to shorten this timespan. During this dilation, contractions will last for 20–90 seconds, be profoundly intense and painful and can occur anywhere between 10 minutes and 30 seconds apart.

Your natural instinct with regard to breathing, and the training you will have received through your antenatal care and yoga classes is never more important than at this stage. The desire to push down and expel the baby is at its strongest, but pushing too early can tear the cervix and lead to difficulties. Your midwife will be very experienced and supportive, leaving you with little

doubt as to how your breathing should be. Do not worry!

Pain relief

Delivering babies is painful. Pain is relative and some mothers are better equipped anatomically and physiologically than others to handle the discomfort. But nobody has a pain-free birth unless they have a very high-level meditation technique!

RECOMMENDATIONS

General Advice

- *Use the self-hypnotherapy techniques taught to you for the pregnancy. Use acupressure techniques (see over).*

  BL31 (bladder 31) – a tender spot at the base of the spinal column approximately one hand-width above the buttocks in the mid-line. Please note that the use of these pain relief points may shorten contractions and therefore should be used only at the point in time when pain is most severe, otherwise labour may be prolonged.

  ST36 (stomach 36) – four finger-widths inferior to the knee cap and one finger outwards.

  BL60 (bladder 60) – in the depression half-way between the outer ankle bone and the Achilles tendon, level with the most prominent point of the ankle bone.

Homeopathic

- *Use Chamomilla 6 (four pills every 15min) for intolerable pains, especially associated with the back. If fear or shivering is present, consider Aconite 6 (four pills every 15min).*

Orthodox

- *Do not be ashamed or embarrassed to ask for pain relief.*
- *Use the 'gas' (nitrous oxide) as much as you like.*
- *If these measures are not effective then do not hesitate to ask for an epidural. It may take some time for the anaesthetist to arrive, so call for the best friend you will ever have, sooner rather than later!*

The delivery of the head is the most difficult and time-consuming part of this second stage. Hopefully the process will be swift, but delays can occur. The most unpleasant aspect is the sensation that the perineum (the area between the vagina and the anus) is tearing. This is not often the case and the use of the mixed Arnica, Calendula and Urtica cream beforehand generally reduces the risk. The midwife will be applying considerable pressure in this area to avoid tears.

> **RECOMMENDATION**
>
> **General Advice**
> • Make sure that the midwife is aware of the sensations you experience and encourage her to give more support or apply more pressure.

DELIVERY – SECOND STAGE OF LABOUR

Now we are getting down to it, the waiting is nearly over. There may be a break between the first stage and second stage, especially in a first pregnancy, and if this is the case, rest.

The second stage starts when the cervix is fully dilated and ends with the delivery of the baby.

Delivery position

There is no correct or incorrect position to deliver a baby. Instinct combined with particular and individual anatomy will make this decision for you (see over). The principal options are:

Shiatsu Points for use through Delivery

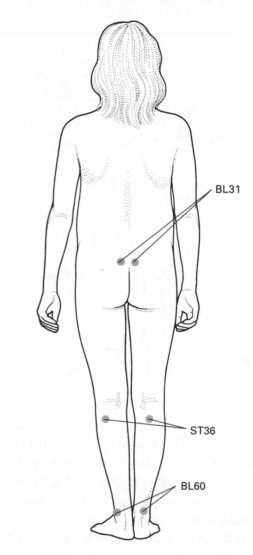

Have your partner apply pressure to the above acupressure points.

Stages of Delivery

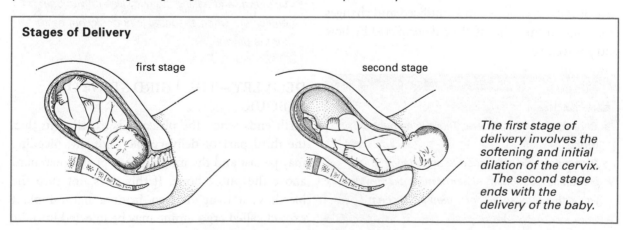

first stage

second stage

The first stage of delivery involves the softening and initial dilation of the cervix. The second stage ends with the delivery of the baby.

Delivery Positions

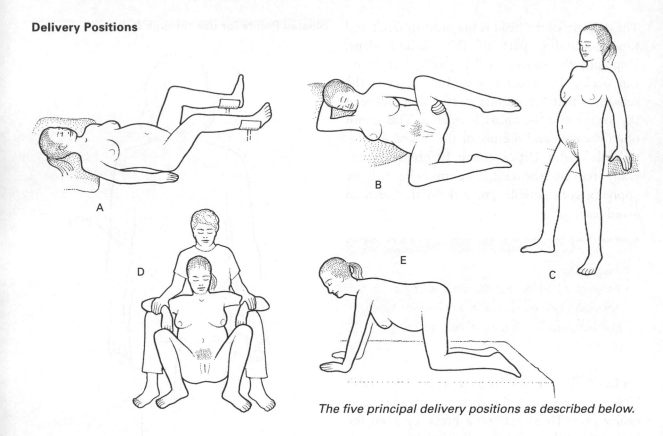

The five principal delivery positions as described below.

A Lying semi-prone on your back with feet together and knees apart or feet in stirrups;

B Lying on either side with the upper leg raised;

C Standing with buttocks supported against the bed;

D Squatting, using your partner's knees and thighs as an 'armchair' support;

E On the knees leaning against the bed or on all fours.

Any of these positions can be utilized and changes from one to the other will be determined by how you are feeling.

RECOMMENDATIONS

General Advice

- *Choose your atmosphere. There is no right or wrong.*
- *Be comfortable with those in attendance. If grandmother, mother, sister or milkman provide you with the most support, then invite them to be present. Do not crowd out the midwife, however!*
- *Unless there is a medical reason, avoid monitors. The presence of modern medical technology creates the perception of the possibility of something going wrong. Both Mum and Dad already have their fears, especially in a first delivery where they are launching into the unknown, and asking the midwives only to use equipment when essential is not risky but better for the psyche.*

DELIVERY – THE THIRD STAGE OF LABOUR

Birth ends when the placenta is expelled in this, the third part of delivery. Occasionally, bleeding may persist and the midwife may push down hard above the pubic bone. If this does not stop the bleeding, a drug derived from a natural plant extract called ergotamine may be injected into the mother's arm. This causes the uterus to contract and applies pressure to the bleeding vessel, thereby stopping the haemorrhage.

The midwife will gently push any blood that is in the umbilical cord towards the baby and within a couple of minutes the cord, which actually pulsates, will come to rest. At this time the midwife will cut the cord by placing two clamps near the baby's tummy and cutting in-between. The clip nearest the baby will remain in place anywhere up to 24 hours or so before the cord closes off completely and the remnant drops away, leaving a sealed umbilicus or belly button.

Occasionally bleeding may occur and, if too prominent, ergotamine may be injected to encourage uterine contractions.

RECOMMENDATIONS

General Advice

- *Follow the midwife's instructions and if any problems have arisen let the professionals get on with their tasks.*

Homeopathic

- *The remedy Secale cornutum 30 should be taken every hour for three doses to encourage uterine contraction.*
- *Rehydrate as soon as it is comfortable to drink water. Any persisting soreness should be treated with Bellis perennis 30 every 3hr.*
- *Arnica 200 should be taken every 12hr for six doses, to deal with the inevitable physical and mental strain.*

The baby

Instinct will take control for both mother and baby. The baby will either rest or seek the nipple and the first feed is extremely important because it provides a special type of milk called colostrum, which aids digestion. Baby's breathing will be very smooth and natural and is stimulated by the cooler temperature and will not need the

Umbilical Clamp

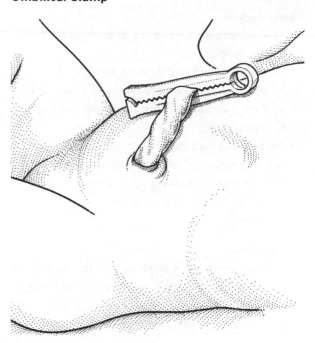

Umbilical clamp in place.

much-heralded slap on the bottom. This is not a nice way to start life and the midwife should be asked not to do this. Nowadays, most midwives wouldn't consider it, but some die-hards may habitually use the technique!

The First Feed

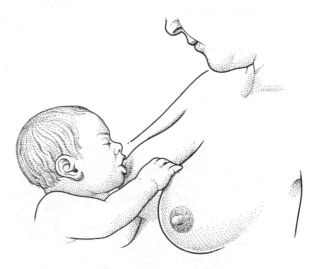

The baby should be allowed to suckle as soon as possible after birth.

General Advice

- *Allow baby to suckle as soon as possible but do not force the point.*
- *Refuse antibiotics in the baby's eyes and, in preference, when baby has finished his first feed squeeze a few drops of breast milk into the eyes to cleanse them.*
- *The baby will have bonded with his mother well before delivery and possibly even with the father through hearing his voice. Time spent together at this early stage is very worthwhile.*

Supplemental

- *Until all controversy has passed, do not give the vitamin K injection. There may be some problems with this vitamin in injectable form and it can promote a tendency to jaundice.*

PHYSICAL PROBLEMS AFTER DELIVERY

Most physical problems that might arise because of pregnancy are covered in this book under their own heading because they may occur at other times as well. For example, mastitis is more common through lactation but because it can occur elsewhere it is covered in its own section. A few problems are specific to postpregnancy and these are mentioned below.

Engorged Breasts

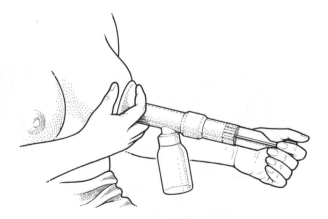

Expressing milk using a pump.

Episiotomy

Occasionally tears will occur in the perineum, simply because the baby is fractionally too large and the stretch of the vagina is too little. There is not much that can be done at the time although the repair process afterwards can be hastened and the appropriate techniques are mentioned below.

Iatrogenic – 'caused by the physician' or, in this case, the midwife – episiotomy is sometimes required. The process involves injecting local anaesthetic (although this is frequently not required) and a surgical incision is made back from the vagina towards the anus. It is a messy and bloody procedure that can be quite a shock if the delivering mother and attending partner are not aware of this. Done properly, the area is stitched up after the delivery and does not cause complications. It is sometimes safer to have an iatrogenic episiotomy rather than allow nature to create its own tear, although a natural tear is thought to heal quicker. Should an episiotomy of any sort occur, the following recommendations should be followed after the delivery.

General Advice

- *Splash alternate hot and cold water over the area for two minutes four times a day until healing is complete.*

Homeopathic

- *Use the homeopathic remedy Bellis perennis 6 (four pills four times a day) until healed. If the wound has not completely resolved or discomfort or discharge prevail after five days, then bring the problem to the attention of your gynaecologist, health visitor and complementary health practitioner.*

Herbal/natural extracts

- *Apply Arnica or Calendula creams to the area and flush the vaginal vault with a dilute solution of Arnica or Calendula fluid extract.*

Painful nipples

Whilst this can happen through chafing at any stage of life, painful nipples are most commonly associated with suckling.

RECOMMENDATIONS

General Advice

- *A tablespoon of olive oil with the juice of half a lemon can be applied four times a day (but wash off before feeding) at the first hint of nipple soreness. If the nipples have a tendency to crack, this should be done twice a day as a prophylactic.*
- *It may be necessary to express milk by hand or pump to give the nipple time to heal away from baby's mouth.*
- *Nipple guards (transparent plastic covers) may be used until the problem has resolved.*

Homeopathic

- *Cracked nipples will benefit from the homeopathic remedy Graphites or Silica, potency 6, taken every 2hr at the onset and reduced to every 4hr once healing has started.*

Abdominal muscles

More than anything, a pregnancy causes abdominal muscles to stretch. In an ideal situation a pregnancy would be started with good abdominal musculature because this will return much more easily to its pre-pregnancy state.

RECOMMENDATION

General Advice

- *Exercise as frequently as possible through the early part of pregnancy, with gentle abdominal exercises, and return to these as soon as you are capable after the delivery.*

Engorged breasts

Engorged breasts occur for two reasons: because the production of milk exceeds the demand and use, and because of engorgement of the breast tissue by excess fluid, encouraged by the persisting high levels of female hormones.

RECOMMENDATIONS

General Advice

- *Ensure that the baby gets all the milk he or she desires; any excess should be expectorated by hand or pump and kept for up to 12hr in the fridge. This might allow Dad the opportunity of a feed and give Mum a rest.*
- *Soak the breasts in a hot bath or apply hot flannels or heat pads. Occasionally, ice wrapped in a flannel may benefit if heat does not.*
- *Acupuncture and herbal treatments may be of benefit in recurrent problems and a practitioner could be consulted.*

Supplemental

- *Supplements may help breast fluid retention and can be taken without unduly influencing mother's milk. The mother should use the following: Vitamin B_6 (50mg), Evening Primrose Oil (1,000mg two or three times a day) and zinc (15mg before going to sleep).*

Homeopathic

- *The homeopathic remedies Phytolacca 6 or Natrum muriaticum 6, taken every 15 min, may help.*

Orthodox

- *The use of paracetamol is acceptable as a last resort but should be taken after the baby's feed so that the body can metabolize it before the baby's next meal.*

Stretch marks

The increased size of the abdomen through pregnancy can stretch the skin and create a scar-like appearance.

RECOMMENDATIONS

General Advice

- *Prevention is the best bet and application of olive oil with lemon juice (half a lemon squeezed into a tablespoonful of pure virgin olive oil)*

may make a difference.
- *Gentle massage regularly may increase blood flow and recover the overstretched elastin fibres.*
- *Return to abdominal exercises as soon as the baby is delivered and Mum is up to it will help.*

Supplemental
- *Vitamin E oil may also benefit if applied regularly.*

Herbal/natural extracts
- *A Calendula- and Arnica-based cream (if a mix is not found, use one of each) applied four times a day.*

Breast-feeding

Many women find it difficult or unpleasant to breast-feed and I am reluctant to make the statement 'breast is best' for the sake of those mothers who may take on an element of guilt or unworthiness. But ...

Nature has been at breast milk formulation for millions of years, as opposed to the pharmaceutical industry who have done a good job over the last 40 years. Breast milk contains a variety of nutrition that is well balanced for a human baby. Formula preparations come close but most use cow's milk as their matrix, which is harder to digest and, despite complex formulation, does not contain everything that breast milk does.

The breast milk also contains high levels of immunoglobulins, which are part of the baby's first line of defence against infection, and breast milk is not capable of creating an allergic or intolerant response. Eczema, asthma and hay fever are less common in breast-fed babies and studies have shown that there may be a slight increase in the breast-fed baby's IQ. Colic is often associated with an allergic response and therefore breast babies may suffer less.

Mother and baby may bond slightly more if the child is suckled, and breast-feeding is much more convenient as far as travelling and the need for equipment is concerned. Sterility is not a problem, of course. An even greater advantage for the mother may be that there is a decreased risk of breast cancer in mothers who feed their babies by the breast longest.

Not enough breast milk

It is not infrequent for a mother to find that her baby is still hungry after a feed. This is often because there is not enough milk. This may be due to dehydration or deficiencies in the mother's diet or simply because of exhaustion.

RECOMMENDATIONS

General Advice
- *Ensure a water intake of at least three-quarters of a pint per foot of height to be drunk throughout the day.*
- *Try to get as much sleep as possible.*

Nutritional
- *Ensure a well-balanced diet or discuss suitable supplements with a complementary medical practitioner.*

Herbal/natural extracts
- *The herb Galega officinalis may be used: a teaspoonful of fluid extract three times a day in milk sweetened with a teaspoonful of honey. (Galega may bring down sugar levels.)*

Weaning

There is no set time to wean (introducing foods other than breast milk) but a good guideline is when the child is not getting enough from mother's milk, which is recognized by the child failing to put on weight or remaining hungry after a feed.

The breasts will still produce milk and engorge if the milk is not expressed. This can make weaning an uncomfortable period.

RECOMMENDATIONS

General Advice
- *If the choice is available, breast-feed for at least four months after the birth.*

- Cut down by one feed per 24hr over one week.
- See **Engorged breasts.**

Herbal/natural extracts

- Try to obtain some jasmine: in fluid extract, essential oil or even from the garden. Three drops of the extract or oil should be rubbed into the breasts, or the flowers should be steeped in water for 24hr and a teaspoonful drunk three times a day.

- Do not involve timid or young children who may not understand what is going on.
- There is plenty of love to go around. Continue to distribute it evenly.
- Baby is going to take plenty of knocks in life, so do not be too critical of a sibling's apparent rough handling. Baby has just come through quite a trauma and it can handle a push and a poke.

THE FATHER AND SIBLINGS

Fathers will at some stage realize how useless they are during a delivery. Massaging and pushing a few acupressure points does not really seem like sharing the burden and the pain that the mother is suffering. Fathers, please do not be too disheartened. Every little bit helps and 'being there' means a lot.

Many deliveries nowadays have older siblings present, the benefit of which very much depends upon the character of that child. A timid or young child who may not understand the process should not be involved because the apparent anguish of their mother will be very hard to comprehend. Remember that children are very self-centred and a young child will assume that the mother is in pain because of something that he or she is doing.

However, it is important to introduce the newborn to a sibling as soon as possible. It is hard to conceive that love is not a finite emotion and siblings may fear that the more people there are, the less Mum can love each one. Logic sticks its oar in and it is extremely important that a sibling feels that the baby is as much a part of them as it is a part of Mum and Dad. Bonding should actually start early on in pregnancy and children should be introduced to the baby as soon as possible. There will inevitably be some jealousy and it is important not to criticize an older sibling for this emotion.

RECOMMENDATIONS

General Advice

- Involve family members from the start of the pregnancy, and especially at the birth, where possible.

AFTER DELIVERY

The first month or so after delivery is an exhausting time both psychologically and physically. Although it sounds harsh, one must remember that pregnancy is in fact a parasitic infestation and the baby will have drained a lot of nutrients from mother whilst growing and will continue to extract goodness through the breast milk. Mother, meantime, is having her sleep disturbed and is having to adjust to a completely new lifestyle. Whether it is the first or twenty-first child, the situation will be no different.

RECOMMENDATIONS

General Advice

- Talk to friends and relatives who have been through the situation before.
- Read as much about newborn babies as possible and realize that the experience is well-documented and that anything you are going through has been gone through before and there is someone out there with experience enough to help.

Nutritional

- High-dose multivitamins, preferably natural food state, along with a strict adherence to five portions of fresh, organic fruit and vegetables daily should replenish the system within two weeks. Discussions with your complementary medical practitioner may be needed if recovery has not been achieved by then.

POSTNATAL DEPRESSION

There is a marked drop in hormone levels as soon as the baby is delivered and the subconscious will register this and notice that there is something 'wrong'. In fact things are simply different but the brain will translate this into an anxiety or a depression. There is also a certain sense of anticlimax when parents realize that the delivery was in fact the start of a lifelong commitment and not just the end of a nine-month event. Tears will come easily; anger and irritation will be prominent but often counteracted with bouts of great joy and the tears that also go with that. Dad will feel this as well but most definitely will suffer the brunt of Mum's depression and mood swings.

All this should pass within a few days and it is only if it does not pass, that a condition known as postnatal depression needs to be considered. Unrecognized or untreated, this condition may go on for years. I have had patients who have gone through several pregnancies and spent decades in a postnatal depression without realizing that this was the case.

RECOMMENDATIONS

General Advice

- Always feel free to speak to a counsellor with regard to any unwanted emotional state but especially so after a birth. Friends and family will try to say what they think you want to hear and resolution of depression is much slower if dealt with that way.
- Never accept that 'she should be over it by now'. Chemical shifts may be permanent unless readjusted.
- Persistent depression should be dealt with by a complementary medical practitioner and counsellor: definitely one who has had children, and preferably a woman.

Supplemental

- Take a multimineral/vitamin supplement at twice the daily recommended dose because depression may be associated with deficiencies.
- Take phenylalanine (an amino acid) at three times the recommended dose on any proprietary package for three days and reduce it to twice the dose for up to two weeks.

Homeopathic

- Consult a homeopathic physician for a suitable remedy.

Herbal/natural extracts

- Consider using Bach flower remedies, paying particular attention to Larch, Pine, Elm, Sweet Chestnut, Willow, Star of Bethlehem, Oak and Crab Apple. These are all excellent for despondency or despair. If the emotion seems to be about responsibility, consider Chicory, Vervain, Vine, Beech and Rock Water. Take a few minutes to read about these in a suitable booklet and pick the most appropriate.

Orthodox

- Artificial oestrogen has been shown to be beneficial when taken sublingually. Before trying this, make sure that other avenues have been explored and consider the use of natural oestrogens first.

CHAPTER 3

INFANCY AND CHILDHOOD

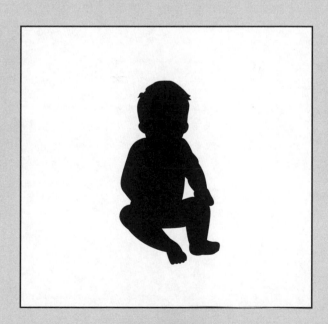

INFANCY AND CHILDHOOD

All things being equal, children, and infants in particular, have remarkable powers of recovery if left to themselves. Medical intervention should be sought in only a few of the common childhood conditions. Conversely, a sick child can deteriorate very rapidly. The skill of good parenting is to know which conditions should be treated at home and when you should seek expert consultation.

I hope that all alternative practitioners will agree when I say that our training with regard to children is generally poor. I am very grateful that I spent large chunks of time, when I was in medical school and after, in paediatric wards. The principles with which a child is treated are much the same as those of an adult but children are much more sensitive, especially to complementary medicines, and can go downhill at a rapid rate. Practitioners who have not had children themselves and who lack teaching or experience in dealing with children can underestimate the speed with which a child can develop a serious problem. This creates a paradox for parents. We would like our children brought up as drug-free as possible but we need to be wary that an alternative practitioner may not have the experience to deal with our child. We wish to avoid medication but do not wish to miss a diagnosis.

> **RECOMMENDATIONS**
>
> **General Advice**
> - *Do not hesitate to obtain the opinion of an experienced GP or paediatrician if your child is not well.*
> - *Once you have established that the child is not seriously ill, utilize alternative treatments for 24hr before subscribing to orthodox medicines.*

RECOGNIZING AN ILL INFANT

Parents, especially first-time parents, often have the preconception that symptoms represent illness and not repair. A whining infant may be uncomfortable but, as a general rule, is not ill. Infants with conditions that require treatment are generally:

- floppy
- sleeping a lot
- not interested in their food
- motionless
- persistent with their symptoms

A child who may be screaming and fractious interspersed with periods of normality, is generally likely to recover quickly. Fevers up to 100°F, blocked and running noses, coughs and most rashes may seem aggressive and worry the parents but if the child is up and about, rarely does this indicate a severe condition.

> **RECOMMENDATION**
>
> **General Advice**
> - *If you have any doubts whatsoever, obtain your doctor's opinion.*

GENERAL

ACCIDENTS

An accident, by definition, is supposedly out of our control and is an event that occurred purely by chance. This may not always be the case. An accident-prone child may have medical conditions that are treatable. For example, more road traffic accidents occur in the early hours of the morning and 2 hours after lunch. This strongly suggests that tiredness and hypoglycaemia (low blood sugar) are instrumental. Certain diets predispose to hypoglycaemia and accident-prone children may well have too much refined sugar in their diets.

Children who feel under pressure to perform may also overextend their capabilities and bodies to impress demanding friends and family, and this can be dealt with from a psychological angle.

Hyperactivity, usually diet-related, brings to mind the adage 'act in haste, repent at leisure'. This is often the case with injuries to overactive children. Poor concentration may result in accidents and may be directly related to dietary deficiencies and food intolerances.

RECOMMENDATIONS

General Advice
- *If diet is not in question, seek the opinion of a child psychologist or art therapist.*
- *Suspect additive/preservative sensitivity leading to hyperactivity in accident-prone children.*

Nutritional
- *Reduce sugars and obtain dietetic advice from a nutritionist for any accident-prone child. Food intolerance/allergy testing may be required.*

The treatment of individual accidents should be undertaken by reference to specific injuries elsewhere in the book.

ASPHYXIA

Asphyxia is the inability of an individual to breathe due to obstruction of the airways. *See* **Resuscitation of Infant or Child**. This is a procedure that all adults should learn.

BIRTH DEFECTS (CONGENITAL ANOMALIES)

The tragedy of the arrival of a child with an unexpected birth defect is indescribable. Fortunately, prenatal (during pregnancy) techniques using blood tests and ultrasound now make this unexpected surprise less frequent. However, the diagnostic abilities of modern science have simply shifted the dilemma to an earlier stage, and the problem still has to be faced.

Defects that are life-threatening may lead to a discussion on terminating the pregnancy (*see* **Termination of Pregnancy**) or create a discussion on the difficulties (or blessings) of all that will arise.

There is little that complementary or alternative medicine can do to alter the physical structure of a child but support can be given to the shocked psyches of parents, especially mothers. Holistic beliefs would hold that defects that were forged at conception would have been created by defective sperm or eggs, and avoidance of these is encouraged by being in good health before fertilization occurs. This is discussed in the section, **Physical Preparation for Conception**, in chapter 1. Defects formed after fertilization are due to the condition within the womb throughout the pregnancy and are predominantly caused by what is taken in by the mother, specifically ingested toxins, which include smoking, alcohol, drugs (both prescribed and recreational), insecticides, pesticides and household cleaning chemicals. Furthermore, from a mental outlook, a controlled study of 3,560 pregnant women who had been exposed to serious psychological life events found a marked increased risk of foetal defects. Orthodox medicine, on the other hand, can now perform intricate operations whilst the foetus is developing within the uterus, and structural anomalies may be correctable.

Biochemical defects, neurological deficits and problems associated with that part of the pregnancy or delivery after ultrasound has stopped being used, are unlikely to be detected until the infant is born.

Conditions such as Down's syndrome (*see* opposite), spina bifida and others are discussed in their own sections in this book. Chromosomal abnormalities that cause physical growth or mental retardation are so numerous (and thankfully rare) that they are beyond the scope of this book. However, the orthodox world often describes the

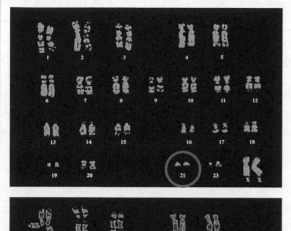

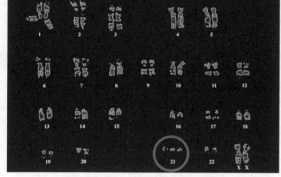

Down's syndrome is caused by the presence of an extra chromosome (circled above).

brain-calming chemicals may benefit the child and keep him or her as one of the one in five who do not have fits.

The Eastern philosophies, particularly the Hindu religion, consider the concept of karma. It may be necessary for an individual to suffer neurological or structural handicaps in order to learn lessons that bring them closer to their God. In the same way that a spontaneous miscarriage may be a blessing conferred by a spirit who needed only a short incarnation, a handicapped child may teach parents many emotional lessons from dealing with shock, disappointment, anger and frustration to a deeper level of understanding, responsibility and most surprisingly, joy. So often, the more severe the handicap, the more the individual is surprisingly free of negative emotions such as anger, hatred, guilt. It may take many lifetimes to achieve the state of joy and innocence that the mentally handicapped can take as a norm.

RECOMMENDATIONS

General Advice

- *Always undergo the safe investigations of pregnancy. Ultrasound and blood tests are essential because forewarned is forearmed.*
- *Consult a professional with experience in dealing with parents of congenitally compromised children. There is so much support, love and expertise out there that this battle need not be fought alone.*
- *Consult with an experienced complementary medical practitioner to ensure that nutrition during pregnancy and the nutrition of the infant are at an optimum, because many conditions are exacerbated by deficiency or toxicity.*
- *Spend time with a spiritual or religious teacher and remember to glean the most from the difficulties that are associated with a child with birth defects. Lessons come in many guises.*
- *Check for pesticides and other toxins in the bloodstream of both parents to determine*

symptoms and explains to the parent the percentage chance of progression to a variety of symptoms.

For example, the rare condition known as Angelman's syndrome (caused by a chromosomal defect) will cause epilepsy in 80 per cent of children around the age of two years. Hyperactivity is another major symptom. The orthodox world offers no suggestions but a more holistic view may surmise or hypothesize that as the child grows and receives more sensory input, the nervous system may become overloaded. If the child has a tendency to hyperactivity in any case, this may be the cause of epilepsy. Presumably 20 per cent of children who do not have fits have some neurochemical mechanism that suppresses this hyperactivity. No studies can prove this suggestion but perhaps homeopathy, herbal medicine and supplemental medicine to encourage the production of serotonin, dopamine and other

whether this may have been the cause of a defect that might affect future pregnancies.

- *A meditation technique or course of psychological counselling is strongly advised to reduce the potential for birth defects and it should be considered of primary importance in those who have had birth defects in previous pregnancies.*

Homeopathic

- *Homeopathic remedies both for the parents and the child can have a profound effect on both the psychology and the physical problems.*

CHICKENPOX

Chickenpox is created by a member of the herpes viral family known as *varicella*. It is a self-limiting disorder (meaning that it will clear itself up without medical intervention) and shows itself as a red rash with characteristic clear or yellow fluid-filled pimples. There is usually an associated mild fever, general malaise and loss of appetite but the worst symptoms are generally the irritation and itch.

The holistic consensus of opinion is that chickenpox, along with measles and possibly mumps, is a useful childhood infection triggering responses in the immune system that help to fight more serious infections at a later stage.

The incubation period (the time when someone is infectious) is generally thought to be one week prior to the arrival of the rash and for the first five days thereafter.

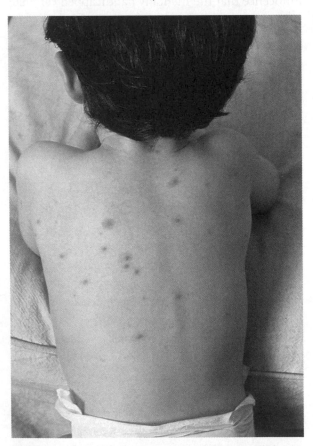

Chickenpox on the back of a two-year-old child.

RECOMMENDATIONS

General Advice

- *If in doubt about the diagnosis or if the pimples and rash are very aggressive or persistent, contact your complementary medical practitioner or GP for advice. Unfortunately, the orthodox world has little to offer other than antihistamine-like topical applications.*
- *Add one tablespoon of sodium bicarbonate to one pint of water and apply with a silk material to the irritated areas. You may concentrate this, if there is no response, to as much as three tablespoons per pint of water but ensure that there is no stinging effect by trying it out on any small cut or scratch you may have before applying it to a child. If the child is old enough to talk, you can apply it directly and ask!*
- *A cool bath with ten tablespoons of sodium bicarbonate can be relieving.*
- *Severe cases should be dealt with by a doctor or specialist in complementary medicine who has experience of this condition.*
- *See* **Herpes**.

Supplemental

- *The following supplements can be administered per foot of height: Beta-carotene (1mg), vitamin C (500mg in divided doses throughout the day) and zinc (2.5mg before bed).*

Homeopathic

- *Consider the homeopathic remedies Rhus toxicodendron or Pulsatilla. A simple technique is to try first one and then the other (potency 6 every 2hr) until improved and then reduce to every 4hr until the rash goes.*

Herbal/natural extracts

- *If a lesion becomes infected, apply Arnica, Calendula or Hypericum cream.*

Orthodox

- *Antihistamine compounds can be used to reduce the itch if complementary techniques are not beneficial.*

COLDS

A cold, supposedly so named because of the incorrect assumption that they occur because of cold weather or being cold, is in fact an infection caused by any of around 120 viruses known as rhinoviruses (after the Latin *rhinus* for nose).

There is, in fact, no such thing as a cold; it is a collection of symptoms: headache, sinus pain, running nose, blocked nose or sore nose, sore throat, cough, aching, general lethargy and tiredness. The cold is therefore a combination of a number of these symptoms.

We are further away from finding a cure for the common cold than we are for cancer, and I suspect that this will continue to be the way because the cold viruses mutate and change and our immune systems are not capable of keeping up with the speed of alteration, so we cannot fight these viruses easily. Interestingly, as we get older our colds become less frequent as we build up our immunity to the 120 rhinoviruses.

Colds rarely need medical intervention, although advice from a homeopath as to the correct remedy and the attention of your GP for too frequent or recurrent colds (to rule out anything underlying or nasty) may be required.

Colds are often the body's method of triggering its seasonal defence mechanism and we should all expect and 'enjoy' a cold at the start of winter and at the arrival of spring.

RECOMMENDATIONS

General Advice

- *Avoid heavy exercise. The concept of sweating out a cold is not correct.*
- *Ensure good hydration by drinking twice as much water as you normally do. The mucus and sweat will double your insensible water loss.*
- *'Starve a fever and feed a cold' is an accurate adage and, provided your cravings are healthy, go with them.*
- *Nasal washing with mild saltwater solutions can speed up the process of decongestion and the removal of the virus.*
- *Do not consider the use of decongestants, either topically sniffed or taken orally, because this will stop the immune system's destruction of the virus and increase the chances of more serious infections, such as middle-ear infections, labarynthitis, sinusitis and even meningitis.*

Nutritional

- *Good old chicken broth soup replenishes fluids and provides protein for repair. The chicken cartilage may actually have an antiviral effect as well.*

Supplemental

- *Consider the use of high doses of vitamin C, vitamin A, bioflavonoids, zinc and magnesium at doses twice those recommended on the packaging and taken with food. Zinc should be taken at a dosage of 5mg per foot of height before bed.*
- *Zinc lozenges, usually 2mg per tablet, sucked every two hours may prevent the onset of symptoms and/or shorten the longevity of a cold.*

Homeopathic

- *Review from your favourite homeopathic manual the following common homeopathic remedies: Allium cepa, Gelsemium, Bryonia, Pulsatilla, Dulcamara and Mercurius. Once the correct remedy is selected, use potency 6 every 2hr.*

Herbal/natural extracts

- *The herb Echinacea can be taken in doses recommended on packaging.*
- *Ginger drinks (with honey and lemon) made from fresh root ginger (half-inch chopped up) and hot water should be drunk and the steam inhaled.*
- *Elderberry, either in capsule or liquid form, tastes quite nice and so it can be used with children. Initially use the maximum recommendation on the packaging.*
- *The African potato (Hypoxis rooperi) has been found to contain phytosterols, glucocides and hypoxoside that may support the immune system.*

COMPUTERS AND VISUAL DISPLAY UNITS (VDUs)

With the advent of computers reaching every child, either in the home or at school, we must be wary of problems that may be associated with them and are, as yet, not well documented.

Like televisions, computers emit a radiation that may be harmful. The intensity of the emotions and the time spent at the computer are known to induce problems with eyesight, headaches and psychological symptoms such as depression, lack of concentration and insomnia.

The radiation from computers is emitted from all around the machine, not just the screen. The use of a protective shield may be beneficial to the user but of no consequence to those sitting close by.

RECOMMENDATIONS

General Advice

- *Ensure that the position of the screen is suitably set in relation to the chair in which you sit, to avoid structural and postural problems.*
- *Ensure that natural light hits the eyes by placing the computer with its back toward the windows.*
- *Use a screen that cuts down the computer's emissions.*
- *Try to use the computer only in short bursts of up to half an hour, with at least a 10–15min break before returning.*

- *Place a screen between yourself and the back of any other computer in your proximity.*
- *Allow as much distance between the computer and yourself as your vision will comfortably allow.*
- *Persistent users of computers should take suitable antioxidant supplements daily to counteract the mild free-radical production that radiation will create.*
- *See **Radiation**.*

DOWN'S SYNDROME

Down's syndrome is named after a physician in the 19th century who recognized a syndrome of mental retardation, atypical faces and various other physical changes, including a single palmar crease. Children with Down's syndrome can resemble the Mongol race, thus the outdated term Mongolism.

This genetic condition is caused by an extra gene being present from conception. A medical term for Down's syndrome is, therefore, Trisomy (three) 21, because it is this 21st chromosome that is trebled (*see* page 61).

A pregnant woman, especially if over the age of 35, will be offered or actively encouraged to have certain tests performed to rule out abnormalities, predominantly Down's syndrome. These tests include a blood test known as the 'Triple Test', which is checking for particular proteins in the bloodstream that, if found, can give strong evidence that further investigation is required. The Triple Test is not, by any means, definitive in itself. Further investigations include ultrasound where, specifically, a pad of fat is sought on the back of the embryo's neck. More invasive procedures such as amniocentesis (where a needle takes a small sample of the fluid surrounding the baby) or chorionic villus sampling (a similar procedure taking some cells from the baby's side of the placenta) are accurate but carry up to a two per cent risk of introducing infection or causing abortion. It is of paramount importance for parents to establish whether or not they would seek the

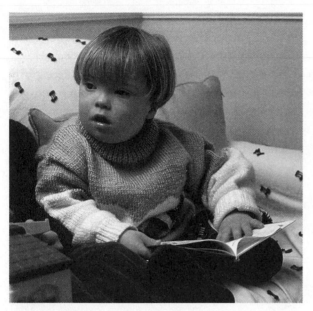

Child with Down's syndrome.

termination of a Down's pregnancy. The risks of the test procedures and the negative attitude of many towards Down's babies makes these tests unnecessary intrusions if parents would not choose to abort.

I have had the privilege of looking after many Down's children through my years of practice. Whilst different, Down's children are generally happy and loving participants of any family unit. Many have IQs capable of functioning in society and few have aggressive or unpleasant tendencies. I wish I could say the same for all 'normal' children.

There is increasing evidence that Down's children are not fatalistically destined to a poor-quality life by their gene malformation. Nutritional and dietetic supplements alongside naturopathic medicine, both herbal and homeo-pathic, may make a profound difference on both cognitive and physical development.

What seem to have been overlooked for decades are the subtle biochemical and metabolic changes that may lead to ill health, poor mental and physi-cal abilities, and growth. Now, researchers are finding that Down's individuals have specific defi-ciencies and certain enzymes that make them less capable of dealing with compounds that we may look upon as mild toxins or even as nutrients.

RECOMMENDATIONS

General Advice
- *Establish as soon as possible, by working with a complementary medical practitioner with expertise in this field, the functioning of the thyroid and thymus.*
- *Establish through a complementary medical practitioner the levels of stomach acid and digestive enzyme.*
- *Cranial osteopathy, osteopathy, physiotherapy and, when the child is old enough, the Alexander Technique, polarity therapy and yoga will all be markedly beneficial both physically and mentally.*

Nutritional
- *Establish any food allergies. Pay special attention to gluten found in wheat, cow's products and specifically lactose (milk sugar).*
- *Isolate and replenish any deficiencies, paying special attention to minerals (including zinc) and amino acids.*
- *Avoid fluoridated water, smoked foods, smoke from cigarettes, algae supplements and Ginkgo biloba. These compounds affect the Down's genetics in a variety of ways but specifically by suppressing the thyroid and the body's defence systems.*

Homeopathic
- *A constitutional homeopathic remedy should be chosen and changed as the child develops through consultation with a homeopath. The homeopathic remedies of Thymus and Thyroidinium, both at potency 3 or 6 given daily in conjunction with a constitutional remedy, should prove to be highly beneficial.*

Orthodox
- *Once a pregnancy is recognized, establish whether a termination would be your preferred choice should your baby have Down's. If not, then avoid the investigations.*

- *All Down's children should be under the care of a paediatrician specializing in this condition. Surgical or orthodox drug intervention may be necessary early on because defects in the heart, lungs and other organs may need to be corrected.*

- *Contact your local Down's Syndrome Association and obtain more information from, probably, the world's leading alternative-thinking Down's syndrome specialist: Dr Jack Warner, The Warner House, 1023 East Chapman Ave, Fullerton, CA 92631, USA. Tel: 714 441 2600.*

DREAMS AND NIGHTMARES

Dreams and nightmares occur at all ages but I have put it in the 'Childhood' chapter because of the frequency with which a child will bring a nightmare to the attention of its parents. They can be particularly disturbing and interfere with sleep patterns, but, to an infant or young child, this may not be so damaging because sleep will be caught up. For adults, whose life structure may not allow them to sleep as much or as long as they would like, frequently disturbing dreams or nightmares may be a health hazard.

Dreams, pleasant or otherwise, are neurological impulses that pass into the conscious centre from the sensory receptor areas of the brain. The speed with which the brain can transmit these impulses is very rapid and an epic dream lasting several hours may actually be imprinted through the conscious centres within seconds.

A dream may be the brain's attempt at reflecting upon an event or trauma and may be used by the subconscious to help sort out problems. A frightening movie before bed may create images as the brain tries to sort out whether it should be concerned at the recently raised levels of 'fear chemicals' such as adrenaline.

Past-life therapists may consider dreams to be carried over and their relevance may be of great import in certain therapeutic techniques. Although much study has been made of dreams, their significance is still poorly understood both from an orthodox scientific or an Eastern philosophical point of view. From a health stance, their only relevance is if they are disturbing sleep.

The contents of a dream do not necessarily reflect an underlying angst. It is hypothesized, for example, that dreaming of death will represent a marriage or birth. These associations are not strictly founded on any scientific studies but on the anecdotal evidence of people who have studied dreams for years. It is more likely that the brain will try to create either an answer or an escape for the consciousness. Ayurvedic physicians from India would consider the dream from the point of view of its *dosha–vata* (space and air), *pitta* (fire) and *kapha* (earth and water): a pitta nightmare may often be violent or heat-filled; tidal waves or drowning may represent excess kapha; and flying may be a vata excess. A tidal wave may also represent being overwhelmed by events beyond the individual's control and may give a pointer to the area of the psyche that needs to be confronted.

RECOMMENDATIONS

General Advice
- *Review your life structure and change stress patterns.*
- *Counselling by a psychotherapist with an interest in the relevance of dreams may be of great use if no obvious anxiety is apparent.*

Nutritional
- *Avoid stimulating foods or compounds that affect the nervous system, for at least 6hr before going to sleep. These include caffeine, alcohol, cigarettes and other drugs. Foods containing amines, such as chocolate and cheese, are also culprits.*

Homeopathic
- *There are hundreds of homeopathic remedies associated with scores of different dream/nightmare subjects. The best remedy is chosen by reference to a homeopathic Materia Medica or a homeopathic prescriber. The*

remedies Aconite, Arsenicum, Belladonna and Nux vomica should all be reviewed for children who are having nightmares. Potency 30 before bed for five nights should do the trick. Please refer to your preferred homeopathic manual for the best remedy.

Herbal/natural extracts

- *The flower remedy Rockrose and good old Rescue Remedy are both useful if taken 1hr before bedtime.*

DYSLEXIA

Dyslexia is an impairment of an individual who once knew or would be expected to know how to read or understand letters and/or numbers. A normal IQ differentiates this difficulty from those who have, say, brain damage or a low IQ.

Dyslexia is commonly overlooked. It ranges from a mild inability to differentiate between, say, the letters 'p' and 'q' or the numbers 6 and 9 to the transgressional dyslexia between the letter E and 3. Speech is normal but written words or letters may be transposed.

In itself, dyslexia is not necessarily a great problem but its social consequences, especially if not detected, can be devastating. A child may find himself/herself ridiculed in class and create an abhorrence of letters and numbers. This not only affects the child's academic standards but can lead to social withdrawal and difficulties in making friends. Children who are ridiculed in class may choose not to participate in sports for fear of more humiliation. Therefore early motor skills may be denied, adding to a further sense of inadequacy.

Any parent who finds their child overly shy, withdrawn, reluctant to participate in group activities, fearful of school or avoiding books and numbers should immediately consider dyslexia. The human being is remarkably adaptable and will often find defence measures, such as becoming unruly at school – a useful tool in avoiding facing up to dyslexia. Because of this, dyslexia may not be discovered until a later age, possibly even into adulthood. I mention this because it is never too late to use the available treatments with great success.

RECOMMENDATIONS

General Advice

- *Discuss the matter with the child's teacher or headteacher, who should have good knowledge of this condition.*
- *There is strong evidence that certain deficiencies may cause or enhance dyslexia. Discuss with a nutritionist any suitable dietetic changes and supplements: use more zinc, lecithin and amino acids, which are used in neurotransmission; above all, beware of dehydration.*
- *There are well-established remedial techniques and, in severe cases, special schooling that will enable a dyslexic to function perfectly normally in society.*
- *Any child who avoids letters and numbers and is particularly shy, antisocial or falling behind in school should be investigated for dyslexia. Any association of these characteristics with clumsiness should also be investigated.*
- *Referral through your GP or the local dyslexia organization to a specialist psychologist in this area is a prerequisite.*
- *Specialized training programmes, remedial exercises and training techniques can be practised in special units and also taught to parents to perform at home.*

Homeopathic

- *Homeopathic remedies, chosen according to the constitution of the child, are potentially beneficial.*

FALLS

A fall can occur at any age, of course, but I have chosen to mention it in the childhood chapter because persistent or frequent falls may be due to deeper problems of lack of concentration, dis-coordination and a general tendency to be accident prone (*see* Accidents).

A fall may result in a bruise, fracture or emotional shock, all of which may be associated with blood loss and internal organ damage. Each of these areas needs to be reviewed in the specific section in this book.

Conditions such as diabetes, hypoglycaemia and the use of drugs (prescribed or otherwise) may be a reason for an individual to fall.

RECOMMENDATIONS

General Advice
- *Any obvious injury, loss of consciousness or change in character of an individual who has fallen needs to be reviewed by a doctor.*
- *An osteopathic opinion should be obtained following any serious fall because other parts of the body may take the strain off an injured part, leading to problems at a later date.*

Homeopathic
- *Any injury can be treated with the homeopathic remedy Arnica, at potencies 6–12, every 2hr.*

FEVER

Fever in a child requires a little more attention than it does in an adult because a persisting or very high fever may cause febrile convulsions (*see* Convulsions). Normal body temperature for all ages is around 37°C, or 97.6°F.

Understanding the cause of a fever is a prerequisite to its treatment, but one must remember that fever is a friend. Most bacteria and viruses are inhibited by high temperatures: certain defensive chemical reactions occur in the body at a faster rate in the presence of fever and it is established that the chemicals produced create the fever. Suppressing a fever from within is therefore unwise and one should only attempt to keep the body cool externally without stopping the actual chemical reaction, as this is less likely to hamper the immune system.

Fever may be an early warning for a serious underlying infection. Children old enough to express themselves may give some clues, but infants with a persisting high fever need to be assessed by a physician.

RECOMMENDATIONS

General Advice
- *Any persisting, recurrent or very high fever should warrant a medical opinion. Specific treatment against, say, an infection should be initiated either from a complementary or orthodox point of view.*
- *Keep the child in light cotton if sweating or remove clothing if dry.*
- *Apply cold compresses to the neck, stomach and ankles.*
- *Remember that a fever is generally a friend, whether it is curing or warning, and should be treated as such.*

Homeopathic
- *Homeopathic treatment needs to be aimed at the symptoms, and reference to your preferred homeopathic manual is required. Pay specific attention to the remedies Aconite, Arsenicum, Belladonna, Gelsemium and Mercurius.*

Orthodox
- *It is not advisable to use herbal remedies in children unless you are absolutely certain of the strength and quality. Orthodox preparations such as paracetamol for children should be employed if the temperature rises above 39°C or 101°F. By this stage, however, medical advice should have been sought.*

Rheumatic fever

Rheumatic fever is characterized by pains in the joints, fever and general malaise following a streptococcal infection usually of the throat. The pains in the joints occur because of a reaction (antigen complex reaction) between the bacteria and the body's defence mechanism.

The body recognizes the infection and sends out antibodies to attack the bacteria (the antigen) and in some cases this triggers an inflammatory response that affects the joints and frequently the heart valves. The complexes can affect the delicate tissues of the kidney, and a sore throat with associated kidney symptoms (*see* **Sore throats**) must be treated as urgent.

The orthodox approach is to use antibiotics at the first sign of a streptococcal sore throat but alternative measures initially may be just as effective. If heart or kidney effects are suspected (associated chest pains, irregular heartbeats or heart sounds) then treatment must be considered as urgent. Prolonged use of penicillin is still considered by many orthodox practitioners to protect against re-infection of damaged heart valves. Antibiotics will also be encouraged if any operative procedure, including dental work, is to be performed.

RECOMMENDATIONS

General Advice

- *Sore throats, and streptococcal sore throats in particular, should not be taken lightly and complementary medical treatment should be initiated swiftly. See* **Sore throats**.
- *Ensure good hydration, especially if there is any kidney involvement.*

Supplemental

- *Commence the child on the following supplements in divided doses throughout the day: vitamin A (1,000iu per foot of height) or beta-carotene (2mg per foot of height); vitamin C (500mg per foot of height); vitamin E (150iu per foot of height); and zinc (5mg per foot of height before bed).*

Homeopathic

- *If rheumatic fever is confirmed, consult a homeopathic practitioner but initiate the use of the remedy Streptococcin 30 every 4hr.*

Herbal/natural extracts

- *Use Echinacea (dried root) 200mg per foot of height. Please note dry powdered extract is not the same as dried root and should be given at ¼ the dose.*

Orthodox

- *At any suggestion of chronic damage to the heart valves (this is diagnosed by a doctor), seek advice from a complementary medical practitioner with regard to homeopathic or herbal cover through adolescence as an alternative to daily use of penicillin. More than two attacks, despite alternative or complementary treatment, warrants the use of prophylactic antibiotics to protect against serious damage and consult a complementary specialist to get advice concerning the side effects of these drugs (see* **Antibiotics***).*

Scarlet fever

Scarlet fever is so called because of the bright red appearance of an individual with a fever. This is caused by a streptococcal infection and is often associated with a sore throat. As the risk of this condition developing into rheumatic fever is slight, but nevertheless real, my recommendations are found under the section on rheumatic fever.

GROWTH

DELAYED GROWTH

Delayed growth in a child can occur at any stage and is defined by falling below a set height or weight, as shown in the charts (overleaf).

It is very important to note that a child's size may be dependent upon their genetics, inherited from their parents. A child with small or light parents may not necessarily be underdeveloped and it is important for each individual to be assessed from this point of view. Growth is governed by good nutritional input and also by a variety of hormones. Specifically, growth hormone (from the pituitary gland) thyroxine and insulin levels

Growth Assessment

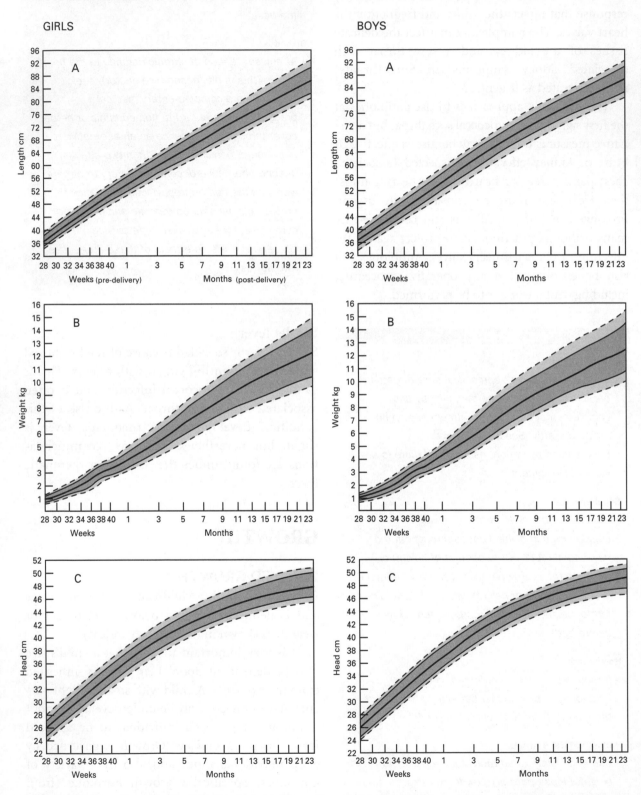

The charts show the ideal length (A), weight (B) and head size (C) of girls and boys over the first two years.

must all be in balance. Malabsorption or malnutrition will deprive the child of proteins, vitamins, minerals and trace elements, all of which are essential to correct growth.

RECOMMENDATIONS

General Advice

• *If worried about developmental failure or if your child does not correspond to the charts, then please consult your GP.*

Nutritional

• *Once serious underlying conditions such as pituitary problems, diabetes, thyroid or malabsorption problems have been ruled out, consider the advice of a nutritionist.*

Homeopathic

• *The homeopathic remedy Silica, potency 30 twice a day for three weeks (or a higher potency as prescribed by a homeopath), encourages absorption and, therefore, growth in cases of poor nutritional intake.*

GROWING PAINS

This non-medical term has crept into use because of its accuracy in describing the symptoms. Pains are constantly felt by children as their muscles and ligaments stretch in response to the growth of their bones. Growing pains may also be related directly to muscular cramps and some adjustment of dietetics, hydration and supplementation generally deals with the problem.

Pain may be located and persistent at the part of the bone that actually grows. This is usually at either end of the bones. It is rare for these pains to be indicative of anything serious, although severe or persistent pain should be reviewed.

Children who grow too rapidly are prone to growing pains and a markedly rapid growth may indicate underlying hormonal dysfunction that will need to be reviewed by a physician or paediatrician.

RECOMMENDATIONS

General Advice

• *Massage, heat or ice (depending on which soothes) and the application of Arnica cream should be relieving.*

• *Persistent discomfort should be reviewed by an osteopath and brought to the attention of a doctor only if osteopathic care and advice does not help.*

Nutritional

• *Increase the calcium and magnesium intake through sesame seeds, nuts, vegetables, fish and chicken, or supplement with a suitable calcium/magnesium compound supplying the recommended daily allowance (RDA).*

Homeopathic

• *Depending on the symptoms and their site, a homeopathic remedy should be chosen from your preferred manual or via a homeopath.*

HYPERACTIVITY AND ATTENTION DEFICIT DISORDER (ADD)

I am sure that parents have noticed hyperactivity in their children ever since the homo sapiens erected onto two legs. Parents today will notice periods where their children are more active or overexcited than at other times. Learning appropriate responses takes time and is the cause of the 'terrible twos'.

I believe that one must be careful not to label a child overactive when the problem may be parental intolerance. Overactivity must be disruptive, persistent and preferably recognized by a third party such as a teacher. There is a strong correlation, especially in America, between hyperactivity and attention deficit disorder (ADD). Attention deficit disorder may be present without hyperactivity and is characterized by a short attention span, poor concentration, an inability to finish projects and an ease of distraction. It is important to differentiate between this and the absences seen in petit mal epilepsy (*see* **Epilepsy**).

It is worth noting that both hyperactivity and ADD may continue beyond childhood and when it does so it is termed 'residual attention deficit disorder'. The causes are much the same and are well researched. It is thought to affect approximately three per cent of the population although – and this is why it is very important to establish diagnosis – some studies have suggested hyperactivity in up to 20 per cent of the population.

Food additives, of which, believe it or not, there are over 5,000 in the USA, have been clearly cited as a cause for these syndromes. It is important to understand that the term additives includes not just colourings but also include thickeners, preservatives, flavourings and many others. Artificial 'anti-oxidants' are being confused by the public as being healthy additives because antioxidants have come to prominence in dealing with cardiovascular and cancer problems. Please do not be fooled. Individuals buying foods predominantly from supermarkets may be ingesting up to 15g of additives per day.

Low blood sugar (hypoglycaemia) is a major contributing factor to hyperactivity and ADD, predominantly caused by taking in refined (white) sugars that are absorbed rapidly, and which cause a large insulin response that in turn lowers the blood sugar level. Any hyperactive child who behaves in such a way an hour or so after eating is probably taking in too many carbohydrates.

Food allergies are a major consideration and an individual correlation between poor behaviour and specific foods can be made by keeping a list, noting any changes with particular foods.

Lead poisoning has been shown to be responsible for bad behaviour and therefore this and other metal or environmental toxins should be considered as possible causes of ADD.

RECOMMENDATIONS

General Advice
- *Discuss the matter of a hyperactive or suspected ADD child with teachers, a counsellor experienced in these matters or a local group.*
- *Consider the possibility of metal poisoning or other toxins such as pesticides.*

- *Consider art therapy if the problem persists and assessment through an art therapist who specializes in problems with children.*

Nutritional
- *Remove refined carbohydrates (especially white sugar) and all processed foods from the diet.*
- *Consider food allergy testing or keep a very clear diary of foods eaten and the child's behaviour.*
- *Consider the possibility of nutritional deficiencies. It is possible that deficiencies in certain amino acids (tyrosine, tryptophan or phenylalanine), as well as a lack of certain minerals such as zinc or iron, may all be contributing factors, if not the cause.*

Orthodox
- *A medical opinion may be necessary if none of the above considerations work but, because orthodox medicine is pharmaceutically oriented, a first-line treatment may be a drug such as methylphenidate hydrochloride, known as Ritalin. This option should be used as a last resort. Ritalin might, although I have no evidence to support this, go on to show itself as an addictive drug and require persistent use. If so, in later life it could lead to a dependency on tranquillizers.*

JAUNDICE OF THE NEWBORN
(*See* **Jaundice** in chapter 5.)

Jaundice of the newborn is frequently seen in newborn infants within the first five days of life. It usually clears within the first two weeks and is due to the incomplete development of a chemical pathway within liver cells, which results in a decreased ability to bind bilirubin (one of the breakdown products of blood cells) with a particular acid. Normally, once this binding has taken place, the waste products are passed into the gallbladder and expelled into the bile, which gives the stool its normal brown colour. If this process does not take place, the amount of bilirubin rises and flows back into the bloodstream, is deposited around the system and causes the yellow discolouration of the skin.

The condition is usually mild and self-limiting without any unpleasant symptoms for the infant but occasionally the problem can persist. Premature infants may be more prone to a longer-lasting, more severe deposition of bilirubin, which can lead to a condition known as kernicterus. This condition is one of severe neurological deficit or even death, caused by degeneration of the nerve cells in the brain due to irritation by the bilirubin.

Another serious condition that causes jaundice in the newborn is erythroblastosis fetalis. This occurs when the blood of the infant contains an antibody from its mother that attacks the infant's own red blood cells.

RECOMMENDATIONS

General Advice

- *Treatment is unnecessary unless the condition is serious, in which case an experienced medically-trained homeopath should be consulted.*
- *A healer may help speed up the process of a return to normality.*

Homeopathic

- *The infant should be given the homeopathic remedies Lycopodium 30 and Ferrum metallicum 30 in fluid form alternately every 3hr through the initial illness and twice a day for two weeks after a recovery is made.*

Orthodox

- *A jaundiced infant is usually spotted before he/she leaves hospital. For those who develop it after they arrive home or after home deliveries, it is imperative that a paediatrician is advised of the situation.*
- *A child who is born yellow or jaundiced may have been suffering with blood incompatibility. The paediatrician at the hospital will diagnose this through a blood test. Treatment is rarely necessary but the child will be kept in hospital and a blood transfusion may be required.*
- *Ensure a full discussion with the paediatrician before a subsequent pregnancy is undertaken.*

ABO and Rhesus blood incompatibility

A child may be born jaundiced and the parents may be told that the child and mother have incompatible blood types. This is caused by two conditions known as ABO and Rhesus incompatibility and is triggered when the baby's blood cells are different from those of its mother's womb and some of the baby's blood cells escape through the placenta into the mother's bloodstream. The mother's defence mechanism recognizes this as a foreign body and forms antibodies against it. These pass back through the placenta and attack the baby's blood cells. Interestingly, the effect is not a big problem in the first child but any subsequent baby with a blood group foreign to its mother will find that it enters the womb of an individual whose immune system is primed to attack its red blood cells. This is why it is important to know the blood group of a mother.

Most people know about the blood groups A, B and O. Making a complicated situation simpler, if you are blood group A you will have antibodies to blood group B, and vice versa. If you are blood group O you are said to be a universal donor, meaning that you can give your blood to anyone. Group O does have antibodies to both A and B but the amount given to someone in a transfusion is minimal. There is another group, AB. People who are blood group AB are universal recipients because they have no antibodies to either group A or group B.

Blood Group Compatibility				
	A	B	AB	O
A	✓	✗	✗	✓
B	✗	✓	✗	✓
AB	✓	✓	✓	✓
O	✗	✗	✗	✓

To make it even more complicated, there is another major red blood cell protein known as Rhesus factor. You either have this (Rhesus positive) or you do not (Rhesus negative). If a baby has Rhesus factor but the mother does not, the mother will form antibodies against this blood cell protein and, as I have mentioned above, will attack it. Rhesus incompatibility is a more common finding and is treated by giving the mother a large injection of Rhesus protein after the infant has been born. The mother's antibodies attack the protein and effectively get 'mopped up'. This injection, known as anti-serum D, may be given prior to or early on in subsequent pregnancies in an attempt to protect the unborn infant. It is generally a successful technique, although problems may arise.

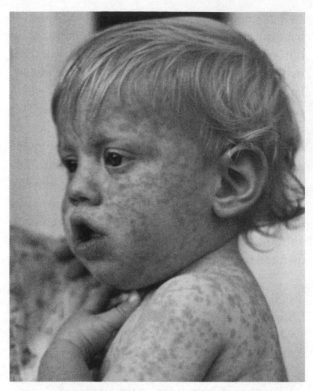

The red rash and raised spots symptomatic of measles are clearly visible.

RECOMMENDATION

Orthodox

- *Please discuss the matter of anti-serum D with your midwives and paediatrician. There is some concern that the manufacturing process does not guarantee injections free of infections such as the 'mad cow disease' organism, HIV or hepatitis. This association has only recently been considered but may become more prominent in the near future.*

MEASLES

Measles is a highly contagious disease typified by fever and a red rash with raised spots. Measles very often causes a cough, runny nose, lethargy and tiredness, and, depending on the areas that the virus attacks, conjunctivitis and irritation in and around the genitals. Typically, spots are seen in the mouth; these are known as Koplik's spots, which usually turn up on day two or three of the infection. The rash usually appears on the fourth day, often starting on the neck and spreading to other areas. The rash may persist for two to four days.

In itself, measles is rarely a serious condition, although children who are immunosuppressed may find the condition fatal due to the secondary conditions and complications. Undernourished children or those with underlying immune weakness may contract bronchitis, pneumonia, otitis media and a rare form of encephalitis (inflammation of the brain). It is these serious conditions that have encouraged the Western world to lay a strong emphasis on vaccination programmes.

At this time I am opposed to the automatic vaccination of all children. *See* **Vaccinations**, where I discuss the measles vaccine in detail.

RECOMMENDATIONS

General Advice

- *See* **Vaccinations**.
- *The irritation of the rash will be soothed by applying a sodium bicarbonate solution. Add one tablespoon of sodium bicarbonate (baking soda) to one pint of water. Iced water may be more soothing.*

- *Discuss the matter with a complementary medical practitioner, especially if the symptoms are severe or the child is particularly unwell.*

Supplemental

- *Beta-carotene (1mg per foot of height given with a meal or in a child's bottle up to three times a day) is protective of infection of mucous membranes such as in the eyes and the lungs. It should certainly be used if any symptoms of conjunctivitis, vaginitis or bronchitis are present.*

Homeopathic

- *The homeopathic remedy Pulsatilla 6 can be given every half-hour, and in particularly irritating cases the remedy Rhus toxicodendron 6 can be given at the same frequency.*

Orthodox

- *Diagnosis is made clinically, although blood tests may be used in more serious cases. Interestingly, because of the vaccination programme, many GPs may qualify and enter a General Practice without having seen measles. Consult Grandma!*

MOTION SICKNESS

Motion sickness can occur at any age but is most troublesome in children. Humankind was not designed to travel at speeds greater than a run and so the advent of the use of animals and machinery to take us at far greater speeds is not ingrained in our nervous system. The movement of objects passing us, in combination with irregular movements within the vestibular canal or balance centre in the inner ear, creates an unusual and unexpected neurological impulse state within the brain. The response is to attempt to stop us and a very good way to do this is to make us feel sick. As we age and become more used to travelling our brain accepts that this is not a dangerous situation and therefore the need for nausea diminishes.

RECOMMENDATIONS

General Advice

- *See **Nausea**.*
- *Persevere with the travel because the body and brain will adjust eventually.*
- *Avoid strong smells of food or tobacco whilst in transit and ensure adequate fresh air.*

Homeopathic

- *The homeopathic remedy Cocculus indicus 6 can be taken every 15min whilst in motion and every 2hr prior to the intended journey, starting the day before. Other remedies include Tabacum and Rhus toxicodendron.*

MUMPS

Mumps is a viral infection that affects glands throughout the body but predominantly the salivary glands under the jaw and the parotid gland in front of the ear. It is an infectious disease spread by coughs, sneezes and by physical contact; it is more common in hot weather and is sometimes associated with a fever. Lifelong immunity is usually conferred after an attack. In a healthy individual mumps is a short-lived problem, usually lasting about ten days, through which time the individual is infectious. Unfortunately, mumps takes two to four weeks to develop and the child has probably been spreading the infection throughout this period.

Rarely do complications occur but the older the individual, the more likely the possibility of infection of the testes, brain or pancreas, which can lead to very serious conditions.

Vaccination is routine and encouraged by the orthodox world, but consideration for vaccinations in general should be made before these are given (*see* **Vaccinations**).

RECOMMENDATIONS

General Advice

- *See **Fever**.*

Nutritional

- *Avoid flavoursome food that encourages salivation and thus increases pain.*

Supplemental

- *A multivitamin – vitamin C and Beta-carotene – should be given at three times the RDA for the age or size of the individual.*

Homeopathic

- *The homeopathic remedies Belladonna, Aconite, Mercurius, Hepar sulphuris calcarium and Phytolacca should all be considered via your preferred homeopathic manual. Potency 6 should be taken every 2hr through the acute phase.*
- *If an individual has been exposed to mumps, protection may be afforded by taking the homeopathic remedy Parotidinum 30, twice a day for two weeks.*

POLIO

Polio is the abbreviation for the disease known as poliomyelitis. It is a common viral disease that usually runs an asymptomatic or mild course, characterized by upper respiratory or gastrointestinal symptoms. The virus may progress to involve the central nervous system and result in either a non-paralytic or a paralytic form of the disease. Poliomyelitis is endemic (meaning that it lives within populations) and has epidemic flare-ups (there is a maximum frequency for this from July to September in temperate zones). As with most transmittable diseases, it is spread by coughing but also by the oral–faecal route (a carrier with polio in the bowel may prepare food without washing off the virus after their last visit to the toilet). Faecal contamination of water and flies are other vectors.

Immunization against polio is available for those in the Western world but for the majority, their own immune system is their only defence. As with all contagious diseases, the health of the individual is the deciding factor on whether polio will come and go and confer a lifelong immunity or strike and create the feared neurological result.

Subclinical polio occurs in 95 per cent of those infected. The immune system fights the battle and the infection may not have been recognized. This form is a mild non-specific illness causing cough or flu-like symptoms or a gastrointestinal disturbance such as diarrhoea.

The non-paralytic form is a meningitis-like illness (*see* **Meningitis**) causing fever, headache and a stiff neck. Less than one per cent of individuals infected may have the paralytic form, which starts with a headache, general illness and muscular pains. Fever, neck stiffness and muscle tenderness may be present. This then leads to severe muscle pains, an inability to move the parts affected and, if the brain is contaminated, difficulty in swallowing and talking. At worst, respiratory paralysis may occur in five per cent of these rare cases, usually due to complications of respiratory paralysis. Patients showing even very severe paralysis may make a reasonable recovery over two years. Only in occasional instances does a permanent paralysis remain.

RECOMMENDATIONS

General Advice

- *See* **Vaccinations**.
- *See* **Influenza** *and* **Herpes simplex**, *because the basic antiviral advice given for these conditions should be followed for polio.*
- *If meningitis is the outcome, see* **Meningitis**.
- *Through the recovery phase, osteopathy, chiropractic, Rolfing and Feldenkrais have been shown to benefit.*
- *If any residual paralysis remains, the Alexander Technique, polarity therapy, yoga or Qi Gong (Chi Kung) should be studied.*
- *Marma therapy and neurotherapy, branches of Ayurvedic physical therapy, can be used also.*

Homeopathic

- *Recovery will benefit from constitutional homeopathic repair and as soon as a diagnosis is made use the remedy Lathyrus 30, four times a day, until a more suitable remedy may be chosen.*

PUBERTY

Puberty is the period at which the sexual organs become capable of exercising their function of reproduction. Increases in androgens (male hormones, the most well known of which is testosterone) and the female hormones (predominantly oestrogen and progesterone) create character changes. A boy will find that his voice deepens and muscle development increases, around the shoulders in particular. Erections become more frequent and seminal discharge will accompany orgasm. Girls will start their periods and develop a rounding of features, especially over the hips. The breasts will start developing at a faster rate.

Delayed puberty

The timing of these events is generally one year before or after the age at which the parent of the same sex went through their puberty. A delay beyond two years and an absence of puberty after the age of 15 years is considered a delayed puberty. Small children and those who are undernourished may find their puberty delayed. Chronic illness and the use of steroids in conditions such as asthma may also prevent puberty.

RECOMMENDATIONS

General Advice

- *If puberty has not occurred by the age of 15 years, consult with a physician, who may refer the child to a paediatric specialist.*
- *Consult a homeopathic practitioner for a suitable constitutional remedy.*
- *If no underlying disease is apparent, test for nutritional deficiencies through blood and hair analysis under the care of a naturopathic specialist, and correct any nutritional deficits.*
- *Consider some form of counselling, preferably art therapy, because a delay may create a marked lack of self-confidence at a very important time of the development of the psyche. Regardless, be extremely supportive as a parent and do not dismiss the child's anxieties.*

Precocious puberty

Should symptoms of puberty occur early, some concern may need to be dispelled. As arbitrary cut-off figures, girls showing signs of puberty before the age of 8 and boys before the age of 10 should be taken to a paediatric specialist. We come across those children who are mature beyond their years both mentally and physically and this may simply be a normal but early development. Musical and mathematical 'geniuses' may simply be children who have developed faculties before the expected age. These are not to be considered a disease process. Social chastisement may occur, however, and this needs to be addressed.

Extremely rarely, tumours of the pituitary gland may produce hormones that stimulate early periods or excessive growth (*see* **Gigantism**), but these can be ruled out by blood tests and, if necessary, brain scans.

RECOMMENDATIONS

General Advice

- *Excessive growth or other early developmental milestones should be assessed by a suitably qualified practitioner or paediatrician.*
- *Moral support must be given by parents to support a child who may be 'different' to his or her peers. Counselling, preferably art therapy, can be utilized.*
- *Early periods may lead to a tendency to iron and protein deficiency, which may inhibit growth. Increased growth or development usually corresponds to an increased appetite, but nutritional foods containing proteins, vitamins, minerals and trace elements must be encouraged and supplements given if the child is a pernickety eater.*

Homeopathic

- *Consult a homeopath for a constitutional remedy.*

RUBELLA (GERMAN MEASLES)

Rubella or German measles is an innocuous infection causing a mild fever, lethargy and a characteristic rash. This rash initially starts on the face and neck, spreads to the trunk and limbs, is characteristically bright red and is often accompanied by rose-coloured spots on the palate and the throat. The rash usually lasts a few days and may be associated with stiff joints and swollen glands. The true diagnosis can only be made through confirmation of a blood test, but most GPs are experienced enough to make a clinical diagnosis. The virus may be contracted and incubated for 14–21 days and the patient is infectious for about one week before and up to one week after the appearance of the rash. In principle, however, German measles is not a problem to an individual.

The danger with rubella is that, more than most viruses, it has an ability to cause malformation in the developing foetus. This makes it a dangerous infection to contract whilst pregnant. The orthodox world with its predilection for vaccination and its disregard of the possibility of risks or dangers associated with this form of treatment used to encourage all teenage girls to have a rubella vaccination. Recently, in a vain attempt to eradicate the disease, all children between the age of five and 15 years are automatically being given rubella vaccinations in combination with measles and mumps. This MMR vaccine is discussed and vilified in the section on vaccinations (see **Vaccinations**).

RECOMMENDATIONS

General Advice

- *Treatment for the symptoms of rubella is similar to that of measles (see **Measles**).*

Orthodox

- *Seriously consider the need to vaccinate your children but, for rubella in particular, girls reaching the age of procreation can have a blood test to check for immunity (very often the infection is contracted unknowingly in earlier years) and if natural immunity has been formed no further action need be taken. If not immune, then the vaccination should be considered (see **Vaccinations**).*

SLEEPLESSNESS

A full discussion on insomnia may be found in chapter 5 (see **Sleep problems**) but in children sleeplessness is rarely a disease process.

Most infants and children will sleep as required although the pattern may not fit in with the parents. A baby may feed every 2–3 hours through the night and by sleeping in bursts for 2–3 hours through the day has its necessary sleep quota (anywhere up to 16 hours) and is perfectly all right. This may leave parents in tatters and very often convinced that their child does not sleep.

Sleeplessness is influenced by colic and the inadvertent ingestion of stimulants either due to food allergy or drinking mother's milk, which may contain caffeine or other stimulants, such as drugs of abuse if the mother partakes.

RECOMMENDATIONS

General Advice

- *Accepting that the most common causes for an infant's disturbed sleep pattern are hunger, colic or discomfort from, say, a soiled nappy, then change, feed and comfort the child.*
- *Ensure that the environment is neither too hot nor too cold and that the child's bed covers are suitable for the temperature. A quilt in summer or a sheet in winter may be inappropriate.*
- *Remember that infants and children are learning constantly and overattention to the slightest complaint will teach them an inappropriate way of attracting attention. If a child seems to be exploiting the parents' anxieties, leave him/her to cry for 5min, then give comfort until settled and leave the room. Next time, wait for 10min. Repeat this process and you may find that the child falls asleep whilst whining. Experience will quickly develop and most parents will be able to differentiate between an attention-seeking wail and a cry associated with a true problem.*
- *Parents should feed their baby, even if it means waking the baby, before they go to bed.*

• Paradoxically, an infant or child may sleep poorly because of overtiredness. Try putting baby to bed 15min earlier and you may find that baby sleeps longer. If this trick does not work, try the common sense approach of allowing the child to stay up later.

• Avoid putting the child to bed within 2hr of the last meal (in the case of an infant or a child that falls asleep after eating, do not awaken the child of course) and avoid exciting or vigorous activity within that time.

Homeopathic

• An irritable baby will be soothed by the homeopathic remedy Chamomilla, especially if the child is teething. Coffea 6, three doses on the hour starting 1hr before bed time may help an overexcited child.

• For children over the age of two years, Nux vomica 200 on three consecutive nights followed one week later by one dose of Sulphur 200 can be magical! If the child responds after any of the doses of Nux vomica, hold off on the sulphur until the pattern is once again disturbed. This process may be repeated up to once a month but if it does not work consult a homeopath for a more specific remedy.

Herbal/natural extracts

• A chamomile tea sweetened with very little honey, if necessary, may be soporific.

SPEECH

The ability to speak is a combination of anatomical and neurological co-ordination in conjunction with learned responses. From as early an age as possible parents must 'teach' children by correlating objects with words. The intricacies of language develop as the child grows and concepts such as verbs and adjectives come into play.

Development of speech

In the first month, baby communicates using guttural sounds and crying. By the second month the child will start to vocalize, making cooing noises and vowel sounds, but continues to communicate mostly by crying.

The third month will see an attempt at communication by squealing and focusing on an individual. Consonant sounds start and the child may repeat combinations of syllables. At this point the child will derive some pleasure from vibrations felt in the lips and be enthusiastic about his/her gurgles.

In the fourth and fifth months the child will be having long 'conversations' by combining vowel sounds with consonant sounds. Babbling will increase, especially if the child is spoken to.

The sixth and seventh months will see a marked increase in phonetics. The child will start to babble whilst performing a simple task or having things done to him/her, such as getting dressed.

By the seventh month the child will be using vocalization to attract attention and will start talking louder if ignored.

Around the eighth and ninth months the first words will come forward – Dada and Mamma are usually the first. (Fathers, do not take umbrage if

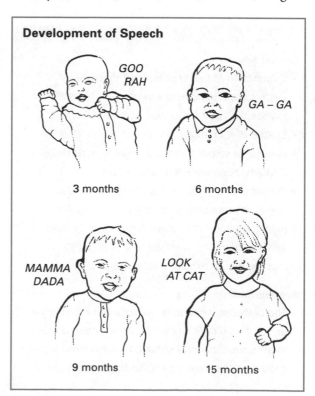

Development of Speech

GOO RAH
3 months

GA – GA
6 months

MAMMA DADA
9 months

LOOK AT CAT
15 months

your partner's name is uttered first! Mamma is actually easier to say than Dada and is often heard a lot more in the first few months of life.) Between the tenth and fifteenth months an infant will start to use meaningful one- and two-word sentences: 'Dada gone' and 'More toast' are common examples.

By 15 months to two years an improvement is seen, to the point that meaningful sentences will come forward. 'Look at birdie' and 'Pasta on floor' are clear indications of the child using language accurately.

Between the age of two and three years full sentences are formed, and in the latter stages conversation should be possible.

After three years of age egocentricity arises and the terms 'I' and 'Me' increase.

Any problems with hearing or vision will impede development but it is important to remember that these months are only guidelines and leeway either side by at least 2–3 months should be allowed before the child is considered to be surprisingly advanced or delayed.

RECOMMENDATIONS

General Advice

- *If your child is falling outside of these basic guidelines, a paediatric assessment is essential to establish hearing, vision and mental ability.*
- *Ensure that constant communication with both visual and verbal aspects is kept at a maximum through these early formative years.*
- *Do not sound or behave critically if a child is failing to pronounce correctly or is not calling objects by the right name. Criticism can cause introspection and shyness at this early age, much more so than at a later stage.*

Supplemental

- *The orthodox world may overlook the importance of nutritional deficiencies in development and a multivitamin/mineral should be considered for children once they are off the bottle or breast.*

Stammering and stuttering

A stammer is one of several irregularities of speech marked by involuntary halting, repetition of words or smaller segments, transposition or mispronunciation of certain consonants or a combination of any of these defects. A stutter is speech-marked by an intermittent inability to enunciate a phonetic segment of one syllable without repeating it, straining to overcome the block, or both.

Stuttering is common among children until the age of five years, but beyond that the majority of stutterers will carry the difficulty into adulthood. About one per cent of adults have a stutter or stammer. This tends to run in families and is more prevalent in males and left-handed people.

If a stammer or stutter starts in a child, the chances are that it is a habit and is very often associated with stress. An onset in adulthood is generally a sign of an injury or disorder to the central nervous system.

Everybody may stammer under pressure because the neck muscles and particularly the vocal cords become tense and less controlled in an embarrassing or awkward situation. This is not a problem unless it is interfering with social life, in which case treatment is required.

RECOMMENDATIONS

General Advice

- *Adult onset of any speech difficulty should be assessed by a neurologist.*
- *A child may benefit from the counselling of an expert in this field, who should also deal with the parents. At a later age, relaxation and meditation techniques should be taught.*
- *Test for metal toxicity. Copper and lead have been shown to be a problem and other metals have similar effects.*

Supplemental

- *Zinc deficiency may be relevant and can be counteracted by taking 5mg of zinc per foot of*

---

height each day before bed for two weeks. If this resolves the problem but it returns, then assume that there is a lack of zinc in the diet or poor absorption. Seek guidance from a nutritional expert.

Homeopathic

- *Many homeopathic remedies may be utilized, depending on the type of speech difficulty. Review the remedies Stramonium, Agaricus muscarius, Cuprum and Arsenicum. Potency 30 three times a day of a suitable remedy taken for one week may make an impact.*

Herbal/natural extracts

- *The Bach flower remedy Trumpet Vine is useful for speech difficulties whilst speaking in public.*

SUDDEN INFANT DEATH SYNDROME (SIDS or COT DEATH)

Sudden infant death syndrome (SIDS), more commonly known as cot death, is the most tragic of occurrences. Approximately three in 100,000 children each year will be found lifeless for no apparent reason. These deaths most commonly occur in the winter months and usually between the ages of two and four months.

There are several factors associated with cot death that are accepted throughout the orthodox world and others that are suggested through alternative sources.

Orthodox associations

- Smoking. The association is startling and it is the most important of all known factors. Maternal smoking during or after pregnancy and those smoking around a pregnant mother or baby may cause up to two-thirds of cot deaths.
- Infants sleeping face down in cots. This may be made worse by certain fire-retarding materials, although the suggestion has not been substantiated.
- Infections, particularly chest infections, whether they are mild or serious.

- Genetic predisposition creating either a fault in the part of the brain that tells the body to breathe or enzyme deficiencies that prevent the availability of energy from food.
- Overheating or exposure to cold.
- Excessive caffeine intake during pregnancy.

Alternative possibilities

- Medicines such as those used in treating colic or decongestants.
- Antibiotics when used to treat infections.
- Food allergy or intolerance.
- Recent vaccination.

Prevention is the key and as many safeguards as possible should be encouraged.

RECOMMENDATIONS

General Advice

- *Place an apnoea blanket under the child. These are easily obtainable, although expensive, and are special blankets that register the child's movement. If the child stops breathing an alarm sound will go off, which may awaken the child and will alert the parents, provided that an inter-room sounder is utilized if the parents or child's guardian are out of earshot.*
- *Cover all cot mattresses with a plastic sheet.*
- *Ensure an even temperature with fresh air in the child's room.*
- *Ensure that the child sleeps on his/her back. Even children sleeping on their side have a higher incidence of SIDS.*
- *Clothing and bedding must be well-fitting because anything loose may slip over the baby's head. Infants should not use duvets until after one year old. Bedding should be securely tucked in.*
- *For this more than any other condition – absolutely **no** smoking through pregnancy, around the child or even in the same house as an infant.*
- *Avoid caffeine during pregnancy.*
- *Pay special attention to any child on orthodox medication. If the apnoea blanket/alarm system*

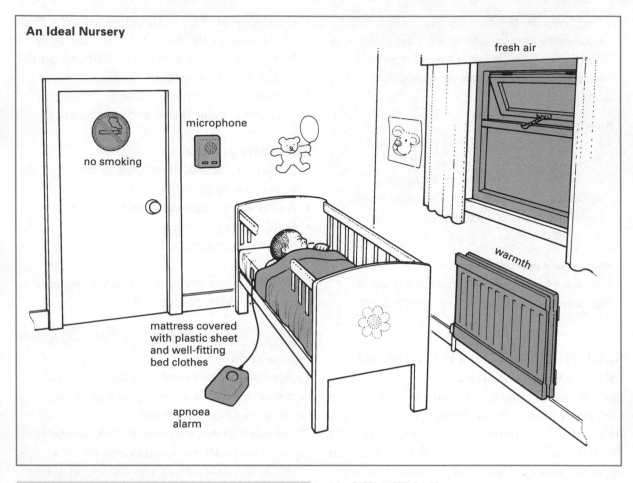

An Ideal Nursery

fresh air

microphone

no smoking

warmth

mattress covered
with plastic sheet
and well-fitting
bed clothes

apnoea
alarm

*is not utilized, a child with an infection may be
best preserved from SIDS by sleeping in the
same bed as the parents.*

If this tragedy has occurred within your family or
circle of friends it may be worth considering the
Hindu philosophy that we are reincarnated as part
of a long cycle of attainment, understanding and
teaching. A spirit that enters the body of a child
who does not live for long is considered to be a
very advanced soul who only needed a short
incarnation and was principally here to teach sadness and loss to those around. Such a visitation is
considered a blessing and although this cannot
touch the pain created by such a tragedy, I have
found that it may give some meaning to the pain
and sorrow.

VACCINATIONS

There are major confrontations between holistic
medicine and modern Western medicine, but
none is more contentious than the matter of vaccinations. As usual, there is no right or wrong
answer but particularly in the case of vaccinations, there is no reason to believe that
vaccinations are correct and safe for all. When
dealing with undernourished and immunosuppressed masses such as in the troubled states of
Africa, the vaccination programme probably
saves millions of lives each year. Of interest, however, is a well-documented report on the use of
vitamin A instead of vaccinations against
measles, which showed an unequivocal comparative success rate between the two treatments with
regard to preventing undernourished children
from developing measles pneumonia, a serious
and often fatal condition. This trial has, to my

knowledge, not been repeated, basically because vitamin A costs next to nothing whereas a vaccination costs a substantial amount. Studies cost money and there is no advantage for pharmaceutical companies to spend money on studies that invalidate the use of their products. All governments are advised by specialists, often on the payroll of pharmaceutical companies, so the truth is hard to get to. Personally, I am unsure of what that truth is.

There is a lot of information on the pros and cons of vaccinations but the negative information is rarely fed to the overburdened and busy GP. The subject demands a book to itself and this section mentions a publication that I recommend be read by all parents and travellers before considering vaccinations.

I make special mention of the measles vaccine later because the government in Britain in 1994 vaccinated eight million children between the ages of five and 15 years with, in my opinion, no true care or concern of the down side. The powers that be boasted that they had saved 50 lives and over 3,000 hospital admissions, but reports that were leaked to the popular press six months later suggested that the expected epidemic (the official reason for doing this mass vaccination programme) may never have occurred and there may have been up to 1,500 adverse reactions to the vaccination reported. There have been several reported cases of autism and the same number of a Crohn's-like disease in children that have been directly attributed to the measles vaccination. These are only the reported cases and may represent the tip of the iceberg because GPs might not yet be correlating the onset of these conditions with the measles vaccination. At the time of writing there is a powerful and contentious debate going on between a research fellow at the Royal Free Hospital, London and senior scientific colleagues. There has been a study of 12 cases of autism that suggest a direct correlation to the MMR vaccination and this adds substance to the reports

mentioned above. A 30-year follow up from 1964 onwards showed that infection with measles before the age of three significantly lowered the risk of asthma. The research has suggested that the measles virus might confer protection against asthma by altering the immune response for years ahead. Studies such as these are rarely brought to the public's attention and we all have to balance the benefit of protecting a child against measles if it increases the risk of asthma at a later date.

The principle of vaccination is the administration of a very small amount of either dead or non-functioning virus, which causes the body to respond by forming antibodies. If an individual comes into contact with the live virus the body will have memorized it as having been present before and the antibodies will attack the invading agent and kill it. Usually vaccines are given by injection (the exception is one of the polio vaccines, which is given orally). Theoretically, this is a sound method of defence.

There is, however, a consensus of opinion in the holistic medical world against the use of vaccines. There is some concern that the process of manufacturing these vaccines allows entry into the body of proteins that, being similar to our own, cause the body to form antibodies against ourselves. There is also the hypothesis that by stimulating the body in this artificial way the natural response is in some way diminished. Introduction of these infections directly into the bloodstream by injection also bypasses primary defences found in the mucous membranes and skin. The body, therefore, produces an antibody defence but none other.

Some diphtheria, tetanus and pertussis preparations (DTP), and some HiB vaccines outside of the United Kingdom, contain a mercury based compound Thiomersal. This has been added to vaccines since its initial use in the 1940s as an anti-microbial compound. Frequent vaccinations using this agent may lead to a cumulative mercury overdose and therefore expose the individual to a known toxin. (*See* **Environmental poisons**).

Add to this the fact that vaccinations caused problems when they were first used and, even up to 1992, when two of the three types of measles vaccine were taken off the market because of adverse side effects, vaccinations have proved to be risky. Until 1995 I advised parents of children and those considering travelling to utilize vaccines but also to take homeopathic remedies at the same time in an attempt to counteract any adverse effects and also stimulate the body to a better response against the agent in the vaccine. I have, however, recently read a considerable amount about the matter of vaccination and my advice now is different. Please read on.

I have, at this time, chosen not to vaccinate my children and, unless more information comes my way, I will avoid their coming into contact with vaccinations.

These are my views; they may be right or wrong. Please may I ask everyone to obtain and read *The Vaccination Handbook* (published by WHAT DOCTORS DON'T TELL YOU) and make their own judgements. Copies may be available through me or my clinics or by calling WDDTY on 44 (0) 171 354 4592 with a credit card number. This publication gives an overview that I think is very accurate.

Basically there is strong evidence that vaccines:

- Do not work as well as we are told.
- Have greater risks attached than we are told.
- May be more dangerous than the disease itself in well-nourished, healthy children.

If asked by a parent or intended traveller about vaccinations, I ask them to read *The Vaccination Handbook* and then I support whatever decision they wish to make, whether using homeopathic remedies either with or without regular vaccination, and am fully behind their decision. I do not recommend an individual to take or avoid vaccinations.

Should I vaccinate my child?

This question boils down to a parent asking themselves the following question: is my child or my child's place in society more important? If vaccinations are carrying an unexpected and unassessed risk then they should be avoided. However, statistically it can be argued that vaccinations do reduce the incidence of disease when given to large populations. The view I take is that children who are liable to be susceptible to infections need vaccinations whereas those who are healthy do not.

A parent, I think, should be able to give an affirmative ('yes') to the following questions and if they can they should not vaccinate their child. On the other hand if any of these questions bring forward a negative ('no') answer then the child should be vaccinated.

- Is my child well nurtured, in a clean and hygienic environment, and likely to stay in such an environment?
- Is my child well nourished and am I aware of his/her nutritional requirements?
- Is my child in good health and genetically predisposed to stay that way?
- Am I an observant parent with the time and and knowledge to notice a depreciation in my child's state of health?

If any of these questions received a negative answer, it is possible that with some education from a nutritionist or naturopath the answer may become 'yes'. If all the answers are 'yes' then seriously consider not vaccinating the child. If any of the answers are 'no', look to vaccinate but follow the advice in this section.

RECOMMENDATIONS

General Advice

- *If an individual or a parent feels that they cannot fulfil the above recommendations, or if the individual or child is in an immuno-compromised state or will be unavoidably subjected to infection, then I feel that the use of a vaccination is less likely to cause a problem than the contraction of a disease and vaccinations should be taken.*

- *Ensure that an individual or a child has no underlying condition that may pre-dispose him or her to the effects of childhood illnesses.*
- *Visit a nutritionist to establish good individual and family nutrition.*
- *Discuss matters of hygiene with a complementary medical practitioner.*
- *If considering the use of vaccinations, ensure that there are no previous reactions to other vaccines, eggs, and that there is no current serious illness. Vaccinations may cause reactions or provoke a reduced immune response.*
- *A bi-yearly visit to a holistic practitioner and a regular doctor to establish good health.*

Homeopathic

- *If taking regular vaccines, use the homeopathic remedy that corresponds to the disease process. This should create a body response to the infection should it be introduced by a faulty vaccine (see **Homeopathic inoculations**).*
- *If vaccines have been given in the past, take three doses of Thuja 200, one each night. If a vaccination has actually caused a reaction, use the remedy Natrum muriaticum 30 four times a day for one week. Both of these remedies are reported as being able to deal with the 'ill-effects of vaccinations'.*

If you are going to vaccinate

If an individual chooses to take a vaccination or to give them to his/her children it may, theoretically, be best to prepare the body beforehand. The following recommendations may prevent the individual from overreacting to the vaccination, prepare the individual for the invasion of animal proteins used in the manufacture of the viral vaccines and also avoid the reaction of a vaccine to which the individual may be allergic.

RECOMMENDATIONS

General Advice

- *Ensure that the individual is in good health with no underlying acute problems, such as a cold or fever, before giving a vaccination.*
- *In the case of children, delay the vaccinations until six months old, allowing the immune system some time to develop without administering a potent immune stimulant.*
- *Try to find a physician who will give one-tenth of the dose of the vaccine two weeks prior to giving the vaccine proper. Theoretically, this allows the body to prepare for the more major reaction and will pre-empt any aggressive reaction.*
- *Give vaccinations as single doses, ie do not give Measles, Mumps and Rubella all at once but separately. Leave at least two weeks between taking vaccinations and preferably three months, so that the body is not subjected to 'overload'.*

Homeopathic

- *Use the homeopathic remedy Thuja 200 prior to any vaccinations, along with specific homeopathic preparations for the vaccine itself (see **Homeopathic inoculations**).*

Homeopathic inoculations

There is no such thing as a homeopathic vaccination. At best, homeopathic remedies may create a response lasting a few months, but certainly not a lifetime. Remedies tend to protect the body against particular infections and if you are subjected to that particular infection then by taking the equivalent homeopathic inoculation your body may well produce a strong immunity.

There is no good scientific evidence that homeopathic remedies confer immunity. However, some studies have been done largely on the Indian subcontinent. These studies show that certain remedies created immune responses but we cannot be certain that the antibodies against these diseases did not form simply because the individual children were exposed to the infection because it was endemic (prevalent in the area). Government statistics (not truly acceptable scientific evidence) do show that homeopathic remedies can act as vaccines and there is evidence of lower levels of infection in groups that have received the correct homeopathic treatment.

I hypothesize that the use of a remedy in a child who will come into contact with the natural infection will bolster their immune system at that time. A remedy will not cause an immunoglobulin (antibody) response. However, if an individual contracts an infection within, say, one month of taking a suitable homeopathic remedy, the immune response may be much swifter and more effective and therefore set us a lifelong immunity without the child even knowing the infection had been contracted. I must stress that this is all theoretical. If I extend this hypothesis, then the use of homeopathic remedies just prior to taking orthodox vaccinations may create a better response and, possibly, protect against the potential side effects or an immune system overload.

The chart below gives the suggested remedies for childhood infections. (A similar chart can be found for the homeopathic equivalent support for travellers' vaccinations in the section on travel.)

Condition	Remedy*
Diphtheria	*Diphtherinum* 200
Hepatitis (A, B and others)	*Lycopodium* 200 and *Chelidonium* 200
HiB (*Haemophilus influenzae* B)	*See* **Meningitis**
Meningitis	*Belladonna* 200 and *Iodoformum*
MMR (Measles, mumps and rubella)	*Pulsatilla* 200
Polio	*Lathyrus* 200
Tetanus	*Hypericum* 200
Tuberculosis	*Tuberculinum* 200

Whooping cough (pertussis)	*Pertussin* 200

*All these should be taken five days apart, starting one month before the first vaccination is given.

The measles vaccine

I make special mention of the measles vaccine because of the recent mass vaccination programme that occurred in Britain in 1994.

Interestingly, but not surprisingly from a financial point of view, the powers that be are recommending that the vaccination programme is repeated because more than the estimated numbers of children have not shown a positive response and have not developed immunity. I discuss below a strong argument against continuing these mass vaccinations.

At the moment, if an epidemic were to strike the country approximately 50 children would be expected to die and over 3,000 would be hospitalized with serious complications. (I mention here that there is no correlation between the health of the child and the type of child who may succumb to measles. All children, whether well-nourished, nurtured and loved or those less fortunate, are bracketed together.)

In 1994, eight million children were vaccinated. Four million of those were girls between the age of five and 15 years. The minimum of children who did not respond to the vaccine is estimated at ten per cent. This means that 400,000 girls are not immune to measles. Over the next ten years these 400,000 children are unlikely to come across measles because it has been eradicated from 90 per cent of their peer group. They will therefore not be able to develop natural immunity.

Let us assume that over the next ten years 25 per cent of those children not immunized will bear their own child; 100,000 infants will therefore be born to mothers who carry no immunity to measles. The antibodies (immunoglobulins) that defend against measles pass from the mother's bloodstream into their baby's while still in the womb and will protect infants for up to six months. Breast-fed babies will also receive antibodies but in the 100,000 infants born to mothers who are not immune, no measles protection will be conferred.

Every paediatrician in the country will tell you that measles in an infant is far more serious and potentially far more lethal.

There may be a 90 per cent reduction in the chances of contracting measles because we have vaccinated the herd, but are we protecting the interests of those 100,000 infants in the generations ahead?

Finally, after all the orthodox pressure applied to parents, the number of cases of measles in children who were vaccinated doubled in 1994.

RECOMMENDATIONS

General Advice

- *Pay heed to the notes above.*
- *Breast-feed as long as possible.*
- *Vaccinate as late as possible.*
- *Only consider 'measles parties' if the original child has a mild case and your child is healthy.*
- *Remember that many infections such as rubella can be tested for by a simple blood test.*
- *Follow the medical press with regards to the research into the possibility that MMR vaccine causes inflammatory bowel disease and autistic-like states.*
- *MMR is linked to a bleeding condition known as ITP (idiopathic thrombocytopenic purpura). It is worth remembering that measles itself can also cause this problem – as can any high fever.*

THE HEAD AND NECK

THE EARS

CARE OF THE EARS

The ears do not require a lot of care and concern because, generally, they are adequately protected. It is important to keep the ears warm and covered as they have little protection from the cold or excessive sun and, as the blood vessels to the ear are very small, damage may take time to repair. Sunburn and gangrene are not uncommon in extremes of weather and the use of protective covering such as sun-blocks and ear muffs should always be considered.

The ear canal is lined by small hairs called cilia, which meticulously flick outwards dirt and debris that enter the canal. Different people will create different amounts of secretion, which, if in excess, can block the canal and is known as ear wax (*see* **Ear problems**).

Cleaning of the ear should be done daily using mild soap and water, cleaning only the external or pinna part of the ear. The use of ear-buds (small balls of cotton on the end of sticks) may cause more harm than good. The insertion of anything into the ear can push dirt, wax and infection deeper into the ear and is unlikely to be of any great benefit because the cilia will do the job.

The need for the protection of the ears from loud noises is becoming more apparent as younger people are experiencing auditory loss (deafness) at an alarmingly increasing rate. This has been associated with the advent of loud popular music but more so with the widespread use of personal stereos. Loud noises cause vigorous vibrations that, in turn, cause small abrasions around the ear ossicles, which slowly but surely scar and reduce the mobility of these middle ear bones. Conductive deafness is the outcome, which may not be repairable (*see* **Conductive deafness**).

EAR PROBLEMS

Problems with the ear can occur at any age but they are most frequently associated with children. The reason for this is probably twofold. Firstly, the middle ear (the most common area to cause problems) is much smaller and therefore easier to affect and, secondly, children are more prone to mucus production and coughs and colds, which

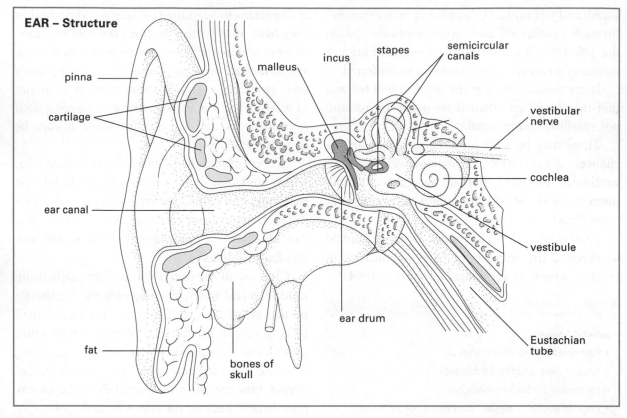

EAR – Structure

pinna

cartilage

ear canal

fat

bones of skull

malleus

incus

stapes

semicircular canals

vestibular nerve

cochlea

vestibule

ear drum

Eustachian tube

can block the narrow Eustachian tube (the channel between the middle ear and the throat).

Anatomically and medically speaking there are three parts to the ear:

- The pinna and outer canal make up the outer ear.
- The middle ear, including the stapes, incus and malleus (which are the ear bones or ossicles).
- The inner ear comprising the cochlea, which contains the fluid through which sound waves are transmitted to the auditory nerves.

Problems must therefore be divided into which part of the ear is affected and treated accordingly.

ACHES AND PAINS
Outer ear
Pains in this part of the ear are usually caused by the cold, trauma, infections or foreign bodies. Eczema of the external ear may often lead to infection and treatment of this dry skin is necessary. Common sense is the initial treatment, including warming of the pinna, removal of foreign objects (*see* **Foreign body in the ear**) and application of soothing balms.

RECOMMENDATIONS

General Advice

- *Apply common sense, especially with regard to the removal of foreign objects (see **Foreign body in the ear**).*

Homeopathic

- *An inflamed external ear associated with cold wind may be successfully treated with Aconite 6, one dose every 2hr.*
- *Review the remedies Petroleum and Graphites if there is eczema associated with the external ear discomfort.*

Herbal/natural extracts

- *Topical application of Arnica or Calendula creams may be curative.*

Middle ear

Aches and pains in the middle ear are usually associated with infection or trauma caused by loud noises.

It is well accepted throughout the orthodox medical world that approximately 50 per cent of ear infections are caused by viruses. The pain is the same but the use of antibiotics (ineffective against viruses) should be limited to infections that are caused by bacteria. The persistent use of antibiotics in ear infections leads to resistant strains and recurrent infections. I recommend that antibiotics are used only when a problem is very severe and preferably after the GP has taken a swab of any discharge and sent it to a laboratory for confirmation of the presence of bacteria. The use of an antibiotic may weaken the individual's immune system and prolong the problem (*see* **Antibiotics**).

RECOMMENDATIONS

General Advice

- If there is discharge, keep the outside of the ear as clean as possible but do not attempt to clear the ear canal.

Homeopathic

- If there is discharge associated with the pain, whilst awaiting the laboratory report on the swab that should have been taken by your doctor or practitioner, consider reviewing the following homeopathic remedies: Pulsatilla, Hepar sulphuris calcarium, Chamomila, Silica and Belladonna.
- Earache without discharge requires reviewing the following homeopathic remedies: Allium cepa, Gelsemium, Belladonna, Magnesia phosphorica.

Herbal/natural extracts

- One or two drops of mullein oil can be instantly relieving and potentially curative. This can be repeated every 3 or 4hr if required.
- With or without discharge, opening of the Eustachian tube is beneficial because it allows drainage of any catarrh in the middle ear. This is best achieved by inhalations of Olbas or lavender oil (one drop in a bowl of steaming water) or inhaling the steam from a ginger tea (chop half-inch of ginger root in hot water).

Orthodox

- Earache that is severe or persistent should be assessed by a GP. If the GP recommends an antibiotic, ask if it is possible to take a swab (it may not be feasible if there is no discharge) and ask the GP's opinion on whether he/she is convinced that it is not viral.

Inner ear

Pain emanating from the inner ear is difficult to assess and an infection of this part of the ear requires specialist attention.

RECOMMENDATIONS

General Advice

- Follow the advice of an ear, nose and throat specialist.

Homeopathic

- Gain the advice of a homeopath based on these symptoms.

BLEEDING FROM THE EARS

Bleeding from the ear is potentially a serious matter that requires a medical opinion to illuminate the cause. A small visible scratch with a little blood loss is not relevant and can be treated with common sense but any bleeding that comes from within the canal or deeper and is not caused by an external cut must be seen by a physician.

RECOMMENDATION

- All bleeding from the ear must be dealt with by a physician (unless from a visible, accessible cut).

EAR WAX

See **Care of the ears**.

Certain children have a predisposition to wax

build-up and regular review by parents, gently pulling the ear lobe down and forward will allow visual access. If in doubt, please ask your GP to have a look.

RECOMMENDATIONS

General Advice

- *Do not attempt to clear out the ear by inserting any objects.*
- *Proprietary ear wax-softening solutions available from chemists are safe and more effective than naturopathic compounds. Warm olive oil may be used, however, with some effect.*
- *Please do not use ear wax candles at any age, and especially not in children.*

Nutritional

- *Reduce mucus-forming foods such as dairy produce, refined foods and especially white sugar.*

Orthodox

- *Persisting wax may need to be 'washed out', which should be done only by experienced medical practitioners, especially in children. Before this you may have success with proprietary drops and supporting the child's head in a comfortably hot bath with the ears below the water line.*

FOREIGN BODY IN THE EAR

It is not uncommon for small children, in particular, to lodge small objects in the ear canal. If these are not easily removed, do not attempt to do so without medical attention.

RECOMMENDATIONS

General Advice

- *An easily visible and removable object can be dealt with by fingers or blunt tweezers. If there is any resistance, either from the child or the object, take the child to hospital.*
- *One or two drops of castor oil, olive oil or even vegetable oil on the way to the hospital may alleviate the problem sooner.*

'GLUE' EAR

Glue ear is not strictly a medical term although it has entered the vocabulary. It is characterized by a thick mucus/catarrh that coagulates within the middle ear and is then unable to travel down the Eustachian tube. This thick syrup prevents the ear bones or ossicles from vibrating in response to sound waves and therefore leads to conductive deafness. The problem is compounded in youngsters who may not hear their teachers, parents or peers and therefore it can lead to poor academic standards, disobedience and poor sociability. A child may be incorrectly labelled retarded in extreme cases.

The thickened catarrh can also act as a medium for the growth of bacteria and fungi, thereby predisposing the child to recurrent infections. Glue ear is most frequently associated with:

- Poor hydration (allowing the catarrh to become thick and tenacious).
- Excess mucus production (associated with mucus-forming foods such as white sugar).
- Poor immune system response (encouraging the production of mucus as a defence process).

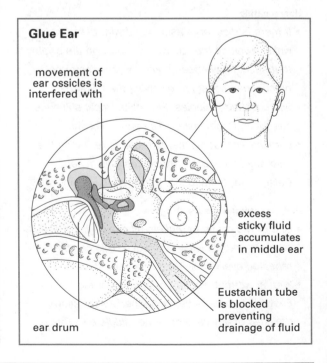

Glue Ear

movement of ear ossicles is interfered with

excess sticky fluid accumulates in middle ear

Eustachian tube is blocked preventing drainage of fluid

ear drum

• Food intolerance/allergy (particularly dairy products).

One of the most important causes is passive smoking. A child living in a home where a parent smokes is 50 per cent more likely to have glue ear. Parents, please note that even if you do not smoke in the presence of your child it may still be a problem because the cigarette toxins settle on carpets, curtains and furniture, they are then inhaled when the child moves around the room.

RECOMMENDATIONS

General Advice

• *The diagnosis of glue ear needs to be established by a practitioner looking at the external eardrum and seeing a level of fluid in the ear. Try the following alternatives before using decongestant or operative options.*

• *Consult a complementary medical specialist to ensure that the child has a sound and effective immune system.*

• *Ensure that adequate water is being drunk. Aim at one pint of water per foot of height per day. Juice and other fluids are not the same as water.*

• *Do not allow the child anywhere near an environment where smoking has occurred.*

• *See* **Otitis media** *and* **Catarrh**.

Nutritional

• *Remove mucus-forming foods such as dairy products, refined foods and especially white sugar. Food intolerance/allergy testing by bioresonance or blood analysis is recommended.*

Homeopathic

• *If the child is catarrhal, use the homeopathic remedy Allium sativa. For chronic catarrh associated with ringing or noises in the ear, consider Causticum, Chenopodium or Calcarea carbonica. All these homeopathic remedies can be used at potency 6, three doses a day for two weeks, in association with the necessary restrictions discussed in the previous recommendation.*

Herbal/natural extracts

• *The use of Olbas or lavender oil inhalations as a decongestant may open the Eustachian tube, and in conjunction with good rehydration making the catarrh less viscous, may allow the 'glue' to drain.*

Orthodox

• *If treatment is not effective, then the placing of small plastic tubes (grommets) through the eardrum under anaesthetic is a surgical option. See* **Operations and surgery** *if this is required. Prior to this, a GP may recommend decongestants but I have not seen these work well.*

INFECTIONS OF THE EAR
Middle ear (Otitis media)

Diagnosis of a middle-ear infection can only be made with the use of an otoscope in the hands of an experienced professional. If the doctor diagnoses an ear infection, ask the following questions.

• Can the doctor see fluid behind the eardrum?
• Does the doctor have strong grounds for believing that the infection is bacterial?

General practitioners are becoming less swift to prescribe an antibiotic for what may be a viral infection, but this does often occur unnecessarily (*see* **Antibiotics**). A red eardrum with no fluid behind it is not likely to burst nor have any permanent damage done and naturopathic treatments could be employed for 24 hours before an antibiotic is used. An eardrum that has burst and allowed the fluid to discharge is *not* a permanently damaging event in most cases. The infection will be able to leave the body and usually the eardrum heals perfectly.

RECOMMENDATIONS

General Advice

• *If you suspect an ear infection (the infant is pulling at the ear), visit your GP.*

Homeopathic

- *Homeopathic remedies are often very effective. The most commonly prescribed are Aconite, Belladonna, Pulsatilla and Silica. Refer to a homeopathic manual to select the best treatment.*

Herbal/natural extracts

- *If the GP is not insistent, then apply two drops of mullein oil or warm olive oil, four times a day to both ears.*

Orthodox

- *If the GP recommends antibiotics, ask the reasons why a bacterial infection is suspected.*
- *If the GP is ambivalent regarding whether the infection is bacterial or viral ask the GP if waiting 24hr may be dangerous.*

If the problem has not resolved over 24 hours, consult a naturopathic practitioner; and if 24 hours later the problem persists, then consider using antibiotics.

Outer ear

Occasionally the outer ear may become irritated, red or scaly.

RECOMMENDATIONS

General Advice

- *Bring any persistence to the attention of a naturopathic physician.*
- *Keep the outer part of the ear clean.*

Homeopathic

- *Select a homeopathic remedy dependent upon the symptoms from your preferred homeopathic manual. In the meantime, give Pulsatilla 6, two pills every 2hr.*

Herbal/natural extracts

- *Two drops of mullein oil four times a day.*
- *Give the child the herbal remedy Echinacea at a dose recommended for children on the packaging*

or obtain advice from a local pharmacist or naturopathic practitioner.

Orthodox

- *Avoid antibiotics. General practitioners are still too quick to prescribe for what may be a viral infection. Many reports in top medical journals suggest that antibiotics should only be used after a definitive diagnosis of a bacterial infection has been made.*

RUPTURE (PERFORATION) OF THE EARDRUM

Rupture of the eardrum, also known as perforation, is associated most commonly with middle-ear infection or trauma. Middle-ear infection causes pressure outwards, which is markedly painful until the eardrum bursts and the pain is relieved. Discharge and small amounts of blood are the characteristic symptoms. Trauma, usually from loud blasts or a slap with an open hand, causes the eardrum to burst inwards, which is characterized by a very severe and sharp pain followed by a dull ache.

Hearing may or may not be affected, depending on the cause, size of the tear and associated damage to the ear ossicles.

RECOMMENDATIONS

General Advice

- *Any suggestion of the above symptoms should be taken for review to your doctor.*

Orthodox

- *Small tears or perforations will generally repair without problem but larger tears may require the expertise of surgical repair.*
- *In the case of rupture caused by infection, antibiotics may need to be used because homeopathic or naturopathic therapies may work too slowly and the infection may worsen the rupture or destroy the eardrum. It may be easier for a complementary practitioner to deal with the side effects of the antibiotics than to repair a potentially serious eardrum injury.*

THE EYES

CARE OF THE EYES

The eyes, like most organs in the body, do not need particular attention because they are capable of maintaining their own well-being. However, the eyes are less well-protected than many other organs in the body, and much more open to the environment. They are remarkably delicate and sensitive and therefore demand a little more respect than other organs.

RECOMMENDATIONS

General Advice
- *Ensure adequate sleep and rest.*
- *Avoid the use of eye drops unless specifically required. Tears are the eyes' best cleanser and protector.*
- *Consider the use of corrective lenses (glasses or contact lenses) for any visual defects.*
- *Rest the eyes through the day by using the palming technique (see **Palming**).*
- *Each morning and evening, splash the eyes 20 times with hot water and 20 times with cold water to encourage fresh blood flow.*

BLACK EYE

A black eye is not strictly a problem of the eye but of the surround. The skin of the face attaches around the eye socket (orbit) such that any bruising that occurs cannot drain further than around the eyes. Trauma to any part of the head from the lower part of the orbit upwards and backwards that causes bleeding will gravitate downwards and form blue/black rings around the eyes.

RECOMMENDATIONS

General Advice
- *Any head trauma that leads to damage or pain of the eye or concussion must be reviewed by a doctor.*

- *The long-established practice of placing raw steak over a black eye generally seems to reduce the severity and the longevity of discolouration but I know of no scientific reason why this should be the case!*
- *Swelling in association with a black eye will be relieved by ice packs. Avoid prolonged contact with excessive cold to the eyeball itself.*

Homeopathic
- *The homeopathic remedy Arnica, potency 6 or 12, can be used every hour for three doses and then every 4hr until discomfort is relieved.*

CONJUNCTIVITIS

Conjunctivitis can occur at any age but is most commonly found in children because of their frequent touching of eyes and eyelids and the highly infectious nature of most of the bacteria and viruses that cause conjunctivitis.

Conjunctivitis is characterized by redness, grittiness or burning and occasionally swelling of the lining of the eyelids.

See **Blepharitis**.

RECOMMENDATIONS

General Advice
- *Bathe the eyes in milk, preferably breast milk if available.*

Supplemental
- *Beta-carotene (2mg per foot of height) in divided doses through the day will speed recovery.*

Homeopathic
- *Review the homeopathic remedies Rhus toxicodendron, Staphysagria, Arsenicum album, Aconite and Mercurius.*

Herbal/natural extracts
- *Consider the use of Euphrasia (eyebright) mother tincture by applying one drop to an eggcup full of water (preferably boiled and then cooled). This can be placed in an eye bath or applied with a*

dropper. Bathing the child's eye with cotton wool soaked in this solution and then gently but firmly prising open the eyelids will allow some of the fluid to enter.

DISCHARGES FROM THE EYES

The eyes of babies are frequently associated with discharge. A not infrequent reason is a blocked duct that drains the tears from the eye through a small tube into the nose. Sometimes this nasolacrimal duct remains closed and requires surgical opening. A persisting watery or discharging eye should be looked at by a specialist.

Mild redness of the eyelids, red veins in the white of the eye, a discharge that is coloured (yellow or green usually) or persisting crusting can be treated initially at home.

A discharge from the eye usually represents a conjunctivitis (*see* **Conjunctivitis**), infection of

the lacrimal gland or ducts or, more rarely, causes such as an embedded foreign body in the eyeball.

General Advice
- *Breast milk, carrying natural immunoglobulins, can be dropped into the eye four times a day. Standard cow's milk can be used in the same way.*
- *Any eye condition persisting for longer than 24hr should be seen by a professional.*
- *Any painful or persistent discharge should be reviewed by a GP.*

Nutritional
- *Persisting eye infections may be an early indication of allergies or food intolerances and this possibility should be mentioned to your naturopathic physician.*

Homeopathic
- *The homeopathic remedy Rhus toxicodendron 6, one pill every 2hr, can be administered.*
- *Specific homeopathic or herbal treatment can be used, depending on the cause. Remedies to review are Pulsatilla, Kali bichromicum and Mercurius.*

Herbal/natural extracts
- *Do not use chemical preparations or naturopathic herbal solutions without the support and advice of a naturopathic practitioner, although a weak solution of chamomile tea can be tried and is soothing and effective.*
- *Cleansing the eyes with a diluted Euphrasia (eyebright) solution can be employed.*

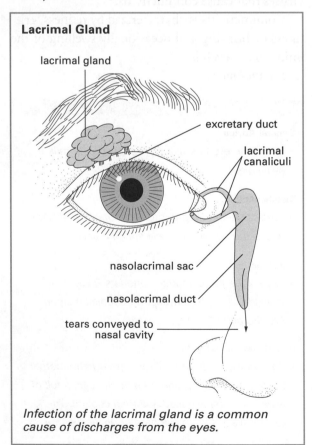

Lacrimal Gland

lacrimal gland

excretary duct

lacrimal canaliculi

nasolacrimal sac

nasolacrimal duct

tears conveyed to nasal cavity

Infection of the lacrimal gland is a common cause of discharges from the eyes.

DOUBLE VISION

See **Double vision** in chapter 4.

Establishing double vision in an infant or child before he/she can speak or show signs, such as bumping into door frames or trying to pick up an object by grasping the air beside it, is nearly impossible. Any suggestion of a visual defect, which also includes responding to Mum's face whilst looking at her ear, should be brought to the attention of a physician or optometrist immediately.

See **Squint** if you notice that your child's eyes point in different directions.

DRY EYES

Chronic dry eyes may represent underlying disease such as sarcoidosis and other autoimmune conditions. These need to be treated appropriately after diagnosis from a doctor or eye specialist.

Acute dry eyes may be treated with the recommendations below, provided that relief and cure are forthcoming within a short period of time.

RECOMMENDATIONS

General Advice
- *Persisting or painful dry eyes must be reviewed by a doctor.*
- *Ensure good oral hydration by drinking at least three pints of water per day.*
- *Avoid eye make-up or, if this is unavoidable, ensure that it is thoroughly washed off as often as possible and certainly do not leave eye make-up on through the night.*

Homeopathic
- *Persisting cases may respond to homeopathic remedies and the following should be reviewed: Sulphur, Petroleum, Silica and Causticum.*

Herbal/natural extracts
- *Avoid artificial tears, which contain chemicals, and in preference use milk or Euphrasia eye drops.*

EXCESSIVE WATERING OF THE EYES

The lacrimal glands produce tears that should drain through a small hole and tube in the corner of the eye that leads into the nasal passage.

Up to 50 per cent of children may be born with a blockage in this duct and less than two per cent have a permanent blockage requiring surgical intervention. Older children and adults may have a foreign body or inflammation from infection or trauma creating a blockage.

RECOMMENDATIONS

General Advice
- *Trauma, injury or infection should be reviewed by a complementary medical practitioner with knowledge in this area and an eye specialist's opinion should be obtained if treatment does not resolve the problem within a matter of days.*
- *Gentle massage from the corner of the eye down the side of the nose may relieve the blockage.*

Homeopathic
- *The homeopathic remedy Silica is effective in dealing with infected or blocked drainage ducts. Silica 6 should be taken every 2hr.*

Orthodox
- *Trauma to the side of the nose or infection may require more urgent treatment and a medical opinion should be obtained, although antibiotics should be avoided until alternative measures have failed.*

EYELIDS

The eyelids are a remarkably important part of the body. They are protective and busy (blinking every 5–8 seconds).

They are coloured to attract attention and similarly this may reflect the health of an individual. Darkened or swollen lower eyelids are a reflection of anything from tiredness through water retention to kidney problems. Many people are born with darkened or swollen eyelids and will maintain them through their lifetime and this is not an indication of ill-health, but a development of 'bags' under the eyes should be reviewed by a complementary medical practitioner initially. The Eastern philosophies of medicine correlate the colour under the eyes to our energy stores, specifically kidney energy.

Inflammation

Inflammation of the external eyelid is a common site for eczema (*see* **Eczema**).

Inflammation of the internal aspect of the eyelid is conjunctivitis (*see* **Conjunctivitis**).

> **RECOMMENDATIONS**
>
> **General Advice**
> - *See* **Eczema** *and* **Conjunctivitis**.
> - *Resist applying any make-up to this area until a treatment course has been set.*

Lumps

Lumps on or in the eyelids may simply be a reflection of the skin condition, such as a wart or a pimple, but are best reviewed by a physician because of the potential spread of infection into the eye and also because of conditions such as skin cancers that may appear anywhere. Lumps that are specific to the eyelids are meibomian cysts or xanthelasmata.

Meibomian cyst (Chalazions)

Meibomian glands are found in the rim of the eyelids and produce a secretion that contains many immunoglobulins and protective immune factors. These glands have small ducts that can become blocked, which leads to the secretion being unable to leave and causes a swelling along the eyelid rims. Rarely are these painful but they do have a tendency to become infected and may develop into styes (*see* **Styes**).

Very often meibomian cysts will reabsorb, but if not, treatment may be required.

> **RECOMMENDATIONS**
>
> **General Advice**
> - *See* **Styes** *below.*
>
> **Homeopathic**
> - *The homeopathic remedies Staphysagria or Thuja can be used at potency 6, four pills every 3hr for five days.*
>
> **Orthodox**
> - *Surgical intervention by ophthalmic surgeons is rarely required but a growing, cosmetically unacceptable or painful meibomian cyst should be seen by such a specialist.*

Styes

Styes usually occur as a red, itchy or painful swelling caused by bacteria proliferating in an eyelash root cell or a meibomian cyst.

Styes are usually self-limiting but recurrent infections may require medical examination for underlying problems such as diabetes or other immunosuppressant conditions.

Styes commonly found in children are often to do with mild malnutrition and occur during growth spurts.

> **RECOMMENDATIONS**
>
> **General Advice**
> - *Bathe the eye in milk.*
> - *Hot and cold compress application can bring the boil to a head and allow easier discharge.*
> - *Ensure correct hygiene by washing your hands because styes tend to be very easily transmitted.*

Stye on Eyelid

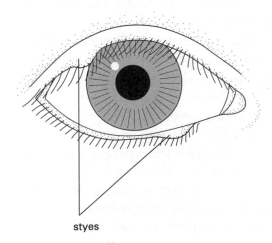

styes

Twitching eyelids

A twitch anywhere is representative of a trapped, irritated, inflamed or damaged nerve. This may occur in the central nervous system (brain or spinal column) or at the neuromuscular junction. Most twitches are short-lived and of no consequence, but others may be a warning or a result of nerve damage or, more commonly, deficiencies.

FOREIGN BODIES AND SUBSTANCES IN THE EYE

Foreign bodies

A foreign body that is not easily removable by flushing the eye with fluid from a dropper bottle or blinking in water in an eye bath or the palms of the hand or by a clean piece of tissue paper

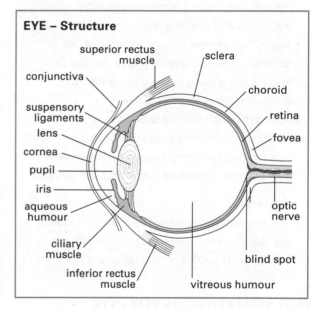

EYE – Structure

superior rectus muscle
sclera
conjunctiva
choroid
suspensory ligaments
retina
lens
fovea
cornea
pupil
iris
optic nerve
aqueous humour
ciliary muscle
blind spot
inferior rectus muscle
vitreous humour

must be taken to a doctor. Any object that is embedded in the eyeball or is causing bleeding in the conjunctiva and is not removable by fingers must, once again, be dealt with by a medical practitioner. It is unwise to use instruments such as tweezers because the sensitivity of the eye makes the patient very jumpy and further damage probable.

Homeopathic

- *Commence the patient on Aconite 6, two tablets every 10min, and gently massage the other eyeball through the eyelid because the eyes move in conjunction with each other and the gentle movement may dislodge the object.*

Foreign substances

RECOMMENDATIONS

General Advice

- *Identify the foreign substance that has infiltrated the eye, keeping any bottles available for inspection by a doctor if necessary.*
- *Regardless of the acidity or alkalinity of the compound, the eye should only be flushed with water under a gently running tap or from a dropper bottle of water or saline.*
- *After a thorough flushing with water, any remnants of an acidic substance should be counteracted by bathing the eye in milk. An alkaline substance should only be washed out with water.*

Homeopathic

- *The homeopathic remedies Apis and Belladonna, potency 6, can be given every 15min until the discomfort is settled or medical advice is sought.*

INFLAMMATION OF THE EYES

Inflammation of the eyelids is known as conjunctivitis (*see* **Conjunctivitis**). Inflammation of the eyes themselves falls into two divisions: iritis, (inflammation of the iris); or scleritis (inflammation of the whites of the eyes).

Both iritis and scleritis may be associated with underlying conditions such as autoimmune disease or venereal disease, and a persistence in either of these problems must be investigated fully as soon as possible.

Iritis

The symptoms of iritis are pain and redness around the central coloured part of the eye.

This is often associated with visual disturbance, such as blurring, photophobia, aching eyes or headaches. Persistent iritis requires medical attention because the inflammation can cause a blockage of the channels between the anterior and posterior 'humours' (fluids), which can lead to an increase in pressure known as glaucoma. Damage to the iris may affect vision (very rarely causing blindness) and encourages the development of cataracts.

RECOMMENDATIONS

General Advice

- *Very severe or prolonged (longer than 4hr) iritis should be seen by a doctor.*

Homeopathic

- *Use the homeopathic remedy Aconite 6 every 15min at the onset of an attack.*
- *Consider the homeopathic remedies Euphrasia, Mercurius corrosivus, Rhus toxicodendron, Arnica and Hamamelis by referring to your preferred homeopathic textbook.*

Herbal/natural extracts

- *Bathe the eye with milk or Euphrasia eye drops every hour.*

Scleritis

Scleritis is a less serious condition than iritis although, if left untreated, this red, dull aching of the white of the eye may run the risk of affecting the retina at the back of the eye or even perforating it, running the risk of the loss of fluid from the eye or allowing infection in.

RECOMMENDATIONS

General Advice

- *A persisting scleritis or one that is particularly painful should be reviewed by a physician.*

Nutritional

- *Food allergy and allergy to airborne matter must be excluded if the problem persists.*

Homeopathic

- *Aconite 6 should by taken every 2hr.*

Herbal/natural extracts

- *Use milk or Euphrasia eye drops as frequently as every 3hr.*

INJURIES TO THE EYE – *See* **Black eye** *and* **Foreign bodies and substances in the eye.**

Injury to the eye occurs from a direct blow, from penetration of the eyeball by a foreign object or from foreign matter on the surface.

Any crush or penetrating injury must be tended to by an eye specialist. Injuries that cause leakage of fluids from the eye into the bloodstream can trigger an antibody response that could cause the body to attack the other eye. This may lead to blindness and needs to be considered and treated immediately.

RECOMMENDATIONS

General Advice

- *If common sense and simple procedures can remove a foreign object from the eye, then proceed. If not, seek medical attention immediately.*
- *The injured eye should be covered and gentle pressure applied if there is marked bleeding. Avoid pressure if a foreign body has penetrated the eye.*
- *Ice wrapped in a flannel may be applied if it is soothing.*
- *A patch or blindfold over both eyes may prevent the other, non-injured eye from moving quite so much. Because the eyes move in unison, as little movement as possible is preferable.*
- *Any persistence of discomfort or visual disturbance should, once again, be examined by an eye specialist.*

Herbal/natural extracts

- *Bathing the eye in milk or Euphrasia may be relieving.*

Pain in the eyes

RECOMMENDATIONS

General Advice

- *Any pain that does not have an obvious cause or does not fall into any of the categories mentioned must be reviewed by a doctor.*
- *Once a diagnosis has been established, treat accordingly.*

Homeopathic

- *Use Aconite 6 every 10min for an eye pain whilst awaiting diagnosis.*

Palming

Palming is one of the Bates' eye exercises designed to give the eyes a rest. The eye muscles, perhaps more so than any other muscles in the body, are constantly in action and therefore tire more easily. This is why when we are tired we find it difficult to keep the eyes open.

The technique of palming allows the eye muscles to relax thoroughly because the technique excludes any light entering the eyes, thereby allowing complete dilation of the pupil, which is the equivalent to full relaxation of the pupillary muscles:

- Keeping the eyes open, place the palms of the hand over the eye sockets.
- Move the palms until no cracks of light can be seen around the edges.
- Stare straight ahead for 3 minutes, blinking as required.
- After 3 minutes close the eyes, remove the palms and open the eyes, ensuring not to look directly into bright light.

SQUINT OR STRABISMUS (LAZY EYE)

The definition of strabismus is an abnormality of the eyes in which the visual axes do not meet at the desired objective point. Put more simply, it means that one eye will be fixed on an object whilst the other is looking elsewhere. This is due to uncoordinated action of the extrinsic ocular

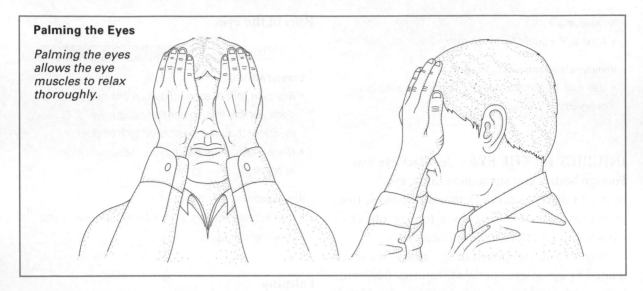

Palming the Eyes

Palming the eyes allows the eye muscles to relax thoroughly.

muscles, which control eye movement.

A squint in an infant is hard to assess because very often the eyes move independently for the first three months. If a child has apparently got convergent or divergent eyes after three months, then a specialist opinion is recommended. At a young age, two visual pictures will be sent to the ocular part of the brain and this is very confusing. The brain will select one, not the other, and the eye whose vision is being rejected will effectively become useless. This is known as a lazy eye and is the reason why expert advice is needed.

A squint developing at a later age (including those that develop in adulthood) may be associated with more serious conditions, such as diabetes, neuromuscular conditions like myasthenia gravis or even brain tumours.

RECOMMENDATIONS

General Advice

- *Any suggestion of a squint should be reviewed by an ocular specialist.*
- *Specific eye exercises, such as Bates' methods, can be utilized before surgery is contemplated.*

Homeopathic

- *The homeopathic remedies, Gelsemium, Hyoscyamus, Belladonna, Stramonium and Zinc*

may all be useful at high potency over a period of two weeks. Prescribing should be done by a homeopath for the most benefit.

Orthodox

- *Techniques such as patching the eye may be less common with the advent of more accurate eye surgery. This includes tightening or releasing the muscles around the eye to allow a better control.*

THE NOSE

Nasal congestion occurs in infants because they have no concept of 'blowing their noses'. Unless they are too wriggly, the very careful use of a cotton bud can relieve congestion from the lower part of the nostrils. Infants spend a lot of time lying flat, which allows gravity to pull the catarrh to the back of the nose. Prop the baby up as much as possible.

RECOMMENDATIONS

General Advice

- *Leave well alone. The problem will resolve by itself despite the apparent discomfort that the child is suffering.*
- *Nose bleeds in infants should be checked by a paediatrician or suitably qualified practitioner.*

Herbal/natural extracts

- *In severe cases hold the child on your lap by a table. Place a few drops of lavender oil, elder flowers, Euphrasia or a mixture of rosemary and thyme in a bowl of steaming water and place a towel over yourself, baby and the bowl. Stay there for a few minutes while the steam and oil acts as a decongestant.*
- *Two drops of lavender oil or chamomile oil on the pillow may be effective or one of the orthodox decongestants can be used, but if the child is taking a homeopathic remedy this will be nullified if the preparation contains camphor, menthol or mint of any sort.*

CATARRH

Catarrh is the medical term for mucus found in the upper respiratory tract – sinuses, nose and throat. Catarrh is an essential part of good health because it contains antibodies and white blood cells that attack invading viruses, bacteria and fungi. Catarrh is also produced when the body is trying to rid the membranes of toxic substances such as pollutants, excess dust and also in response to foreign proteins such as plant pollen. The orthodox approach to troublesome catarrh, usually associated with colds, is to try to suppress this useful excretion, whereas the holistic approach is to encourage its production so that the cause of the excess mucus can be eliminated.

RECOMMENDATIONS

General Advice

- *Try to encourage the production of catarrh if the symptoms are mild.*
- *Persistent catarrh may be an allergic response. See **Allergies**.*
- *Ensure good hydration, drinking at least one pint*

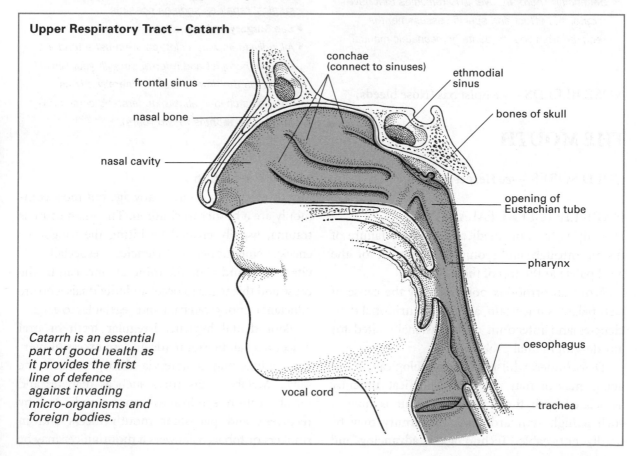

Upper Respiratory Tract – Catarrh

frontal sinus

nasal bone

nasal cavity

conchae (connect to sinuses)

ethmodial sinus

bones of skull

opening of Eustachian tube

pharynx

oesophagus

vocal cord

trachea

Catarrh is an essential part of good health as it provides the first line of defence against invading micro-organisms and foreign bodies.

of water per day per two feet of height in addition to your normal fluid intake. This dilutes down the catarrh, making it easier for the body to blow or cough out.

Nutritional

- Excess catarrh can be reduced by eliminating dairy products, alcohol and sugar from the diet until the condition has improved.

Supplemental

- The following vitamins and supplements can be of benefit if taken as prescribed, with food, per foot of height: vitamin A (1,000iu), vitamin C (500mg) and zinc (2.5mg).

Homeopathic

- Homeopathic remedies can encourage the production of catarrh and, depending on the colour, consistency, amount and time of day of production, a suitable remedy can be most beneficial. There are over 200 remedies that have a catarrhal effect and specific assessment is required from your favourite homeopathic manual.

NOSE BLEEDS – *see* Epistaxis (Nose bleeds)

THE MOUTH

COLD SORES – *see* Herpes simplex

HARE LIP (CLEFT PALATE)

Hare lip is the non-medical term for a failure of fusion through embryonic development of the hard palate at the top of the mouth.

From an orthodox point of view the cause of cleft palate is uncertain, although nutritional deficiencies and infections are occasionally cited for any developmental problems.

Deformities, whilst being psychologically damaging, may or may not have a physical difficulty associated with them. Surgical repair is now at such a high standard that a deformity may be hardly noticeable. Technology is advancing and

repair of serious cleft palates can be done *in utero* (with the baby still in the mother's uterus). Severe deformities can lead to problems with speech and, more seriously, with the inhalation of food that is difficult if not impossible to chew. Such deformities must be repaired.

RECOMMENDATIONS

General Advice

- Cranial osteopathy will help post-operative healing and also correct any imbalances in the cranial bones.

Nutritional

- Have a consultation with a nutritionist to discuss the possible deficiencies that may be present in any developmental abnormality.

Orthodox

- Cleft palate is diagnosable through ultrasound of the foetus in utero. Discuss the possibility of surgical repair as soon as possible.
- See **Surgery and operations**.
- All individuals with a cleft palate must attend a speech therapist and referral through your GP will advise on the time to start. Generally it is as soon as a child is able to understand commands (around 18 months to two years).

MOUTH ULCERS

Mouth ulcers can occur at any age but most commonly are a bother to children. The main cause is trauma, usually created by biting the tongue or cheek. Nutritional deficiencies, especially of vitamins A and C or the mineral zinc, can be the cause and this tends to occur in individuals who are reluctant or not given fruit and vegetables to eat.

Poor dental hygiene, irregular teeth or oral braces may all be traumatic and an excess of mercury fillings may irritate via absorption into the saliva. Metabolic disorders such as diabetes and malabsorption syndromes can be indicated by recurrent and persistent mouth ulcers and in smokers or tobacco chewers a mouth ulcer may be the sign of an oral cancer.

Food allergy or intolerance may trigger any inflammatory or degenerative process and may need to be considered; sharp, acidic or spicy foods may aggravate rather than cause problems.

RECOMMENDATIONS

General Advice

- *Ensure good dental hygiene and regular check-ups from the dentist.*
- *Do not eat quickly and avoid talking whilst eating as this encourages biting of the tongue or cheeks.*
- *Mouthwashes with warm salty water with or without Calendula fluid extract will speed up healing.*
- *Persistent ulcers should be brought to the attention of a complementary medical practitioner, who should check for diabetes, malabsorption syndromes, leaky gut syndrome, food allergies and specifically oral candidiasis (thrush), which is not uncommon in bottle-fed infants and individuals who are run down.*
- *Keep a food diary and see if there is any obvious food intolerance/allergy.*
- *Gluten is associated with mouth ulcers in those with Coeliac disease but may have an effect in others.*

Supplemental

- *Scientific studies have shown that deficiencies in iron, folic acid and vitamin B12 may cause ulcers, so supplementation with these at doses recommended on the product label would be beneficial.*
- *Deficiency in the mineral zinc can cause ulcers. Take 2mg per foot of height each night before bed.*
- *Bioflavinoids taken at the doses recommended on the product label may heal and give symptomatic relief.*

Homeopathic

- *The homeopathic remedies Mercurius and Arsenicum should be reviewed, although other homeopathic remedies may fit the symptoms and reference should be made to your preferred homeopathic manual.*
- *Beryllium metallicum potency 6 four times a day, increase to potency 30 if there is some effect but it is slow.*

Herbal/natural extracts

- *Clove oil applied to the lesion will sting but will give considerable relief. Dilute down in olive oil if the initial application is unpleasant.*
- *Mouth washing with Wild Strawberry tea or, if available, the Chinese herb Sheng ma, and then swallowing the solution, three times a day, may be curative.*

Orthodox

- *Aspirin-containing gels may be used in the short term quite effectively.*

THE TEETH

The tooth is made up of an outer, hard, enamel coating below which is a layer of dentine, which forms

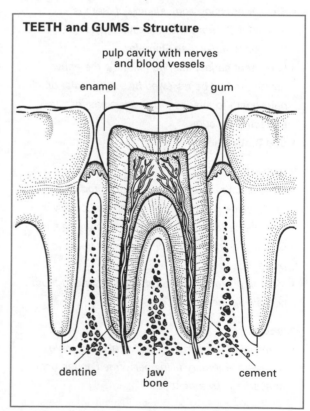

TEETH and GUMS – Structure

pulp cavity with nerves and blood vessels

enamel

gum

dentine

jaw bone

cement

the bulk of the tooth and is a hard, elastic, yellowish white substance. This is embedded in a cement that resembles bone in structure and whose action is to anchor the tooth. The cement is attached to periosteum tissue (that covers the jaw bone). The tooth is divided into the crown (that above the gum), the neck (that at the level of the gum) and the root (which is embedded into the jaw).

CARIES

Avoidance of caries (holes in the enamel of teeth) is dependent upon good oral hygiene and dietetics. Caries are produced by trauma or because of production of acid from bacteria that exist in the mouth. This acid breaks down the hard enamel and dentine and reaches the inner pulp. It is this that causes toothache because the pulp contains the nerve fibres.

RECOMMENDATIONS

General Advice
- *Regular brushing and cleaning of teeth is essential. A fluoride toothpaste should only be used once a day (see **Fluoride**).*
- *Persistent caries, despite following the above advice, should be reviewed by a nutritionist or naturopath to assess if the saliva has lost its protective function.*
- *See **Toothache**.*

Nutritional
- *Good calcium intake through dairy products, meat, chicken and fish, nuts and particularly sesame seeds is required from an early age.*
- *Chewing on raw fruit and vegetables helps to prevent caries.*
- *Most importantly, avoid refined sugars and foods containing them.*

Orthodox
- *Removal of the infection and sealing the hole with a non-mercury filling performed under local anaesthetic by a dentist.*

FILLINGS

Dental fillings can be required at any age but the risk of fillings and the potential number are both increased in childhood.

There is much controversy about the use of mercury in tooth cavity-filling substances called amalgams. At present the British Dental Association refuses to accept that mercury from fillings is a problem but most physicians associated with environmental or nutritional medicine consider mercury to be a problem (*see* **Mercury poisoning**).

Cavities in the teeth need to be filled with non-mercury fillings.

RECOMMENDATIONS

General Advice
- *Ensure six-monthly visits to the dentist and have any fillings repaired.*

Homeopathic
- *Prior to the visit, regardless of whether any dental work will be done, take homeopathic remedy Arnica 6 four times a day starting the day before the visit.*

Orthodox
- *If fillings are known to be required insist on non-mercury fillings, and, if this is not possible, change your dentist.*
- *If mercury fillings are in place visit a practitioner who uses a bioenergetic diagnostic device such as a Bicom or Quantum CI computer (see **Bioresonance**) to establish whether mercury is a problem within your system. Alternatively, a red blood cell mercury level can be obtained. If toxicity is the case, then a sympathetic dentist needs to be found who will remove all amalgam fillings and replace with non-mercury composite.*

FLUORIDE AND FLUOROSIS

Fluorosis is the medical term given for fluoride poisoning. Ingesting or inhaling any fluorine-containing compound is potentially lethal. Very small amounts can be handled by the body but not so well by bacteria. This is the reason why individuals in Western societies are forcibly, and without option, fed fluoride. Fluoride is placed in our water reservoirs, our processed foods and even our vitamin supplements. Most famously it is advertised as an important additive to our toothpaste. This latter addition is encouraged because of the association of decreased dental caries when fluoride was initially introduced at higher levels into our food chain.

Unfortunately, studies have shown that tooth decay diminished at the same rate in areas where water was not fluoridated. Consider the healthy teeth of young Caribbean children who have not been introduced to enforced fluoridation. One might like to note that these children often chew constantly on wild cane, which does not have the same decaying effect on the teeth that our Western refined sugar has.

The argument that fluoride destroys bad bacteria is correct but unfortunately it is not specific and it creates considerable damage to our own beneficial bacteria. The amounts that are forced upon us do not take into account the levels of fluoride that we take in through our food, and therefore potentially toxic levels of fluoride may affect all of us. Some individuals have a specific allergy or an oversensitivity to fluoride and they are particularly susceptible to conditions such as fluorosis of the teeth or bones, causing increased caries or tendency to fracture. Fluoride has also been noted (and the information suppressed by the big businesses that provide fluoride and introduce it into our food chain, such as food manufacturers and water suppliers) to cause biochemical changes in the body, birth defects and cancer.

Toxic levels may be created by taking in water that contains ten parts of fluoride per million parts of water. The recommended dosage for 'good dental health' is four parts per million. A fractional error in contaminating our water supply may lead to poisoning and no mention is made of those people who may have a higher level of fluoride in their diet from such foods as tea,

seafood, some meats and green vegetables. Children often enjoy the taste of toothpaste and swallow it, and many vitamins may have fluoride as part of their constituents.

It should be noted that few areas in the UK have the water supply fluoridated but it is worth asking about your area.

RECOMMENDATIONS

General Advice

- *An individual who has a well-balanced diet including seafood and tea, and who uses fluoride-containing toothpaste should have a reverse-osmosis water filter installed to remove the excessive fluoride from tap water.*
- *An occasional drink of tap water will quite adequately provide the flouride we need.*
- *Use a fluoride-containing toothpaste once a day only.*
- *Ensure good exercise to maintain bone density strength.*

Homeopathic

- *Consider a bi-yearly use of the homeopathic remedy Fluoricum acidum 200 (one dose) to encourage the body to fight against excess fluoride.*

GRINDING TEETH (BRUXISM)

Teeth grinding occurs for two reasons, neither of which are confined to childhood but it is most frequently noticed at this age. This predisposition most commonly occurs in those under stress. The masseter (jaw) muscles are very sensitive to stress, as is shown by the obvious clenching of those who are concentrating or are angry. Most frequently this occurs at night.

The second reason is not well supported by scientific evidence but is anecdotally accepted as a possible calcium deficiency. The body is aware of the calcium levels in the teeth and tries to make it available by grinding. Most commonly this occurs in children rather than adults and during sleep rather than whilst awake. Teeth grinding can be associated with threadworms and any symptoms such as an itching anus or excessive appetite with no weight gain should be noted.

RECOMMENDATIONS

General Advice

- *Establish any emotional causes and deal with them appropriately. Basic counselling may be most beneficial.*
- *A consultation with a cranial osteopath may relieve tension in the jaw muscles.*
- *If the tendency is persistent please review the individual case with a complementary medical practitioner.*

Nutritional

- *Add in a calcium supplement or take sesame seeds and dairy products, provided that there is no allergic or intolerant association.*

Supplemental

- *Use chelated zinc (3mg per foot of height) before bedtime.*

Homeopathic

- *The homeopathic remedy Arsenicum album 6, four pills before bed, can be most effective. Also refer to the remedies Zinc, Phytolacca, Calcarea phosphorica and Silica.*
- *If bruxism is associated with threadworms, use the homeopathic remedy Cinchona 6.*

Orthodox

- *A dentist's opinion may be required if grinding is persistent and may suggest a protective cover put on at night to prevent wearing down the teeth.*

ORAL HYGIENE

It is best to start an infant's oral hygiene as early as possible. A small gauze pad or soft cloth should be wrapped around your finger, moistened and used to massage the gums. This helps teeth break through and gets the baby used to teeth cleaning.

Infants should not have fatty foods or refined sugars introduced to their diet. In fact it is quite feasible to avoid artificial sweeteners until the child attends the home of a less conscientious parent which may not be until the age of two or three years. Refined sugars encourage bacterial growth and if a sweet food is ingested a gentle gum or teeth rub with chamomile tea will encourage salivation and wash the sugars out.

PLAQUE AND TARTAR

Plaque is a collection of bacteria that adheres to the enamel of teeth and tartar is a build-up of a calcium compound that itself adheres to teeth. The plaque lives within tartar and slowly, but relentlessly, eats away at the gum, encouraging infection, tooth decay and loss of teeth.

RECOMMENDATIONS

General Advice

- *Proper dental hygiene and regular de-scaling by a dental hygienist is essential.*
- *Using specialized brushes that get between the teeth or dental floss is good hygienic practice. This is even better if started at a young age before gaps clearly form between the teeth where food can stick and encourage bacterial growth.*

SENSITIVE TEETH

Sensitivity to hot or cold is a common manifestation and is generally caused by the exposure of nerves in the gum or the pulp of the tooth.

RECOMMENDATIONS

General Advice

- *Ensure that general care is taken as advised above to avoid tooth or gum damage.*
- *Regular dental check-ups (at least every six months) and specific attention to a sensitive area may seal the exposed nerves.*

Homeopathic

- *The homeopathic remedy Natrum muriaticum 6 can be taken four times a day. Sensitivity to cold may respond better to Silica 6, four times a day.*

Herbal/natural extracts

- *Application of clove oil directly onto the area by dipping a cotton bud into the essential oil may help. Be careful not to allow too much clove oil onto the area because this will irritate the tongue. Application twice a day over a period of ten days will, potentially, numb the nerve permanently.*

TEETH DISCOLOURATION

The overuse of fluoride through toothpaste, water and tablets was a common factor, especially in the children of dentists, 30 years ago. Nowadays fluoridation is controlled and this mottled appearance is no longer seen commonly. The same effect may be produced by the use of tetracyclines (aggressive antibiotics). Smoking, chewing tobacco and excessive ingestion of red wine (not all that common in young children!) may stain teeth at an older age.

The most common cause of discolouration is the yellowing that occurs from teeth that are not cleaned. Certain infections may cause a grey white patchy discolouration, the most common of which are whooping cough and measles.

RECOMMENDATIONS

General Advice

- *Ensure that regular cleaning takes place.*
- *Regular visits to the dentist or the dental hygienist for removal of debris will benefit.*

Homeopathic

- *The discolouration from infection may be removed by using the nosodes (homeopathic remedies made from the causative agent) Pertussin for whooping cough and Morbillinum for whooping cough and measles respectively. Use potency 6 or 12 twice a day for one week.*

TEETHING

Teething is a term that describes the arrival of the milk teeth (the first set of teeth) in an infant. This usually occurs anywhere from before birth to the age of three years. Typically the first tooth will arrive at around six to eight months and the full set will be exposed around the 30-month mark. The breaking of the gum is a painful experience and it is not surprising that infants are often inconsolable as they go through this period. There is usually marked excessive salivation and, less frequently, a red rash that resembles the aftereffects of a smack around one or both cheeks. A fever may be noted, either by the child feeling hot or by a thermometer, and a general malaise or lethargy may be observed. Diarrhoea is often associated.

Gently feel the gums for protrusions and, if possible, look for any redness or swelling. If there is no evidence of teething, do not assume that any symptoms are due to teething, but consider other possible problems.

A teething fever is generally mild. A temperature over 100°F (38°C) is unlikely to be caused by teething.

RECOMMENDATIONS

General Advice

- *Give the child something hard to chew on, preferably a carrot or a piece of apple but otherwise an artificial 'teether'. The colder these objects are, the more relieving it will be.*
- *Gentle massage around the jaw may reduce inflammation.*

Homeopathic

- *The use of the homeopathic remedy Chamomilla 6, one dose every half-hour if the child is particularly upset, otherwise twice a day throughout the period of teething.*

Herbal/natural extracts

- *Two drops of clove oil in eight drops of olive oil applied to a ruptured gum is very soothing. Test it on your own tongue. It should tingle, not burn. Dilute with more olive oil if necessary.*
- *Catnip, lime flowers or chamomile teas throughout the day can be very soothing.*

TOOTHACHE AND DENTAL PAIN

Toothache is either created by exposure of nerves in the gum or the pulp of the tooth. Cleansing and debriding (removing) of tartar and plaque (*see* **Plaque and tartar**) is essential to remove the base of the bacterial infection that has produced the acid that has decayed the area.

RECOMMENDATIONS

General Advice

- *Visit a dentist at the earliest opportunity to cleanse the area and isolate the inflamed nerves.*
- *Prepare a mouthwash from a cup of water with a teaspoon of salt and a teaspoon of Arnica fluid extract. Force this through the teeth at a temperature that is soothing or comfortable.*
- *A persistent toothache may be associated with sinusitis or an osteopathic lesion in the neck or jaw that may be pinching the trunk of the nerves supplying the jaw. An osteopath may be very effective.*

Homeopathic

- *The remedies Arnica 6 or Hypericum 6 may be taken every half-hour if the discomfort is bad, before the dentist is seen.*
- *Please refer to your preferred homeopathic manual for a more suitable remedy based on the type of toothache, the site and its sensitivities.*

Herbal/natural extracts

- *The application of clove oil via a cotton bud dipped in the essential oil and applied just to the sensitive area. Do not use too much clove oil because this will cause stinging of the surrounding tissue.*

THE GUMS

A lot of dental work is needed not specifically because of the teeth but due to poor health of the gums. The gums are a specialized, tough mucous membrane that covers the jaw bone and lower aspects of the teeth. Maintenance of the integrity of the gums is essential to avoid tooth decay and jaw bone problems.

There is mounting evidence that pockets of infection found within the gums may be responsible for disease in other parts of the body. The principle concern is that parasites, bacteria and viruses can settle in this area, live comfortably and multiply profusely. These germs can then enter the bloodstream directly or be continually swallowed causing problems throughout the digestive tract.

CARE OF THE GUMS

Infections of the gum are often difficult to treat because the bacteria can find their way into deep recesses around the tooth root, well-protected from the mouth's natural antibodies found in the saliva and also from oxygen, which is often detrimental to bacterial growth.

Plaque is a thin transparent film of bacteria on the surface of the teeth that live comfortably despite the body's natural defence mechanisms and slowly but surely eat into the gum tissue. It is this plaque that needs to be destroyed.

RECOMMENDATIONS

General Advice

- *As early as possible, teach your child to brush the teeth with a circular motion, ensuring that the bristles travel between the teeth.*
- *The toothbrush should be as hard as the gums will accept without bleeding.*
- *Toothpaste (without fluoride) or sodium bicarbonate can be used as a tooth cleanser, although the brushing action with lightly-salted water is the most beneficial aspect of gum care.*
- *Regular mouthwashes with salt water being forced between the teeth is highly recommended.*
- *Avoid the use of a mouthwash. The antibacterial action kills the good bugs as effectively as it kills the bad bugs and has little effect on the hard*

barrier of protection of the plaque. The outcome is the loss of good bacteria rather than the bad.

- Ensure regular chewing of raw vegetables or hard fruit, which encourages blood flow into the gums.
- Chewing on liquorice sticks (fresh, not sweetened) is most beneficial.
- Regular flossing between the teeth with cord or a wooden stick is recommended.

Nutritional

- Avoid refined sugars or ensure teeth brushing and gum cleaning (the same thing) after any sweet meal. Natural sugars do not have the same bacterial support, as is noticed by the healthy teeth in Caribbean children whose sweeteners come from raw cane rather than refined sugar.

Supplemental

- The gums, like all body tissues, are dependent upon good nutritional and vitamin intake. The gums are particularly sensitive to vitamin C deficiency.

RECOMMENDATIONS

General Advice

- See **Care of gums**.
- Ensure that your toothbrush is neither too hard nor too soft.
- Persisting bleeding of the gums, despite the above measures, requires investigations by your GP or a holistic-minded dentist.
- Use a toothpaste with homeopathic Arnica or Calendula twice a day. Use an Arnica or Calendula fluid extract – 1 teaspoonful in a cup of water already containing $1/2$ a teasponful of salt. Use this as a mouthwash and forcibly push this through the teeth.

Nutritional

- Consult a complementary medical practitioner or nutritionist to ensure that you are not missing any vital nutrients.
- It may be necessary to investigate this through blood, sweat or hair analysis.

Bleeding gums

Gums bleed due to overenthusiastic brushing, poor hygiene due to not cleaning the teeth and gums, deficiencies and diseases such as diabetes, those effecting blood clotting, and other rarer conditions. The term gingivitis is given to gums that are inflamed, spongy and tend to bleed easily.

Gingivitis

Gingivitis is the medical term for inflammation of the gums. The underlying cause is generally infection, although deficiencies, including low intake of vitamin C, may also cause it. Pregnancy can trigger gum inflammation as can the oral contraceptive pill. The hormones dilate blood vessels and alter cells in the lining of the gums. Treatment

Dental Hygiene

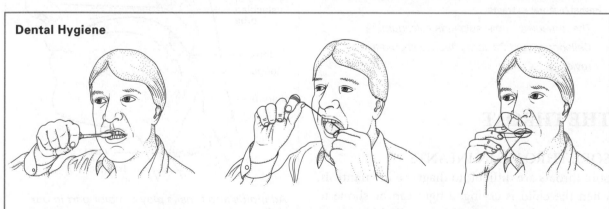

brushing with a circular motion　　flossing with an up and down motion　　mouthwashing with salt water

depends on the cause and a holistic dentist or a complementary medical physician should assess persisting gingivitis. For treatment, *see* **Bleeding gums** and **Gum infections**.

Gum infections

Pockets of bacteria, fungi, yeasts and viruses can settle deep in the gums and cause problems both to the oral cavity and, if swallowed or absorbed into the bloodstream, throughout the body. Regular review by your dentist is essential to avoid this.

RECOMMENDATIONS

General Advice

- *Gentle brushing around the area and dental flossing of the gap above the infection (very gently) in association with a salt water mouthwash will often clear up gum infections.*
- *Toothpaste containing myrrh, cloves, cinnamon and bee propolis (avoid if you have allergic reactions to bee or wasp stings) can be curative. If the toothpaste is not available, application of the essential oils can be useful in both clearing the infection and reducing the pain. Painful infections are particularly relieved by clove oil.*
- *See* **Care of the gums**.

Supplemental

- *Suitable doses of vitamin C, zinc and magnesium should all be taken with any gum infection.*

Herbal/natural extracts

- *The remedies Hepar sulphuris calcarium, Belladonna and Calcarea fluorica should all be reviewed.*

THE THROAT

SORE THROATS IN INFANTS

Sore throats are difficult to diagnose in infants. If, when the child is crying, a light can be shone to the back of the throat, redness or discharge (pus) may be visible.

RECOMMENDATIONS

General Advice

- *Try the child on warm or cold drinks to see if either is soothing.*
- *Breast milk must be encouraged.*

Supplemental

- *A multivitamin, preferably recommended by a health practitioner, can be administered.*

Homeopathic

- *The homeopathic remedies Aconite, Baptisia, Kali bichromicum, Kali muriaticum, Mercurius and Phosphorus should all be referred to. One pill of potency 6 every 2hr will often clear up a sore throat in an infant.*

ADENOIDS AND TONSILS

The adenoids and tonsils are lymphatic glandular tissue found at the back of the nose at the top of the throat. They should be there. They are the

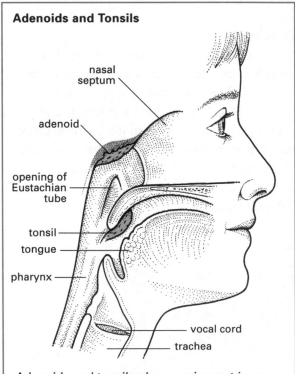

Adenoids and Tonsils

nasal septum

adenoid

opening of Eustachian tube

tonsil

tongue

pharynx

vocal cord

trachea

Adenoids and tonsils play a major part in our defence against infections.

home to numerous white blood cells that kill infections. Children are particularly prone to nasal and throat infections and the adenoids and tonsils are a main part of the defence mechanism.

Until the 1970s it was commonplace for the adenoids and tonsils to be removed, quite often for no reason. Nowadays, most ear, nose and throat specialists and paediatricians agree that removal should be a last resort.

Recurrent inflammation and an excess of thick mucus result in enlargement of these glands, leading to snoring, a nasal-sounding voice and sometimes partial asphyxia. The problem is not the adenoids and tonsils but the child's immune system being ineffective and allowing persistent or recurrent infections.

RECOMMENDATIONS

General Advice
- *Ensure good water intake. This thins the mucus.*

Nutritional
- *Reduce or remove white sugar and excessive sweet things from the diet. These thicken the lymph which blocks the glands.*

Supplemental
- *Ensure good diet and supplement with multivitamins if the child has persistent infections. Obtain naturopathic advice before being threatened by antibiotics and operations.*

Homeopathic
- *Review the following homeopathic remedies through your manual: Belladonna, Calcarea carbonica, Hepar sulphuris calcarium, Pulsatilla and Silica.*

CHOKING

An inhaled object or incorrectly swallowed food may block the trachea (windpipe) leading to choking, which, if fully obstructive or persistent, can be fatal.

Choking in an infant or child

- As soon as evidence of choking occurs, try to remove the object with your fingers from the back of the throat. Do not waste time trying to view the object.
- If you cannot reach the object, pick the child up by the feet and whilst upside down apply firm slaps with the palm of the hand between the shoulder blades. If the child is too heavy, then place him/her head down over your knee or thigh and repeat the slaps.
- If this fails then the Heimlich manoeuvre should be employed (*see* **Heimlich manoeuvre**).

QUINSY (PERITONSILLAR ABSCESS)

The tonsil is a collection of lymphatic tissues within a capsule at the back of the mouth. An infection that does not drain may become an abscess, which has been named quinsy after the surgeon who first described it.

A patient will complain of a severe sore throat usually associated with fever and, on examination, a tonsil (it is usually one-sided) will appear enlarged and inflamed. There is usually swelling around the area and a mass may be seen (although often it is not because the abscess may be tucked behind the tonsil).

RECOMMENDATIONS

General Advice
- *See **Sore throats** for complementary treatments.*

Supplemental
- *Take twice the recommended dosage of a good-quality acidophilus (yoghurt bacteria tablets) product for five days longer than the antibiotic.*

Orthodox
- *A quinsy should be treated with antibiotics once diagnosed. This condition may obstruct the airways or eat into the close-lying carotid artery if left unattended.*

'STREP' THROAT

A streptococcal sore throat is a frequent diagnosis that can actually only be made accurately once a swab is taken of any discharge from the tonsils or back of the throat, and found to be growing the bacteria *Streptococcus*.

The symptoms, which are most common in childhood but can occur at any age, are: sore tonsils and back of the throat; difficulty in swallowing; and, if the tonsils are particularly enlarged, difficulty in breathing. Fever, either dry or sweating, loss of appetite, lethargy and swollen external neck glands are all part of the picture.

RECOMMENDATIONS

General Advice

- *See* **Sore throats** *and* **Tonsillitis**.

Homeopathic

- *Pay attention to the homeopathic remedies Hepar sulphuris calcarium, Belladonna and Streptococcus by referring to them in your preferred homeopathic manual.*

Orthodox

- *Request a throat swab, especially if the individual is being threatened with a course of antibiotics.*

TONSILLITIS

Inflammation from infection of the tonsils is dealt with in chapter 4.

THE CHEST

ASTHMA

Asthma is the broad term given to shortness of breath caused by narrowing of the bronchial tree (the main airways in the lungs) due to contractions of the muscles in the tubes and by excess excretion of the normal mucus production. This mucus is often thicker than normal and causes plugs in the already narrowed airways. Asthma can be acute or chronic and range from mild to severe. Minor upper respiratory tract infections can cause temporary asthma and simply may last for the few days of infection. Asthma attacks may be triggered by other lung irritants, such as airborne pollution, fog and humidity as well as certain intolerances to food, which can be very specific. Interestingly, one study found that children exposed to the chemicals from their mother's cigarette smoke while in the womb also had decreased lung function after birth. It is well established that paternal smoking or being in a smoky environment through youth decreases lung capacity and function. Common triggers include caffeine, chocolate, cow's milk products, wheat, oranges, nuts and eggs.

There has been a sixfold increase in childhood asthma in the last 20 years. Many hypotheses are put forward, the most recent being that food hygiene and a decline in childhood infections may be at the root of the increase. A large study in Italy showed that those exposed to infections in early childhood may prevent the development of atopy (genetically predisposed disorder of the immunity) and that without these infections asthma (and rhinitis) are likely to be worse. I suspect that a genetic predisposition must be triggered by several factors, including air pollution, food (pollutants such as preservatives, additives and pesticides), an increase in our refined sugar intake, our increased use of vaccinations and antibiotics and climatic changes such as the loss of the ozone layer. Asthma must never be underestimated. It is a lethal condition and can come on very swiftly, causing fatal airway obstruction, especially in children. Doctors are very swift to diagnose asthma and encourage the use of bronchodilators (drugs that relax the muscle spasm and reduce mucus production), such as salbutamol.

Recognizing asthma

The power of pulling air into the lungs through the diaphragm and intercostal (rib cage) muscles is much greater than the power available to exhale. Asthma is actually most often caused by an inability to remove the carbon dioxide from the lungs rather than a difficulty in getting air in.

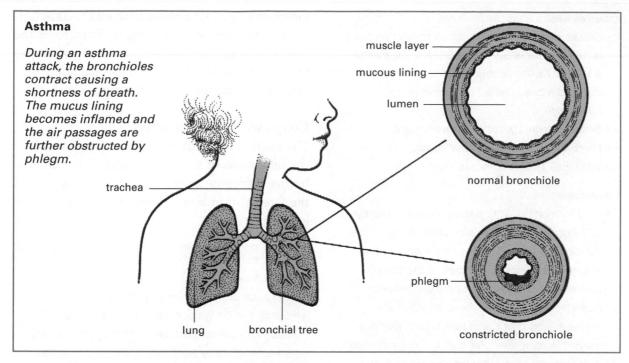

Asthma

During an asthma attack, the bronchioles contract causing a shortness of breath. The mucus lining becomes inflamed and the air passages are further obstructed by phlegm.

muscle layer

mucous lining

lumen

normal bronchiole

trachea

phlegm

lung   bronchial tree

constricted bronchiole

In mild to moderate asthma, therefore, you will see individuals pursing their lips in an attempt to blow out the trapped air. This and a respiratory rate of more than 15 inhalations per minute are the immediate tell-tale signs. A rattling in the chest, most easily heard through a doctor's stethoscope, is usually present as the air is forced past the mucus plugs. However, asthma does not demand rattling. Wheezing is much more common, again caused by air being forced past the mucus obstruction.

Moderate to severe asthma will have all these signs plus a noticeable amount of panic on the part of the sufferer. Any suggestion of dizziness, blacking out or blueness around the mouth needs to be treated as a medical emergency.

Self-help for asthma is limited but works on the following principles:

• Removing triggers
• Learning breathing techniques
• Dealing with acute attacks

Removing triggers

It is important to keep a journal or list of attacks. This should include times and recent events, foods and drink taken in the previous 24 hours and stress factors. If asthma attacks are occurring in conjunction with any particular input or event, these can be eliminated. Triggers such as coughs and colds require a naturopathic opinion on why the immune system is behaving incorrectly.

Learning breathing techniques

These are not applicable until the child is old enough to understand and learn different patterns. This is discussed in chapter 4.

Dealing with acute attacks

RECOMMENDATIONS

General Advice

• *At any sign of asthma bring the patient to the attention of your GP. In mild to moderate cases, resist the immediate use of bronchodilators until you have consulted with a naturopath.*

• *If attacks are occurring in association with stress situations, then a child psychologist, preferably an art therapist, should be consulted.*

• *See* **Asthma** *in the Young Adult chapter.*

Supplemental

- *Ensure that any child with an asthmatic tendency is taking extra vitamin B_6, vitamin C, magnesium and zinc. The amount is variable, depending on the child's size, and is best prescribed by a naturopath.*
- *Beta-carotene 1000iu per foot of height.*
- *Chromium 10mcg per foot of height.*
- *Vitamin D 100iu per foot of height.*

Homeopathic

- *Take the homeopathic remedy Aconite, potency 6, 12 or 30, two to four pills every 10min, if the attack comes on suddenly; take Arsenicum album 6, four pills every 15min if the child is better with warm drinks, for attacks between midnight and 3am that are associated with restlessness; take Carbo vegetalis 6, four pills every 15min, if worse for talking and associated with a cough; take Natrum sulphuricum 6, four pills every 10min, for attacks that come after 3am and when the child is holding the chest.*

Herbal/natural extracts

- *Mix and keep aside the essential oils of lavender and chamomile. Place a few drops in steaming water and apply to the collar of the child or use as a steam inhalation. See **Nasal congestion** for the technique.*

Orthodox

- *At any suggestion of a moderate to severe asthmatic condition, take the drugs and obtain a complementary medical view afterwards.*
- *Avoid giving pain killers such as aspirin and non steroidal anti inflammatories but especially paracetamol (calpol) to asthmatics as it may worsen asthma.*

COUGHS

Coughs and colds in infants are usually self-limiting and require little, if any, treatment. Remedies should be considered if a cold persists for longer than three days or the child is particularly unwell, in which case a physician should be consulted.

A cough, whilst distressing to listen to, is the body's way of eliminating unwanted substances from the bronchial tree (the pipes leading to the lung tissue) and the alveoli (the lung tissue).

Cough with a sudden onset

The sudden onset of a cough may be caused by the inhalation of a foreign object. If the child is having difficulty in breathing, becoming red in the face or even blue, assume that an object has been inhaled.

RECOMMENDATIONS

General Advice

- *Have somebody call an ambulance.*
- *Gently but firmly open the child's mouth by applying a pincer pressure to the jaw muscle and shine a light into the throat. If an object can be seen, try to extract it using your fingers. The use of an instrument such as tweezers should only be used if the child is asphyxiating (unable to breathe) or is blacking out.*

Loose coughs

A cough that sounds catarrhal is usually associated with the production of excess mucus and is related to a cold. Unless the child is asthmatic, these coughs may last for weeks, especially through the winter season, but are associated with a healthy, happy and functional child and should not be taken too seriously.

RECOMMENDATIONS

General Advice

- *Avoid dehydration by encouraging water intake because this keeps mucus from becoming too thick or tenacious.*

Nutritional

- *Avoid cow's products and refined sugars because these encourage mucus production.*

Homeopathic

- *Refer to the remedies Antimonium tart, Sepia, Nux vomica or Pulsatilla, although others may be indicated.*

Herbal/natural extracts

- *A few drops of the oil of aniseed, cinnamon or hyssop can be used as an inhalation. See **Nasal congestion** for the technique.*
- *Fresh ginger or thyme can be chopped and used as an inhalation as above.*
- *One drop of lobelia per year of age in water or diluted juice, three times a day, can be most beneficial.*

Dry coughs

Dry coughs may indicate more serious problems, such as whooping cough, laryngitis, croup and tracheitis. A dry cough of sudden onset should alert one to the inhalation of a foreign object. Most dry coughs are viral and can be treated as follows.

RECOMMENDATIONS

Supplemental

- *Vitamin C, 100mg per foot of height three times a day.*
- *Vitamin A, 300iu three times a day (for children aged six months or older). Give 100iu three times a day until six months old.*

Homeopathic

- *A homeopathic remedy should be chosen from all the symptoms. Initially, however, the following remedies are masters at the quick cure: Aconite for a hard barking cough of sudden onset in a restless infant: Belladonna if the child is red, hot and has bursts of coughing that distress it particularly; Drosera if the child is being sick with the cough; and Sticta if the cough has a ring to it and is worse at night. Any of these should be given at potency 6 every 15min for 1hr and, if improvement is forthcoming, every 2–3hr until the child is better.*

Herbal/natural extracts

- *Steam inhalations with linseed, liquorice or mullein oils, using the technique described for nasal congestion.*

CROUP

A dry cough that persists for longer than three days or disturbs the child's sleep for more than two nights should be brought to the attention of a health practitioner. Croup is a spasm of the vocal cords and will improve if steam inhalations are encouraged. Boiling a kettle in the child's nursery is an effective initial treatment. The dry cough of croup is alarming and inhibits the child's breathing and *must* be brought to the attention of a physician *immediately*. A croupy cough is always associated with breathing difficulties and sounds like the call of a crow. It has a vibrant ringing quality, almost as if the child is calling whilst coughing.

RECOMMENDATIONS

General Advice

- *Avoid giving the child anything by mouth in case an anaesthetic has to be given to pass an intubation tube.*

Homeopathic

- *Give Aconite 6, Hepar sulphuris calcarium 6 and Spongia 6 in rotation every 5min. If the child is not improving within half an hour, call the doctor or take the child to casualty.*
- *If the child settles, contact your health practitioner as soon as possible, continuing to alternate the Hepar sulphuris calcarium and the Spongia every half-hour.*

SUFFOCATION

Suffocation is the interference with the entrance of air into the lungs, which, if it persists, will result in asphyxiation.

Resuscitation of Infant or Child

Heaven forbid one ever should have to perform this technique, but all adults should know the procedure. The following steps are worth practising on a large doll or teddy bear:

(a) Lie the child flat.

(b) Gently tip the chin back until the throat is stretched straight.

(c) Ensure that any obstruction at the back of the throat is removed.

If the child has not responded to this, then proceed to step (d):

(d) Place your mouth over the infant's mouth *and* nose.

(e) Look at the child's chest.

(f) Breath until the child's chest expands. *Do not blow hard or for too long because this will over-expand and possibly damage the child's lungs.*

(g) Count to three and repeat, stopping every five breaths to see if the child has started to breath spontaneously.

If the child has not responded after five inhalations, proceed to step (h):

Resuscitating a Child

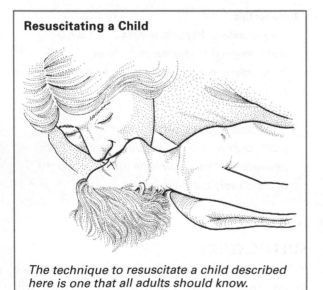

The technique to resuscitate a child described here is one that all adults should know.

(h) Place two fingers to the side of and just above the Adam's Apple. A pulse should be felt. If there is no pulse, place the forefinger and middle finger of one hand onto the child's breast bone (sternum).

(i) Apply pressure until firm resistance is felt and repeat five times.

(j) Repeat steps (d) to (f) five times and then return to pushing the sternum five times. Alternate this until the child revives or the ambulance arrives.

Once the child has revived, give him/her one pill of Arnica 6 every 10 minutes. Nothing else should be given by mouth in case the child requires an anaesthetic.

RECOMMENDATIONS

General Advice

• *Pay special attention to the covering of a child, ensuring that it cannot entangle bedclothes around the head.*

• *Be wary of pets, especially cats, that may rest on the warmth of the baby's body.*

• *See* **Asphyxia**.

WHEEZING

Wheezing is a high-pitched sound created by inhaling or exhaling through a narrow tube. The narrowing may be caused by muscular contraction such as in asthma or by an inflamed mucous membrane as in asthma, bronchitis and pneumonia. If associated with crackles, the narrowing may be due to mucus production or fluid secondary to pulmonary oedema.

RECOMMENDATION

General Advice

• *See* **Asthma** *earlier in this chapter and in chapter 4 for tips on how to open the tubes and breathe more freely.*

WHOOPING COUGH

Whooping cough is characterized by spasmodic coughing bouts that can last up to 1min. As the child draws in breath there is the recognizable 'whoop', which is often associated with the expectoration of thick mucus and often vomiting. It is caused by a highly infectious bacteria known as *Bordetella pertussis*, which causes an inflammatory process within the air passages.

Whooping cough is a prolonged illness that develops over a two-week period and lasts up until six weeks. It is not a particularly dangerous condition unless contracted in the first year of life, when the coughing spasms not only interfere with feeding but are exhausting. A prolonged spasm may result in an inability to breathe, causing asphyxiation with brain damage or death. This is extremely rare and can, of course, happen with any infection.

Whooping cough is associated with the production of much mucus, which may plug airways rendering them ineffective or causing the lung tissue beyond to collapse.

A diagnosis is made by hearing the characteristic whoop, but this is not necessarily present. Culture can be made from a swab or sputum and antibodies may be measured.

There is no orthodox antibiotic that attacks this unusual organism so treatment is based on treating the symptoms, although the orthodox medical world would give antibiotics to prevent a secondary infection. One holistic concern is that by taking out some of the necessary healthy body bacteria we are reducing the competition and the ability to digest and absorb, thereby leaving the individual with a reduced immune system capacity.

Whooping cough is known to occur in epidemics and when it does it is generally quite aggressive because through our use of vaccinations we have been breeding more difficult strains to attack. The vaccination question is particularly relevant in the case of pertussis because, like all vaccinations, there is a positive and a negative aspect. The pertussis vaccine developed in the 1960s had a very high incidence of causing epilep-tic fits and, potentially, brain damage. Many GPs at that time quite rightly became reluctant to administer the vaccine, and this fear was passed on to generations of parents and doctors taught by this group.

The pharmaceutical industry has gone to great lengths to purify the vaccine and claims that it is quite safe now. The evidence suggests otherwise. There are many reports of continued problems and strong evidence to support the ineffectiveness of the vaccine. Some studies and plenty of anecdotal evidence, including comments from paediatricians, suggest that children vaccinated against whooping cough will actually fare worse than those who are not, should they contract the infection. It appears that the immunization is only partially effective but it convinces the body that it already has a defence mechanism and thereby delays the immune response. This continues to be a controversial subject but then so were the side effects of the measles vaccine until strong evidence of high risk was finally brought to light in July 1997.

Whooping cough needs to be treated aggressively and home treatment is not necessarily the best form. However, the help of a complementary medical practitioner is invaluable because if the condition persists it can lead to a weakened lung, which may give rise to problems throughout life.

RECOMMENDATIONS

General Advice

- *See* **Coughs**, **Colds**, **Pneumonia** *and* **Fevers**. *Treat appropriately.*
- *If the child (or adult) is old enough and can appreciate the teaching of a breathing technique, a yoga, Qi Gong (Chi Kung) or meditation teacher should be able to give instructions.*
- *Bed rest is essential, along with good nutrition and the supplements recommended for coughs or pneumonia should be reviewed (see* **Coughs** *and* **Pneumonia***).*

- *The child should not return to school until well, even if there is a likelihood of falling behind. Firstly, the child may be contagious and, secondly, running around will make things worse and probably lead to more chest infections over the next formative years, leading to more missed school time.*

Homeopathic

- *Administer the homeopathic remedy Drosera 30 every 2hr if a whooping cough is suspected.*
- *Use Drosera 200 as soon as symptoms alleviate, one dose each night for five nights. This potency may also be administered nightly for five nights if whooping cough is known to be in the area or your child's school.*
- *If Drosera does not seem to be controlling the situation, the next remedy to try is Pertussin 30 given every 3hr. It would be best to consult a complementary medical specialist with homeopathic and herbal knowledge sooner rather than later.*

Herbal/natural extracts

- *Lobelia fluid extract, one drop per foot of height in a small amount of warm water, should be given three times a day and a teaspoonful placed in steaming water for inhalation.*
- *Comfrey root, mouse ear and sundew (Drosera) are all established herbal treatments and should be discussed with a herbalist for the correct dosages. It is not wise to dose a whooping child without expert guidance.*

THE DIGESTIVE SYSTEM

ABDOMINAL PAINS

It is very difficult to differentiate which part of an infant's body is in pain, although babies have a tendency to pull or touch areas that hurt. Once children can communicate, life is a lot simpler. Abdominal pain is very often the culprit. In a non-talking child, wait for a quiet moment and gently push on the abdomen. A painful tummy will usually trigger crying again. Persistent crying requires a doctor's opinion but once abdominal pain is diagnosed the following tips may be helpful.

Colic

Incidentally, colic is twice as likely in young babies whose mothers smoke, and breastfed infants are less likely to be colicky than bottle fed ones when their mothers smoke.

RECOMMENDATIONS

General Advice

- *If the following alternative suggestions do not resolve an infant's or child's abdominal pain within a few hours, contact a general practitioner. Any severe pain, or if the child is clearly unwell, do not delay but get a medical opinion immediately.*
- *'The Colic Carry'. Place the baby on your forearm, chest down and legs either side of your elbow with the head in the palm of your hand. Walk around. Honestly, this makes a big difference!*
- *Tummy patting. Cup your hand and gently pat baby's tummy. Trapped wind is often the cause and a few moments of this followed by burping the baby over your shoulder will help.*
- *Consider a consultation with a cranial osteopath.*
- *Mothers should not smoke.*

Nutritional

- *Assume a food intolerance. Breast-feeding mothers should cut out spices, caffeine, onions and excess white sugar. If this does not seem to help then specific food intolerances, including dairy produce, should be eliminated (see **Food intolerance**). Older infants and children should be considered for food restrictions (see chapter 7).*

Homeopathic
- *Refer to a homeopathic manual and consider the remedies Arsenicum album, Chamomile, Carbo vegetalis, Coloccynthsis, Nux vomica and Silica.*
- *High-dose homeopathy should be considered and a consultation arranged.*

Herbal/natural extracts
- *Weak chamomile tea can be used at all ages, but if the problem is not resolved through such a drink, stop administering anything in case an anaesthetic is required.*

Orthodox
- *Pharmaceutical colic medicine and paracetamol may be used as a last resort, although there is some level of toxicity created by these compounds and a possible association with SIDS (cot death).*

Abdominal migraine

Migraines are generally associated with headaches. The cause of most migraines is dilation of the blood vessels in the brain and this can occur in the abdomen, especially of children. Usually associated with food intolerance or stressful situations, the advice relating to head migraines is also suitable here.

Mild viral infections that cause lymphatic gland activity (as is commonly felt in the neck of patients with infections) can occur in the large number of lymphatic glands in the abdomen. A stomach ache associated with glands in the neck, under the arm or in the groin should be suspected as inflamed lymph glands.

RECOMMENDATIONS

General Advice
- *See **Abdominal pains and migraine**.*

Homeopathic
- *Refer to a homeopathic manual and consider the remedies Belladonna, Calcarea carbonica, Kali carbonicum and Phytolacca, all good glandular remedies.*

Appendicitis

The appendix is thought to be vestigial (a part of the body no longer a necessary organ). It is, in fact, a collection of lymphatic tissue about the size of your own little finger. It probably plays a minor role in the defence mechanism of the bowel. In

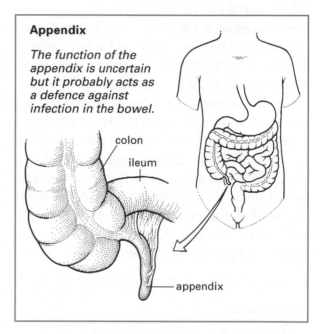

Appendix

The function of the appendix is uncertain but it probably acts as a defence against infection in the bowel.

colon

ileum

appendix

some unfortunates, the appendix can become inflamed and cause appendicitis.

Appendicitis is characteristically a sharp pain on the right lower abdomen. It is characterized by 'rebound' tenderness. If you push on the tender area there is not as much pain pushing in as when you let go. This sign is pathognomonic for an inflamed lining of the bowel and requires immediate hospital attention. Appendicitis can start with a pain around the tummy button but usually migrates down into the right iliac fossa, as that area is medically termed. There is often a mild fever and the individual will be off their food and may have diarrhoea.

RECOMMENDATIONS

General Advice
- *With any persistent stomach ache or any suggestion of rebound tenderness, have the child seen by a doctor.*

Intussusception

Intussusception is a surgical problem found more commonly in boys than girls and usually around the first eight months after birth. For some reason the bowel folds in on itself much like a telescope.

The characteristics are a limp child who screams with pain at intervals, associated with the contractions of the bowel. A child with intussusception is ill. In-between bouts of pain they are likely to be floppy and inert. Vomiting may occur but a characteristic red, jelly-like stool is almost diagnostic. A hard lump may be felt in the child's abdomen, most commonly in the lower right quarter, and the child will be distressed if any pressure is applied to this point.

COELIAC DISEASE

Coeliac disease is characterized by weight loss, undigested greasy stools and any disorders

Intussusception

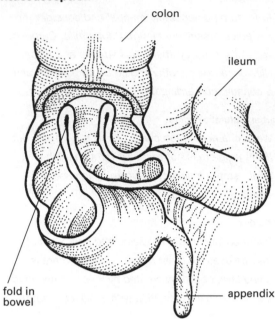

colon

ileum

fold in bowel

appendix

showing deficiency such as stunted growth, poor learning ability and recurrent infections. Diagnosis of this condition is, however, only made through very specific blood tests and biopsy of part of the small intestine called the jejunum. This process requires the patient to swallow a metal capsule on the end of a wire and when the capsule is in the right part of the small intestine, as defined by X-ray, the capsule is opened, grabs part of the mucosal lining, is closed and withdrawn with the biopsy sample. It is not a particularly unpleasant test, other than you have to sit there with a wire hanging from your mouth and the discomfort of the instrument hanging down your throat. It may take several hours for the capsule to reach the jejunum but usually this occurs within one or two.

The condition is caused by a sensitivity to one of the proteins in gluten called gliadin. This protein, found predominantly in wheat but also in rye, oats, corn (maize), buckwheat, rice and millet, causes a type of inflammation in specific individuals that makes the small intestine swell and become incapable of proper absorption.

The condition is most commonly genetic, being passed down family lines. The genetic fault seems to be created by an incorrect defence or immune response affecting the lining of the bowel that comes into contact with gliadin. The need to treat this condition is paramount because there are associated problems with the thyroid, rashes and psychiatric disturbances such as schizophrenia. More disturbingly, there is a higher incidence of diabetes and cancer in untreated coeliac patients.

RECOMMENDATIONS

General Advice
- *Coeliac disease can only be diagnosed in a specialist unit but any suspicion must be referred through your GP for investigation.*
- *Coeliac societies in your area can be found through your GP and they can help with diet programming and finding support groups.*

Nutritional
- *Once a diagnosis of gluten sensitivity has been established, all gluten-containing foods must be avoided. The list above gives the main foods in question but millet, corn and rice should only be avoided until the problem has settled because their level of gliadin is negligible.*
- *Milk and milk products should be eliminated initially because the condition is often associated with milk intolerance.*
- *Keep a very close eye on pre-prepared foods or on foods eaten out, because many foods such as sauces, ice cream, soups and alcoholic beverages contain gluten products.*
- *See **Food intolerance**. Any small intestinal inflammation can lead to poor digestion and the absorption into the bloodstream of large molecules, which in turn lead to an immune response. It is worth having a food allergy/intolerance test performed through blood investigation or by the use of Vega/bioresonance computers.*

Supplemental
- *Intravenous nutritional supplementation is of benefit in severe cases and can be utilized initially because the exclusion treatment may take several weeks to prove effective.*
- *High-dose oral antioxidants, particularly beta-carotene, may correct nutritional deficiencies swiftly.*
- *The compound papaine, found in papaya, specifically digests wheat gluten and up to 1,000mg taken with meals may allow those with mild coeliac disease to tolerate small amounts of gluten.*

Herbal/natural extracts
- *Herbal treatments and homeopathic remedies should be prescribed by an expert in those fields.*

DIARRHOEA

Diarrhoea in childhood is not an uncommon ailment while infants develop their bowel flora and habits. Also children have a tendency to put anything and everything into their mouths. One must never underestimate the effects of serious, profuse or chronic diarrhoea because malabsorption, malnutrition, dehydration and infection may all be associated.

In principle, diarrhoea should not be considered a bad thing. Most often diarrhoea represents the body's attempts to throw out some toxin – either a food that disagrees or a bacteria or virus, the most common of which is *Campylobacter*. Allowed to run its natural course, a few bouts of diarrhoea with or without abdominal pain will clear within a matter of hours or a couple of days and nothing needs to be done other than a simple homeopathic remedy and ensuring good hydration by keeping up the water intake.

Persisting diarrhoea in an infant may be associated with conditions such as coeliac disease (allergy to wheat) or other food allergies. The orthodox world, whilst having a clear definition and picture of wheat allergy, seems reluctant to accept that other foods may cause the same problems. It is worthwhile remembering this and obtaining a complementary medical practitioner's suggestions before ending up following a drug-orientated orthodox approach. Incorrect bowel flora can show itself as persistent diarrhoea and often follows the use of an antibiotic, immediately or up to six months later. Unfortunately, much of our food is treated with antibiotics and chemicals, especially with meats, and gut dysbiosis (alteration of our bowel flora) can occur quite unwittingly due to the ingestion of these chemicals.

RECOMMENDATIONS

General Advice

- Severe, persistent, bloody or mucousy stool is an indication that a doctor's opinion is required.
- Any diarrhoea that persists beyond 48hr or is associated with pain, pallor or a change in the character of the child should be reviewed by a GP.
- Ensure good rehydration. The smaller the child, the quicker dehydration can set in. Rehydration should occur with a mixture of fluids to ensure glucose and nutrient intake. Alternating some water then half an hour later some diluted fruit juice, water then some soup, water with a pinch of salt in rotation should do the trick. Try to match any output (including any water loss through sweat if fever is associated) with the amount taken in. Avoid milk and other cow's produce except live yoghurt, which may be of benefit.
- Avoid anything too sweet as this will pull water into the bowel and make the diarrhoea worse.
- Estimate the amount of diarrhoea and replenish with the same quantity of fluids. Dilute juices are acceptable but water is best.
- Obtain the opinion of a complementary medical practitioner with a knowledge in nutrition, homeopathy and/or herbal medicine before taking orthodox medicine.

Nutritional

- Allow the child to eat by instinct. If the appetite is good then try to encourage foods that will 'mop up' poisons, such as wholegrain bread, pasta and rice, but avoid anything with refined sugar, caffeine or an excess of 'binding' foods, such as eggs.

Supplemental

- Use probifidus as a live yoghurt culture to encourage the growth of the body's normal bowel flora.

Homeopathic

- Refer to your preferred homeopathic manual and pay attention to the remedies Chamomilla, Carbo vegetabilis, Nux vomica, Mercurius and Arsenicum album. These can all be used safely at potency 6, two tablets every 1–2hr.

Herbal/natural extracts

- A weak chamomile tea can be very soothing and replenishing. Stir in a teaspoonful of honey per half-pint of fluid and a pinch of salt (it should not be possible to taste this) to replenish some glucose for energy and for salts that invariably have been lost.

GASTROENTERITIS

See **Gastroenteritis** in chapter 5.

Gastroenteritis in children can be particularly serious because the fluid loss due to diarrhoea in small beings may be rapid and cause dehydration and biochemical changes rapidly.

A typical causative organism is *Campylobacter*, which can be fatal in undernourished children although is usually not severe in well-nourished Western children.

RECOMMENDATIONS

General Advice

- Any persistent diarrhoea or vomiting should be referred to a physician who should be encouraged to check the stool for Campylobacter urgently. Severe cases should be treated with antibiotics and a complementary medical

practitioner consulted to deal with the effects.
• Follow the guidelines in chapter 5 on gastroenteritis and diarrhoea in this chapter.

ITCHY ANUS (PRURITUS ANI)

Not an uncommon problem in children and this can occur at any age. The principal causes are the laying of eggs by parasitic infestations, usually worms (threadworms, roundworms or tapeworms). Candida (thrush) infection, especially for infants still in nappies, trauma, eczema or piles (haemorrhoids – very unusual in children) may all be responsible.

One commonly overlooked possibility is that of food allergies.

RECOMMENDATIONS

General Advice

• Examine the anus first thing in the morning because eggs are laid at night. See **Worms**.
• Persistent itching should be reviewed by a physician for a clear diagnosis and reference made to the relevant sections in this book.
• Keep the area dry with non-medicated talcum powder.

Homeopathic

• The homeopathic remedy Aesculus 6 may be taken four times a day.

Herbal/natural extracts

• Hamamelis fluid extract diluted in iced water and applied to the rectum may be very soothing.
• Calendula cream may be of benefit but only applied for a few minutes each day.

LEAKY GUT SYNDROME (INCREASED INTESTINAL PERMEABILITY)

The small intestine acts like a selective sieve, allowing into the bloodstream only the breakdown products of digestion. Larger proteins, carbohydrates and fats are kept out permitting only the amino acids and short chain peptides (from proteins), monosaccharides or disaccharides (from carbohydrates), and small chain fatty acids (from fats) to enter the bloodstream. If anything larger is absorbed into the bloodstream, the body may set up an allergic or immune response. From that time on, if not treated, the body may recognize those basic foods as bacteria or viruses and, potentially, set up an attack.

Anything that inflames the bowel may cause leaky gut syndrome. Parasitic, fungal or yeast, bacterial and viral infection are often responsible. The most frequent causes are anything that diminishes the bowel's natural flora. These include antibiotics, either prescribed by the doctor or found inadvertently in processed foods. Chemical toxins such as pesticides, preservatives and additives may also be culprits.

Stress produces an acidic response from the stomach that can alter the bowel pH level and this may have an effect and excess adrenaline cuts down the blood flow to the bowel, reducing oxygen and nutrients, which causes deterioration of the bowel wall.

A study has drawn a connection between rheumatoid arthritis and a leaky gut and even the orthodox world has published a review supporting the possibility that multiple sclerosis is associated with the body recognizing protein sequences in foreign substances which resemble the body's own, thereby causing an attack on the nervous system. Other conditions with evidence of being caused or worsened by the presence of increased intestinal permeability are: inflammatory bowel disease (IBD), ankylosing spondylitis, Crohn's disease, allergic disorders such as asthma, hay fever and eczema, schizophrenia and migraine.

Testing for a Leaky Gut

The orthodox medical world does not yet recognize this as a medical condition. There are laboratories in the USA and one in the UK that test for this condition using a very simple method. A solution of inert (indigestible) molecules is drunk and the urine is then collected over the next six hours. A sample of this is sent to a laboratory. A certain percentage of the small molecules should have passed through the gut wall into the bloodstream and been filtered out by the kidneys into the urine. The larger molecules should not have got through, but instead pass out with the faeces. The presence of any large molecules in the urine indicates increased intestinal permeability – leaky gut syndrome.

At this time, instructions and collection kits can be sent to an individual (*see* details page 713). Once the sample is collected, it is sent directly to a laboratory and results are usually available within seven days.

RECOMMENDATIONS

General Advice

- *Test for a leaky gut. If a leaky gut is established, and symptoms of ill health can be associated with this condition, then treatment is a prerequisite for a return to good health.*
- *Test for bowel candidiasis, parasites and normal bowel flora.*

Nutritional

- *Remove anything that may irritate the bowel wall. This includes anything that may cause symptoms of indigestion or bloating.*
- *Specifically, stop using alcohol, refined sugars, spicy foods and caffeine.*
- *If candida or other yeasts/fungi are present, consider an anti-fermentation diet (see **Anti-Candida diet**).*

Supplemental

- *High dose acidophilus, preferably different strains each month for 3 months. Follow the product instructions – they are often to take 2 billion organisms (2 capsules) with each meal.*
- *L glutamine and/or glutathione 500mg three times daily for an adult and half the quantity for those aged 5 to 12 (below age 5, consult a physician).*

- *Any compound that can deliver oxygen to the bowel such as specialized clay or stabilized oxygen will help.*
- *A quality mixed antioxidant twice daily.*

Homeopathic

- *A choice of remedy should be made on the symptoms rather than on a diagnostic label.*

Herbal/natural extracts

- *Take advice from a qualified herbalist about extracts that kill E. coli and other 'bad' bacteria and parasites, but leave other bowel flora alone. Consider Berberis, Uva ursi, and Wormwood.*

Orthodox

- *At this time there is no established orthodox treatment.*

MALABSORPTION

The orthodox medical world recognizes malabsorption as an 'all or nothing' syndrome that occurs at any age but is most often seen in children. It is due to deficiencies in enzymes or oversensitivity of the immune system. An example of the former is lactose intolerance, where the body does not form the correct enzyme to break down milk sugar. Oversensitivity occurs in conditions such as coeliac disease where the body attacks gluten found predominantly in wheat and most other grains.

I believe that there is a considerable grey area where many individuals may not absorb a variety of nutrients from the bowel usually because of food intolerance creating inflammation in the small intestine.

Any symptoms ranging from mild tiredness and depression through to major malabsorption syndromes will cause failure to thrive or grow and decrease learning abilities. Physical illnesses will follow but are generally not the symptoms that bring malabsorption to a parent's or physician's attention.

Malabsorption may occur because of a failure of the body to produce the right digestive juices. Achlorhydria is an accepted orthodox condition describing an inability of the stomach to produce hydrochloric acid. In fact, diminished production of this acid may have a profound effect on absorption. The alternative medical world is aware of this not uncommon problem and specific tests can be done to establish if low acid concentration is present. Most digestion occurs because of enzymes produced by the pancreas. A deficient pancreatic exocrine function (an exocrine gland is one that produces a substance that does not pass directly into the bloodstream) is another factor well-recognized by complementary practitioners and will also cause malabsorption due to a poor ability to break down the foods.

RECOMMENDATIONS

General Advice

- *Any developmental delay or failure to thrive must be reviewed by a paediatrician. Specific blood tests can be obtained to establish which foods or nutrients are not being absorbed.*
- *Any history of antibiotic use or bowel disturbance may suggest leaky gut syndrome. Specific treatment under the care of an experienced complementary medical practitioner to deal with allergic responses and to correct the imbalance in the bowel is required.*

Supplemental

- *Replenishment of deficiencies may make a difference if high-strength supplements are given but this may not make a difference if the body is incapable of absorbing. Intravenous administration is rarely required but may be considered.*
- *Please note that hydrochloric acid and pancreatic supplementation should only be administered to children under medical supervision.*

Homeopathic

- *Genetic deficiencies in enzyme production are unlikely to be treatable but constitutional homeopathic prescribing by an experienced homeopath may make a difference.*
- *The homeopathic remedy Silica encourages*

absorption and should be taken at potency 30 twice a day for two weeks. If a response is noted increase the potency to 200 for three nights and repeat monthly if the effect wears off.

Orthodox

- *Enquire about non-invasive investigations of hydrochloric acid and pancreatic enzyme production (see **Gastrograms** and **Pancreatic exocrine tests** in chapter 8).*
- *If required or if non-invasive tests are not available, try a hydrochloric acid supplement a few minutes before each meal. If a warm glow occurs, then reduce the amount or strength of the acid supplement.*
- *There are two types of naturopathic pancreatic supplement that may be tried if non-invasive investigations are not available: the first stimulates the pancreas to produce more enzymes and is generally made out of a selection of herbs; the second is usually an extract from the pancreas of an animal and acts directly on foodstuffs. Follow the instructions on the packaging as instructed by the practitioner.*

PYLORIC STENOSIS

Food is mixed with acid in the stomach and is passed through a valve known as the pylorus into the duodenum, the start of the small intestine. Some children are born with a congenital thickness of this valve, which causes a narrowing (stenosis).

A child or infant will show a characteristic projectile vomit due to the stomach compressing harder in order to force food through the stenosis but, in fact, pushing food up past the much weaker oesophageal stomach valve. The vomit is generally fermented food. The infant will not be growing and will be persistently hungry, therefore whining. The child may only want very small feeds because discomfort occurs if the stomach is filled and a diagnosis of constipation may be falsely suggested because the child only passes small amounts infrequently.

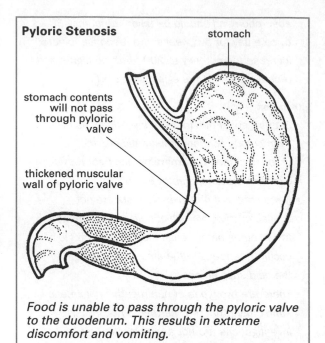

Pyloric Stenosis

stomach

stomach contents will not pass through pyloric valve

thickened muscular wall of pyloric valve

Food is unable to pass through the pyloric valve to the duodenum. This results in extreme discomfort and vomiting.

On occasions a knot may be felt in the upper part of the abdomen below the sternum (chest bone).

RECOMMENDATIONS

General Advice
• *Any failure to thrive or a persistently uncomfortable child must be reviewed by a doctor or paediatrician.*

Nutritional
• *Nutritional deficiencies may have set in and a consultation with a nutritionist postoperatively is recommended to ensure a well-balanced high-calorific diet.*

Orthodox
• *Pyloric stenosis requires an operative procedure (see Operations and surgery).*

STOMACH UPSETS – *see* Gastroenteritis, Diarrhoea and Abdominal pains.

VOLVULUS
When the bowel develops, a mesh known as the mesentery is attached to the 30 feet of intestine. This provides blood vessels to and from the bowel walls and also contains the nerves and lymphatic systems. This mesentery should be a fairly tight sheet but in rare cases may develop loosely, thereby not functioning as a fixator of the bowel. This allows the bowel to twist upon itself and may occlude the lumen, the space inside the intestine, and in severe cases, this will compromise its circulation. This most commonly occurs in the sigmoid colon (lower part of the bowel) and can occur at any stage of life. Pain and symptoms of obstruction, such as bloating and constipation, arise and if not fixed quickly can result in bowel ischaemia and gangrene.

RECOMMENDATIONS

General Advice
• *Any abdominal pain that is severe or persistent must be reviewed by a doctor.*

Orthodox
• *Volvulus requires surgical repair (see Operations and surgery).*

WORMS
Infection of the intestine in human beings is a mild problem in Britain and other Westernized countries, but can be chronically debilitating in the tropics.

Roundworms (nematodes) and threadworms (pinworms)
These white worms can grow up to a centimetre long and are found specifically in children all over the world. They live in the colon and rectum and travel down to the anal margin to lay their eggs, usually at night. The result is an itchy anus, which is the principal symptom. Irritability and insomnia are other factors.

Worms may be seen in the faeces or even protruding from the anus and a simple diagnostic procedure is to place a piece of adhesive cellophane (such as Sellotape) across the anus and, folding the adhesive sides together, take this sample to a

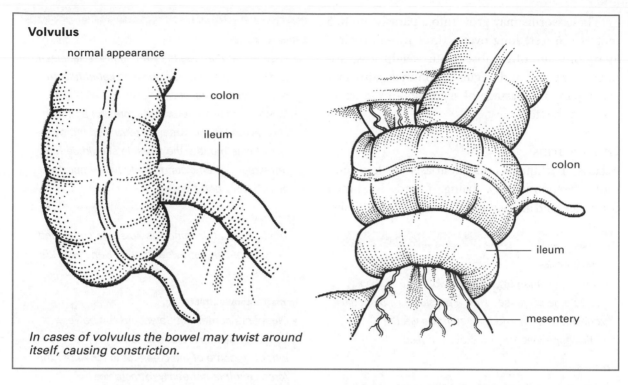

Volvulus

normal appearance

colon

ileum

colon

ileum

mesentery

In cases of volvulus the bowel may twist around itself, causing constriction.

laboratory or GP's surgery for examination under a microscope. The eggs may be visible.

Whipworms

These are very common parasites, with the worms growing up to half a centimetre in length and tending to attach themselves to the first part of the large bowel. Symptoms are extremely uncommon unless a child is malnourished, when bloody diarrhoea or rectal prolapse may actually occur.

Toxocariasis

This is not to be confused with toxoplasmosis, which is a parasitic infection also contracted from cats and specifically dangerous in pregnancy.

This condition is an accidental infection from cat or dog faeces. The worms do not develop in humans but if the larvae are ingested they travel via the bloodstream into major organs, where they die causing obstruction of blood vessels.

Tapeworms (cestodes)

Tapeworms normally share two hosts: the worm living in the intestine of one organism and the larvae normally in the muscles of another. In human beings the most common tapeworms are *Taenia saginata* and *Taenia solium*. The former exists in beef and the latter in pork.

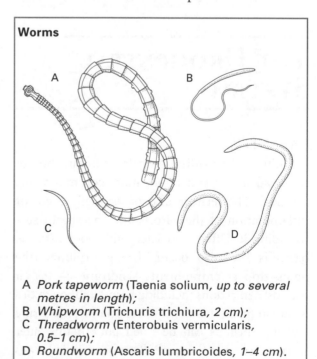

Worms

A

B

C

D

A *Pork tapeworm* (Taenia solium, *up to several metres in length*);
B *Whipworm* (Trichuris trichiura, *2 cm*);
C *Threadworm* (Enterobuis vermicularis, *0.5–1 cm*);
D *Roundworm* (Ascaris lumbricoides, *1–4 cm*).

These worms may grow into a parasite up to 5 metres (26 feet) long over a three-month period. Symptoms are often absent but weight loss, disturbed appetite and vague abdominal pains may accompany the passage of segments of the worm noted in the stool.

Other worms

Ascaris, Trichinosis and Filoariasis are less common, predominantly being found in hotter countries, and are beyond the scope of this book.

RECOMMENDATIONS

General Advice

- *Any symptoms suggestive of worm infestation should be discussed with a physician who should check the anus and take samples via the stickytape method and stool samples.*

Orthodox

- *Treatment with orthodox antihelminthic drugs is safe and recommended. Remember that the whole family group and possibly the school class should be treated as well.*

THE UROGENITAL SYSTEM

BALANITIS

Balanitis is the medical term for inflammation of the head of the penis and, more commonly, the foreskin. The term is also occasionally used for inflammation of the clitoris and the sheath surrounding it. Often associated with poor hygiene, balanitis can also occur through trauma (the penis–zipper entrapment syndrome – as it sounds!), infections including herpes (although this is rare in infants) and, most importantly, make sure diabetes mellitus can be ruled out. In this latter situation, sugar in the urine allows bacteria and yeasts to multiply rapidly causing irritated inflammation.

RECOMMENDATIONS

General Advice

- *Ensure that the area is clean and that nappies or underwear are dry. Use non-medicated talcum powder in abundance.*
- *Slowly, but surely, retract the foreskin as the child ages. Do not force the retraction but by the age of nine months the foreskin should be fully retractable. Then clean this VIP (very important place) every bathtime.*

Homeopathic

- *The homeopathic remedies Apis, Mercurius and Causticum can be reviewed and given every 2hr at potency 6.*

Herbal/natural extracts

- *Ointments containing Calendula can be very soothing. Being careful and tender, try to introduce some of the cream or lotion under the foreskin if it is not easily retractable.*

Orthodox

- *Persistence of inflammation should be reviewed by a GP and in rare circumstances circumcision may need to be considered (see **Circumcision**).*

BEDWETTING

Urinating in the bed is only a problem if it occurs beyond a certain age. This age is very variable. About 10 per cent of children will still be wetting the bed at five years of age and intervention and treatment should only be considered if the child is still wetting the bed after the age of seven or eight years. Occasional bedwetting can occur in association with fevers and urinary tract infections in children and adults of all ages. Incontinence associated with old age is discussed elsewhere (*see* **Incontinence**).

Children should understand the concept and feeling of a full bladder at about the age of two years. Control and requesting to go to the toilet should occur by three years of age and control at night follows on from that.

Most commonly bedwetting is associated with stress. This may be apparent or subconscious and may be associated with the child or the atmosphere in the home or school. Children are extremely intuitive and problems between parents, however well disguised from the child, may often be the cause. Infections (bacterial or parasitical, such as worms), diabetes and food intolerance can all be physical causes and need to be ruled out before psychological causes are assumed.

RECOMMENDATIONS

General Advice

- *Have a urine sample checked by your local GP.*
- *Ensure that the child does not drink too much fluid within 2hr of bedtime.*
- *Ensure that the child urinates before bed and awaken the child to go to the toilet again prior to your going to bed.*
- *A visit to the osteopath, chiropractor or craniosacral therapist can be instantly curative if there is any structural imbalance in the lower spine or pelvis, which in turn puts pressure on the nerves to the bladder.*
- *Electro-acupuncture may help treat bedwetting in children who do not respond to other therapies.*

Homeopathic

- *Provided that there is no obvious physical cause, consider the following homeopathic remedies by referring to your homeopathic manual: Plantago, Equisetum and Kreosotum. A less well-known remedy and therefore difficult to read about is Ilex paraguayensis. Use potency 6, four pills nightly for three weeks and if improvement is not persistent obtain higher potencies until resolution is achieved.*

CIRCUMCISION
Male circumcision

Circumcision is the removal of the loose skin (known as the foreskin) found at the head of the penis. The medical reasons for circumcisions include a narrow opening (*see* **Phimosis**), balanitis (*see* **Balanitis**) or trauma such as the penis–zipper entrapment syndrome (self-explanatory!). There are no other medical reasons to perform this traumatic surgery. There is no benefit with regard to cleanliness provided that good hygiene is followed and the foreskin is retracted at bathtime. There is no sexual enhancement one way or the other, although an uncircumcised penis may be slightly more sensitive.

Religious reasons need to be respected, although some of the techniques of circumcision are only little short of barbaric and run high risk of complications, which at worst can lead to penis amputation and enforced gender changing in children. To perform circumcision without good hygienic preparation, preferably in a surgical unit, or without anaesthetic, is medically and, in my opinion, morally unacceptable. The concept that infants do not remember pain is unproved and the effects on a child's psyche when pain is created, apparently with parental approval, may have much deeper and more profound effects in the long term.

Circumcision for cosmetic reasons, like any self-mutilation on narcissistic grounds, should be considered only after time spent with a counsellor and assessment of the effects that social pressures, usually from advertising, have created. I am considerably against circumcision for anything other than medical reasons without available alternatives.

The foreskin is a protective sheath that may be of use if left attached and its removal can offer no benefit. The argument that the foreskin allows the harbouring of potentially infectious material such as human papilloma virus (genital warts) or other infectious agents is not acceptable provided that good hygiene is followed.

RECOMMENDATIONS

General Advice

- *Unless recommended by a GP, do not circumcise.*
- *If any complication whatsoever or however mild appears, such as swelling, bleeding or redness, please contact your doctor without hesitation.*

Herbal/natural extracts

- *If circumcision is to go ahead, then prepare the*

---

area by applying an Arnica or Calendula (or both) cream at least three times a day five days prior to the operative procedure.

Orthodox
- *See **Operations and surgery**.*

Female circumcision

Certain cultures remove the protective hood from around the clitoris and, unbelievably, remove the clitoris itself.

This barbaric act is unconscionable and potentially extremely risky both from a health point of view and a psychological one.

RECOMMENDATIONS

General Advice
- *Endeavour to do your best to avoid this operation.*
- *If unavoidable, ensure that the poor individual is prepared for an operative procedure by following the guidelines in this book.*

PHIMOSIS (NON-RETRACTABLE FORESKIN)

Occasionally children are born with a constricted foreskin that does not allow for retraction. This can cause constriction over the exit of the urethra, which can create an obstruction to the outflow of urine. This can create a ballooning under the foreskin with a high-pressure stream through the small, narrowed outlet.

RECOMMENDATIONS

General Advice
- *Do not try to force back the foreskin, because this will lead to tears and potential infection.*

Orthodox
- *The situation should be reviewed by a specialist because an operative procedure, including circumcision, may be required.*
- *If an operation is considered, see **Circumcision**.*

UNDESCENDED TESTICLE

The testes develop within the abdominal cavity through the foetal stage. They travel down into the scrotum either just before birth or within the first few weeks after. As they descend, they bring with them blood vessels, lymphatic vessels and nerves and travel down the inguinal canal.

In some cases, for no known reason, the testes fail to descend. This is sometimes associated with short vessels that do not stretch, thereby impeding descent.

The testes hang away from the body and the scrotum because they function at a lower temperature than the body would provide. Failure to descend or entrapment within the inguinal canal will prevent maturity and the ability to produce sperm.

RECOMMENDATIONS

Homeopathic
- *Undescended testes by the age of one year may be treated by the homeopathic remedy Clematis 200, one pill each night for three nights. If there is no effect over the next month then use the remedy Aurum metallicum 200, one dose each night for three nights.*

Orthodox
- *Surgical intervention may be necessary and this is usually performed after the age of three years. See **Operations and surgery** if this avenue is to be taken.*

STRUCTURAL MATTERS

ACHES AND PAINS

All children have aches and pains. The term 'growing pains' is often bandied around and refers to the stretching of tendons and ligaments created by the child's growth. There is rarely anything to worry about although persisting discomfort, especially around joints, should be brought to the attention of a physician. Certain deficiencies and dehydration can cause mild problems and need to be corrected.

RECOMMENDATIONS

General Advice

- *Do not underestimate the power of a kiss on the injured part.*
- *Gentle heating and massage of the area will help.*
- *Dehydration is a common cause of aches and pains. Ensure that your child is drinking enough water, very diluted juice or herbal teas. Aim at half a pint per foot of height per day.*
- *Persisting pain without an obvious cause should be reviewed initially by an osteopath or chiropractor. If relief is not forthcoming then a paediatrician should be approached.*

Supplemental

- *Minor deficiencies of calcium, magnesium, zinc and copper can all be culprits for aches and pains. A good diet should be adequate but sometimes mineral supplementation is beneficial.*

Herbal/natural extracts

- *Chamomile tea can be very soothing.*

Please note that any aches and pains that are altering the child's gait (walking) should be assessed by an osteopath or other body worker specializing in children.

BROKEN BONES AND FRACTURES

See chapter 4 for the principal information on fractures.

Children heal quickly but have a tendency to misbehave whilst having a broken bone, which can lead to a delay in repair. It is important to maintain a watchful eye. Fractures that occur near the growing points of bones need to be monitored by orthopaedic specialists. Definitely see an osteopath to encourage alignment to take the pressure off the opposite side of the body. Remedies can be used as for young adult fractures but *do not* administer a comfrey remedy to a child.

THE FEET

CARE OF THE FEET

The feet may be considered phenomenal when one reflects on exactly what they do and the way we treat them. We cram them into tight socks, shove them into often ill-fitting shoes and pay scant regard to their hygiene despite their use and tendency to sweat in their cramped environment. We then stand on them, walk with them and with each step place our entire body weight on the three

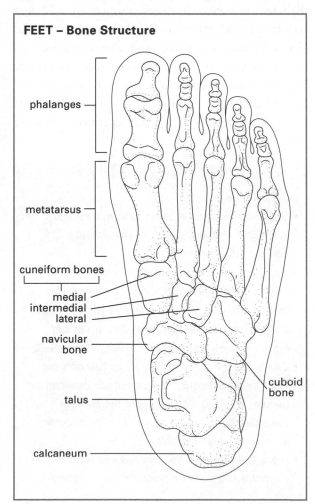

FEET – Bone Structure

phalanges

metatarsus

cuneiform bones

medial
intermedial
lateral

navicular
bone

talus

cuboid
bone

calcaneum

square inches that we call the ball of our feet. The feet contain small blood vessels that, when we are standing, have the effect of gravity pulling blood into them and then we get surprised when our feet swell! The bones and muscles, despite the weight they carry, tend to be very resilient and rarely cramp but infrequently do we spend any time relaxing these hard-working parts of our body.

The Eastern philosophies also consider the feet to be our connection with Mother Earth but rarely do we spend time with our feet directly on the ground. I find it interesting that the masters of yoga will spend time upside down and in the lotus position with the soles of the feet facing the sky, thereby creating a potential connection between our 'soles' and heaven.

Any diseases of the arteries through smoking, diabetes or a genetic predisposition to cold feet require special attention to the feet because the blood vessels are small and any occlusion, as found in the above conditions, can discourage healing. Diabetics in particular may have neurological deficits and therefore not be aware of damage to their feet; special attention must be paid to this area.

RECOMMENDATIONS

General Advice
- *Spend as much time as possible in bare feet, preferably with some of that time allowing contact with the earth.*
- *Ensure that socks and shoes are loose fitting.*
- *Ensure cleanliness of all parts of the body but pay special attention to the feet and between the toes. This is a very comfortable area for warmth and moisture to encourage bacterial and fungal growth.*
- *Careful cleaning and drying, especially between the toes, is essential. The use of non-medicated talcum powder is encouraged if the feet are sweaty or if any length of time is to be spent in socks and/or shoes.*
- *If possible spend a few minutes each day with the soles of the feet exposed to direct sunlight.*

- *Any injury should be treated with respect. The blood vessels in the feet are small and injuries may not receive a good blood supply.*

ATHLETE'S FOOT

Athlete's foot is characterized by a red, itching and peeling skin generally between and around the gaps in the toes. This is created by a fungus usually (*see* **Tinea versicolor**), although secondary bacterial infection can make the condition worse.

Most commonly contracted from damp changing room or swimming room floors, the condition usually responds to good foot hygiene.

RECOMMENDATIONS

General Advice
- *Treatment is often unnecessary if the basics of foot hygiene are followed (see* **Care of the feet***).*
- *Always keep the feet dry and use non-medicated talc.*
- *Spend as much time barefoot as possible, keeping in mind that these fungal infections are transmittable.*

Herbal/natural extracts
- *Tea tree oil, applied in a concentrated oil and then dried with a hair dryer, is beneficial.*
- *Rub crushed garlic onto the affected areas, leave for 20min, wash off and dry thoroughly. Calendula ointment can be used similarly.*
- *For resistant infections, apply grapefruit extract twice a day for one week.*

Orthodox
- *Avoid orthodox preparations if possible. They can lead to resistant strains of fungus that are harder to clear up.*

CLUB FOOT – *see* Talipes

FLAT FEET

The inner, middle aspect of the foot is supposed to have an arch. There is no particular amount of arching that is healthy or unhealthy but if this part of the anatomy rests flat on the ground then the individual has flat feet. This is not a problem unless there are pains in the feet, a persistence or occurrence of discomfort in other parts of the body, especially the lower back and lower limb joints, or if running is painful or ungainly.

The arch of the foot is created by the muscles and ligaments around that part of the anatomy. As these tighten and develop the arch is raised. A child's foot is very often flat and the arch will develop once the child is walking.

RECOMMENDATIONS

General Advice

- *Treatment for flat feet is not required unless any of the above criteria for discomfort are apparent.*
- *Correct-fitting shoes with a raised arch will be fitted and prescribed by podiatrists who should be consulted.*
- *Discomfort will be relieved by reflexology and a cranial osteopath, osteopath or chiropractor should by consulted if there are pains elsewhere.*
- *Walking barefooted and specific foot exercises can be discussed with the podiatrist.*
- *If there is any alteration of gait when walking or running, then a visit to an Alexander Technician to discuss posture is recommended.*

FUNGAL INFECTIONS OF THE FEET – *see* Athlete's foot

HOT OR BURNING SENSATIONS IN THE FEET

This is a surprisingly common symptom often found in individuals who have had the symptom all their lives and take it for granted. Indeed, there may be no particular disease process associated and it may simply be an awareness on the part of these individuals.

Certain diseases such as multiple sclerosis, other neurological conditions and diabetes may all create neurological damage that sends impulses to the brain, indicating heat in the area, even though there may not be anything excessive.

Burning feet may be an indication of nutritional deficiency, particularly folic acid, vitamin B_{12} and other vitamins within the higher complexes.

Eastern philosophy may consider that heat in the feet is an indication of a block in the lower chakras, thereby causing excess energy to remain in the lower limbs.

RECOMMENDATIONS

General Advice

- *Persisting heat or burning sensations in the feet should be assessed by a medical practitioner to rule out serious underlying conditions.*
- *Sometimes, but rarely, cold applications on a persistent basis may make a difference.*
- *If the above treatments do not relieve the situation then some form of energy release under the hands of a healer, acupuncturist or Shiatsu practitioner may release a block in the pelvis allowing the energy to flow more freely and relieve the pressure on the feet.*

Supplemental

- *Take three times the daily recommended dose of any zinc and B complex (ensure that it contains vitamin B_{12}) for at least three weeks.*

Homeopathic

- *Discuss the problem with a homeopath because many remedies have burning feet as part of their symptom picture but correlation with the individual's constitution as a whole is more likely to find the right remedy.*

SHOES

The selection of shoes is extremely important, as is ensuring that socks are not too tightly fitting. Tight-fitting shoes will alter the very delicate bone structures in infants' feet and the same can be said up until growing has stopped at the age of 20 years or so. Shoes should be measured both for length and width, be comfortable and lined with natural material to avoid sweating.

Many persistent backaches, whether neck or lower back, are created by malalignment of the pelvis, which, in turn, can be created by one leg being longer than the other. This is corrected by accurately fitted inner soles or additions to the heel and external soles of shoes.

RECOMMENDATIONS

General Advice

• *Ensure that shoes are fitted by accurate measurement of a child's feet and not by fashion consciousness.*

• *Ensure, to the best of your ability, that shoes are made out of natural materials and that the inner lining allows 'breathing' and sweat absorption.*

SWEATY FEET

Sweaty feet, like hot or burning feet, are not necessarily an indication of ill-heath and may simply be a genetic predisposition.

RECOMMENDATION

General Advice

• *See* **Hot or burning sensations in the feet**.

TALIPES (CLUB FOOT)

This condition is present at birth and is character-ized by one foot or both feet being angled inwards and pointing downwards. Medically speaking, club foot can also represent an outward and upward deformity of the ankle and foot.

RECOMMENDATIONS

General Advice

• *Assessment is best made by an orthopaedic surgeon.*

• *Doctors, chiropodists, and some osteopaths and chiropractors will be able to show parents massage techniques that may correct this condition. The use of Arnica cream whilst using this technique is beneficial.*

• *Splinting may be necessary.*

Orthodox

• *Surgical intervention is sometimes required. If so, see* **Operations and surgery**.

THE SKIN

BITES
Human and animal

It is not uncommon for anyone to be subjected to the bite of an insect, animal or human being. I talk about bites in the chapter on childhood because bites tend to occur more often at this age. Treatment is, however, similar for all age groups.

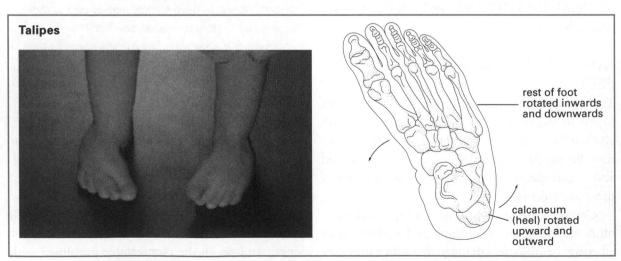

Talipes

rest of foot rotated inwards and downwards

calcaneum (heel) rotated upward and outward

A bite is of no consequence unless it breaks the skin. Once this has occurred and the outer protection of the body has been breached, however minor the abrasion may appear, treatment is essential. Human bites are particularly problematic because the mouth carries many viruses and parasites that are extremely aggressive. The same can be said for animal bites, the most infamous of which is the bite of an animal carrying rabies. Insect bites (as opposed to stings – *see* **Stings**) may well inject poison into the area at the same time. Reptilian (snake) bites and their associated venom vary appreciably in danger but all need medical attention.

General Advice

- *Any bite that breaks the skin should be assessed by an orthodox physician, preferably in an accident and emergency department.*
- *With any bite, flush the area immediately with running water and soak the injury in a heavy saltwater solution (five tablespoons per pint of water) with any available antiseptic but preferably five teaspoonfuls of Calendula and/or Hypericum lotion.*
- *Human bites are notorious and must be flushed out immediately. The same can be said for other animal bites.*
- *In dealing with a snake bite, ignore everything that you have seen in cowboy movies. Do not use a tourniquet and if you are going to suck the poison out of the wounds do not cut it first and do not consider this procedure if you have any obvious cuts or sores in the mouth. Keep the victim resting because activity will increase the heart rate and move the poison around the body quicker.*

Homeopathic

- *If there is any suggestion that the animal is rabid, obtain the homeopathic remedy Hydrophobinum, potency 30, 12 or 6, and take one dose every 10min as soon as it is obtained.*

Do not delay going to the hospital, however.

- *You will be advised to have a tetanus injection and whether you do or do not have one, use the remedy Hypericum, potency 30, 12 or 6, four pills every 15min for the first hour and then every 2hr for three days.*

Herbal/natural extracts

- *Apply Arnica, Calendula and/or Hypericum or Urtica creams.*

Orthodox

- *If bitten by an animal or insect, try to capture it or at the very least memorize close details of it. Antivenom serum is very specific and being able to remember the markings on a snake is of vital importance to the emergency team.*

BURNS

Burns are liable to occur at any time but are most worrying in children. A six-inch square area of a burn on an adult may represent two per cent of skin damage but on an infant it may represent up to 20

Skin Percentages

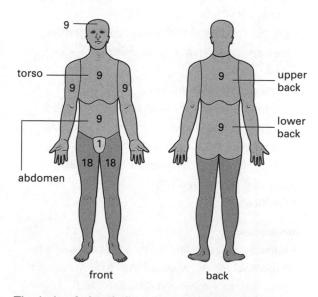

front   back

The 'rule of nines' gives the percentages of the surface area of skin for each section of the adult body. However, the results are not the same for children due to their differential growth rates.

per cent. The skin is essential for many processes including protecting from germ invasion and holding fluid in the body. Loss of skin through burning can allow fluid loss very rapidly. The greater the area of skin that is damaged, the greater the fluid loss and the larger the risk to the individual.

Burns are described as:

- **First degree** when only the superficial layer of skin is damaged.
- **Second degree** when the superficial and middle layers are involved but the deep layer where reproduction of the skin occurs is still intact.
- **Third degree** when the skin, including its basal layer or skin manufacturing layer, is destroyed.

Third-degree burns, if they are small, may have skin growth from around the area but if they are too large they will require skin grafting.

RECOMMENDATIONS

General Advice

- *Any burn that breaks the skin or weeps should be assessed by a GP.*
- *Any burn greater than three per cent of the body area should be viewed in an emergency department.*
- *Apply cold water immediately.*
- *Contrary to many old-wives' tales, do not apply butter or oils (the area will fry) and do not burst blisters.*
- *Do not remove clothing from a burned area unless it falls away easily.*
- *See* **Sunburn***.*

Homeopathic

- *Consider the remedies Arnica and Urtica urens for superficial burns, Arnica and Kali bichromicum for second-degree burns and Causticum and Hypericum if the pain of the burn persists. Take potency 6 of any of these every 10min.*

Herbal/natural extracts

- *Arnica, Calendula or Hypericum fluid extracts should be applied, three tablespoons to a pint of water.*
- *Apply Aloe vera, Calendula, Hypericum or Urtica gels or lotions continuously.*

CHAFFING

Although chaffing can occur at any age, it is most commonly found in children because their intolerance of cold when they are playing outside seems to be greater. Chaffing is a medical term for the breakdown of the superficial layers of the skin, allowing dryness and cracks to appear due to a combination of dryness and cold.

RECOMMENDATIONS

General Advice

- *Avoid using moisturizers, chapsticks, etc, because this leads to a dependency in that part of the body. In severe conditions where the elements are unavoidable, such as when skiing or sailing, then short-term use is acceptable.*
- *Skin is best moisturized and healed from within, so ensure good hydration and suitable nutritional intake in the form of fruit and vegetables.*

Supplemental

- *If damage has occurred, administer the following supplements in the dosage suggested per one foot of height: vitamin A (1,000iu), vitamin C (500mg), vitamin E (100iu) and zinc (2.5mg). These should be given in divided doses with meals.*

Herbal/natural extracts

- *The use of Arnica or Calendula creams for short periods is effective and acceptable.*

CHILBLAINS

Chilblains are painful swellings usually found on the extremities, such as toes and fingers. In severe cases the swelling may cause the skin to break down and secondary infection may compound the problems.

Chilblains are caused by poor peripheral (capillary) circulation and are brought about by the affected part becoming cold. The skin is more likely to break down if the area is damp as well. Principally this is a problem with the circulation as a whole and topical intervention may be of benefit, but a deeper look at the miasm or chronic tendency of the individual and their ancestors to have poor circulation is a much more profound treatment.

RECOMMENDATIONS

General Advice
- *In acute cases ensure that the area stays warm. It is a fallacy to believe that socks and shoes necessarily keep the feet warm. Tight-fitting footware will actually impede circulation and make the problem worse. Loose woolly socks in slightly oversized shoes are a must for sufferers.*
- *Gentle warming with warm hands or other dry, warm applications can be most relieving.*
- *Rotating the arm at the shoulder or the foot at the knee will pull blood into the peripheries.*
- *In adults only, a tot of alcohol daily can increase peripheral circulation. An excess of alcohol will create a rebound effect causing initial increase in circulation but a latter and prolonged decrease.*

Homeopathic
- *The homeopathic remedies Petroleum 6 and Agaricus 6, one dose every 2hr, may be beneficial in acute cases but prolonged or chronic conditions require a homeopathic prescription based on the individual as a whole.*

Herbal/natural extracts
- *In persistent or mild conditions of poor peripheral circulation, high doses of cayenne pepper extract and then lowered maintenance doses can be beneficial if taken over three months or more.*
- *If the chilblains are causing itching when warmed, a cream containing Calendula, Arnica and Urtica can be most soothing.*

CHONDYLOMATA – *see* Warts and verrucas

COLD SORES – *see* Herpes simplex

CRADLE CAP

Cradle cap is characterized by crusty patches on the scalp created by an over-production from the scalp (and skin) of the natural oil known as sebum. The sebum dries over and under the skin, which is why picking or trying to remove the unsightly condition will inevitably lead to bleeding and the possibility of secondary infection.

A study of 11,458 children showed an uncomfortable 50 per cent correlation between infants with cradle cap going on to develop atopic eczema. This means that any parent whose baby has cradle cap should be wary of their child developing eczema and take suitable precautions where possible. (*See* **Eczema**).

RECOMMENDATIONS

General Advice
- *Frequent shampooing (even if there is not much hair) will speed up the process. If there is hair, do not shampoo more than three times a week because this will take out the natural oils.*
- *One teaspoon of lemon juice in two tablespoons of olive oil applied to the scalp twice a day may help.*
- *Do not pick.*
- *Gentle massage and brushing with soft bristles will encourage faster flaking.*

CUTS AND ABRASIONS

These can occur at any age, of course, and the treatment is much the same.

RECOMMENDATIONS

General Advice
SEVERE CUTS
- *Remove any debris or dirt with fingers or tweezers as soon as possible.*
- *Heavy bleeding should be stemmed by applying a clean material to the wound with suitable*

pressure. Medical assistance and assessment should be obtained as soon as possible.

- *Rarely, if localized pressure is not stemming the blood flow then occlusion of the artery higher up the limb may be considered by tying any material tightly. This should not be done except in exceptional circumstances.*

MINOR CUTS

- *Clean the wound with water, preferably previously boiled, but tap water or stream water is perfectly acceptable.*
- *If bleeding is persistent, obtain a medical assessment in case a stitch is required.*

Herbal/natural extracts

- *Apply a Calendula-based cream. Take Arnica potency 6 every half hour for three doses and then every three hours until pain has resolved.*

ECZEMA (DERMATITIS)

Eczema is a simple term for what is a complicated condition. Many people have their own idea of what eczema is but, medically speaking, it is characterized by irregular skin patterns with various characteristics. Eczema may be nothing more than a dry scaly patch of skin or it may be characterized by redness, swelling, cracking and dry or exudative lesions. This damaged skin is more open to infection and therefore there may be associated pimples or pus.

Contrary to popular belief, eczema is not always a longstanding or chronic condition and may occur as an acute condition arising as quickly as it may disappear. By definition, eczema has no recognized orthodox cause and, strictly speaking, any rash that resembles eczema that has a known cause, such as topical irritants, staphylococcal infections or food/drug allergy reactions, should be referred to as dermatitis. Very often, lay-medical books will refer to dermatitis and eczema as the same thing.

Despite eczema occasionally being exudative of clear fluid (serum), the main characteristic is dryness and redness. Eastern medical philosophies consider eczema to be a condition of excess heat, although the serum may be an attempt to correct the problem, in which case this form of eczema would be considered to be 'damp heat'. Alternative therapies are therefore geared towards finding the cause of this excess heat and removing it. There may be genetic predispositions to eczema (as there is in asthma and hay fever) and in these cases the eczema is known as *atopic* eczema.

Hahnemann, the father of homeopathy, formulated the medical belief of the presence of deep-seated tendencies or problems he called miasms (*see* **Homeopathy**). One of these miasms was known as the psoric or psora which is manifest by skin eruptions, and Hahnemann believed that $7/8$ of all chronic illnesses were ascribed to suppression of skin conditions. Indeed, in the centuries before the advent of the suppressive effects of steroids, many diseases showed themselves initially through the skin. As homeopaths fervently believe in the transmission of a disease process from one generation to the other until treated effectively, skin conditions and particularly eczema are looked at as a problem of the

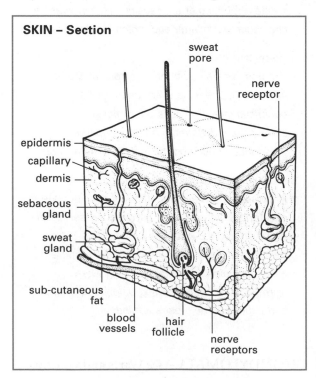

SKIN – Section

sweat pore

nerve receptor

epidermis

capillary

dermis

sebaceous gland

sweat gland

sub-cutaneous fat

blood vessels

hair follicle

nerve receptors

internal working of the body rather than as an actual problem with the skin and frequently 'passed on' from generation to generation.

The skin is certainly a remarkable organ having many functions. It is directly or indirectly related to most other organs and systems in the body and therefore when dealing with a skin problem one must look closely at the body as a whole. The skin acts as protection and contains many of the facets of the immune system; it can absorb and excrete, performing functions similar to the lung and the kidneys (sweat and urine are very similar in composition); and the skin can transform sunlight into chemicals that are both protective and essential to our well-being, such as melanin (our tanning process) and the production of vitamin D (essential for our survival).

The skin is also a reflector of our emotional state, becoming, for example, pink with embarrassment, red with anger and white with fear. The skin, therefore, according to Eastern philosophies, reflects the inherent energy of the heart, lung, liver and the nervous system because all of these organs have associated emotional states.

When the skin misbehaves, therefore, the answer may be an associated underlying condition affecting any of our organs.

RECOMMENDATIONS

General Advice

- *Eczema must be treated holistically and as far as possible without suppression. Very often the condition is so severe that steroids or natural equivalents are necessary, but they should be used only in conjunction with a complementary medical view and then only sparingly.*
- *A tablespoon full of sodium bicarbonate in a pint of warm or cool water (depending on which is most soothing) may reduce the itch.*
- *Ensure that no chemicals, including medicated soaps or shampoos, come into contact with the skin. Water, glycerine soaps or aqueous cream should be the only cleansers.*

- *The close connection of the psyche with the skin requires that stress management techniques are employed. If the patient is old enough, then psychotherapy, hypnotherapy or techniques such as neurolinguistic programming (NLP) should be instigated. If the child is too young, then massage techniques should be employed. It is important to understand that a child's stress may be a reflection of the anxiety levels within the house and that unhappy parents or siblings may need counselling in order for the child's skin to clear up.*
- *Low levels of hydrochloric acid in the stomach, i.e. hypochlorhydria, is a common finding in patients with eczema. This decreased ability to break down foods may lead to the absorption of larger food molecules, leading to allergic responses. Tests to check for hydrochloric acid secretion are available through a complementary medical practitioner and should be checked.*

Nutritional

- *Eczema may be a reflection of food intolerance or allergy. Assessment through Vega or bioresonance computers, as well as blood tests, is recommended in resistant cases.*

Supplemental

- *The following vitamins and supplements should be taken in amounts recommended by a specialist: vitamin A, vitamin E, copper, flax seed and gamma-linoleic acid.*

Homeopathic

- *Review eczema with a homeopathic practitioner in conjunction with a Chinese or Tibetan doctor. Remember, however, that many herbal treatments, although effective, are plant steroid-based and may be suppressive.*
- *In acute eczema the homeopathic remedies Psorinum, Calcarea carbonica and Graphites can be used at potency 6 every 2hr until your complementary medical specialist is consulted.*

Herbal/natural extracts

- *Dry eczema can be treated and protected from infection by the use of Calendula or Urtica creams, vitamin E cream or non-medicated petroleum jelly extracts.*
- *A base massage oil may have Roman chamomile, lavender or neroli essential oils added, which can be soothing if not curative.*
- *Extracts from the fruit and bark of the Kigelia africana tree can be applied topically.*

IMPETIGO

This bacterial infection, usually caused by a staphylococcal bacteria, is most commonly found in children but can occur at any age. It is generally an indication of a weakened immune system because staphylococcal bacteria are usually commensal (they live on us without any harm being caused). Use of antibiotics or antiseptic creams and lotions can lead to resistant strains that are tougher for the body to deal with and often result in a staphylococcal or impetigo infection.

It is important to recognize these blisters, which appear in a red rash, burst and form a brown crust, because impetigo is highly contagious and can spread rapidly. It is most often seen on the face but can occur anywhere.

RECOMMENDATIONS

General Advice

- *Any aggressive, painful or fast-spreading rash should be assessed by a complementary medical practitioner and then reviewed by a doctor if the condition does not respond to complementary medicine. Antibiotics may need to be used.*
- *Remember the highly contagious nature of impetigo and ensure good hygiene and that the infected party uses separate towels. No school until the infection has completely cleared.*

Supplemental

- *The following supplements should be given per foot of height in divided doses throughout the day with meals: beta-carotene (2mg), vitamin C (1g) and vitamin E (100iu). Zinc should be given at a dose of 5mg per foot of height before bed.*

Homeopathic

- *Insist upon a skin swab and consider using the homeopathic nosode (the remedy made from the bacteria), potency 30, every 2hr until improvement is seen and then four times a day until better.*
- *Specific homeopathic remedies can be chosen depending on the symptoms, and a constitutional remedy should be administered via a homeopath.*

Herbal/natural extracts

- *Apply a Calendula lotion to the area every 2hr. Do not use an oil-based cream because the bacteria prefer a moist environment. Do not use antiseptic solutions such as TCP which will kill off the good bacteria around the lesion that are competing with the bad bugs.*
- *Manuka honey is a wild honey produced in New Zealand and it is proven to have antibacterial, antiseptic and anti-inflammatory properties. It has been shown to be effective in tests against methicillin-resistant staphylococcal aureus (MRSA) infections. Look out for Comvita manuka honey – it is a better tested and more effective product.*

LICE

Lice are parasites found predominantly in children, contracting it from classmates, but they can be found in all age groups. Different types live in different parts of the body, such that the head louse is a different species to the pubic louse (crabs). These parasites lie flat on the skin, attaching to small capillaries, and cause itching, redness and occasionally bleeding because of aggressive scratching.

Lice lay their eggs at the base of body hairs and attach them with a tenacious cement.

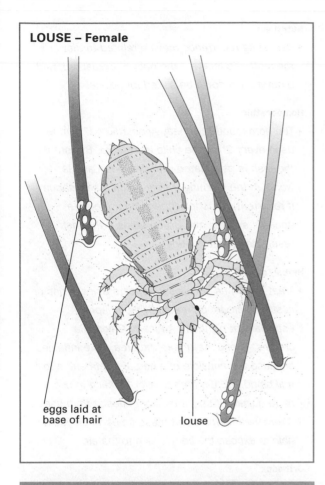

LOUSE – Female

eggs laid at base of hair

louse

Herbal/natural extracts

- *Take 100ml of almond oil and put in 10ml each of lavender, eucalyptus and bergamot. Apply to the scalp and hair and cover with a shower cap overnight. Wash out thoroughly the next morning and follow the combing instructions below.*
- *A citrus fruit extract, if available, has proven effective in trials.*

MOLLUSCUM CONTAGIOSUM

This is a common viral infection, most commonly found in children, and it is characterized by one or more dome-shaped nodules with a dip (punctum) in the middle. These often shiny, wart-like lesions are usually without symptom, but they may be itchy or irritating. Secondary infection can occur due to scratching, but these spots generally come and go, lasting a few weeks or, occasionally, up to a year or two.

They are quite contagious (hence the name) and spread around schools and families swiftly. They tend to be a cosmetic rather than a medical problem.

RECOMMENDATIONS

General Advice

- *Alternative therapies may be beneficial and should be considered before the use of any proprietary solutions. Government health and safety laboratory tests have shown that the active ingredient, malathion, is readily absorbed into the system by the scalp and may affect developing nervous systems.*
- *Comb with a metal nit comb twice a day for a period of two weeks. Electric nit combs are now available which cut down on the time involved since the lice are killed on contact.*
- *All members of the family or close social group (such as class mates) should be treated.*
- *Malathion and permethrin, the most common chemicals used as insecticides now, have failure rates of 64 per cent and 87 per cent respectively.*

RECOMMENDATIONS

General Advice

- *Try and keep covered and advise contacts of their being contagious.*
- *See* **Warts**.

Homeopathic

- *Thuja potency 30 taken twice a day for ten days may trigger a healing response.*

Herbal/natural extracts

- *Apply thuja tincture, enough to cover the whole spot, twice a day for three to four weeks. If there has been no effect after that time it is unlikely to be beneficial.*
- *Apply collodial silver to the sponge of a sticky plaster and cover the warts for seven nights.*

Orthodox

- *There is no orthodox topical cream applicant but*

the lesions can be 'cored' – taking out the centre of lesion that harbours the virus. This should only be done by medically trained practitioners under sterile conditions.

NAPPY (DIAPER) RASH

All children will develop rashes in the area of the groin and buttocks at some point. Indeed, if an adult were to spend time in moist underwear, as is often the case after a workout at the gym or other exercise, rashes and the associated irritation or discomfort would become apparent all too soon.

Nappy rash is a red, irritating and occasionally spotty condition found in and around the areas covered by the nappy. It is caused by ammonia in the urine and digestive juices from the faeces irritating the skin.

It is important to differentiate this common rash from more persistent and irritating conditions such as *Candida* (thrush) or bacterial, viral or fungal infections. Occasionally secondary infection from normal skin bacteria or skin fungi will worsen the situation. Infection by *Candida* (thrush) is not uncommon.

A persisting or frequently recurring rash may be indicative of more serious conditions such as diabetes.

RECOMMENDATIONS

General Advice
- Any rash that does not respond to the suggestions below after 48–72hr should be seen by a physician for a firm diagnosis.
- Allow the baby to spend as much time as possible without a nappy on.
- Change nappies frequently and ensure that the area is cleaned three times a day using water or simple non-chemically treated soaps.
- Use non-medicated talc liberally before bed and with every other nappy change throughout the day.

Nutritional
- Persisting recurrence may be related to diet or the mother's intake if the baby is breast-fed, and a nutritionist could be asked for advice.

Homeopathic
- The homeopathic remedy Anacardium 6 can be used every 2hr if the child is irritable, Bovista if the rash is associated with diarrhoea and is worse in the morning, Hepar sulphuris calcarium if recurrent, Rhus toxicodendron if the area appears swollen and Urtica urens if the rash resembles a nettle sting.

Herbal/natural extracts
- Treat a rash as soon as it appears using a zinc or caster oil cream before applying a nappy, especially at night. Try Arnica or Calendula creams. These may make the area more inflamed because the principle of a herbal treatment is to pull blood into the area to allow healing to occur more quickly. If this is the case, desist from use. Clean the creams off at these times when you are able to expose the baby's skin to the air.

Orthodox
- Most irritant rashes will benefit from the application of zinc oxide creams. These should be used with the knowledge that they are barrier creams and a generous application is required. These creams do not need to be rubbed in but are left on the surface.
- The use of creams containing benzyl compounds is acceptable if natural products are not dealing with the problem.

RINGWORM

Ringworm is an infection of the skin, hair or nails by a variety of fungi, although most commonly one called *Tinea*. These produce a red circular lesion with raised borders and a normal or slightly pale-coloured centre, which is in fact healed skin. It is this ring-like appearance that gives the condition its name because there are no worms involved!

Ringworm

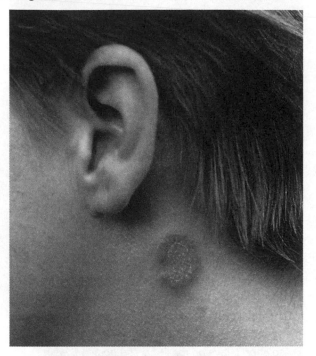

If the condition affects the scalp, alopecia (bald patches) can occur; *Tinea* is also one of the skin fungi that cause athlete's foot, groin rashes and other lesions in moist areas.

Ringworm has no species preference and will pass through pets as easily as through human beings. It is quite contagious and, left to its own devices, may persist and irritate for weeks.

RECOMMENDATION

General Advice
• See **Fungal infections**.

SCABIES

This is a contagious disorder that is caused by a little mite and is characterized by intensely itching lesions that can take many shapes. The itch is often markedly worse at night because the female insects burrow beneath the skin to lay their eggs, which causes the irritation.

Areas of the body that are most commonly affected are between the webs of the fingers and wrists, but it can appear anywhere.

Identification is by recognizing the characteristic burrows, which are a few millimetres to one centimetre long, wavy and with a little lump at one end. The body mounts an immune response against this mite, as it would to any other infection, and therefore the more often an infection is contracted, the more aggressive the response can be. A patient who has never had scabies before may remain symptomless for anywhere up to one month, by which time a large area may be infected.

Unrecognized, the irritation may continue and the itching will lead to the possibility of secondary infection, an eczema-like condition and a persisting and profoundly irritating rash.

Investigation is usually done by a GP, who will recognize the characteristic lesions and may be able to spot the mites with a magnifying glass. It is possible to remove a parasite from a burrow with a pin and look at it under a microscope. Skin scrapings may also be examined in this way.

RECOMMENDATIONS

General Advice
• *All clothes need to be thoroughly cleaned if they have been worn within a week. Mites generally do not live longer than 3–4 days away from the skin and one week is allowing a good safety margin.*
• *Please note that all members of a family, and possibly a school group, should be treated.*

Homeopathic
• *The homeopathic remedy Sulphur 6, taken four times per day, is often effective although it may exacerbate the irritation and cause a flare-up of any other underlying skin conditions.*

Herbal/natural extracts
• *Lavender oil is a well-established and longstanding treatment, probably working in the same way as proprietary drugs. A quantity in the bath or directly applied if the area infected is small may do the trick, but it needs to be repeated twice a day for five days at least.*

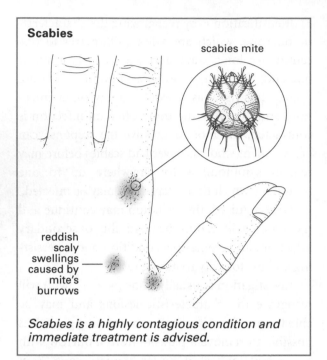

Scabies

scabies mite

reddish
scaly
swellings
caused by
mite's
burrows

Scabies is a highly contagious condition and immediate treatment is advised.

Orthodox

- *Orthodox lotions are effective and, if the skin is not particularly damaged, are unlikely to be absorbed at a rate that a healthy body could not deal with. Treatment is swift and efficient, although repeated use of the chemicals might be necessary whilst the remaining eggs hatch.*

SCALDS

A scald is damage to the skin caused by hot fluids and should be treated as for any burns (*see* Burns).

SPLINTERS

A splinter is a small shard of any material that embeds itself in the skin. These are generally painful and worse if the area where the splinter has embedded has any pressure applied to it.

RECOMMENDATIONS

General Advice

- *Any puncture wound may have debris or a splinter beneath the skin surface that may be invisible. Any puncture wound that continues to hurt should be examined by a doctor.*
- *X-ray investigation is only beneficial if the splinter is made of metal, because most other materials will not appear radio-opaque (visible on X-ray).*
- *Any attempt to remove a splinter should be done with the correct implements, such as a pair of fine tweezers. The use of a needle to break the skin over a splinter to allow access for the tweezers is acceptable if the splinter is not buried too deep. All equipment should be sterilized in boiling water over a naked flame for at least 1min. (Do not hold the other end of the metal instrument whilst sterilizing it.) Alternatively, a dilute solution of a disinfectant may be used but this needs to be washed off with boiling water before applying to the skin.*
- *Squeamish children (or adults!) may try applying the adhesive part of a sticky plaster to a visible splinter. Leave on for 48hr. The body will eject the foreign object at the rate of skin growth and this may adhere to the sticky plaster which, when removed, will pull the splinter out.*
- *Do not hesitate to visit a doctor, who will have all the equipment to remove a splinter and be able to offer a local anaesthetic as well.*

Herbal/natural extracts

- *Use an Arnica- or Calendula-based cream before and after.*

STINGS

A sting is usually provided by an insect and differs from a bite by injecting a chemical that causes burning, pricking or … stinging! Most commonly, stings are given by wasps, bees and the mosquito group, which includes gnats. Less common are the more dangerous stings from hornets. Certain marine animals such as jellyfish and types of coral may also impart a sting.

The injected irritant directly affects the nerve endings but also breaks down cells that release histamine-like chemicals that attract blood into the area. Rubbing and scratching the site tends to spread the poison and make the situation worse.

General Advice

- *The best treatment is avoidance and the use of insect repellent in areas of infestation.*
- *Apply a cold or ice compress as soon as possible.*
- *Vitamin B$_6$ (50mg at dusk) may repel mosquitoes and the application of pyrethrum solution will ward off most insects.*
- *Remove any residual part of the insect or its sting as quickly as possible using sharp fingernails or tweezers. Do not use teeth or suck out the toxin as a more aggressive reaction may take place in the mouth. Remember that certain insects will leave a sting and the poison sacs pumping in the wound.*

Supplemental

- *In multiple or aggressive stings, papain or bromelain supplements should be taken at three times the recommended product dosage for three days.*

Homeopathic

- *The homeopathic remedies Ledum or Apis mellifica can be taken at potency 6 every 5min. The more red and inflamed the sting, the more the preference would be for Apis.*

Herbal/natural extracts

- *Stay inside and apply directly to the sting any of the following tinctures: Calendula or tea tree oil for gnat and mosquito bites; Arnica or lavender for bee stings; and Arnica or Ledum for wasp or hornet stings.*
- *If the above are not available or do not work, try applying the juice from a potato by pressing a freshly cut potato over the area. If this has not worked within 2min, use an onion.*

WARTS AND VERRUCAS

A wart is an overgrowth of skin triggered by a viral infection in the basal (growth) layer. Depending on where they are, a wart may be soft and fleshy (such as in the vagina) or firm (as found on hands and feet). A verruca is a wart found in the hardened tissues of the soles of the feet.

Nutritional

- *At the onset or arrival of a wart, increase your vitamin A and zinc intake via orange and green vegetables or through supplements (twice the recommended dosage).*

Homeopathic

- *Homeopathic remedies are beneficial and, depending on the type, should be selected from Thuja, Nitric acid, Dulcamara and Causticum.*

Herbal/natural extracts

- *Apply Thuja tincture, garlic or caster oil for several days underneath a bandage. If this is impractical, then apply the compounds frequently through the day. Ask a complementary medical practitioner if the wart is internal.*

Orthodox

- *Liquid nitrogen may be applied by a doctor to freeze off the warts and preparations may be available over the counter at a pharmacy but should only be used if other treatments have failed because the chemical treatments damage the surrounding skin and lead to a higher incidence of recurrence.*

THE NERVOUS SYSTEM

CEREBRAL PALSY

Cerebral palsy is a disorder of movement originating *in utero*, in infancy or in early childhood. Most often the damage to the brain that causes this problem occurs during birth due to a lack of oxygenation or, more rarely, by infections of the brain, seizures or maternal drug abuse during pregnancy.

The extent of the brain damage varies and may be mild or may leave the infant incapacitated, unable to communicate and possibly unaware of his/her surroundings. Uncontrolled movements, aggressive behaviour patterns, blindness, deafness and an inability to speak are some of the more serious problems.

Eastern philosophies consider the birth of an incapacitated child to be part of that individual's soul karma. We all, at some point in our cosmic cycle, have to go through a period of incapacity and dependency on others. The karma of the parents is also that of a lifetime of servitude to a distressed physical body and mind. I find that it helps to discuss the inevitable trauma that befalls the family of a cerebral palsy victim by discussing matters from a more ethereal and spiritual angle. Very little pleasure can be derived from the necessity of caring for a severely debilitated child but then a connection between two souls is not dependent upon physical or material means, and caring for a soul in a distressed body can be a very loving and enlightening experience. To give is often considered a greater pleasure than to receive, and if one can focus on this, then caring for a cerebral palsy case should be considered a blessing.

RECOMMENDATIONS

General Advice
- *Contact a local cerebral palsy group to share with other families your grief, joys and experiences.*
- *See **Paralysis** and **Birth defects**.*
- *Ensure that cranial osteopathy or craniosacral therapy is tried for at least six to ten sessions since profound changes in an individual can be seen.*

Nutritional
- *Consult with a nutritionist and a homeopath because correct supplementation and homeopathic medication can be of great benefit, although not curative.*

CONVULSIONS

Convulsions, commonly termed seizures or fits, are an involuntary occurrence of muscular spasm or contraction. There are two types of convulsion: clonic, characterized by alternate contraction and relaxation; and tonic, which is a continuous contraction or spasm.

Convulsions can occur due to any insult on the nervous system, which leads to it sending out massive impulses instructing the muscles to behave incorrectly. Convulsions are most commonly associated with a loss of consciousness.

Occasionally convulsions will occur in association with high temperatures, most commonly in young children below the age of two years. Other causative factors are epilepsy, infections such as meningitis or encephalitis, an adverse drug reaction or food allergy, or lesions such as tumours in the brain.

RECOMMENDATIONS

General Advice
- *Have somebody call an ambulance. This request can always be cancelled if the convulsions are minor and/or short-lived.*
- *One convulsion or fit does not represent a serious condition in most cases, but all fits should be reported and examined by a doctor. Referral to a neurological specialist is sometimes required.*
- *Do not restrict someone having a convulsion. Instead, clear the area of solid objects and protect the patient by surrounding with cushions or other soft objects.*
- *If blood is seen to be coming from the mouth, this may be due to biting of the tongue and firm but careful opening of the jaw with an instrument surrounded by a handkerchief or cloth is acceptable.*
- *If associated with fever, use cold compresses or a lukewarm bath to lower the temperature (see **Fever**).*
- *Recurrent fits must be assessed by a doctor. If no serious underlying cause is present then an*

Cranial Osteopathy

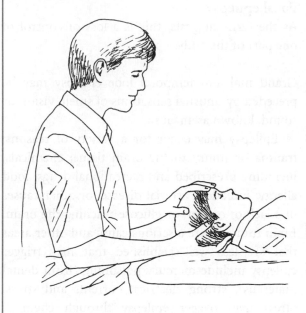

frontal occipital hold

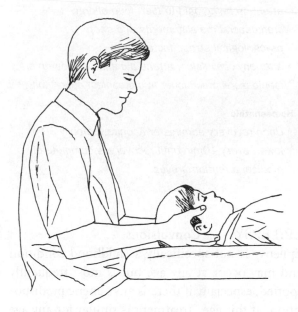

palpation of splenoid motion

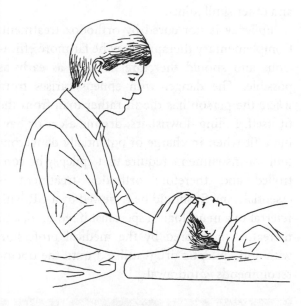

frontal base hold

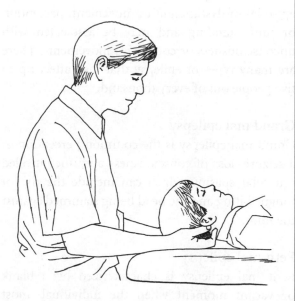

cranial base release

Cranial osteopathy is a gentle technique in which the bones of the skull are manipulated.

It is especially useful with children and can help treat a wide range of symptoms.

assessment from a complementary medical practitioner is recommended, with special attention being paid to diet, food allergy, craniosacral malalignments and deep psychological stress factors.

• *After any convulsion, attend a cranial osteopath or craniosacral practitioner at the earliest opportunity.*

Homeopathic

• *Upon recovery administer Aconite, potency 30 or lower, every 10min until recovery is complete or medical attention arrives.*

EPILEPSY – *see* Convulsions

Epilepsy is not specifically a childhood condition and may occur at any age but is most frequently spotted, especially if there is any genetic predisposition, at this age. Treatment is similar for any age group.

Epilepsy is a disorder created by excessive nerve discharges in the brain. These manifest episodes of dysfunction in movement, perception or understanding and may be associated with unconsciousness or convulsive movements. There are many types of epilepsy that may affect up to five people out of every thousand.

Grand mal epilepsy

Grand mal epilepsy is the common perception of a seizure: loss of consciousness and uncontrolled muscular spasms, which can include the risk of tongue biting and the head being slammed against the floor.

Petit mal epilepsy

Petit mal epilepsy is characterized by a blank or vacant moment when the individual, most frequently a child, is unresponsive. Repetitive movements may be apparent.

Temporal lobe epilepsy

This must be considered if there is a temporary loss of awareness, confusion or disorientation and auditory or visual hallucinations.

Focal epilepsy

As the term suggests, this is a loss of control of one part of the body.

Grand mal and temporal lobe epilepsy may be preceded by unusual sensations of smell, vision or sound, known as an 'aura'.

Epilepsy may occur for a variety of reasons: trauma or injury to the brain tissue; chemicals, including prescribed and recreational drugs; food allergy; infection; arterial disease; or other causes of a lack of oxygen or glucose reaching the brain. Brain tumours are a serious cause and other areas that are less well-established that may trigger epilepsy include mercury poisoning (from dental materials), strong electrical currents and stress. Stress may trigger epilepsy through chemical effects of adrenaline and other catecholamines but may also tighten the muscles around the skull leading to cranial osteopathic lesions of the jaw and other skull joints.

Epilepsy is not cured by orthodox treatment. Complementary therapies may be far more efficacious and should therefore be used as early as possible. The danger with epilepsy arises from *where* the person has the fit rather than from the fit itself. Falling downstairs, driving a car or having a fit when in charge of potentially dangerous tools or instruments require that epilepsy be controlled and therefore orthodox treatment is essential. Any fit should be reviewed by a GP, with referral to a neurological specialist if required, and thereafter monitored by the medical profession with anti-epileptic drugs utilized until the doctor recommends withdrawal.

RECOMMENDATIONS

General Advice

• *Any suggestion of epilepsy needs to be fully investigated by a specialist in neurology to rule out any serious cause.*

- Supervision and the avoidance of any dangerous situations, such as cooking or operating machinery, must be avoided until the problem is solved.
- Craniosacral work, the Alexander Technique and polarity therapy should all be considered.

Nutritional

- A set diet from a nutritionist with knowledge of this area is essential. Avoidance of sugar, caffeine, alcohol and artificially sweetened food (saccharine and aspartame) should be strictly adhered to. Canada is currently pioneering a specific nutritional treatment known as the Ketogenic diet, which may become an essential aspect of the treatment of epilepsy.
- The brain produces many anticonvulsant chemicals, the most prominent of which is adenosine. This is blocked by theophylline-containing drugs often used by asthmatics. Tea should also be avoided therefore.

Supplemental

- To encourage the body's natural anticonvulsants, an alternative practitioner should be consulted to prescribe the correct dosages of specific amino acids, namely taurine and gamma-aminobutyric acid. High-dose vitamin B complex is also necessary.

Homeopathic

- Constitutional homeopathic remedies are essential and a homeopath should be consulted.

Herbal/natural extracts

- Herbal treatments are available as anticonvulsant therapy, but today's drugs are well-established, generally safe and probably better to use.

Orthodox

- Orthodox medical treatment should be utilized if fits have become frequent, although one fit does not make epilepsy. Alternative treatments may be considered following diagnosis of the cause but should not exclude the possible benefits of orthodox drug treatment.

MENINGITIS

Infection of the lining of the brain known as the meninges can be characterized by a mild persistent headache through to violent pain with coma and, if not treated swiftly, death. There is often an associated photophobia (dislike of or pain from light) and an almost characteristic neck stiffness that differentiates meningitis from migraines and other headaches.

Recognizing meningitis in an infant may be impossible without medical expertise. An inconsolable child clearly in pain that is worsened by attempting to dip the chin onto the chest or a child who is markedly fevered or becomes floppy or unresponsive must be considered possibly to have meningitis and rushed to the hospital.

One particular type of aggressive meningitis is caused by a bacteria called meningococcal bacteria which can be very swift in its effect. Meningococcal meningitis can kill a child within 4 hours. A headache associated with a rash that does not blanch when a glass is pressed onto it is meningococcal meningitis and must be treated by antibiotics via a hospital or doctor immediately. This rash characteristically appears on the thighs.

Meningitis can occur at any age but I mention it in the childhood chapter because of the swift and severe nature should it strike at this age. Most meningitis is caused by viral infection and tends not be particularly dangerous. The pain is hard to control but the condition is usually self-limiting and rarely leaves any sequela. Bacterial or fungal meningitis is much more serious and can lead to persistent neurological deficits.

RECOMMENDATIONS

General Advice

- Any persistent or severe headache must be reviewed by a GP or accident and emergency department.
- Contact your complementary medical practitioner for advice on treating with alternative medicines

alongside orthodox treatment rather than trying to deal with this problem without expert guidance.

Orthodox

- A lumbar puncture will be required for a firm diagnosis, along with blood and urine examination. More intense investigations, such as CAT scans, may be required and none of these should be refused.
- Viral meningitis will not respond to an antibiotic but secondary infection may make the situation worse and, especially in a child, orthodox medication should not be refused.

MENTAL HANDICAP

The term mentally handicapped refers to those individuals who, for any reason, have damage to the brain causing a marked debility in mental function. There are several scales used throughout the world to measure mental handicap and these finer definitions are best left to the experts.

Mental handicap affects two parties: the individual who, very often, is quite unaware or disturbed by the abnormality; and those who care for them. Most helpful advice needs to be given to the latter, who may have had no training or expectations – only fears – of being placed in such a position.

Mental handicap can vary in severity from mild, such as is often the case in conditions such as Down's syndrome (see **Down's syndrome**), to the severely handicapped who may be further hampered by physical inabilities or sensory loss, such as those with cerebral palsy, post-traumatic injury or those with the sequela of infections such as meningitis. All levels of handicap can benefit from complementary medical treatment to some degree.

RECOMMENDATIONS

FOR THE INDIVIDUAL

General Advice

- Ensure that hygiene and sanitation are at a premium. Those who cannot care for themselves

are more likely to contract infections.
- Do not isolate anyone with a mentally handicapped state. Social interaction, kisses and cuddles have a profound effect on the biochemistry and psychology of all individuals.
- Ensure that the highest quality accessories are made available. In particular, pay attention to the mattress, seats or wheelchairs. Sores are notoriously difficult to heal in individuals who may scratch or play with an injury or who are confined to a position that applies pressure to the damaged area.
- Never underestimate the level of understanding of a mentally handicapped individual. As there is a fine line between genius and insanity, the mentally handicapped may have a marked sensitivity to negative emotions and, as much as any of us, need to be surrounded by laughter, joy and music. Children make excellent companions for the handicapped because they are before the age where we adults have introduced prejudices.
- Frequent cranial osteopathy or craniosacral therapy along with healing may make a profound difference, especially if the individual is in any way aggressive or seems disturbed.
- Ensure that exercise is undertaken where possible. Swimming is best and most swimming pools will have set times and facilities for the handicapped.
- Regular massage or Shiatsu is essential for those who are incapacitated by their handicap.

Nutritional

- Consult with a nutritionist because minor deficiencies can cause major problems and correct supplementation may dramatically alter the general well-being of the mentally handicapped.

Homeopathic

- Consult a homeopath to assess a suitable constitutional remedy, which can enhance a sense of well-being and, theoretically, prevent infections.

FOR THE CARER

General Advice

- *Remember that you are not alone. There are many in your situation and many groups in all areas of mental handicap. Individual discussion with counsellors or group therapy is essential.*
- *Ensure that you have home help if possible and that you spend time away. Feelings of guilt for leaving the individual will only reduce well-being on both sides and encourage feelings of guilt in the handicapped person. Remember that emotions are not only perceived at a mental level but also on a spiritual one.*
- *Ensure that regular exercise is taken. All too often one forgets to allow time in which to maintain physical well-being.*

Homeopathic

- *Have consultations with a homeopath or naturopath, whose remedies will help to maintain the spirits through difficult times. The use of constitutional remedies, good nutrition and Bach flower remedies can be beneficial in both the short and the long term.*

TETANUS

Tetanus is a disease caused by a poison produced by a bacterium known as *Clostridium tetani*. It is characterized by severe painful muscle spasms which is often noticed initially as difficulty in chewing, discomfort in the jaws and aching in the neck and back. These symptoms led to its common name 'lockjaw'. If untreated, the problem may lead to difficulty in breathing and swallowing. *Clostridium tetani* forms spores, which are found in soil and particularly in the faeces of animals. This bacterium is very resistant to climatic changes and will survive drought or flood.

The bacterium will enter the body through an injury, which may be no more than a scrape, and multiply locally. The toxin from *Clostridium* enters the bloodstream and travels to a specific part of the nervous system that normally blocks muscular activity. With this inhibition diminished, muscles tense up.

The symptoms develop any time from two days to several weeks later, and if left untreated may last up to ten weeks. Complications can arise because of a loss of respiratory muscles and the effect the toxin may have on the heart muscle and the muscles within the arteries.

Treatment of tetanus is difficult because the antibiotic (usually penicillin) may kill the bacteria but does not remove the toxin. Tetanus immunoglobulins are available in serious cases. These are antibodies taken from other humans that are specific against tetanus. The prognosis in cases of tetanus is dependent upon the well-being of the individual and the medical care available. Most cases of tetanus are mild but some may be fatal.

Vaccination against tetanus – *see* Vaccinations

Tetanus vaccine is usually given in combination with diphtheria and pertussis (whooping cough) and is known as DPT. There are reports of convulsions, collapse, sudden infant death syndrome (SIDS) and even encephalitis and anaphylaxis, and it is very much up to an individual or the parents of a child to decide whether or not to vaccinate against tetanus. The holistic consensus of opinion would be that an individual with a good immune system would not have a problem in fighting tetanus and the chances of contracting tetanus must be put into the equation. Picking up *Clostridium* in cities, for example, is rare. One must balance what is called the risk–benefit ratio, considering that adverse reactions do occur with the vaccine.

General Advice

- *A cut or graze at risk of Clostridium infection should be thoroughly cleansed and debrided (dead tissue removed). A hospital may be necessary for this to be done completely. Any dirt in a wound needs to be removed.*

Homeopathic

- Give the homeopathic remedy Hypericum 30 every hour for 3hr and then every 4hr for three days. Following this, take one dose of Hypericum 200.

Herbal/natural extracts

- Immediately apply a solution of Hypericum at a dilution that just tingles but does not sting. This should be repeated every 15min for 1hr.

Orthodox

- Antitetanus serum should be given by a doctor.
- Consider systemic penicillin if the wound was inflicted in an area where animal faeces may have spread.
- A tetanus vaccine will be offered by any orthodox physician but will have no benefit to the possibility of an infection for at least two or three weeks.

PSYCHOLOGICAL MATTERS

AUTISM

Autism is a clinical entity quite distinct from childhood schizophrenia. The principle difference is that autism manifests itself from early infancy whereas childhood schizophrenia more or less follows normal behaviour during the first two years of life. It is characterized by a collection of psychological symptoms ranging from body rocking, withdrawal from social situations, little if any language development and repetitive, often self-damaging, actions.

The cause of autism is poorly understood from an orthodox point of view. Autism is biologically determined and associated with brain dysfunction. Recent research has shown that low levels of sulphates may interfere with the metabolism of certain proteins and have a particular effect on autistic children. Sulphur-containing foods should be encouraged. The best sources are beans, fish, eggs, cabbage and beef.

There is considerable evidence that food allergy has a strong link and in some cases may be the underlying cause of autistic characteristics. It is, in my opinion, essential to rule out any food allergy and food intolerances using specific blood tests and the less scientifically validated bioresonance techniques. Food exclusion diets are risky as deficiencies may ensue and deficiencies, as mentioned above, may be very relevant in autism.

There is also some correlation between autism and the presence of *candida*. *Candida* is a normal yeast commencal (one normally found in the bowel flora) but if it over grows or becomes abundant then many problems can ensue. Autism is possibly one of them.

There are many techniques being used with a variety of success in autism. Art therapy, music therapy and specific learning techniques are constantly being developed and are available locally in the UK by contacting the National Autistic Society.

In 1997 a researcher at the Royal Free Hospital in London noted that children who had been given the Measles, Mumps and Rubella (MMR) vaccination were at increased risk of developing an inflammatory bowel condition similar, if not actually, Crohn's disease. This has been associated with an increase in autism. The complementary medical world had been aware of this association for quite some time. (*See* **Vaccinations.**) A change in character of a child or any signs or symptoms of autism developing within a few months of an MMR vaccine should arouse suspicion.

RECOMMENDATIONS

General Advice

- Discuss the matter with your doctor, an art therapist and the National Autistic Society.
- Introduce the child to a cranial osteopath.
- Test for candida using either a stool test or a blood test for gut fermentation (a lab test where a sweet drink is taken and 1hr later a blood sample is drawn to test for alcohol which is produced by gut yeasts). Preferably, use both.

- *Undergo both food allergy and food intolerance testing.*

Nutritional

- *All autistic children should have their sulphate food input increased (as listed above).*
- *Increase foods containing sulphur, such as beans, fish, eggs, cabbage and beef, and give a daily dose of MSM. Give the recommended dose on the packaging depending on the child's age.*

Supplemental

- *Ensure that the child is on a high-dose multivitamin tablet that includes zinc and manganese.*

Homeopathic

- *Homeopathy should be utilized but requires a specialist prescription.*
- *If a vaccination is considered a possible cause, discuss high-potency Thuja and Natrum muriaticum (both homeopathic remedies that may have an effect on the adverse effects of vaccinations) with a homeopath.*

BEHAVIOURAL PROBLEMS

It is very difficult to define a badly-behaved child. So much depends on the objective attitude of the parents and their view of their child. To establish if a child has a behavioural problem requires the following criteria to be met.

- The parents, close friends and, if the child is of school age, a teacher must all express concern.
- The child must display some antisocial or self-harming behavioural patterns, such as aggression or self-inflicted wounds, inappropriate behaviour with regard to a particular situation, excessive crying or irritability, poor food intake, or cruelty to animals.

Bad behaviour may not be a psychological problem. It has been established that many deficiencies and some toxicities can create a problem. Studies in the prison population have shown that slight alterations through the use of supplemental medicine can have a profound effect on the behaviour of prisoners and this hypothesis has been supported by several small studies on children.

Toxins, especially lead and therefore, by inference, other heavy metals such as mercury, may cause an effect. Refined sugars and other aspects of poor nutrition may lead to hypoglycaemic states, which can create irritability and therefore poor behaviour. All of these aspects must be taken into consideration.

RECOMMENDATIONS

General Advice

- *See Hyperactivity and Attention deficit disorder.*
- *Rule out dyslexia. See Dyslexia.*
- *If a behavioural problem is established and the matter is not one of ill-discipline, then I recommend art or music therapy for all child psychological problems.*
- *If response is not forthcoming with the above treatments and therapies, there are specialized behavioural clinics with which the child psychologist or your GP will be able to put you in touch.*

Nutritional

- *Remove processed foods: foods containing high sugar or salt content, additives, preservatives and caffeine.*

Supplemental

- *Many psychological problems are created by deficiencies. Ensure that the child is getting the following supplements in divided doses each day in combination with a well-balanced diet: zinc (2mg per foot of height); multi-B complex as recommended by a nutritionist or pharmacist; vitamin C (1g per foot of height); and any trace element supplement as recommended for the weight and age of your baby by the health food shop or pharmacist.*

Homeopathic

- *Homeopathy is marvellous if the correct remedy is chosen. It is preferable to be accurate and therefore the use of a homeopath is required.*

LEARNING DIFFICULTIES

There are a broad range of reasons why a child may present with difficulties in learning. The age at which the child appears deficient is also very relevant. An infant who is slow to talk or perform expected tasks may have an unnoticed deficiency in hearing or eyesight or may be exhibiting mental handicap. Not achieving developmental landmarks needs initially to be assessed by a paediatric psychologist.

In older children, handicaps and autism (childhood schizophrenia) should be apparent and need to be dealt with appropriately. If obvious causes are not apparent, then conditions such as dyslexia, attention deficit disorder (ADD) and poor nutrition need to be considered. Deficiencies in B complex, zinc and various amino acids can impair learning ability. Most of us have some hidden talent and, taking this concept to an extreme, all of us may be a genius at something if given the time, space and training. If your child is proving slow at languages but adequate at mathematics, then education and not medicinal support is required.

RECOMMENDATIONS

General Advice
- *As a parent, do not try to diagnose your own children. Seek help from a child psychologist if you have any doubts about your child's development or learning abilities.*
- *If a problem is diagnosed, then treat appropriately, but slow learning may be improved by cranial osteopathy and art or music therapy.*

Nutritional
- *If you have any doubts about the child's nutrition, talk with a dietician.*

Supplemental
- *Ensure that the child's diet is well balanced and if you have a pernickety eater, give daily supplements for those food groups that may be missing.*

Homeopathic
- *Without doubt, the correct homeopathic constitutional remedy will benefit and should be selected by a trained homeopath.*

TOILET TRAINING

Toilet training may be a messy matter but it is rarely an illness or a disease process that requires treatment. Girls tend to potty train quicker than boys but each individual will come out of nappies at their own rate. A problem should only be considered if a child is still soiling after the age of about four years.

The usual cause of delayed toilet training is because the child does not feel uncomfortable in a wet or soiled nappy. There is very little that can be done about this other than gentle persuasion. Criticism or punishment will only help to delay matters further, be used as an attention-seeking device or cause the child to withhold and become constipated.

RECOMMENDATIONS

General Advice
- *Toilet training should start as soon as the child is old enough to understand verbal instructions.*
- *Aim for daytime potty-use initially and then moving on to the toilet thereafter.*
- *Urination should be trained first and defecation afterwards.*
- *Night-time training should follow in reverse order, encouraging the child not to soil the nappy but expecting a wet nappy each morning. When the child is old enough, try to have them pass urine before bed, when the parent goes to bed (which necessitates awakening the child) or if the child awakes in the night.*
- *Thoroughly congratulate the child on successful use of the potty or toilet but never criticize them for failing. Explanation of the situation as the child gets old enough to understand is ample critique.*
- *Bedwetting is usually not a training problem and is discussed in its own section (see **Bedwetting**).*

YOUNG ADULT

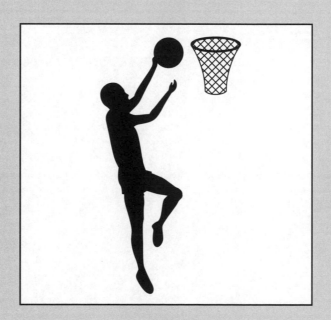

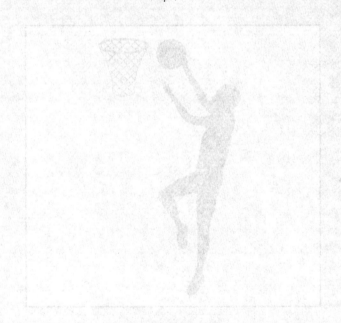

CHAPTER 4

YOUNG ADULT

GENERAL

ALLERGIES

See also **Food allergy and intolerance** *and* **Food allergy testing.**

An allergy is an inflammation triggered by the interaction of a foreign substance (called an antigen) with the body's defence system. The body has specific white cells that produce chemicals called immunoglobulins, which attach to an antigen and make them recognizable to other defence cells, which then envelop them or destroy them. This reaction is constantly going on throughout the system and is only termed an allergy when the body, by mistake, is overreacting.

The word allergy is commonly used to refer to the running, itching and red nose of a hay fever sufferer. This is correct but allergic reactions can cause symptoms depending on the area of the body the inflammation is affecting. A reaction can be triggered by an antigen or allergen being inhaled, ingested or coming into contact with the membrane. Symptoms can occur anywhere in the body and include skin rashes, asthma, gastrointestinal problems, mood swings, lethargy and tiredness. In fact, any set of symptoms anywhere in the body *may* be created by allergy. There are four types of allergic reaction as defined by medical science.

- Type 1 is called *immediate onset allergy reaction*. Here, immunoglobulin E attaches to an allergen and causes several body defence reactions. These include the release of histamine, free radicals, lysosomal enzymes and other complicated chemicals. These compounds are produced to attack a foreign substance but they unfortunately and inadvertently damage the local host tissues. The symptoms are felt because these chemicals and reactions cause digestion of cells, increase the blood flow and make capillaries more 'leaky' to allow the defence system to get to the area affected. These chemicals also cause constriction of the blood vessels leaving the area in order to stop further spread of the foreign substance, to close down the bronchial (lung) tree and to increase mucus production.

- Types 2 and 3 allergic reaction are reactions differentiated by *biochemical* changes and do not have the same immediate or aggressive effect as type 1. They develop within a few hours and may show up as anything from a mild rash or wheeziness to not being noticed at all.

- Type 4 is known as *delayed onset allergy* and may take up to 72 hours to develop. Being delayed does not reduce the severity, and this allergic response may be as severe as immediate onset but is more commonly noticed as a mild reaction or not noticed at all. Delayed onset or type 4 allergy is commonly associated with foods and may well give rise to chronic conditions such as cancer or diabetes, although this hypothesis has not been fully established.

There is a holistic consensus of opinion that allergy will occur when the body is already primed to fight something else. Everybody comes into contact with pollens and house dust mites but not everybody overreacts. There are certainly genetic tendencies but many families will have some allergy sufferers when other members have no problems, even though they share the same genetic traits. The overresponsive system is generally battling a condition elsewhere, knowingly or otherwise. Hay fever sufferers (who may also have eczema or asthma, as this triad is not uncommon) may struggle because they have an allergy to some food or other input without which they would not react to pollen.

There is strong evidence to suggest that allergies are linked to the psyche. In a well-known study of a psychiatric patient with multiple personalities the allergies would change as each personality took control. Another example was illustrated by an artificial flower triggering hay fever. Hypnosis can achieve the same effect.

One may often hear the term atopic used in conjunction with allergic responses such as atopic eczema and atopic asthma. This simply refers to the predisposition or genetic tendency for that individual to have allergies. There is evidence that the development of allergic tendencies in later life may be predisposed by the oestrogen levels fed to a foetus by its mother. One study, for example, has shown that girls who start having periods at an early age tend to have higher levels of oestrogen throughout their life, especially through pregnancy. Other factors, such as the mother's diet while pregnant, especially the intake of peanuts, wheat and milk, might all be relevant.

Atopic allergic reactions have been considered to have a genetic element but recent developments have suggested that atopy may also be associated with exposure to common childhood infections. Recent studies have shown that men with antibodies to viral infections and those who had older siblings (leaving them more prone to being introduced to childhood infections) had less atopic allergic responses. This suggests that the more the body learns to fight infections when younger, the less likely it is to overreact as in the case of allergic responses. The prevalence of allergies such as hay fever, asthma and eczema has greatly increased over the last 30 years. This, interestingly but not surprisingly to a holistic practitioner, coincides with the increased use and advent of vaccinations, which has possibly reduced the body's need to activate an immune response early in life, thereby increasing allergic tendencies. This may mean that we need to reconsider the automatic vaccination of children against measles, mumps and rubella, for example, because the lives we save or improve by protecting against measles may not compensate for the damage and deaths caused by asthma at a later age.

Treatment is, therefore, to illustrate any sensitivities or toxins specific to that sufferer and also to alleviate the symptoms. Never underestimate the potential danger of an allergy. We have all had contact with or heard of people having anaphylactic reactions, sometimes lethal, to eggs, peanuts or bee stings.

Tests for allergies

Testing for allergies can be performed using the following routines:

- Skin testing
- Hair analysis
- Blood allergy testing
- Bioenergy computer techniques
- Avoidance and restrictions

Skin testing

Small or dilute amounts of suspected allergens are pinpricked under the skin's surface. The body's allergic response will occur if immunoglobulins are present in the system. Dilutions are made of the reactive substances to give an idea of how strong the allergic response is. A technique of desensitization (enzyme-potentiated desensitization) can be used once this diagnostic process has isolated the culprits (*see* Recommendations below).

Hair analysis

This is a poorly proven way of testing for allergy but the principle is sound. If the body has poisons in the system it may well choose to eliminate them by combining them with the inert keratin that makes up hair. By taking a hair sample and combining it with immunoglobulins against particular foods, for example, reactions will take place that can be studied under the microscope or in a more sophisticated manner by computer. One may hypothesize that if there is a reaction to the compound in the hair there may well be a reaction in the body, because the body seems to be throwing this particular substance out.

Be wary of hair allergy testing that uses radionics (a pendulum technique) since this has not been shown to be accurate and can lead to aggressive restrictions that have no scientific basis. This does not mean that radionics are not accurate but that they need to be put into the context of a broader and more established allergy assessment.

Blood allergy testing

See **Food allergy testing** in chapter 8.

This is generally performed using accepted and scientifically proven techniques, the most available and sensitive being Enzyme-Linked Immunosolvent Assay (ELISA). It is a complicated technique involving competition between the body's antibodies and specially 'labelled' antibodies. In principle, your blood's serum will be mixed with a laboratory solution and then passed through a special machine that checks for the presence of a fluorescent dye, which will attach itself to the serum if an antibody/antigen (allergy) reaction has occurred. Many of these tests are qualitative (will tell us whether there is any reaction) but a few are quantitative (will tell us how strong the reaction is) and the latter are very helpful in determining which foods may be troublesome. This method of testing can be used for inhaled pollutants but having this information may not alter any treatment programme because it is often not possible to change the air that we breathe other than by moving to a different location.

Bioenergy computer techniques

Computers such as the Voll and Vega machines have now been surpassed by Bioresonance, Bicom and Quantum computers, all of which are capable of measuring electromagnetic changes in the system in response to stimuli such as specific foods and airborne allergens. The individual is attached to the computer, a small electromagnetic current is passed through the system and either different compounds are added to the circuit via the computer or the computer has within its own structure the energetic resonance or vibrations from the electrons from a multitude of substances. These techniques are becoming more available and, although not accepted by the orthodox

scientific world, I believe they are very accurate and effective investigations.

Avoidance and restrictions

This is not strictly a test but may prove to be a very clear and concise manner of illustrating the foods to which you may be allergic. To test this, make a list of any foods you suspect make you feel unwell, any foods you crave and any foods you eat frequently. Eliminate all of these and set up a five-day dietetic plan that does not repeat any of the foods you are going to eat. Stick to this rotation diet for one month and then introduce one of the 'forbidden' foods every five days to see if there is a reaction. If your list of suspected allergens is long or you seem to be cutting out a major food group then this technique should only be undertaken with the supervision of a nutritionist.

Causes of a predisposition to allergy

As I have mentioned, there certainly are genetic tendencies within families but many substances act as a trigger that can predispose any of us to allergic responses.

Principally the problems of allergy will arise when foreign matter, usually protein, gets into the bloodstream or the body is battling some other problems and therefore, being already primed, acts overzealously in defending itself. Very often proteins that should be broken down by the digestive enzymes into smaller peptides or amino acids are absorbed into the bloodstream due to a 'leaky' gut. Something, somehow, affects the mucous membrane in the intestinal tract to allow larger molecules to be absorbed, which are then recognized in the same way as bacteria or viruses. This 'leaky gut syndrome' can occur through infestation with *Candida*, parasites or chemical insult from eating contaminated foods. Poor secretion of the stomach acids and intestinal enzymes, alcohol and certain drugs such as aspirin, antibiotics and non-steroidal anti-inflammatory drugs can all have a detrimental effect. See **Leaky gut syndrome**.

General Advice

- *For any allergic condition other than a mild one, place yourself under the care of a complementary practitioner. The cause of most allergies is often deeply buried and needs expert guidance to illustrate.*
- *Do your best to avoid the allergens that cause your problems. Look broadly and consider fabrics, metals such as nickel, aerosols and the cosmetics you should not be using.*
- *Ensure that you are drinking one pint of water per foot of height per day. Correct hydration is essential for proper immune response but diluting the system can also dilute the allergen and reduce the response.*
- *Acupressure and reflexology points. A point in the web between the thumb and index finger can be very relieving of nasal symptoms.*
- *A nasal washing technique taught by a yoga teacher can be very beneficial for nasal symptoms (see **Nasal washing**).*
- *Be fastidious about the vacuuming of carpets, mattresses and pillows. Curtains should be washed frequently, as should all bed linen. Use allergy covers for mattresses and pillows.*
- *Visit a hypnotherapist or preferably a neurolinguistic practitioner to remove any psychological element.*
- *Enzyme-potentiated desensitization. This technique is performed by few practitioners but can be very effective and should be considered if other therapies have not worked.*

Nutritional

- *Have a food allergy test and eliminate all foods to which you react strongly.*

Supplemental

- *High-dose vitamin supplementation may be effective: vitamin C (1g for every foot of height in divided doses with each meal), vitamin B_6 (20mg for every foot of height) and vitamin B_5 (100mg for every foot of height).*

- *Quercetin (150mg per foot of height) taken with breakfast and hydrochloric acid tablets and pepsin with meals are beneficial.*

Homeopathic

- *Visit a homeopath for an accurate prescription. Minor ailments can be alleviated by considering the use of the following remedies: Allium cepa, Sabadilla, Euphrasia, Apis, Urtica urens and Arundo taken as potency 6 every 2hr.*

Orthodox

- *Avoid orthodox medication except in severe cases until alternative treatments have been used and failed. Orthodox treatments such as anti-histamines block the effect of the body's attempts to cure itself.*

ANAEMIA

The diagnosis of anaemia is made through a blood test. It is defined as a lack of haemoglobin or red blood cells.

Symptoms arise from having a lack of oxygen delivered from the lungs to the body tissues. The symptoms of anaemia can be very subtle but include pallor, general weakness, lassitude and inability to fulfil a normal day's function, unexpected exhaustion on exercise and, less commonly, recurrent infections and nausea.

Causes of anaemia

- Blood loss: trauma, ulcers, heavy periods, haemorrhoids and other internal injuries.
- Inability to make red blood cells or haemoglobin: disease of the bone marrow and toxins such as drugs.
- Disease process: cancer and other chronic diseases.
- Malabsorption: disease of the bowel, malnutrition and food allergies.
- Physiological: pregnancy and the first few periods.

Normal and Anaemic Blood Samples

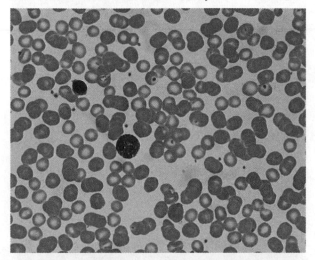

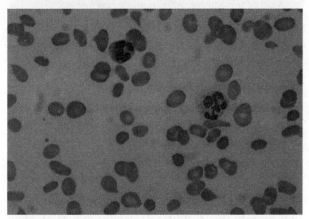

The anaemic blood sample (bottom) shows a much lower number of red blood cells. Many of the remaining cells are deformed. Consequently, the oxygen carrying capacity of this blood is drastically reduced.

All food groups are needed to maintain red blood cell production including amino acids, vitamins and trace elements. Certain compounds are particularly important and are needed in quantity. These are:

Iron: offal, red meat, oysters, eggs (principally the yolks), dried peaches, nuts, beans, asparagus, molasses and oatmeal.

Vitamin B$_{12}$ – offal, red meat, pork and dairy products.

Folic acid: – deep-green leafy vegetables, carrots, liver, beans, rye and cantaloupe melon.

RECOMMENDATIONS

General Advice

- *Establish a cause after a blood test has confirmed anaemia. Many conditions mimic anaemia and a clinical diagnosis is not always accurate.*

Nutritional

- *A pot of plain yoghurt with a teaspoonful of turmeric is an Ayurvedic treatment and is best eaten on an empty stomach any time of the day before the late afternoon.*
- *Ensure good intake of the foods listed above.*

Supplemental

- *Blood tests can identify the cause of anaemia through deficiency and, having established this, supplements can be taken.*
- *Ensure a vitamin C intake of around 1g per meal minimally to encourage iron absorption.*

Homeopathic

- *The homeopathic remedies Ferrum metallicum and Ferrum phosphoricum can help iron-deficiency anaemia and remedies such as Veratrum album, Arsenicum album, Carbo animalis and Cinchona arsenicum should be reviewed to help the symptoms.*

BODY ODOUR (BO)

Everybody has their own specific body odour. The smell should be neither obtrusive nor offensive but nevertheless distinctive. The smell emanates from the sweat pores and is dependent upon the content of sweat and other matters. This is not an unusual problem for many teenagers due to body odour being associated with poor hygiene after exercise. Bacterial activity in association with changing hormones and the predilection of this age group to use chemical deodorants that damage the body's natural flora and allow bad bacteria to produce their toxins and odours on the skin unchallenged. Persistent bad body odour may represent the presence of certain systemic diseases.

Sweat is similar in composition to urine except

for the presence of urea, a nitrogen-based protein waste product. The blood is generally cleansed by the kidneys and rarely has to resort to eliminating through the skin, but dehydration and certain drugs and diseases affecting the kidney can lead to the utilization of sweat as a waste product and thereby alter its smell.

Eating an excess of pungent foods such as garlic or spices may simply overload the system and the sweat absorbs the product with no pathology being present in the system.

Skin bacteria should produce little, if any, odour but certain strains, especially those that have been altered by the use of antibiotics, can produce noxious gases that are experienced as BO. The more sugar in the diet and the moister the environment in which the bacteria live, the more they multiply and these increased numbers create increased odour.

Some hormones have their own smell, such as adrenaline (the smell of fear), and female cyclical hormones actually encourage bacterial growth which in turn may encourage body odour.

RECOMMENDATIONS

General Advice

- *Use only unmedicated soaps and avoid deodorants other than topical applications of essential oils, preferably to the undergarments.*
- *Wear natural fibres that absorb sweat more effectively and change clothes regularly if necessary.*
- *Ensure good hydration by drinking at least a pint of water for every foot of height in divided doses throughout the day. Ensure that more water is drunk if exercise is undertaken or if alcohol and caffeine are drunk as these dehydrate the body.*
- *Ensure good hygiene and regular washing and changing of clothes.*

Nutritional

- *Observe any changes on a daily basis in association with certain foods. Foods such as*

garlic and onions can create a body odour and individuals may be susceptible to particular foodstuffs. Keep a journal and ask a family member or close friend to monitor changes over a period of a few weeks. Correlate this to foods eaten and avoid any suspect foods.

Supplemental

- *Bad bowel bacteria can produce toxins that find their way into the sweat. Use high doses of Lactobacillus acidophilus and Probifidus shortly before each meal. Chlorophyll can be utilized similarly.*
- *Zinc (30mg each night) should be tried.*
- *Poor digestion can lead to an abundance of foods for bacteria, who multiply quicker and produce more toxins. Use hydrochloric acid and digestive enzymes in the amounts recommended on the packet.*

Homeopathic

- *Review the homeopathic remedies Calcarea carbonica and Silica and use potency 6 three times a day for ten days.*

CHRONIC FATIGUE SYNDROME (CFS)

Inexcusably this condition (also known as myalgic encephalomyelitis (ME) and postviral fatigue syndrome (PVFS)) have only been officially recognized by the medical profession in the UK since the summer of 1996. Other countries have been a little bit more open but a large percentage of doctors refuse to accept that this syndrome exists.

The definition of CFS is initially a 'diagnosis of exclusion'. This means that other medical causes must be investigated and eliminated. The symptoms must include fatigue or lethargy causing a 50 per cent loss of physical and social function for at least six months. Four of the following symptoms must also be present:

- **Physical:** sore throat, persistent infections, swollen and/or sore lymph nodes, headaches and pain in muscles or joints.

Herbal Remedies for Chronic Fatigue Syndrome (CFS)

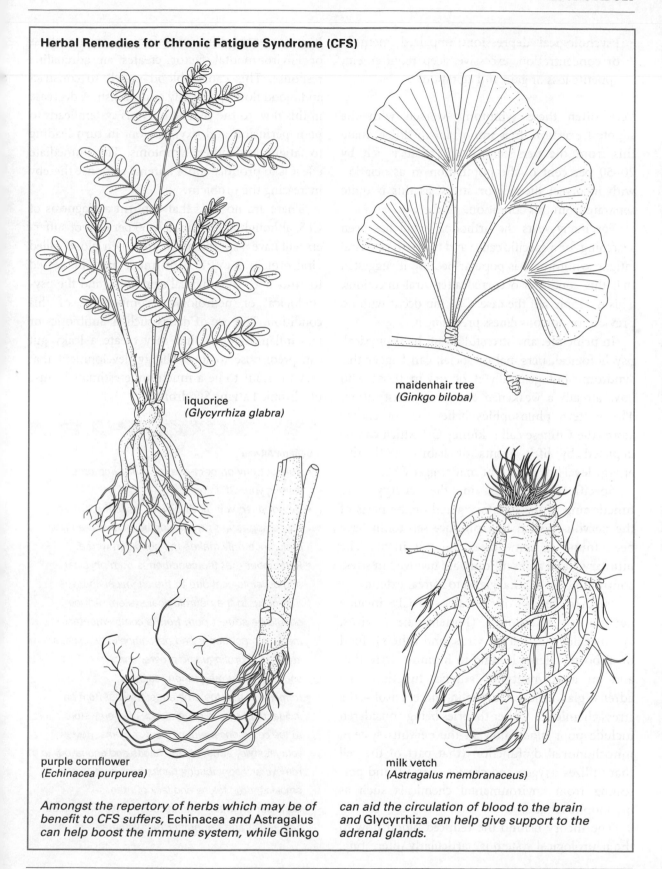

liquorice
(Glycyrrhiza glabra)

maidenhair tree
(Ginkgo biloba)

purple cornflower
(Echinacea purpurea)

milk vetch
(Astragalus membranaceus)

Amongst the repertory of herbs which may be of benefit to CFS suffers, Echinacea and Astragalus can help boost the immune system, while Ginkgo can aid the circulation of blood to the brain and Glycyrrhiza can help give support to the adrenal glands.

- **Psychological depression:** impaired memory or concentration, excessive sleep requirement, appetite loss or gain and agitation.

Very often these symptoms worsen with the slightest exertion. It is important to differentiate this from the persistent fatigue that is felt by 20–50 per cent of the population in association with incorrect lifestyle or stress, as this is quite separate from this condition.

For many years the orthodox world has been searching for a specific cause and the term postviral fatigue syndrome was popular because it suggested that this condition occurred after viral infections. This is simply not the case; CFS can occur with no previous or obvious illness preceding it.

In principle, any stressful event, be it physical, psychological, personal or social, can trigger this syndrome but generally it occurs in those who have already a weakened energy or constitution. The Eastern philosophies believe in an energy store (the Chinese call it kidney Qi) which can be depleted by life's events or habits. With this energy level low any event may trigger CFS.

Specific imbalances in the energy and functioning of the pituitary gland or the parts of the nervous system that produce serotonin have been found in some cases but not in all. The pituitary gland and serotonin are involved in stress controlling the adrenal gland to a great extent.

Further theories of the causes of CFS include persistent infection (Epstein-Barr virus, cytomegalovirus, herpes virus, and others), food or airborne allergy leading to immune activation and an abnormality of adrenal function (the adrenal gland makes adrenalin and cortisol – the stress chemicals). Other theories being considered include poor blood flow in the nervous system, mitochondrial dysfunction (that part of the cell that utilizes oxygen and creates energy), and poisoning from environmental chemicals such as organophosphates.

The theory behind the reduced blood flow to the neurological system is particularly interesting.

It is suggested that an infection, injury, stress or environmental factor creates an adrenaline response. This causes blood vessels to constrict and blood flow apparently to diminish. A decrease in this flow to the central nervous system leads to poor perfusion and oxygenation, in turn leading to fatigue and other symptoms. The immediate effect is to produce more adrenal response thereby increasing the problem.

There are no tests that confirm a diagnosis of CFS, although approximately 60 per cent of sufferers will have a specific protein in their blood called viral protein 1 (VP1). Treatment must be geared towards both the physical symptoms and the psychological or neurological components of this condition. The use of drugs such as antibiotics or anti-inflammatories that may create a leaky gut can predispose to food allergy development that may turn out to be a much underestimated cause of Chronic Fatigue Syndrome.

RECOMMENDATIONS

General Advice

- *Rule out any other cause for your symptoms by visiting your GP initially.*
- *Do not push your body beyond its limits. Unlike, say, trying to get fit, working beyond your body's endurance only makes the condition worse.*
- *Remember that the condition is both physical and physiological due to the chemical changes that occur in the neurological system. Advice should be sought both from a complementary medical practitioner and psychological specialists such as neurolinguistic programmers, counsellors or meditation teachers.*
- *Remember that the problem stems not from an incident but from a general lack of energy store prior to the commencement of the symptoms. Review your lifestyle, stresses and habits and endeavour to remove any contributing habits such as cigarette smoking, drug taking and lack of exercise.*
- *Consider an initial detoxification programme (see chapter 7) and remember that you may feel an*

exacerbation of your symptoms as your body starts to repair.

- *Investigation through your GP or senior complementary health professional is essential to rule out any of the causes mentioned above. Specifically, some complementary therapists will have access to heart stress or pulse pressure monitoring which can help the practitioner to choose the appropriate therapy.*

Nutritional

- *Ensure that your diet is suitable for yourself (see chapter 7). Test for food allergy/intolerance through blood test or bioresonance techniques.*

Supplemental

- *Take twice the recommended daily allowance of the following compounds in divided doses with breakfast and a late afternoon snack (not with your evening meal): beta-carotene, a multi-B complex, vitamin C and zinc.*
- *Maximum recommended doses of adrenal extract and thymus gland extract should be taken.*
- *A recent study has found that the amino acid L-carnitine can be of benefit in reducing fatigue. The recommendation is 1000mg 3 times daily. The only side effect was that 1 in 18 participants developed diarrhoea. If this should happen, reduce the dose until this effect disappears.*
- *There may be a significant folic acid deficiency so take high doses, 500mg per foot of height, daily for 3 weeks to see if there is any benefit.*

Homeopathic

- *Homeopathy can be most effective, depending on your symptoms, and referral to your preferred homeopathic manual or a session with a homeopath to choose a remedy for the symptoms and your constitution is an excellent first step.*

Herbal/natural extracts

- *Ginseng and liquorice may be supplemented with some success. See **Herbal remedies** on previous page.*
- *A mushroom, Coriolus, has been well researched and may have an impact on CFS. Prescription is best carried out by a qualified practitioner, but if available in a shop take the maximum dose recommended for 1 month and then half the dose for the next 2 months.*

Orthodox

- *In some patients, low-dose hydrocortisone reduces fatigue levels in the short term but longer-term studies are still required.*
- *A majority of patients are prescribed antidepressants and as many as 60 per cent of these improve. Whether there is an improvement because the patient feels less depressed or because of an actual therapeutic benefit is still in doubt.*
- *Not strictly orthodox, but a derivative of a morphine (heroin) antagonist, naltrexone, is undergoing research in relation to conditions that effect the nervous system. Prescribed by those physicians in the know this may prove to be a potential cure.*

If you have no response with these supplements within one month, then contact your preferred complementary medical specialist.

CIGARETTES

An entire book could be written about the toxic effects of cigarettes. My experience is that many people do not know a fraction of the detrimental effects that cigarettes can cause, merely assuming that you either get cancer or you do not. Everybody knows somebody in their eighties who has smoked 40 cigarettes a day. This is indeed true, but for every one person who tolerates cigarettes and their poisons, there are 1,000 who do not. Whichever way you look at it, cigarettes are highly toxic and very few of us have the constitution that will allow us to smoke and not develop some disease process, be it mild or terminal.

There are over 3,000 recognized compounds in cigarette smoke. We have no idea of the effect of many of these compounds on the system but we have recognized 16 compounds known to cause cancer and recently, beyond the dispute of the tobacco industry and their friends, one compound, a bendrofluoride, has been shown to trigger cancer changes in lung tissue. The tar in which these compounds are contained is a breeding ground for bacteria and, as the tar coats the delicate lung tissues, allows the bacteria to destroy the air sacs where oxygen is absorbed.

Nicotine is a most highly addictive compound proving even more difficult to withdraw from psychologically than heroin.

Conditions that are smoking-related include:

Sinusitis	Anosmia (loss of smell)
Ear infections	Catarrhal conditions
Taste loss	Recurrent coughs and colds
Conjunctivitis	Poor facial skin
Tooth and gum decay	Laryngitis
Pharyngitis	Recurrent sore throats
Acute bronchitis	Chronic bronchitis
Emphysema (loss of lung tissue)	Heart attacks
Strokes	Gangrene
Stomach and duodenal ulcers	Oesophageal ulcers
Ulcerative colitis	

Cancer is not the most common medical condition created by smoking but of the following list smoking is implicated in increasing the chance of contracting this cancer or is directly related to its onset: cancer of the mouth, tongue, throat, larynx, bronchial tree (lungs), oesophagus, stomach, large intestine, skin and the ovaries.

It is worth remembering that the lungs do not finish growing until we are in our early twenties. Smoking before this time will damage the foundations of the lung and the earlier cigarettes are started, the worse the prognosis.

Passive smoking (inhaling other people's smoke) carries equal risks for those who are sensitive or reactive.

RECOMMENDATIONS

General Advice

- *Do not smoke.*
- *Do not be around smoke.*
- *Do not smoke indoors. Smoke lingers.*
- *Do not smoke anywhere near children or where they live or play.*
- *Do not smoke in front of children – they mimic.*
- *See* **Smoking**.

CLUSTER HEADACHES – *see* Migraines

DEHYDRATION

Dehydration can occur in both an acute and a chronic state: the former is easy to identify and fairly easy to remedy; the latter is insidious, overlooked and, I believe, the cause of many of today's illnesses and conditions.

Acute dehydration

This occurs most frequently in younger adults who overexercise in hot or humid conditions. The athletes we see failing in their excursions due to cramp are usually doing so because of dehydration. The symptoms are obvious in some cases but in others require a little thought.

A sensation of thirst, dry mouth and lips is fairly obvious but overlooked are tiredness, muscular fatigue and cramps, dry skin or cessation of sweating. Later signs of acute dehydration will include dizziness or fainting, rapid heartbeat and confusion or delirium. This usually only occurs when dehydration is very severe, as can be seen in desert movies!

RECOMMENDATIONS

General Advice

- *Avoid dehydration! If you are in a hot climate or performing exercise, ensure a regular or persistent intake of water.*
- *If dehydration has occurred, replenish water slowly. Alternate with salty or sugary solutions, or use specially prepared electrolyte solutions in*

conjunction with water to replace the lost salts and glucose. Use natural sugars, not refined.

- In more severe cases, place the body in a bath or wet cloth and, of course, remove from heat where possible.

Chronic dehydration

Chronic dehydration does not have the same immediate or acute symptoms as described above. It occurs over a period of time when most individuals slowly but surely drink less water than they require and the body adjusts by losing its sensitivity to thirst and learns to live with dry lips, dry skin, muscular aches and pains and a variety of other symptoms described below. This lack of sensitivity is a tribute to the human body's ability to adjust to its circumstances but it may be that this adaptation has led us to deal with an increase in many of the symptoms that plague us, especially in the Western world. These include cancer, asthma, arthritis, eczema, digestive problems and susceptibility to infections.

The biochemistry of the body requires water in most, if not all, of its reactions. Most of these reactions go on within cells that will be reluctant to give up water if less than adequate amounts are taken in regularly. Every cell in the body will protect itself by taking up cholesterol, other fats or lipids and proteins to create a lipoprotein layer around itself. This prevents water leaving the cells but also inhibits water from entering the cells. The biochemical processes continue but, like a stagnant pond, will eventually use up some of the natural energy provided in molecules that can interchange with each other and, although the processes will continue, the natural energy associated with them may not. Meanwhile, the water we take in is not absorbed fully into the cells, our tissues can become bloated and the bloodstream mildly diluted, telling the brain that we do not need water and thereby reducing our thirst and perpetuating the dehydration cycle.

The cholesterol, fats and proteins that are required for this protective process are made by the liver. The liver works overtime and has less availability to deal with the body's general requirements for metabolism, both in breaking down toxins and building up the compounds that we need. More energy is required to keep the liver functioning and therefore less energy is available elsewhere so that tiredness and fatigue become common initial symptoms. The lack of breakdown of toxins puts pressure on the kidneys and poisons get deposited around the body. Much of this poison is taken up by fat stores, which also accommodate the extra fats that the liver is constructing for the benefit of the protective layer of the cells, and so the fat stores increase, as does one's weight. Toxins are dissolved into the fat stores and more water is pulled into these tissues to dilute down these toxins. This again increases the body's retention of water in areas where it should not be held.

The slightly higher metabolic rate created by dehydration encourages the production of free radicals known to promote atheroma, leading to heart attacks, strokes and also cancer.

Lacking water, the body generally concentrates its fluids. The hydrochloric acid in the stomach and the digestive juices throughout the intestine become more concentrated and, whilst this may help digestion overall, it challenges the lining of the bowel leading to inflammation and ulcerative conditions and this inhibits the correct production and multiplication of the body's natural bowel flora.

The higher concentration of acidity is absorbed into the bloodstream and can cause: arthritic conditions; conditions in the skin, such as psoriasis or eczema; and concentration of other fluids, such as in the gallbladder, leading to gallstones.

Need I go on … ?

Put simply, the argument could be made for dehydration affecting many if not most medical conditions in the body. Dehydration is insidious. One must remember that we are losing approximately two pints of water each day in our urine, approximately the same through sweat and about a pint through nasal mucus and stool. This has to be replaced, otherwise we fall into a dehydration pattern.

General Advice

- *Any persistent or recurrent condition of a lack of health or illness requires a review of the body's hydration.*
- *There is no strictly accurate amount that suits everybody. If you are a thirsty person, ensure that your thirst is quenched by water and that any other fluids (tea, coffee, alcohol, juices, etc) are taken for pleasure or effect rather than to quench the thirst.*
- *If you are not a thirsty person then a minimum of half a pint of water per foot of height should be taken throughout the day.*
- *Do not confuse the intake of fluid with the intake of water. You are not rehydrating yourself using anything but water or the most dilute of juices.*
- *Tea, caffeine and sugars (both refined and natural, such as fruit juices) are all potentially dehydrating. Each time any of these are enjoyed, a glass of water should follow within 15min.*
- *Avoid tap water where sanitation is poor or the water is fluoridated (see* **Fluoride***). The installation of a reverse osmotic filter or the use of mineral water should be balanced with one glass per day of tap water in fluoridated areas, unless the fluoride intake through the diet is known to be adequate or fluoride toothpaste is used.*
- *Vary your mineral water because some are higher in some components than others.*
- *Water should be drunk at room temperature or warmer, especially if rehydrating. Iced drinks, whilst enjoyable, are not good for the body and should be limited.*

DIABETES MELLITUS

Diabetes mellitus, commonly shortened to diabetes or sugar diabetes, is a complex condition that arises because the body's metabolism of sugar is impaired, faulty or absent.

Diabetes is often discovered through the simple symptoms of passing urine too frequently and having a persistent thirst. This is caused by too much sugar in the blood being passed through the kidneys into the urine, and water following due to osmotic attraction. Because the individual is passing so much urine, the body recognizes dehydration and drinks more. Excessive sugar in the bloodstream can lead to problems in any organ or system in the body, predominantly by causing arteries to clog up. Unrecognized diabetes can, therefore, cause blindness, kidney failure, strokes, heart attacks and a myriad of neurological symptoms. The problems may take years to develop and therefore a regular screen of the urine and blood is a wise precaution, especially if there are any diabetics in the family. Diabetes has a strong genetic tendency. The tests are simple and accurate. Testing for raised sugar levels (above 140mg/dl or greater than 10mmol/l) is done simply and the same blood sample can measure a particular type of haemoglobin known as HbA, which can be monitored to establish the severity of the diabetes.

There are several types of diabetes, which I classify as follows.

Temporary diabetes

This can occur through pregnancy and is known as gestational diabetes (*see* **Vessel of conception**). Temporary diabetes can also be associated with a variety of ailments such as viral infection, malnutrition, eating disorders and pancreatic disease. Several commonly used drugs can induce diabetes. Most of these conditions will be short-lived or respond when the causative factor is removed.

Non-insulin-dependent diabetes mellitus (NIDDM type 2 diabetes)

The onset of this type of diabetes is usually in

adulthood and is either caused by a mild deficiency in production of insulin from the beta cells in the pancreas or due to cells in the body not responding to the insulin that is being produced, possibly even at high levels. The reasons for this loss of sensitivity are not well-established but it is known that being overweight seems to desensitize the individual to insulin levels; chromium deficiency is also implicated.

Insulin-dependent diabetes mellitus (IDDM type 1 diabetes)

This type of diabetes usually has its onset at a young age. It is possible to be born with this hereditary lack of beta cells in the pancreas or they may be destroyed by virus, autoimmune attack or drugs (medical or from food).

The Eastern philosophies of medicine consider the pancreas to lie under the vessel of conception (*see* **Vessel of conception**) and it may also be the area for the solar plexus, a central yogic chakra. The vessel of conception is an energy line provided for by the parents and therefore a weakness would be, in Western terms, genetic. The advent of diabetes during pregnancy, where the uterus (another organ on this mid-line meridian) pulls energy into itself to feed the child, therefore depriving the pancreas and thyroid of their energy. These two organs control sugar levels and thyroxine levels, both of which can fall, inexplicably, during pregnancy.

Recognizing diabetes

I mention above that the most common symptoms are those of excessive urination and thirst. Increase in appetite, weight loss despite eating, frequent infections and slow healing of simple wounds are all warning signs.

More serious complications such as blindness and stroke occur after years of uncontrolled diabetes and are generally discovered by taking the problem to a physician.

If the basic blood and urine tests are equivocal then a glucose tolerance test is performed: a 75g dose of a sugar solution is given orally and blood samples are taken just before and at half-hourly intervals after ingestion. If the levels of sugar in the blood exceed those expected, then a diagnosis of diabetes is made.

Diabetes is not a condition to be confronted without professional support. Monitoring by your GP or hospital is essential. Consultations with a complementary medical practitioner with training in nutritional medicine should run alongside orthodox monitoring. Uncontrolled diabetes can cause coma and death fairly swiftly, and if treatment is required with insulin the same outcome may occur if too much insulin is injected. Insulin has to be injected because it would be destroyed by the acid in the stomach if taken orally. There are several types of insulin, including those made artificially and those extracted from animals such as the pig. There is some controversy as to which is the best type but your individual specialist will have his or her own protocol and this should be followed until the scientists come up with complete answers. Insulin comes in quick-acting, intermediate and long-acting forms and generally insulin-dependent diabetics will require a mixture.

Do not underestimate diabetes as a disease. It effects over four per cent of the Western population and this number is rising. There is a strong correlation between diabetes and diets high in refined sugar, such as those found in the West. Type 2 diabetes or NIDDM is usually well-controlled through diet and supplementation, and very often complementary medical practitioners will help an individual avoid the insulin-lowering drugs that are all too quickly prescribed by many diabetologists.

RECOMMENDATIONS

General Advice
• *Monitor urinary and blood sugar levels through your GP or hospital specialist. They will explain home-monitoring options, usually by pinpricks*

of blood, nowadays monitored by small computers kept by the bedside. Do not shirk this responsibility.

- *If you are overweight, lose it. Obtain as much help or support as you need but obesity may cause or adversely affect diabetes.*
- *Formulate a personal exercise programme that includes daily yoga. Excessive exercise may cause fluctuations in sugar levels from too low to too high, but yoga has actually been shown to be of benefit to diabetics. Aerobic exercise at the right level is essential to enhance cardiovascular strength as well as being part of a weight control programme.*
- *Reduce stress. Stress creates chemicals such as adrenaline and cortisol that raise blood sugar levels, and again techniques such as meditation have been shown to lower blood sugar levels and give diabetics better control.*

Nutritional

- *Consider the Pritikin diet (see **Pritikin diet**) early after a diagnosis of non-insulin dependent diabetes.*
- *Discuss dietetics with a well-qualified and experienced nutritionist. Ensure that the following areas have been covered: eat low-fat, low-sugar, whole food and avoid refined sugars, flour and any additives, preservatives or other chemicals; avoid cow's milk products, which may be directly responsible for promoting diabetes in some genetically susceptible individuals.*
- *Enjoy garlic, onions and fenugreek in your diet and discuss with a herbalist suitable amounts of anthocyanoside from blueberry or blackberry sources.*

Supplemental

- *Discuss with your nutritionist the correct amounts of chromium, zinc, magnesium and other trace minerals, all of which have an important co-factor relationship in sugar level balancing.*
- *Until glucose levels are stable (and there is*

*strong evidence that the stability is more important than the level) use high-dose antioxidants and follow the advice in the section on atheroma (see **Atheroma**) in an attempt to protect the arteries from clogging up.*

- *Ensure a daily intake of gamma-linoleic acid and omega 3 and omega 6 fish oils.*
- *Quercetin, 100mg per foot of height twice a day, should be added to the use of high-dose antioxidants if there is any suggestion of cataracts, eye or neurological problems.*
- *High-dose antioxidants especially carotenoids, such as beta-carotene, lycopene and zeaxanthin, may protect against the development of diabetes. A formulation combining these, or any of these taken separately at the maximum recommended dose on the package is recommended.*

Homeopathic

- *Homeopathic remedies aimed at the individual's constitution will help, but they need to be given at specific, high potencies and will only be beneficial if prescribed by an experienced homeopath.*

DIABETES INSIPIDUS

This condition is characterized by excessive passing of dilute urine and excessive thirst. It is created by the lack or blocking of antidiuretic hormone made in the pituitary gland.

The causes range from tumour, drug intake (medical, drugs of abuse or others yet to be established), infections and blood loss. It is sometimes associated with heavy bleeding after delivering a child.

RECOMMENDATIONS

General Advice

- *Excessive urination and thirst must be assessed by a physician and if diabetes insipidus is diagnosed, follow orthodox treatments.*

- *Complementary medical treatment should be based on the symptoms, but acupuncture, Shiatsu and yoga are considered to strengthen the mid-line energy that is part of all Eastern philosophies of medicine (see **Vessel of conception**).*

ENLARGED SPLEEN

Any examination of the abdomen will require the physician to push under the ribs on the left side of the body. We are checking for the possibility of an enlarged spleen.

The spleen is basically an organ full of lymphatic tissue and blood vessels. It works as a store for blood and breaks down old or useless red blood cells. Lymphatic tissue, acting like a large lymphatic gland, will swell with infection or any process such as leukaemia that involves the increased production of white blood cells.

An enlarged spleen, therefore, can represent nothing more than a bad viral infection, but may be associated with disorders of the bloodstream and, at worst, cancer.

EXAM NERVES – *see* Nervousness

EXERCISE

Exercise is one of the most important factors in maintaining health. The human being has evolved over millions of years as an ambulatory (walking) creature and anthropologists suggest that 'man' probably walked for 6–8 hours a day much like the period we may work in today's Western culture. Much of the body design is geared towards walking, with short bursts of high energy (running or fighting). Exercise is necessary to

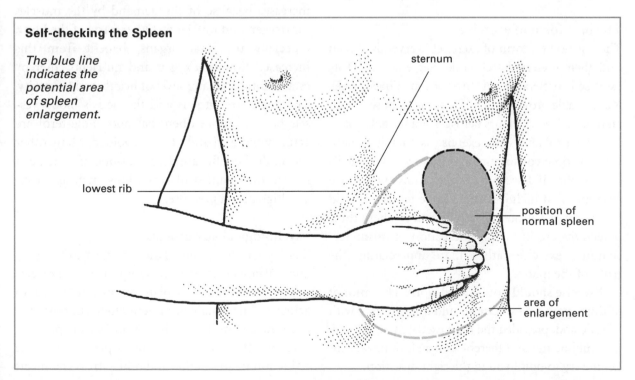

Self-checking the Spleen

The blue line indicates the potential area of spleen enlargement.

sternum

lowest rib

position of normal spleen

area of enlargement

maintain physical as well as psychological well-being. During exercise the body burns up stress chemicals that can inhibit concentration and it has been demonstrated that exercise can enhance creativity and reduce depression.

Western culture has provided an abundance of food and this, combined with our natural survival instinct of storing food in our body, leads to a tendency to obesity. Our ancestors had to work hard to produce, gather or catch their food and calorific input and output seemed to balance. Nowadays this is not the case and with the advent of telephones and take-away food we could exist with very little physical demands.

The outcome of all this is a need to exercise. As a general rule the male metabolic rate, at rest, uses up approximately 2,200 calories and the female approximately 1,700 calories. If you consider that a bowl of cereal and two pieces of toast with butter and marmalade replace up to 800 calories, and a prawn cocktail, meat and two veg followed by an apple pie with cream can add up to over 1,500 calories, you can see that we are generally out of balance. To redress this, we need to exercise.

The best form of exercise

There is no best form of exercise! Everybody should find their preferred technique and enjoy it. Daily exercise is preferable but three or four times a week is acceptable provided that it is of the right sort. Half an hour a day or 3 hours per week is a sensible goal.

'The problem with exercise is that it is hard work, is time consuming and there is no immediate benefit.' If I were to ask an individual to do anything that included these three factors, should I be surprised if there is a reluctance? These three objections are in fact an indication of misunderstanding exercise rather than appreciating the truth of the matter.

Exercise should not be hard work. The amount of time spent on exercise should not interfere with lifestyle and, provided the right exercise is employed, it should be fun and thereby of benefit immediately. Let me try to point you in the right direction.

What is exercise?

Exercise is defined as muscular exertion for the purpose of preservation or restoration of health or the development of physical prowess or athletic skill. This occurs through many mechanisms, both physical and psychological.

Physical benefits

Exercise burns up calories. The body is extremely good at taking in what it needs and it is only when we consciously fight our own instinctive ability to balance our physical exercise with our food intake that exercise can be harmful. By staying within certain boundaries, as described below, exercise controls excess.

When we exercise, our body uses up stress chemicals such as adrenaline and cortisol. Too much stress created by our daily life is thus taken out of the system benefiting health as a whole. Exercise also produces the body's natural opiates known as endorphins and enkephalins. These reduce pain and create a sense of well-being, even euphoria, and benefit the body as a whole. The heart beats faster and the respiratory rate increases because of the demand by the muscles for oxygen and nutrients. Other parts of the body, especially the vital organs, benefit from this increased flow of oxygen and nutrients, thereby establishing a greater level of health and longevity. The heart strengthens and the body's blood vessels become more open. Fat and cholesterol are actually reduced and obesity avoided. Many other metabolic benefits are derived, some of which can reduce the chances of conditions such as stroke and high blood pressure.

Psychological advantages

'Look good, feel good' is most accurate. Our body and self-image are extremely important in directing our confidence, which in turn helps us to achieve. This simple argument alone supports the encouragement of exercise but in fact the production of the body's natural opiates and the reduction in adrenaline and other stress chemicals has a profound effect on our state of mental well-being. Depression is alleviated, anxiety is reduced, addictive tendencies are transferred and sleep patterns are corrected.

Choosing an exercise

The benefit of exercise will only be noticed if around 30 minutes of a suitable standard is undertaken at least three times a week. This is strictly for maintenance and if you are trying to improve your level of fitness more exercise is required.

The exercise chosen should raise the heart rate to a level of approximately 75 per cent of the individual's maximum heart rate. This is calculated by subtracting your age from 220. A 20-year-old should exercise to a level of 75 per cent of 220 minus 20, which is equal to 150. A 60-year-old should reach a heart rate of about 120. Heart rate should not exceed 80 per cent of the maximum level.

Exercise needs to be enjoyed, otherwise enthusiasm will wane rapidly. Those who are competitive by nature will benefit from competitive sports. Those who are not, should choose non-competitive pastimes. Brisk walking is not likely to strain the body, but is time consuming and it may not take the heart rate to its optimum level, but if an enjoyable environment can be found then an exercise-paced walk may be most stimulating and relaxing. It is better to aim at an exercise that fits in with the individual's lifestyle. A mother may benefit by taking her young children to the swimming pool. A busy professional might find 20 minutes on the local gymnasium's treadmill quicker and more convenient.

Do not forget exercises such as dance and cycling which can fit into your entertainment or travel sections of the day. Yoga, Qi Gong, Tai Chi and techniques learnt in a local aerobic class can be used in convenient breaks in the working schedule at home, in the office or whilst travelling. A small floor space can act as effectively as a thoroughly equipped gymnasium once the techniques are understood. Ten minutes three times a day may not be as beneficial as a straight half-hour, but it is better than nothing. Twenty minutes each working day supplemented by 45 minutes at the weekend can transform a body within a month.

A gym instructor will be able to set a suitable programme, and specific machines or gymnasium techniques such as Pilates can help an individual to reach fitness at a rapid rate.

Swimming is heralded as the best form of exercise and, for those who enjoy it, it probably is. It is not weight-bearing and, provided that there are no neck problems, it rarely puts a strain on any part of the system. Swimming, more so than other exercises, helps to control breathing and can be very useful in lung disorders such as asthma.

The body is very much geared towards survival. If weight reduction is necessary then the body will do its best, provided that it is not fed incorrectly. A diet containing the recommended 10–15 per cent fat of its total recommended input (approximately 70 per cent carbohydrate and 20 per cent protein make up the whole – *see* **Nutrition**, chapter 7) will comfortably return a body to its preferred weight. Removing fats and carbohydrates completely will dramatically lead the body into thinking that it is deficient and it will therefore go into storage mode. The next time any amount of fat or carbohydrate is eaten it will be swiftly converted into fat storage. The biochemical adage is that 'fat burns in the flame of carbohydrate'. To break down the fat stores requires energy. In fact, two units of energy are required to release six units of energy stored in fat. If we do not feed ourselves with a certain amount of carbohydrates then fat stores will not diminish. The body can convert protein into energy, but this is not as easy as carbohydrate conversion.

Exercise should be divided into two categories.

Meditative exercise

Clearing the mind while exercising allows a balance of the mind–body connection. The body automatically does this as it supplies oxygen to the active muscles, thus decreasing the availability of oxygen in the brain. It is difficult to concentrate or be creative through exercise therefore. On a busy day when our consciousness spends most of its time from the neck upwards, the strain and mild pain that the body should feel when exercising allows the consciousness to move down and distribute the Qi. Techniques such as Yoga, Qi Gong, Tai Chi, martial arts, calisthenics and simple stretching release blocked energy whilst exercising the muscles. (To stretch a muscle group, a joint must be extended or flexed and this is only created by the work of an opposing, contracting muscle group. Exercise!)

Aerobic exercise

Aerobic exercise is a term coined to describe the increased utilization of air. For aerobic exercise to be most beneficial the heart rate should not exceed an individual's age plus 100, and the respiratory rate must not prevent the ability to answer a question. Of course, both of these parameters will be exceeded in a competitive moment or if pushing the body to achieve a new limit of endurance, such as might be expected from professional athletes, but for the rest of us, exercising within these parameters is wise.

I am a great believer in eliciting expert opinion initially, but this is not necessary. A sensible programme starting, if you are unfit, with a brisk walk is perfectly acceptable. Any sport, competitive or otherwise, should be considered but do not go back to five-a-side football when you are 40 years old if you have not played for 20 years. The mind will remember your previous abilities but the body will have a markedly reduced capability. Any such desire should be reviewed by a coach or gym instructor and a certain level of fitness should be achieved first.

I think that modern gymnasiums are excellent starting points, with their electronic gadgetry combined with basic weights and floor exercises. Any gym instructor will set up a suitable programme that should leave the new exerciser

feeling that they have achieved and want to do more. However, it is wise not to carry on but instead come back tomorrow.

Weight-bearing exercise (especially for women) because of its anti-osteoporosis effect, must take up some of the week's exercise. Floor exercises (most commonly used for abdominal and back strengthening) and swimming are excellent forms of exercise and should be considered a part of the programme, but only a part.

RECOMMENDATIONS

General Advice

- *Like so many things in our lives, getting motivated and remaining enthusiastic are often the hardest parts. Have a look in the mirror. Are you satisfied? Visit your preferred health carer and ask for a basic assessment. Are you jeopardizing your health? Can you keep up with your friends/children? Ask whatever question it takes but initiate a decision to reach an optimum level of health.*

- *Choose a date upon which you will start. For the week prior to this, cut out as many bad habits as possible: smoking, drinking and overeating should be reduced, if not stopped, and a healthy diet initiated.*

- *Ensure that rehydration is at the top of your list by drinking at least half a litre per foot of height per day.*

- *Establish a routine and be as disciplined towards this as one is towards the work routine.*

- *Do not put pressure upon your work or social time. Exercise within your acceptable parameters.*

- *Partake in an exercise that is enjoyable. If none obviously fall into that category, look around and ask friends for their opinion. Golf may be boring until you have a go. Pop into a local gym and try the various machines or resurrect an old school sport if possible. Experiment with different exercises.*

- *Half an hour a day or 3hr a week is an optimum amount of time to be spent on exercise. More should not be considered until a peak of fitness is reached.*

- *There is no preferred time of the day to exercise and each individual should choose by instinct the period of day that suits them. It is not wise to exercise within 1hr of eating because the body is in assimilation mode.*
- *If you have a competitive nature, make a plan of what you want to achieve or take on individuals of your own calibre. Do not overestimate your abilities. Fitness will come quicker than you think and will remain longer if you achieve a high level more slowly.*
- *Do not hesitate to use a professional guide or teacher initially. Never feel embarrassed about asking a physical fitness instructor about setting a plan. They too have their masters.*
- *Regardless of what exercise is chosen, have a lesson or two in yoga, Qi Gong or Tai Chi. They will enhance your abilities in any sport by improving your balance and strength and, more ethereally, helping to control Qi. Enjoy both meditative and aerobic exercises.*
- *Start slowly and build up. As with anything, stop whilst you are enjoying the event rather than pushing yourself through a pain barrier. This is a sure way to remove the enthusiasm and feel degraded.*
- *Stretching before and after exercise is extremely important. The before bit is well-established but even experienced athletes underestimate the importance of stretching after as a 'warm-down'. Keep warm and do not rush the post-exercise shower or bath.*
- *Do not exercise in a state of dehydration. It is better to drink one pint of water approximately 40min before exercise and the same amount over a period of 1hr after exercise.*
- *The meal taken before exercise should be predominantly carbohydrate and light.*
- *Only wear absorbent natural materials when exercising.*
- *Use bodywork techniques such as Shiatsu and massage regularly, especially through the initial weeks of starting an exercise programme.*

FACIAL FLUSHING

Facial flushing may occur because of a medical condition such as fever, a skin condition such as eczema and the taking of certain drugs, including steroids, but in young adults it is most commonly known as blushing. High blood pressure and alcoholism may also create a red face but this tends to be permanent rather than fluctuating.

A blush is a facial arterial response to the hormones created by the nervous system, generally in response to embarrassment. This is a physiological condition and need not be treated unless severe.

A flush of the face may also occur in response to adrenaline-like substances produced with anger. This too is a physiological response and does not warrant treatment.

RECOMMENDATIONS

General Advice
- *Unless particularly severe and causing social difficulties, this is not a condition requiring medical treatment.*
- *Hypnotherapy, meditation techniques and counselling, including the use of neurolinguistic programming, may all reduce the amount of hormone produced in response to embarrassment or, in the case of anger, bring out any underlying subconscious reasons for this overreaction.*

Homeopathic
- *Blushing through embarrassment may benefit from the homeopathic remedies Lachesis or Baryta carbonica taken at potency 200 nightly for seven nights and allowing one month for the full effect to take place.*

Orthodox
- *An operative procedure known as an endoscopic thoracic sympathectomy may be considered. This procedure is done by endoscopic examination and requires the cutting of nerves lying over the second and third rib that are accessed by a small cut in the armpit.*

FAINTING

Feeling faint is a weakness or lack of strength but actual fainting is a temporary loss of consciousness. Generally caused by a lack of oxygen to the brain, fainting may also be induced by low blood sugar, toxins in the bloodstream, such as drugs, occasionally food to which the individual is allergic, or shock.

Evolutionarily, a faint was a survival mechanism. Lying completely still or feigning death apparently encouraged the predator to ignore the 'carcass' in favour of that individual still alive. We are rarely confronted by such life and death situations in modern Western life but we still have the tendency in response to sudden shocks or prolonged anxiety, such as before exams or public speaking.

RECOMMENDATIONS

General Advice

- *An occasional faint may just be a characteristic of an individual and, provided that there is an obvious trigger, no further action need be taken.*
- *Repeated faints without any obvious pathological cause as defined following full medical investigation should be reviewed by a homeopath, nutritionist and cranial osteopath.*

Homeopathic

- *The homeopathic remedies Aconite, Arsenicum album, Sepia and Veretrum album should all be reviewed in a homeopathic manual.*

Orthodox

- *Frequent or repeated fainting requires investigation by an orthodox medical practitioner. Attention should be paid to hypoglycaemia, arterial occlusion and input of drugs or alcohol.*

FEVER (PYREXIA)

See **Fever in children**

Fever should be considered a friend. Fever itself is unlikely to cause any problems to an adult but it is important to assess the underlying cause because a fever may be a symptom of problems such as meningitis, pneumonia or kidney infection.

A normal temperature lies in the range 36°–37°C or 96.8°–98.6°F.

RECOMMENDATIONS

General Advice

- *A persistent or very high temperature (above 41°C or 104°F) should be reviewed by a medical practitioner.*
- *Refer to the relevant section in this book for the treatment of any established cause of a fever.*
- *Ensure good water intake, increasing normal consumption by at least 2 pints of water per day. A fever with sweating may need more. Avoid cold water, preferably drinking room temperature or warm water.*
- *Cold compresses on the forehead, neck, abdomen and ankles will bring the discomfort down whilst leaving the core temperature raised to encourage the immune system response.*
- *Exercise should be kept to the minimum of a short walk in fresh air if the patient feels like it.*

Nutritional

- *Fever diminishes appetite and the saying 'starve a fever, feed a cold' is true for short periods of time. Eat by instinct.*
- *Avoid alcohol, caffeine and other stimulants.*

Homeopathic

- *Refer to your preferred homeopathic manual for suitable remedies, paying special attention to Aconite, Arsenicum album, Belladonna, Bryonia, Gelsemium and Phosphorus.*

Herbal/natural extracts

- *Herbal remedies include extracts from elderflower and peppermint as an equal mix, or chamomile by itself or with yarrow as an infusion taken four times a day.*

FIBROMYLAGIA

Fibromyalgia is not a commonly diagnosed condition and may be poorly understood by many physicians. The signs and symptoms are numerous but 90 per cent of sufferers have severe fatigue, 50 per cent have headaches or migraines, and all will have some or many of the following:

Aching and stiff muscles, anxiety, depression, joint swellings, burning and/or throbbing pains, sleep problems, skin over sensitivity, palpitations and persisting or frequently recurring pain anywhere in the body.

The name 'fibromyalgia' derives from algia, meaning pain, with 'fibro' and 'myo' referring to the fibrous and muscular tissues of the body. It is very much a diagnosis of exclusion meaning that the label is given when no other obvious cause can be diagnosed. It is often mistaken for chronic fatigue syndrome.

The underlying cause is not understood. Hypotheses include viral attack within the central nervous system and, more specifically, the hypothalamus. This is a small area of the brain that controls much of the part of the nervous system that we do not consciously control (the autonomic nervous system) and specifically the blood pressure, sweating, fluid balance, temperature and heart rate. Other causes are thought to be toxins including chemical exposure and possibly vaccinations. Allergies, metal poisoning and possibly parasites are also theoretical causes.

RECOMMENDATIONS

General Advice

- See **Chronic fatigue syndrome** as treatment for the two conditions overlaps.
- Low-intensity exercise such as walking, gentle yoga or Tai Chi will be beneficial. Do not do so much that the pains are worse later on or the next day.
- Acupuncture, especially electro-acupuncture can be beneficial in this condition.
- Consider testing for a 'leaky gut' (see **Leaky gut syndrome**).

Nutritional

- As with any potential immune or inflammatory condition, increase the amounts of antioxidants through fruits and vegetables and essential fatty acids through oily and fresh water fish.

Supplemental

- Calcium 200mg per foot of height.
- Magnesium 200mg per foot of height.
- Vitamin E 75iu per foot of height.
- Vitamin B complex – maximum dose as recommended on product label.
- Anthocyanidins 50mg per foot of height.
- S-adenosylmethionine taken as recommended on the product packaging.

Homeopathic

- A choice of homeopathic remedy depends upon the symptom picture and would be best prescribed by a homeopath.

Herbal/natural extracts

- Glandular extracts (usually from cows) have been shown to be beneficial. Consider adrenal, thyroid and thymus glandular extract.
- Ginger, about an inch of root chopped up, covered with a mug full of boiling water and allowed to cool, can be drunk three times a day as the phenol compounds within can block pain chemicals.

GERMAN MEASLES (RUBELLA)

See **Rubella**.

Attention should be paid by pregnant women who do not know if they have had a previous exposure to or infection by rubella.

RECOMMENDATIONS

General Advice

- See **Rubella** in chapter 3.

Orthodox

- All women intending to become pregnant should have a blood test for previous exposure and current immunity to German measles. If negative, vaccination should be considered (see **Vaccinations**).

GLANDULAR FEVER (EPSTEIN-BARR VIRUS)

Glandular fever is so named because of the association with swollen glands in the neck, axilla and groin (although glands in the abdomen and thorax will also be enlarged but not palpable) in association with a fever. This condition is often recurrent because the causative agent, Epstein-Barr (EBV) virus, is resilient and may hide intracellularly, especially within the liver. (It may cause hepatitis.)

Glandular fever usually appears as a sore throat, fever, malaise and lethargy in association with the above findings. In a healthy individual the problem will last less than two weeks. Recurrence, however, may be every couple of weeks or it may in fact lie dormant for several months. Known in the past as the kissing disease, Epstein-Barr virus is disseminated by kissing, sneezing, coughing and mouth-to-hand-to-mouth contact (shaking someone's hand who may have licked their fingers). Unless one is already immuno-compromised as is the case in AIDS, Epstein-Barr virus is not generally a serious infection although it can cause a non-chronic hepatitis.

Epstein-Barr virus may be responsible for chronic fatigue syndrome (postviral fatigue syndrome) but most frequently appears as a sore throat, muscle pain, loss of concentration and depression with the aforementioned glandular swelling.

RECOMMENDATIONS

General Advice

- A blood investigation known as the Paul Burnell test should be performed on any persisting, resistant or recurring fever. A positive result may be indicative of acute or past infection.

- Epstein-Barr virus (EBV) is a member of the herpes group of viruses (see **Herpes**).
- Persisting affliction requires a complementary medical opinion because it is usually indicative of a suppressed immune system.

Supplemental

- Recurrent infections should be treated with Echinacea or Hydrastis by taking, per foot of height, 100mg of powdered solid extract or three drops of fluid extract in water in divided doses throughout the day.

GUILLAIN-BARRÉ SYNDROME (GBS)

The Guillain-Barré syndrome (GBS) is a neurological condition that is characterized by symptoms ranging from lethargy and muscle weakness to paralysis. In severe cases, paralysis of the respiratory muscles may prove fatal. The aetiology (cause) is unknown and the condition is diagnosed by excluding other causes of the symptoms. There is a strong association between GBS and previous, recent viral infections and recent vaccinations, particularly the measles and polio vaccines.

I believe that this potentially devastating syndrome is multifactorial and will only be triggered if the underlying nervous system is weak. This weakness can be created by persisting physical causes such as food allergy, drug abuse and other unhealthy lifestyles. I believe that stress leading to excessive adrenaline production over a period of time can 'strain' the nervous system and leave it open to such problems as GBS.

RECOMMENDATIONS

General Advice

- Any persisting neurological problem or one involving any form of paralysis must be reviewed by a GP or a neurological specialist. Any problems with breathing make this a medical emergency.
- Besides life-saving first aid, the orthodox world can only offer palliative treatment for GBS.

Consult a complementary medical practitioner with experience in this field.

- *Consider osteopathic or Marma therapy.*
- *Polarity therapy, cranial osteopathy, yoga and the Alexander Technique have, in my experience, all been beneficial.*
- *Strictly review lifestyle because any toxin may be responsible for the underlying weakness. Smoking, excess alcohol and drug abuse may all be culprits.*
- *Sit with a counsellor to discuss any obvious or subconscious anxieties and stresses.*
- *See* **Paralysis**.

Nutritional

- *Ensure that food allergy testing is performed (see* **Food allergy testing***).*

Homeopathic

- *Homeopathic remedies based on the symptoms should be prescribed by a homeopathic specialist. If vaccinations have been taken prior to the onset of GBS, consider using the homeopathic remedy Thuja or Natrum muriaticum, potency 200, morning and night for one week.*

HANGOVERS

This is a section often looked at in health books by the fit and healthy male! It is not that females do not have hangovers, but their health conscientiousness seems to be in the right place. Sorry to disappoint you, but there is no magic cure despite my reading around the subject, especially in parts of my misspent youth.

It is important to understand that a hangover is a 'good thing'. Alcohol in excess is a toxin that can damage many parts of the body, particularly the liver, heart, pancreas, kidney and nervous system. Alcohol is associated with high blood pressure, low blood sugar and diabetes, cirrhosis and neurological problems such as blindness, to mention but a few. The hangover is the body's attempt at warning of our overindulgence and risk. As we age, our liver produces more chemicals to break down alcohol, which is why our tolerance increases but unfortunately our body also adapts and therefore loses its hangover. This is not a good thing because we may be unaware of the damage we are doing and the extra work that our livers are having to perform.

The hangover sensations of headache, lethargy, muscle weakness, diminished concentration, photophobia and an upset stomach are all associated with dehydration and the breakdown product of alcohol and aldehydes.

I do not think it appropriate for a doctor of holistic medicine to give any of the numerous tips he or she may have to reduce a hangover because a successful treatment may encourage people to overindulge with the knowledge that they will not feel the pain. My recommendations are therefore based on helping the body to clear out, thereby minimizing the damage but not necessarily reducing the discomfort.

RECOMMENDATIONS

General Advice

- *Drink a third of a pint of water for every measure of alcohol (half a pint of beer, one glass of wine or one measure of spirits).*
- *Eat before drinking alcohol, even if it is only a small amount. Avoid drinking on an empty stomach.*
- *Do not mix your alcoholic drinks at any session.*
- *Avoid the popular use of 'the hair of the dog'. Whilst making some impact on well-being, it enhances the potential damage. Coffee is also a poor idea because it enhances the dehydration.*
- *Joking apart, frequent hangovers may be an indication of a mild form of alcoholism (see* **Alcohol***).*

Supplemental

- *An individual who indulges and creates frequent hangovers should consider the daily use of a liver support such as milk thistle or other herbal concoctions such as Liv 52.*

- *N-acetyl-L-cysteine 500mg three times through the day after meals can be considered.*
- *Glutathione, best taken as a lozenge or oral spray (as absorption is better through the mouth rather than through the stomach) can be used at levels recommended on the packaging.*

Homeopathic

- *The homeopathic remedy Nux vomica potency 6 can be taken every hour. A more specific remedy choice may be made depending on the symptoms and remedies such as Aconite, Chamomile and Pulsatilla should all be reviewed.*
- *The following can be taken at potency 6 four times a day (if symptoms continue after the first dose you can use these remedies hourly):*
  - *Natrum phosphoricum – especially useful after drinking wine and/or feeling acidic.*
  - *Natrum sulphuricum – if struggling with a dull heavy headache.*
  - *Cocculus indicus – for dizziness, nausea and drowsiness.*

Herbal/natural extracts

- *The National Headache Foundation in the USA has reported that eating or drinking a tablespoonful of honey before and after drinking alcohol can reduce the effects of a hangover.*
- *Boil up a pint of water and add two teaspoonfuls of chamomile, hawthorn, hops and peppermint.*

HEAD INJURY – *see* Concussion

HUMAN IMMUNODEFICIENCY VIRUS (HIV) INFECTION and ACQUIRED IMMUNODEFICIENCY SYNDROME (AIDS)

There are some basic facts to establish:

- Having HIV does not mean having AIDS.
- Human immunodeficiency virus is not proven beyond doubt to be the sole cause of AIDS.
- Having HIV in the system may not need to lead inevitably to AIDS.

Taking these three points into account, it is worth examining potential treatments against HIV and AIDS. The HIV is not a particularly aggressive or fast-replicating virus. It affects different people in different ways, which is why some people can contract the virus and die rapidly whilst others are alive and healthy 15–20 years later. The state of the individual's immune system appears to be very relevant to this observation. Carrying HIV is asymptomatic (without symptoms) but the effects of HIV can be minor or profound.

The virus finds a comfortable home in a subset of the body's white cell defence mechanisms which are commonly known as T-helper cells. They are so called because they are produced in the thymus and help other white cells to be active in the destruction of other invaders such as bacteria, fungi and viruses. Destruction of these cells allows minor infections that would normally not bother the system to become lethal. Once two or more of these infections are present, then the criteria for a 'syndrome' are satisfied and a diagnosis of AIDS is made. If the symptoms are not particularly severe then another term, AIDS-related complex (ARC), is used to describe the symptoms, thus creating a syndrome that is not in itself life-threatening.

Acquired immunodeficiency syndrome, on the other hand is a life-threatening condition. Symptoms can occur throughout the body but most commonly affect the lungs (*Pneumocystis carnii*), the skin (Kaposi's sarcoma and wart infections), the bowel (*Campylobacter*, *Candida*) and the nervous system (a variety of infections). It is found all over the world, very often in people with no HIV infection. This is a pedantic point because the majority of AIDS patients have their condition as a result of the association with HIV.

Many scientists and doctors from all over the world, some very eminent, believe that AIDS is not solely associated with HIV. Very acceptable concepts have been put forward to suggest that AIDS will only manifest when the body's immune system is incapable of keeping the T-helper cells healthy and functional. Human immunodeficiency virus undoubtedly damages this section of the immune system but then so do many other factors. It is feasible that HIV will not be lethal unless associated with other components that damage these T-helper cells. Drugs (both prescription and drugs of abuse), unhealthy lifestyle, infectious diseases such as syphilis, fungi and parasites and environmental pollutants have all been put forward with enough evidence to create scepticism in some scientific areas. Currently there are 29 different illnesses that exist independently, any of which in combination are labelled AIDS, but are these secondary infections possibly part of the cause of the immune system failure?

Many government departments and 'independent' watchdogs are financially supported by the pharmaceutical industry who would like to find a compound or compounds that would kill HIV. This means that authorities and the pharmaceutical industry, generally, do not emphasise the concept of personal health being relevant in fighting AIDS.

Human immunodeficiency virus is transmitted through some body fluids more than others. Theoretically HIV can survive in most body fluids but, in reality, blood and semen appear to be the main transmitting factors. If transmission has occurred through saliva, sweat or other discharges it is extremely rare and not well documented. The virus needs to be transmitted directly into the recipient's bloodstream which occurs through punctures and abrasions in the skin and mucous membranes.

The term HIV-positive does not refer to having AIDS. It has been established that there are two viruses (although many others are suspected), namely HIV-1 and HIV-2, both of which have detrimental effects on the T-helper cell population. The phrase 'HIV-positive' refers to the presence in the bloodstream of antibodies against these viruses. This phrase does not refer to the presence of HIV. It infers that HIV has at some time been present in the bloodstream because the immune system has produced a defence against them. This is of vital importance because it is a qualitative result (a 'yes' or 'no' to infection) and not a quantitative test (how much virus is in the system). More accurate tests, such as the polymerase chain reaction (PCR), measure the amount of virus. The PCR is not routinely done because of the expense and the controversy concerning its accuracy. Measurement of the T-helper cell and specifically the CD4 level indicates the amount of damage to the immune system but is not a good predictor of prognosis because the cell count can rise or fall independent of HIV but very dependent on the other factors that alternative practitioners and many scientists think are relevant to the disease process.

One often hears of the CD4/CD8 ratio. The CD8 T-cells are immune system inhibitors. They are equally important in normal health because they prevent an overreaction in the immune system. Unfortunately, if the normal balance between the CD4 helper cells and the CD8 inhibitor cells is disturbed, then ill-health will arise.

A most fascinating point of interest is that the speed with which HIV multiplies, infects and then destroys T-helper cells is much slower than the normal replication speed of the T-helper cells themselves. One eminent authority has likened the process to chasing an airline jet on a pedal bicycle. As this is the case, how the orthodox world continues to assume that HIV is solely responsible belies logic.

The carriage of HIV and AIDS is not a homosexual disease. The practice of anal intercourse allowing infected semen directly into the bloodstream through the inevitable abrasions in the rectal mucosa has allowed the spread of HIV to move rapidly in this section of society. The virus, which probably originated in Africa, having mutated from a harmless virus, is also transmitted heterosexually and through accidental injury. The vaginal mucosa is much tougher and less prone to abrasions and the vaginal secretions are much more antiviral than many other fluids. Once the 'epidemic' was established and accepted, the 'safe sex' practices of male homosexuals stemmed the increase in transmission in many educated parts of the world. Educated or otherwise, the increase in the spread amongst the heterosexual population is now the world's largest problem. Those who understand about the epidemic have been poorly educated into understanding that heterosexual sex is a danger and in uneducated areas people simply know no better. Contraception is not easily available in many parts of the world and anal intercourse is practised to avoid pregnancy throughout Africa and Asia. The increase of heterosexual HIV carriage is quite alarming in these parts of the world.

Despite hygiene and education being the most likely treatment to work, the orthodox world continues to follow its 'germ' theory and spends billions of dollars researching into drugs that can inhibit the growth of HIV. The drugs AZT and more recently DDI and DDT are highly toxic chemotherapy agents that aim at killing the cells in the immune system on the assumption that this will not allow the virus to survive. Most patients placed on AZT will come off the drug because of its side effects and the main study – the Concord Trial – showed that patients using AZT fare worse than those not taking it. It is disturbing that the authorities who allowed such a treatment to be practised are the same people who block the use of naturopathic treatments for exactly the safety reasons that they bypassed for this far more profitable drug.

Despite the poor outcome of AZT trials, the pharmaceutical industry continues to attack the virus whilst ignoring the common sense approach, which would be to stimulate the human immune system. Having found that the destruction of infected T-helper cells does not prolong the life of AIDS patients, two new drug groups were focused upon: nucleosides inhibit HIV production and protease inhibitors block the chemical process by which HIV enters new T-helper cells, as well as blocking viral replication. Currently, all AIDS and HIV-carrier patients are being 'strongly' advised to use 'triple therapy', which includes taking AZT

with drugs from both of these new groups several times a day. Those who can tolerate this chemical cocktail certainly show good results initially. I say, initially, because long-term studies have not been completed and one must remain sceptical because the initial findings of AZT were equally promising.

Most importantly, before I discuss the options for treatment, be very aware that there are documented cases of HIV infection clearing up. This has been noted in children and was reported most recently in the *New England Journal of Medicine*, 30 March 1995.

A baby boy born prematurely at eight months was diagnosed as having asymptomatic HIV-1 infection. The child contracted the infection from his mother who had had intercourse with a former intravenous drug abuser. The infant was not well due to his prematurity but showed no evidence of AIDS. Blood tests were done on separate occasions and showed the child to be infected with the virus. Blood tests were repeated at frequent intervals and at the age of 1 year the tests proved negative. They could find no evidence of HIV. The child and his immune system had destroyed and removed all evidence of the HIV. The case was finally reported when the child was aged 5 years and when he continued to remain free of disease.

I believe that AIDS is not caused by HIV alone. Without a doubt this virus is detrimental to the immune system and speeds up the process of disease but is not solely responsible for the ill-health associated with AIDS. More relevant is long-term abuse of the body through poor nutrition, environmental toxins in the air and food chain, the chemicals produced by stress, drugs (both prescription and those of abuse) and frequent exposure to infections and the antibiotics with which they are treated.

Treatment recommendations are based on dealing with all these factors.

General Advice

- *Avoid risks. Whether you have contracted the HIV already or not, have 'safe sex'. Oral sex cannot be considered safe if an individual is carrying HIV.*
- *If you have unhealthy habits or lifestyle, make a change.*
- *Do not fight this battle alone. Find a complementary practitioner with knowledge of AIDS and a group or counsellor specializing in this area.*
- *Remove toxins from your life in the form of drugs (including tobacco and excess alcohol) and foods containing steroids or antibiotics (most meats). Spend times in fresh air out of the cities. Do not ignore this good advice, it is essential.*
- *Deal with or come to terms with the stresses in your life. Excess adrenaline is poisonous to the immune system. Do not underestimate the importance of this factor.*
- *Try to avoid antibiotics, steroids in particular, because they damage the immune system. All infections should be given the opportunity to be treated from an alternative angle.*
- *Do not be surprised if alternative practitioners offer a treatment that they claim may be curative. Ensure with a medical practitioner that the treatment is not in itself poisonous and give it a go. It cannot be as harmful as orthodox drugs.*

Nutritional

- *Discuss with either of the above, or a nutritionist, a suitable diet plan. This is absolutely essential to your well-being.*
- *Ensure food allergy/intolerance testing is undertaken through blood tests or by an experienced bioresonance computer technician.*

Orthodox

- *The use of the 'triple therapy' should be considered if good health is not being maintained or blood counts are dropping to low levels. Until long-term studies have been done, I consider these chemicals toxic and should only be used as a last resort.*
- *Consider naltrexone 3mg before bed. This may slow down CD4 T-cell deterioration.*

Dealing with HIV and AIDS is a team process and there is an answer, as in the case described above. Do not give in to the orthodox view of inevitable demise because there is plenty of evidence to suggest that treatment and possible cure are available.

HYPERVENTILATION

Hyperventilation is not specifically defined as an illness but refers to a tendency to overbreathe. There is a natural instinctive tendency to control breath in times of stress. If very frightened we may hold our breath but with moderate levels of anxiety we may have a tendency to overbreathe. This is very often a necessary physiological response and not a problem, as is shown in exercising.

Without wishing to blind the reader with science, the need to hyperventilate or alternatively hold the breath is governed by the level of carbon dioxide in the bloodstream, which is measured in a part of the brain known as the respiratory centre. It is all based on a chemical equation:

$$H_2O + CO_2 \rightleftharpoons H_2CO_3 \rightleftharpoons 2H^+ + CO_3^{2-}$$

Keeping it simple, this equation shows how water (H_2O) and carbon dioxide (CO_2) react to form a chemical chain of two hydrogen ions ($2H^+$) and a carbonate ion (CO_3^{2-}). The hydrogen ions are kept at a particular level to allow the body's biochemical function. Any disturbance requires this equation to flow one way or the other. For example, when we exercise, our muscles produce more CO_2 as a waste product. This CO_2 is blown off by our breathing more swiftly. Because we are throwing out more CO_2, the equation moves to the left and the number of hydrogen ions in the body diminishes. This is a 'good thing' because we are also producing

Hyperventilation

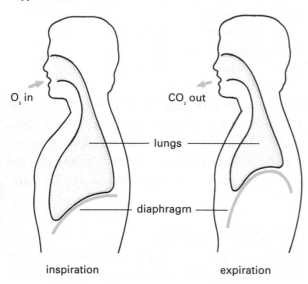

O$_2$ in

CO$_2$ out

lungs

diaphragm

inspiration

expiration

During inhalation the diaphragm contracts making the lungs expand. When exhaling the diaphragm expands forcing air out of the lungs.

more lactic acid from our muscle use and if we did not get rid of the hydrogen atoms in our bloodstream we would become too acidic and many of our biochemical functions would fail.

If you have managed to follow this so far, then the relevance and importance of hyperventilation will be apparent. Hyperventilation most often occurs when we are frightened. We blow off the carbon dioxide causing a loss of hydrogen ions, and what is known as a respiratory alkalosis occurs, which makes us feel dizzy and faint. The time-honoured tradition of breathing in and out of a paper bag causes us to inhale our exhaled carbon dioxide thereby reducing the loss of hydrogen ions and rebalancing our blood acid/alkaline levels (pH). This in turn returns our biochemistry to normal and we stop feeling odd.

The important point of all this is the tendency of many of us to hyperventilate without realizing it. Being under pressure or stress, which so many of us are, constantly causes us to hyperventilate not at a level that causes dizziness and fainting but at a level that alters our blood pH. Living at a persistently mild alkaline level affects the biochemistry of the body and can have profound effects, particularly on the cardiovascular system and lungs. Asthma, heart attacks and stroke are the most researched problems but it is possible that other conditions, including cancer, may result from a persistent state of hyperventilation.

It is difficult to assess whether an individual is hyperventilating because breathing 14 or 15 times a minute is only wrong if you should be breathing 12 times a minute, and symptoms and problems may develop only after many years.

Recognition of chronic hyperventilation is not possible from a clinical standpoint. Orthodox blood tests are of little value because modern science has shown that the biochemistry of the body will take place at a set, narrow band (a pH of 7.34–7.48). The body is very good at maintaining these levels but may be putting a considerable strain on the tissues and cells in controlling this. It is this strain that may cause chronic and serious illness. The use of the Humoral Pathological Laboratory Test and bioresonance techniques may disclose an alkalosis or acidosis and such tests must be considered in chronic illness (*see* **Humoral Pathological Laboratory Test** *and* **Bioresonance**).

RECOMMENDATIONS

General Advice

- *Acute hyperventilation from a shock, fright or an acutely anxious situation can be dealt with by placing a suitable container such as a carrier bag over the mouth and nose and re-breathing the exhaled carbon dioxide.*

- *There will be a tender point either side of the shoulders between the neck and the shoulder tip. Gentle pressure on these will help. There will also be tender points 2 inches either side of the chest bone and 2 inches below the collar bone. Gentle application to these will also help.*

- *Everybody should have training in breathing techniques (see **Breathing**). Yoga, Qi Gong and Buteyko methods are appropriate.*

HYPOGLYCAEMIA

This is the medical term for low blood sugar. The condition of *hyperglycaemia* is better known as diabetes and much is known about this condition. Hypoglycaemia, on the other hand, is poorly documented and is not considered a problem by the orthodox world unless somebody overdoses on insulin or some other form of blood sugar-lowering agent when treating themselves for diabetes.

The holistic consensus of opinion is that hypoglycaemia is far more prevalent and, in my experience, I must agree.

The symptoms of an acute hypoglycaemic attack are dizziness, confusion, blurred or double vision, poor balance, nausea, sweating, muscular lethargy and, at its extreme, fainting. In the case of a diabetic who has overdosed on a blood sugar-lowering agent, the symptoms can come on very rapidly. Individuals who have low blood sugar may find that symptoms are mild, persistent and/or recurrent. They most commonly occur about 1 hour after eating or first thing in the morning.

The main reason for low blood sugar is an overproduction of insulin. The pancreas, under the control of very sensitive sugar-level monitoring systems in the nervous system, produces more insulin when sugar levels rise. Refined or white sugar is absorbed very rapidly and therefore the insulin production is equally rapid, causing blood sugar levels to drop. Having a persistent low blood sugar level or tendency towards hypoglycaemia can cause metabolic changes, especially in the membranes of the body. A low blood sugar level can cause an excess of mucus production and a tendency for muscles to spasm. When this occurs in the lungs or the bowel, problems including asthma and irritable bowel syndrome (IBS) can ensue. Any persisting membrane problem that does not respond to other areas of treatment should be considered as being possibly caused by hypoglycaemia.

Other than an excess of insulin, some conditions within the system can use up blood sugar rapidly. The biggest culprits are infections, especially abnormal bowel bacteria and yeast infections such as *Candida*. Symptoms of hypoglycaemia or chronic diseases of membranes in association with bowel problems may well be *Candida*-related.

It is also worth noting that hypoglycaemia may be physiological, not pathological, as is the case when natural processes use up the available blood sugars in pregnancy and after exercise. More sinister conditions such as cancer, which can also burn up sugars, have to be considered and ruled out.

Some Eastern philosophies place a central energy point or chakra on the midline at the top of the abdomen. This coincides with the pancreas and an energy block that prevents the vital force from moving through that area can interfere with digestion and insulin control.

RECOMMENDATIONS

General Advice

- *A glucose tolerance test, most often used in establishing diabetes, can be used to diagnose hypoglycaemia (see* **Glucose tolerance test***).*

Nutritional

- *A diet high in fibre and low in refined carbohydrates and sugars is essential.*
- *Frequent small snacks throughout the day are better than three larger meals.*

Homeopathic

- *Several homeopathic remedies may match the symptoms and a reference to your preferred homeopathic manual should include reviewing the remedies Phosphorus, Aconite, Veretrum album and Carbo vegetabilis.*

Herbal/natural extracts

- *Herbal treatments may be of benefit but should be taken only under the expert guidance of a holistic practitioner. In the case of bowel bacteria problems, a one-week course of 2 billion acidophilus pre-meals is indicated along with the consideration of the use of capryllic acid under the care of a complementary practitioner.*

INFLAMMATION

Inflammation is the body's response to damage of tissues. If an injury occurs the body will attempt to repair the damage by sending more blood into the area. The blood carries scar tissue-forming cells, oxygen and nutrients necessary for repair and is therefore a 'good thing'. Unfortunately, the increased blood flow puts pressure on the nerves, which are already injured, and therefore the inflammation is painful. In severe injuries there will be a reflex reaction of a severed artery to close off, in which case inflammation does not take place and eventually gangrene sets in.

Inflammation is controlled by the nervous system, which opens or closes blood vessels by a reflex action that may include pathways through the spinal column. The nerves are stimulated by special tissue factors that are released from damaged cells and also by chemicals released from white blood cells that are pulled into the area by the initial nervous reflex. Orthodox drugs generally work by closing down the blood vessels or blocking the chemical reactions of these tissue factors or those within the nervous system.

The orthodox world considers only the symptoms and therefore does its best to suppress inflammation. There are a myriad of lotions and potions that pronounce themselves anti-inflammatory, ranging from aspirin and other non-steroidal anti-inflammatory drugs to steroids. Topical creams made from these drugs are also freely available. These treatments have their place when pain is unbearable but they are, in principle, slowing down the healing process.

RECOMMENDATIONS

General Advice

- *Inflammation is a healing process and should not be suppressed unless out of control. The holistic principle of encouraging the process will lead to a speedier recovery in most cases. This advice must be ignored if the inflammation is of a major organ such as the brain (ie meningitis) heart or kidney. Persistent inflammation*

may be associated with infection and reference should be made to the relevant section in this book.

- *Application of ice in a flannel or cloth will relieve symptoms but will not prevent the purpose of inflammation.*

Homeopathic

- *Reference to your preferred homeopathic manual and the selection of a remedy based on the predominant symptoms can be made, with special attention to Apis, Belladonna, Rhus toxicodendron and Urtica urens.*

Herbal/natural extracts

- *Arnica creams for deep tissue inflammation, Calendula cream for skin reactions and Urtica creams for very superficial inflammation can all be used.*
- *Persistent inflammation can be treated with high-dose vitamins and herbal remedies, but should be done under the guidance of a complementary medical practitioner.*

LUPUS – *see* **Autoimmune disease** *and* **Systemic lupus erythematosus.**

MASTURBATION

When religion sets down a doctrine it usually has a basis in some health or social foundation. I fail to see why religion is almost universally against masturbation. There are no serious health disadvantages and, if anything, it will enhance the desire for sex, thereby increasing the likelihood of procreation. It is interesting, however, that all higher levels of spiritual attainment generally involve celibacy and do not condone masturbation.

The Eastern philosophies, coinciding with Freudian concepts, suggest that sexual energy is a lower form than spiritual energy and perhaps there is some basis in avoiding masturbation and orgasm if trying to attain a higher spiritual level. I actually believe that an orgasm is the pinnacle of both spiritual and physical pleasure and therefore masturbation, in leading to an orgasm, is a simple technique of achieving a glimpse of Nirvana.

Excessive masturbation may cause bruising to the penis or clitoris and masturbation at inappropriate times or places may be an indication of psychiatric disorder but otherwise, from a medical point of view, there are no pros or cons.

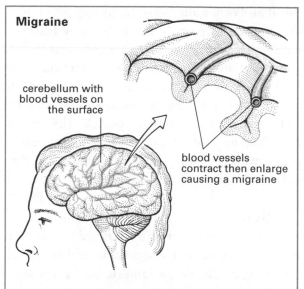

Migraine

cerebellum with blood vessels on the surface

blood vessels contract then enlarge causing a migraine

After an initial narrowing of the arteries in and on the brain, they then dilate and this causes the symptoms associated with migraine.

RECOMMENDATIONS

General Advice

- *There is no medical reason not to masturbate.*
- *Avoid excessive masturbation that can cause bruising and avoid the incorrect use of instruments to enhance pleasure.*
- *Excessive or inappropriate masturbation should be reviewed by a counsellor in case an underlying psychiatric disorder is associated.*

Homeopathic

- *Bruising can be helped by the use of the homeopathic remedy Arnica 6 every 2hr and an Arnica-based cream applied two or three times a day.*

MIGRAINE

A migraine is a recurrent headache that is probably created by changes in the level of dilation of the blood vessels in the brain. Migraines vary in intensity, frequency and duration. They commonly start on one side of the head, spreading to other areas, and are often associated with nausea, vomiting, visual disturbances or other neurological sensations, weakness and even paralysis and mood disturbances. Migraines are often found to run in families and they therefore have a genetic factor.

A classic migraine may last up to 24 hours and 50 per cent of sufferers have warning symptoms known as auras, which can be anxiety, fatigue or any of the neurological symptoms mentioned above that occur before the pain comes on. A type of migraine known as 'cluster headaches' are migraine-like pains that usually localize around one eye and tend to occur in clusters of up to three or four headaches a day over a few days, but only recurring every few months.

Interestingly, one in five men and one in four women will suffer from migraines at some time in their lives. Very often the onset is in childhood. Most migraines start between the ages of 20 and 35 years and generally disappear as we get older.

The jury is still out on deciding which of several possible mechanisms is responsible for causing migraine. Even with the technically advanced use of specialized tests, there is still some debate. There are thought to be several main factors that can trigger a migraine, however.

Stress chemicals such as adrenaline and catecholamines

Stress chemicals cause the release of a chemical called serotonin from specialized blood cells called platelets. This chemical causes blood vessels to constrict, resulting in a reduced oxygen flow to parts of the brain. A rebound defence reflex occurs that causes an increase in blood flow, causing pressure on the nerves and also a release of a substance that triggers pain, known cleverly as substance P.

Food and other allergens, including pollutants

Food intolerance and other toxins may trigger a stress chemical response as described above. A specific group of proteins known as amines that are found in alcohol, chocolate and cheese can all trigger attacks by directly causing vasoconstriction (narrowing of blood vessels). The list of foods that have been found in many trials to cause problems is very long but isolating each individual's food 'triggers' is necessary.

Structural

Any problem that can affect cranial blood flow may be relevant and malposition of the cranial bones, especially the jaw joint (known as the temporomandibular joint), is common.

Hormonal and other causes

Hormonal changes found in a normal female cycle, tiredness, weather changes and eye 'strain' can all precipitate migraines, as can withdrawal from drugs that cause vascular changes. A withdrawal syndrome may occur within a few hours of smoking a cigarette or drinking a cup of coffee and does not always refer to stopping a drug to which an individual is addicted or takes a lot of.

RECOMMENDATIONS

General Advice
- *Keep a concise journal over a period of time that covers at least three migraines. This must include food intake, stress levels, times of the attacks and hours asleep. Try to isolate and alter any obvious causative factors from those mentioned above.*
- *Learn a relaxation technique through yoga, Qi Gong or meditation.*
- *Counselling, hypnotherapy and biofeedback techniques are all beneficial.*
- *Consider cranial osteopathy or craniosacral work to correct any malalignment of the cranial and neck bones.*

- *Polarity therapy and Alexander Techniques to maintain posture may be relevant.*
- *Acupuncture and acupressure (Shiatsu) have been shown to be very effective in reducing the frequency of attacks.*
- *For symptomatic relief, see* **Headache**.

Nutritional
- *Consider food allergy testing but specifically eliminate caffeine, cheese and chocolate.*

Supplemental
- *The following supplements may be beneficial and should be taken in divided doses throughout the day at the recommended dosage per foot of height: Niacin (vitamin B_3), 10mg; Magnesium 100mg; Quercetin 100mg.*

Homeopathic
- *Homeopathic remedies should be chosen based on the symptoms, but pay special attention to the following homeopathic remedies that could be tried, one at a time, at potency 6 every half-hour in the 'aura' stage or every 10min if a migraine starts: Thuja and Spigalia for left-sided onset; Sanguinaria, Rhus toxicodendron and Iris for right-sided onset. Accurate prescribing based on the symptoms is essential, and referral to your favourite homeopathic manual or a homeopathic prescriber is preferable.*

Herbal/natural extracts
- *The herbal medicines capsicum taken at 5mg per foot of height in divided doses throughout the day and feverfew taken at the same levels may be beneficial.*

Orthodox
- *Orthodox drugs are available that work specifically against migraines. These need to be prescribed by a medical practitioner and should be considered only when alternative therapies have failed. Always try to take a minimum dose of a drug and even experiment by halving the dose recommended just in case you need less.*

POLYPS

A polyp is a smooth, round or oval projection from a membrane surface. Polyps may be broad-based or on a stalk. They rarely cause any sensations and are usually discovered on routine examination.

> **RECOMMENDATION**
>
> **General Advice**
> * *Treatment is dependent upon the site of the polyp, ie nasal polyp (see below), bowel polyp or cervical polyp (see relevant section, depending on the site of the polyp).*

SEXUAL PROMISCUITY

There is no right or wrong concerning sexual promiscuity but from a holistic and medical point of view, the subject needs to be broached. The definition of promiscuity is dependent both upon peer and social boundaries. One country may differ markedly from another, governed predominantly by the strength of its religion. Within any geographical distribution peer groups exert an enormous amount of pressure on an individual. The availability of suitable partners, sex and personal attractiveness or, at least, personal self-confidence are all factors in deciding the number of partners that an individual may have.

Medically speaking, promiscuity is defined arbitrarily, but in the West it usually encompasses four or more partners within 12 months.

Physical considerations

The higher the number of partners, the higher the risk of contact with a sexually transmitted disease (STD). Viral infections cover both ends of the medical spectrum. Human papillomavirus (genital warts) and herpes are rarely life-threatening, although the former may trigger cervical cancer in women. On the other hand, human immunodeficiency virus (HIV) is clearly associated with AIDS. Bacterial infection such as gonorrhoea is rarely a problem provided that adequate treatment is available, whereas syphilis is becoming more resistant to antibiotics and, once again, is on the increase. Other infections such as *Candida*, *Chlamydia* and *Trichomonas*, the latter two being responsible for the majority of non-specific urethritis (NSU), are also more prominent in the promiscuous.

Nasal Polyps

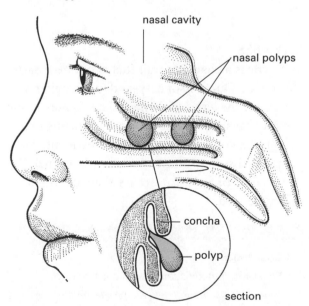

nasal cavity

nasal polyps

concha

polyp

section

Polyps are most commonly found in the nasal lining although they may be present on most mucous membranes. Usually they are benign.

> **RECOMMENDATIONS**
>
> **General Advice**
> * *Promiscuity is a risk and reducing the number of partners is medically advisable.*
> * *Safe sex needs to be practised, principally by using non-penetrative sex or correct use of condoms.*
> * *Prompt attention to any genital irregularity is to be recommended.*
> * *A social conscience that inhibits promiscuity by those that have infections must also be encouraged.*

Psychological considerations

The psychology of sex is a vast subject and beyond the scope of this first-aid book. Sex, designed to be an act of procreation, is used by the human species to reflect many underlying emotions. Anger, aggression and frustration through rape, love and adoration through making love and, arguably, low self-esteem and loneliness may be reflected by promiscuity, which temporarily placates the latter and, through peer adoration, raises the former. Sex is used as a recreation and our sexuality is pinpointed by many forms of advertising as a way to sell products. Our subconscious is constantly alerted by sexuality. Sex is pleasurable and the psyche is geared towards seeking pleasure. Sex is not always exactly what the individual requires but may be the inevitable end-point of the cuddle that was.

RECOMMENDATIONS

General Advice

- *Focus on the reason that sex is being sought and performed.*
- *Reflect, especially if alcohol or drugs are required to enjoy the act. Altered senses usually give altered signals of requirement.*
- *Remember that sex is not the inevitable outcome of any relationship where attraction is manifest. Most longstanding and supportive relationships succeed on other foundations.*
- *Never be ashamed to sit with a professional to discuss any problems of sexuality.*

Spiritual considerations

Spirituality and sexuality in combination create a fascinating subject. Religion, proclaiming in different guises to be the height of spirituality, generally chastises the sexually promiscuous. Spirituality, without religion, generally accepts sexuality as a part of a 'being' and in the case of Tantric yoga actively encourages male promiscuity within certain spiritual confines. If we accept the concept of unity with all living creatures that is expounded by the native Indian peoples of North and South America, we must tie our sexual/spiritual sense to our animal instincts. Many of these cultures believe that we all have a connection to an animal spirit, and universally across the animal kingdom sexual promiscuity is a method of promoting natural selection and the strongest genes for the species.

The most satisfying aspect for the soul is the experience of oneness, wholeness or union. It looks like you unite with another, but it is in fact the removal of the 'sense of oneness' that makes us feel separate, that makes us seek to re-unite. If sexual activity leads only to a heightened awareness of separateness or loneliness, it is not being used properly.

Our spirituality governs or *is* our being. Suppression of any aspect will lead to a suppression of our physical and psychological selves, so clarity of thought and an understanding of our deeper spiritual/sexual selves is essential for good health.

RECOMMENDATIONS

General Advice

- *Spend time in meditation or discussion on the underlying beliefs and energies that motivate a choice of partner or partners.*
- *Consider the concept of a 'soul mate' and ask the question 'do many partners increase or decrease my chances of finding one?'*

SHYNESS

To be shy is a character trait that is not necessarily abnormal. Our personality and upbringing will determine the levels of shyness and it is only if our timidity causes social or personal problems that it need to be considered worthy of treatment. Most people will suffer some shyness but if an inability to socialize or perform occurs then treatment is recommended.

RECOMMENDATIONS

General Advice

- *Behavioural modification techniques through counselling or neurolinguistic programming may benefit but commitment to the course is necessary.*

Supplemental

- *Copper or zinc excess or deficiency may encourage timidity. A hair sample should be taken and deficiency supplemented. If there is an excess, it is necessary to isolate the foods that may be putting too much into the system and remove them.*

Homeopathic

- *Consult a homeopathic Materia Medica and choose a remedy that most matches other psychological and physical attributes of the individual. Pay special attention to the remedies Baryta carbonica, Coca and Pulsatilla.*

Herbal/natural extracts

- *Bach flower remedies, specifically Buttercup and Pink Monkey Flower, may be tried.*

SMOKING AND HOW TO STOP
– See **Cigarettes**

Amongst the 3,000 or so chemicals found in cigarettes lurks nicotine, a strongly addictive substance. Within a few weeks of smoking most people will find their nervous system in need of nicotine to maintain a sensation of well-being. Whilst this is the main reason for addiction to cigarettes, it is also worth noting that tobacco, being a plant, has many compounds in it that the body utilizes. Examples are nickel and cobalt, both of which are necessary for the absorption and utilization of oxygen in the bloodstream. Therefore, when attempting to stop smoking not only does the nervous system recognize that it is missing something but the body may also actually move into deficiency because substances absorbed through the lung are taken in very rapidly and after a while saturate the body's requirements therefore negating the use of the bowel. In other words, if you are getting what you need through the lungs the bowel does not need to work so hard and stops the chemical processes, such that if you stop smoking there may be a lag phase of several days before the bowel again begins to absorbs what you need. This combination of the nervous system recognizing that it is missing something and the bowel not absorbing quickly leads to many people eating more in an attempt to satisfy their cravings. The nervous system lives off glucose so the cravings tend to be for sweets or carbohydrates and therefore people put on weight. This factor is very relevant when it comes to helping people to stop.

Stopping

Many different techniques have been employed over the years to help people stop smoking and most have an element of success. My view, and perhaps the truly holistic view, is to utilize whichever treatments may work and use them in combination. Determining whether somebody is psychologically or physically (or both) 'hooked' leads us to the suggested treatment course.

Psychological treatments
Counselling

It is necessary to establish whether a smoker 'wants' to stop smoking or 'wants to want' to stop smoking. Most failed treatments occur because the individual has no real desire to stop. This must be confronted and a counsellor may be necessary to help decide which level the smoker is at. Counselling or other psychological measures (*see* below) must be utilized to move the smoker into the 'wants to stop' bracket.

Hypnosis

There are two techniques of using hypnosis, which may be used individually or in combination. I have called them suggestive hypnosis and 'part' hypnosis.

Suggestive or suggestion hypnosis involves the individual being hypnotized into a deep state of relaxation and a suggestion that smoking is an uncomfortable or distasteful habit is placed in the subconscious. On returning from the deep relaxed state hopefully the smoker will dislike cigarettes. Allow three or four sessions of this type of hypnotherapy. Success in helping to stop smoking occurs in 10–30 per cent of patients.

Part hypnosis takes the smoker into a hypnotized state and, whilst there, the hypnotherapist will have a conversation with the subconscious 'part' of the person's psyche that is encouraging the habit. Very often smoking starts at an age where acceptance into a group apparently requires cigarette smoking. Not having a cigarette with the 'gang' may lead to being an outcast and the subconscious quickly correlates the nicotine buzz with being accepted and being socially adequate. It is a small step to find that the cigarette is your best friend and will indeed substitute for the group, especially if you did not like the group in the first place! Nicotine, by creating a sense of well-being, may mask sadness, guilt or fear, which is pushed into the subconscious and can be avoided by using the drug. Again, the underlying psychological pull needs to be established and dealt with before smoking can be taken away, otherwise it is similar to removing the crutch from an individual with an injured leg.

Physical therapies

Supplementation therapy

This much underused technique is based on the principle that when we stop smoking the body craves some of the useful compounds that we may absorb through the cigarette smoke. High-dose supplementation may make the availability of these trace elements greater, therefore taking away some of the craving. More useful is the use of intravenous supplementation therapy, which bypasses the slower bowel absorption.

Diet

The use of detoxification diet techniques (*see* **Detox diet**) helps rid the body of the nicotine that will have settled in the nervous system and in fat stores. The quicker the nicotine is out of the system, the quicker the cravings diminish.

Exercise

It is essential in nearly every case to introduce an exercise programme that helps to control breathing and increase oxygen consumption. Smoking reduces the lung capacity and the body's oxygen utilization, which, when increased, will make the individual feel better. Techniques such as Qi Gong, yoga, Tai Chi and basic aerobic exercises are most beneficial.

Breathing techniques

Until recently, techniques of breathing through yoga or Qi Gong were the best methods of retraining the lungs and bloodstream into accepting and enjoying oxygen without toxins. These techniques are still very beneficial if practised correctly, but more recently a Russian doctor named a technique after himself. The Buteyko technique of breathing is, in fact, quite different from yoga techniques. It encourages a shallow breathing that alters the acid/base balance in the body (*see* **Breathing** and the **Lung**) and seems to remove the craving for cigarettes. This technique is becoming more widely available and, whilst the teaching requires several hours of attendance, early research shows it to be extremely beneficial.

Bodywork techniques

The use of massage techniques, especially manual lymphatic drainage or Shiatsu, help in removing the nicotine levels that have settled into the tissues, which, in turn, help to maintain the cravings.

Acupuncture

When used in conjunction with other therapies acupuncture is an extremely beneficial method of removing the craving. Even used by itself, it has proven effective. The acupuncture may be general or auricular (needles in specific parts of the ear).

Nicotine replacement

Nicotine patches, chewing gum or implants are beneficial in non-responsive cases but it must be remembered that the nicotine is still being pulled into the system with all its neurological and addictive aspects. One is not dealing with the underlying addictive tendency, merely shifting it from one compound to another. Eventually the replacement stops and the cigarette craving, not having been dealt with, may well return.

RECOMMENDATIONS

General Advice

- *Establish that you 'want' to stop smoking and not that you 'want to want' to stop smoking. If you do not 'want to want', then visit a counsellor or hypnotherapist initially.*
- *Learn a Qi Gong, Tai Chi or yoga technique. Perform aerobic exercises two or three times a day for 10–15min. If you can find a Buteyko teacher, try this preferentially.*
- *If the going is tough, visit a manual lymphatic drainage masseur or Shiatsu practitioner regularly.*
- *Acupuncturists can treat you regularly or place a 'stud' needle in the ear for days at a time.*
- *Avoid nicotine replacement if possible.*

Nutritional

- *Consider the macrobiotic diet (see chapter 7).*
- *Use a detoxification diet or even consider a week or two under supervision on a health farm.*

Supplemental

- *Take in high levels of multiminerals, trace elements and vitamins for at least six weeks. Consider intravenous supplementation.*

Homeopathic

- *Establish, through reading or a visit to a qualified homeopath, your constitutional remedy and take this at high potency for one month.*

STAGE FRIGHT – *see* Nervousness

SYPHILIS

Syphilis is a sexually transmitted disease caused by a bacterium called *Treponema pallidum*. It is transmitted through any form of intercourse – oral, anal or vaginal – but is more prevalent in the homosexual population following non-vaginal intercourse. Like most sexually transmitted diseases, *Treponema* passes into the tissues of the genitals, rectum or throat via seminal fluid or vaginal excretions entering small abrasions.

There are four stages, at any one of which the body's immune system may overwhelm the infection, or treatment may be applied. The later the stage, the less likely it is that the outcome will be good.

Primary syphilis is characterized by a sore or chancre developing three to four weeks after infection. This sore is hard to heal but will spontaneously disappear about six weeks later. This is not a fixed time schedule and any lesion in the genital or anal area must be regarded with suspicion. Lesions in or around the mouth or throat must also be considered as potentially syphilitic especially in the promiscuous or in homosexuals.

At this stage investigation includes a swab that is placed under a microscope and a technique known as dark-field microscopy is used to identify the bacterium. It is necessary, sometimes, to repeat this as the bacterium may be missed by the swab technique.

Secondary syphilis manifests before the chancre heals or may be delayed for up to a year. Symptoms of a skin rash, sore throat, headache and fever in association with a history of a genital sore must raise suspicion.

Dark-field microscopy is again utilized and by this stage blood tests will be positive for syphilis.

Latent syphilis only occurs if an untreated secondary stage continues. This latent phase is symptomless and is due to the bacterium, for some reason, not replicating but lying dormant. Occasionally small lesions may appear but may not be considered relevant. Blood tests throughout this period of time, which may last a lifetime (the average, however, is 10–15 years), may be negative or only weakly positive.

Tertiary syphilis – the fourth stage – must be suspected in any condition that does not have another obvious answer. The *Treponema* generally attacks the mucous membranes, the skin and arteries and therefore can pass into any system. Ten per cent of untreated syphilis will develop into neurosyphilis, to which it is assumed Henry VIII succumbed, along with many, in the years prior to the Second World War when the introduction of sulphonamide antibiotics offered effective treatment.

Syphilis took a marked decline in frequency after the Second World War but is now on the rise. Injudicious use of antibiotics has led to resistant strains and there are reports of *Treponema* strains that are, along with tuberculosis, proving resistant to all known antibiotics. What may be more worrying is a poorly substantiated but nevertheless growing concern that syphilis is directly related to HIV infection.

RECOMMENDATIONS

General Advice

- *Any genital lesion must be investigated by a GP or specialist in this field.*
- *Choice of treatment should be selected by a complementary medical practitioner using homeopathic and herbal treatments.*
- *Alternative therapies have been used for centuries but should only be used in a complementary fashion now, provided that antibiotics are effective (which they still are in most cases).*

Herbal/natural extracts

- *Topical treatment is rarely needed because these lesions are generally painless but applications of Calendula or Hypericum cream may be beneficial.*

Orthodox

- *Antibiotic use must only be undertaken once the sensitivity of that particular syphilitic strain is established.*

TERMINATION OF PREGNANCY (TOP, ABORTION)

The need for the termination of a pregnancy should be based on medical grounds, such as a risk to the mother's health or life or due to the inevitability of a non-viable foetus – one that will not live beyond a certain point of development *in utero*. In many parts of the West, however, a termination may be considered if the mother might undergo psychological duress or if the child will be born with anything but normality. Many societies do not allow termination at all and others only if life-threatening physical conditions exist.

Termination of pregnancy is an emotive subject but from a holistic point of view it needs to be considered from four angles.

The body aspect

Pregnancy confers a marked change in hormonal profile in women. The well-known female hormones oestrogen and progesterone maintain high levels and, as any woman who struggles with premenstrual syndrome (PMS) will tell you, many changes go on throughout the system. A termination suddenly removes the control mechanism, the body goes through a sudden drop and many of the changes that were taking place will cease, creating some biochemical confusion. These are corrected over a period of time but a variety of symptoms ranging from tiredness, headaches, mood swings, water retention, abdominal pains and skin changes may occur.

A termination is generally performed by inserting a vacuum-like instrument through the cervix into the lumen of the uterus and extracting the contents through a sucking action. The embryo or foetus is pulled out with the inner lining of the uterus. The body has to deal with this injury as well as with the effects of the anaesthetic on the nervous system and liver. Repair of all of these areas is necessary and requires both energy and building materials.

Any operation carries a risk and a problem with the procedure or the introduction of infection into the uterus may lead to illness and sterility if the uterus or Fallopian tubes become scarred.

The psychological aspect

Every individual is different and will relate to the concept of a termination differently. Parental values, religious teachings, social status and peer pressure will all alter the ease or difficulty with which one comes to terms with an abortion. Very few women find the decision easy and this is compounded by the natural fear of a general anaesthetic and operative procedure.

The conflict with social and religious doctrines inevitably creates a dilemma and there is rarely a termination that does not have its supporters and critics.

The spiritual aspect

There is no right or wrong outside of one's beliefs but most human beings have a high respect for life and a termination distinctly goes against that innate pre-disposition. All religions, supposedly derived from spiritual values, will criticize (and in many countries ostracize) a woman who undergoes a termination. A decision must come from the depths of the soul of the individual.

The Hindus profess that a spirit chooses its parents and that a karmic (vital force) connection is made even before conception. A termination severs this bond and, unless the soul returns in a later pregnancy, that experience and energy will be lost, at least for this lifetime. I do not think that the Hindu spirituality is greater than any other doctrine, but looking at the situation from this point of view may alter the perception that a termination is not a deeply spiritual conundrum. It is.

The partner aspect

Sadly, all too often, the male plants the seed and then he leaves. Men who behave in this way claim that it is a natural response and that masculine animals have many mates and that they are simply obeying an acceptable male instinct. Absolute rubbish. This is self-denial designed to alleviate the potential for responsibility that most males fear so markedly in comparison with the female of our species. The truth of the matter is that males in the animal kingdom rarely plant a seed without accepting the responsibility of protecting and nurturing their offspring.

Nevertheless, if this attitude happens to be that of a specific partner then there is little that can be done and, quite frankly, his opinion should be discarded in favour of friends and family who are around to give support; no energy or time should be wasted on chasing the aberrant male.

I would like to think that the majority of partners who find their mate pregnant in a socially unacceptable situation will take an important role in supporting the decision of the woman. A burden shared is a burden halved, they say, and although I do not think that the division is quite 50/50 in the case of a termination, all and any support is beneficial.

RECOMMENDATIONS

General Advice

- *Closely review the spiritual aspects of termination. Only each individual can do this and they should not be led by any social doctrines or pressures. If a connection with the life growing inside is there at all, termination should not be considered.*

- *Psychological considerations may be made easier by asking the question: Do I feel that a termination is the right approach or do I think it is? Always go with your feelings. It is much easier to look back on a mistake and say 'I did what I felt was right' rather than have to deal with 'I did what I thought was right'. Remember that suppression of emotion creates illness, but making a mistake does not.*

- *Remember that a possible side effect of a termination is sterilization. Terminating a pregnancy may lead to a life barren of children.*

- *Consult a counsellor or health practitioner with whom you have a connection. Discuss your emotional state fully and ensure that any decision is reached after complete and absolute discussion by looking at the problem from both sides of the fence.*

- *Do not surround yourself with friends who support only one side of the debate. You may be covering guilt by obtaining moral support for a decision that you are not certain about.*

Orthodox

- *A termination may be performed at an early stage of pregnancy by chemical induction with high doses of progesterone-like drugs. These have the side effects of nausea, vomiting, headaches and other unpleasant symptoms, including abdominal pains, and they work by disrupting the chemical balance required for pregnancy and encouraging contraction of the uterus. Menstruation (a period) is the outcome. If chemical termination is used, see* **Heavy and painful periods** *and follow the advice.*
- *If a termination is to be performed by operative procedure, generally this is necessary after the eighth week of a pregnancy (see* **Operations and surgery***).*

TOXOPLASMOSIS

This is an infection by a protozoan (bacteria/viral-like organism) called *Toxoplasma gondii*, which is widely distributed in nature and can cause foetal developmental problems as well as infections within individuals.

Clinical manifestations of damage include enlarged liver and spleen, blindness, cysts, mental retardation and the development of too large or too small a brain. Problems may be apparent soon after birth or develop later on in life. In the acquired form, a fever with a rash, enlarged glands, enlarged liver and spleen and an inflamed eye may occur. If serious, the infection may affect the brain or the heart.

Toxoplasmosis is spread predominantly by animal faeces and especially those of cats. Owners of dogs and cats should be particularly and specifically wary, especially prior to an intended pregnancy.

In the unfortunate circumstance that a toxoplasmosis blood test shows positive in a pregnant woman, there is a need for further investigation to pinpoint when the infection took place. Toxoplasmosis can have a devastating effect on a foetus in the first trimester. The infection can lead to growth defects, brain damage and death. Once the placenta has formed (usually by 12–13 weeks), it is harder for the infection to get into the baby but transmission does occur and can lead to other damage, including blindness, limb growth retardation and less serious brain effects.

Calculating when an infection took place is therefore paramount because a decision to terminate on medical grounds may be considered. Pinpointing the time of infection is done by taking blood samples from the mother at an interval of at least three weeks apart. A current infection will have a rising level of antibodies against toxoplasmosis, and the amount of antibodies and the speed with which it is being produced give a clue as to when infection took place. The level of antibodies, known as the titre, will remain stable if the infection was from some time ago but will rise if the infection was more recent. If toxoplasmosis is suspected, ultrasound will give a clear definition of any obvious brain damage or limb defects but cannot illustrate conditions such as blindness.

It is currently not common practice in Britain to test pregnant women for toxoplasmosis as a general rule. I think this is wrong and any woman who owns or has been in contact with animals, especially domestic cats, should be tested for antibodies before conception and at the end of the third trimester.

RECOMMENDATIONS

General Advice

- *Prior to becoming pregnant and during a pregnancy a blood test should be done to test for the presence of Toxoplasma.*
- *Consult a complementary medical practitioner for treatment to run alongside orthodox antibiotic care (see* **Antibiotics***).*
- *Your preferred complementary medical practitioner should be consulted to boost the immune system and deal with the possible use*

of antibiotics and, if you are pregnant, to advise you on the best counsellor for the inevitable anxiety that will be present.

Orthodox

- *If any of the main symptoms are present in conjunction with a positive blood test for toxoplasmosis, an antibiotic treatment should be taken.*
- *If pregnant and a positive test is found but no symptoms are present, then consult your obstetrician and ask to be put in touch with the area or national specialist for toxoplasmosis. He/she will be able to advise you on the chances of a problem and also as to the best treatment.*

YEAST INFECTION

Yeasts are a subgroup of fungi in the big scheme of categorization. It seems less emotive to discuss the potential for infestation by yeast rather than suggesting that somebody is infected by a fungus!

The most common fungal infection is thought to be *Candida*, although many other fungi and yeasts live in or on the body surfaces. In their natural place they act as symbionts (both taking and giving some benefit from the host), principally by attacking other, perhaps more dangerous, organisms and also eating available sugars and thereby reducing the amount for other organisms, which, in turn, have their growth inhibited.

Yeast infections are most commonly associated with the vaginal vault, and discharges, discomfort, odours and diseases may result.

Yeast may flourish in the bowel but generally it causes no problems unless the normal bowel flora are reduced and a population overgrowth occurs. The yeasts and fungi of the body tend to produce chemicals that we find toxic and if these increase then symptoms ranging from malaise and tiredness to chronic fatigue syndrome and cancer may evolve.

Yeasts or fungi should not travel around the body and if they are found in the bloodstream

Normal and fungal blood samples

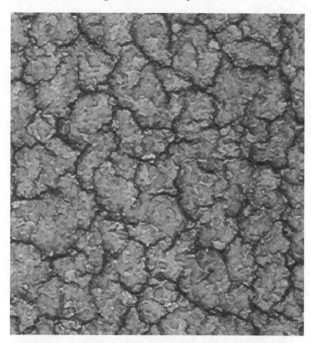

The blood above is a healthy sample while strands of fungi are clearly visible below in this Humoral Pathology Laboratory Test.

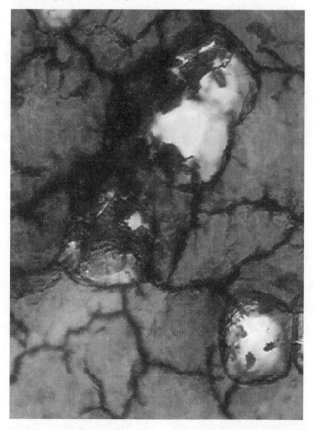

they are usually killed off rapidly or filtered out by the liver and kidney. If they do survive they may travel to major organs and cause serious complications. This is much more apparent in those with an immuno-compromised status, such as AIDS.

RECOMMENDATIONS

General Advice
- *The orthodox world very rarely takes into account the presence of yeasts and fungi and persistent problems should be assessed by a complementary medical practitioner, who should be reminded of the possibility of yeast infection.*
- *Treatment depends on the problem (see Candida and Fungal infections).*

Orthodox
- *Orthodox cultures of urine and stool rarely look for yeasts and sometimes it is worth specifically asking a laboratory to do so.*
- *A Humoral Pathological Laboratory test (examination of blood samples under high-powered microscopy) may show fungal or yeast spores in any body fluid or excreta or the reaction by red blood cells to the presence of fungal toxins.*

YELLOW FEVER

This is an acute viral disease transmitted to human beings by mosquitoes and characterized by fever, jaundice, bleeding tendencies and a slowing down of the heart rate and other neurologically associated problems if the condition is severe.

Vaccination is recommended for those who are liable to come into contact with the infection but, like any vaccine, it has its risks and the benefits must be weighed against these.

RECOMMENDATIONS

General Advice
- *See Vaccinations.*

Orthodox
- *Follow orthodox advice for this extremely dangerous and contagious condition; for complementary medical support, see Fever.*

THE HEAD AND NECK

DANDRUFF

Dandruff, unless very severe, is more of a cosmetic nuisance than a medical problem. Characterized by a flaking of the scalp, dandruff is of no medical consequence unless it is disturbing an individual's social lifestyle or irritating the scalp.

Occasionally associated with more aggressive skin conditions, such as psoriasis or dermatitis (eczema), the cause is either a minor fungal infection, an excess of heat in the system (from an Eastern point of view) or is associated with a lack of water intake (dehydration) and an excess of heat-creating foods or adrenaline-producing stress.

RECOMMENDATIONS

General Advice
- *Wash the hair with a selenium-containing shampoo not more than three times a week for three weeks.*
- *Standing on your head will increase blood flow and should be performed for 10min per day.*
- *Consider chronic dehydration and correct this by drinking $\frac{1}{2}$ pint of water per foot of height per day.*
- *Severe dandruff may be associated with underlying skin diseases and dandruff of sudden onset or not resolving swiftly should be reviewed by a doctor.*

Supplemental
- *Take a vitamin B complex, five times the recommended daily dose for one week. Take zinc (5mg per foot of height) each night for two weeks and flaxseed oil (1 teaspoonful per foot of height) in divided doses with meals.*

Herbal/natural extracts

- *Flaxseed oil can be applied directly to the scalp with gentle massage.*
- *Persisting dandruff should be reviewed by a complementary medical practitioner with experience in herbal treatment who may consider several herbs including chamomile, figwort, rosemary and willow. Shampoos made from any of these may be curative.*

ENCEPHALITIS

The word encephalic means affecting or involving the brain; 'itis' on the end of any word means inflammation. Encephalitis is inflammation of the brain, which is an extremely serious condition and is not one to be dealt with at home. This can occur at any age.

Severe headache and any neurological symptoms such as visual disturbance, numbness, tingling, unsteadiness, dizziness or feeling faint, may all represent an encephalitis and any such symptoms that persist or are associated with drowsiness, loss of consciousness or even coma must be considered.

RECOMMENDATIONS

General Advice
- *Any unexplained neurological symptoms should be assessed by a doctor immediately, especially if loss of consciousness or pain is associated.*

Homeopathic
- *Use Aconite 30 every 15min on the way to the physician.*

HEADACHES

Everybody gets headaches. They occur at any age and their causes are numerous. Most headaches are an indication of fatigue or mild neck muscular tension but others may be an indication of a more serious complaint. Headaches are one of the most common reasons why people see their physician and they account for the largest use of 'over-the-counter' painkillers.

Reasons to consult a physician

Most headaches can be dealt with by using simple home measures but some types of headaches do require a medical opinion. These include:

- Headaches associated with neck stiffness, photophobia (inability to look at light), nausea and/or vomiting.
- Frequent headaches.
- Headaches interfering with normal thinking or enjoyment of life.
- Headaches that persist despite basic treatment.
- Headaches associated with any other neurological problems such as visual, auditory hallucinations, numbness, paralysis, etc.
- Headaches that are controlled only by excessive amounts of painkillers.

The causes of headaches can be broken down into a few main categories:

Fatigue and tiredness, muscular tension of the neck and back, infection (sinuses, gums, ears and other parts of the head and neck), nutritional deficiencies, metabolic disorders such as diabetes or low blood sugar hypoglycaemia, circulatory problems including strokes, high blood pressure and any condition that might cause fever. There is a particular correlation between headaches and bowel problems especially constipation but no obvious orthodox link has been established.

Emotional and hormonal imbalances are common causes especially in adolescent females.

Brain damage or tumours (often the primary fear of a patient with a persisting headache) are rarely an underlying cause.

RECOMMENDATIONS

General Advice
- *Ensure good hydration by drinking ½ pint (¼ litre) of water per foot of height daily.*

- Consider a hot bath to relax muscular tension.
- A gentle exercise, such as a walk or basic stretching, especially of the neck and upper back muscles, may relieve muscular tension.
- Consider learning a relaxation technique if headaches are stress-related.
- Consider regular physical therapy such as massage or Shiatsu.
- Use a screen on your computer monitor and ensure good lighting when doing deskwork.
- The use of an ionizer may be beneficial if in a poorly ventilated room or surrounded by computers and electromagnetic machines.

Nutritional

- Do not allow blood sugar levels to fall. Eat a healthy snack mid-morning and mid-afternoon.
- Keep a food diary and consider the possibility of food intolerance/allergy by correlating headaches with previous meals eaten.
- Avoid too much refined sugar as this encourages low blood sugar levels 2–6 hours after eating it.
- Withdrawal from caffeine can be a frequent cause of headaches, so reduce your intake slowly.

Supplemental

- Consider using the following once no serious cause is established:
  - Magnesium, 100mg per foot of height, taken in divided doses through the day.
  - Niacin (vitamin B1), 10mg per foot of height, taken in divided doses through the day.
  - Quercetin, 100mg per foot of height, taken in divided doses through the day.

Homeopathic

- There are many remedies that should be considered depending on the type of headache and reference to your preferred homeopathic textbook is recommended. All the remedies below should be taken at potency 6 two tablets every half to one hour:
  - For a right-sided headache: Rhus toxicodendron or Iris;
  - For a left-sided headache: Spigelia or Thuja;
  - For a throbbing headache: Natrum muriaticum;
  - For headaches with dry fever: Belladonna;
  - For headaches associated with a cough or a cold: Bryonia;
  - At the start of a headache, if taken within the first fifteen minutes, Aconite.

Herbal/natural extracts

- Feverfew or Capsicum can be considered, but should be taken only at the dosage recommended on the packaging. Orthodox 'over-the-counter' medication is better studied and so potential side effects and risks are established, but this does not make them necessarily safer to use.

Orthodox

- Orthodox painkillers such as aspirin, paracetamol and the non-steroidal anti-inflammatory drugs such as ibuprofen are the pharmaceutical industry's bread and butter. Occasional use is probably not harmful, but be wary of aspirin and the NSAID's potential for causing ulcers in the stomach and small intestine. Try to take any painkiller with a substantial meal. Do not exceed the recommended dosages and remember that there are over 2,000 deaths each year from the use of 'over-the-counter' drugs. Stronger painkillers may be prescribed once investigations as to underlying cause have been completed.

INTRACRANIAL BLEEDS
Extradural haemorrhage

There are several linings to the brain, the outer-most of which is called the dura. A bleed, usually caused by trauma but occasionally by disease of blood vessels or an infection, is known as an extradural haemorrhage.

As with any bleeding vessel the flow of blood may be swift, in which case neurological symptoms, loss of consciousness and headache may be

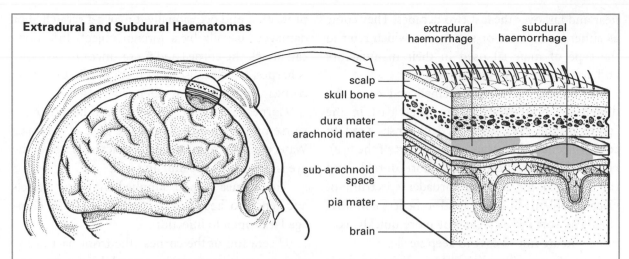

Extradural and Subdural Haematomas

extradural
haemorrhage

subdural
haemorrhage

scalp
skull bone
dura mater
arachnoid mater
sub-arachnoid
space
pia mater
brain

*Extradural and subdural haematomas may form blood clots which put pressure on the brain. The symptoms described in the **recommendations** should be watched out for in anyone who has suffered a blow to the head.*

apparent. A slow bleed, however, may take up to six weeks before symptoms as mild as a change of character may be noticed.

RECOMMENDATIONS

General Advice
- *Any injury or blow to the head, persistent headache or neurological symptoms should be reviewed by a physician.*
- *A telltale sign of an intracranial (within the skull) bleed is one pupil (often on the other side from the injury) being dilated or constricted – but definitely different from the other side and potentially unresponsive.*
- *Any suspicion of a bleed must be examined by a CT scan for safety.*
- *Following a head injury, ensure that friends and relatives keep an eye on behaviour patterns. A change in character anywhere up to six weeks following a blow to the skull needs to be treated as an emergency by a hospital.*

Homeopathic
- *The homeopathic remedy Natrum sulphuricum potency 6 can be used every 15min on the way to the hospital following any head injury.*

Natrum sulphuricum 200 taken each night for three nights can be used following a head injury.

Orthodox
- *Orthodox treatment may be as simple as monitoring but may also include blood-letting following bur-holes in the skull (see **Operations and surgery**).*

Subdural haematoma

A subdural haematoma is a bleed underneath the dura. It behaves and requires treatment similar to an extradural haematoma or haemorrhage.

RECOMMENDATION

General Advice
- *For recommendation and treatment (see **Extradural haemorrhage**).*

THE EYES

CONTACT LENSES

Contact lenses are a remarkable invention that have benefited people with poor eyesight, both near and far, over the last two decades. They come as either hard lenses or soft lenses, which refer to the type of material used in their manufacture and, to some extent, their thickness.

Hard lenses tend to be small and cover the dimension of the pupil (the black part in the centre of the eye), whereas soft lenses tend to cover the entire iris (the coloured part of the eye). Hard lenses are cheaper and more durable and can be used for a much broader spectrum of visual problems but they tend to be less comfortable. The soft lenses wear out more quickly, cost more and are not so easy to keep sterile.

It is of paramount importance that sterility is maintained when the contact lenses are not in the eye. Following your optician's instructions is extremely important to avoid irritation, inflammation such as iritis and conjunctivitis and more serious conditions such as chronic blepharitis. Always wash your hands before removing or inserting your contact lenses and, however experienced you may be, do not rush the process. It takes one misjudged addition or removal to cause potentially permanent eye damage. Please note that contact lens cleaner may have an association with chemical damage to the eyes and must be rinsed off thoroughly.

RECOMMENDATIONS

General Advice
- *The choice of lens should be made in consultation with an optician specializing in contact lenses.*
- *Do not shirk the responsibility of cleaning the lenses.*
- *Clean hands before touching the lens or eyes.*
- *Always thoroughly wash off any contact lens cleaning solution because these may damage the eye.*
- *Antiseptic solutions will also kill off the body's normal and useful bacteria found along the edges of the eyelids.*

CORNEAL ULCERS

The cornea is the transparent part of the eyeball that lies over and protects the pupil. Its job is protection and occasionally it may get scratched or damaged, usually by a foreign object. Infections can attack the cornea and a not uncommon cause is herpes, which causes a branching effect over the cornea and is known as a dendritic ulcer.

Corneal scratches are very painful and made worse by the eyelid rubbing the area as it blinks. Watering and redness are characteristic and the eye is generally kept shut and still.

The cornea is well supplied by blood vessels and tends to heal fairly rapidly but whilst damaged it is open to infection.

Ulceration of the cornea (the front part of the eye) is most commonly caused by trauma but may be associated with rarer diseases and malnutrition. It is a painful and serious condition insomuch that if it is not dealt with properly the pain continues and, if it is associated with illness, blindness may result if the ulceration worsens.

RECOMMENDATIONS

General Advice
- *Any eye injury involving foreign matter should be cleansed with running water if possible (see* **Foreign bodies and substances in the eye***).*
- *A cold compress over the closed eye may give relief.*
- *Any eye injury must be reviewed by a doctor, however slight, and accept a referral to a specialist if necessary (see* **Injuries to the eye***).*
- *General advice includes patching the eye, although recently it has been advised to keep the eye open to the air to allow faster healing.*

Supplemental
- *Severe damage may heal faster by taking beta-carotene (5mg) with each meal if you are over the age of 12 or proportionately less (best prescribed by a nutritionist) if you are younger.*

Homeopathic
- *With any eye injury take the homeopathic remedy Aconite or Hepar sulphuris calcarium potency 6 or 12, four pills immediately and every 15min until you are seen by a medical person.*

- An accurate selection of a remedy from your preferred homeopathic manual is recommended should other symptoms set in (see **Inflammation of the eyes**).

Herbal/natural extracts

- Euphrasia (eyebright) lotion, 1 drop in an eggcupful of water, can be very soothing and antiseptic.

DETACHED RETINA

The retina is the medical term for the layer at the back of the eye where all the visual nerves collect

Detached Retina

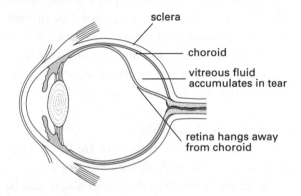

sclera

choroid

vitreous fluid accumulates in tear

retina hangs away from choroid

The retina hangs away from the choroid – the rich layer of blood vessels at the back of the eye.

the light that travels through the lens, cornea and vitreous fluids in the two chambers of the eye.

Detachment usually occurs following injury, surgery, infection or arterial damage such as atheroma in the elderly.

Symptoms of retinal detachment are seeing flashing lights, funny shapes and eventually blindness that starts with the peripheral vision (outer part of your vision) and moves inwards.

RECOMMENDATIONS

General Advice

- Any visual problem should be taken to your doctor or local emergency room immediately. Specific laser treatment may now be used to prevent further detachment of the retina once it starts and the sooner this treatment is provided the better.
- Recurrent detachment needs to be treated by a complementary medical specialist with experience in this field who may use specific homeopathic remedies and high-dose supplementation in conjunction with eye exercises. High-dose antioxidants may be used until the consultation (see **Antioxidants**).

Homeopathic

- On your way to the doctor the remedies Apis or Aconite, potency 6, can be taken every 10min.

DOUBLE VISION

Double vision is created by the optical part of the brain receiving two images at the same time. This occurs because the eyeballs are not synchronized or because of extra impulses being incorrectly transmitted through the nervous system.

Problems can occur from the front of the eye, caused by the muscles of the eye pulling the eyeball in different directions, and from neurological problems of the optic nerve leading to the optical part of the brain.

Trauma, infection, damage to the nerve tracts by growths, diabetes or drugs must all be excluded. More complicated neurological or muscular diseases also need to be eliminated as possible causes.

Remember that the most common cause of double vision is a blow to the eye or head and is liable to be temporary but, as in any visual disturbance that lasts for more than a few minutes, a medical opinion is best sought.

Conditions such as multiple sclerosis or muscular dystrophy may rarely present as double vision and therefore I must emphasize the importance of establishing an underlying cause because naturopathic treatments for even these serious conditions may work better if started early in the course of such diseases.

General Advice

- *Visit a doctor or emergency room for any visual disturbance.*
- *Having ruled out the necessity for orthodox intervention, cranial osteopathy, craniosacral therapy and specific eye exercises such as the Bates eye exercises will be beneficial.*

Homeopathic

- *The homeopathic remedy Arnica should be used if trauma initiated the double vision. Take Arnica 6 every hour until the problem resolves. A persistent double vision, caused by trauma, that has been examined to rule out any other complications may be treated by Natrum sulphuricum 30, four pills four times a day for five days.*

DRY EYES

Dry eyes are more of a symptom than a medical condition, although lack of tears can be associated with disease processes such as sarcoidosis or blocked tear ducts. A persistence of this problem needs to be seen by a doctor.

Most frequently dry eyes are associated with adverse weather conditions or mild conjunctivitis (*see* **Conjunctivitis**).

General Advice

- *Persisting dryness or dryness without obvious cause needs to be reviewed by a doctor.*
- *Rule out an association of dry eyes with smoking, poor-quality air-conditioning or allergies to airborne or food antigens. If associated, try to change the situations.*

Herbal/natural extracts

- *Euphrasia as a diluted fluid extract can be used as an eyebath and can be used as a remedy, potency 6, four times a day.*

Orthodox

- *Artificial tears (available from chemists) can be used in the short term.*

THE MOUTH

DENTAL OPERATIONS

There is a strong predilection amongst many dentists automatically to remove the back molar or wisdom teeth. This, along with trauma and decay of teeth and gums through poor hygiene, frequently leads to the need for dental operations. More unusual situations such as infection in the gums or jaw may need to be pre- and postoperatively treated.

Most dentists would encourage the use of antibiotics in any surgical procedure and especially in people who have a history of heart valve disease (*see* **Rheumatic fever**) or kidney infections. Studies and trials suggest the use of antibiotics in such situations as being warranted. These studies tend not to look at the sequella and are probably done on people with a broad spectrum of preoperative health. Antibiotics (*see* **Antibiotics**) are not necessarily harmless or safe and if they can be avoided they should be. I have always been fascinated by the fact that dentists and doctors are so adamant concerning the use of these antibiotics before dental operations. Very often the bacteria that may be involved in any infection live in the mouth, so why should they only be a problem when an operation is involved? These bacteria are being absorbed into the cuts in the mouth and around the infected area all the time and generally do not seem to cause us any problems.

General Advice

- *Ensure adequate hygiene by cleaning the teeth and gums two or three times a day as soon as any problem is suspected.*
- *Commence mouthwashes preoperatively using Arnica and Calendula lotions or fluid extracts diluted in water. Ensure that the solution is forced through the teeth and not just rinsed around the mouth. This should be done four times a day,*

preferably starting one week before the dental work, but even one wash may be beneficial.

- *It is very worthwhile consulting a cranial osteopath after any dental work since adjustments to the jaw joint will encourage blood flow to the damaged area and avoid the possibility of jaw strain, which can lead to headaches, migraines and other complications.*

Supplemental

- *The following supplements should be used per foot of height: vitamin C, 1g; argenine, 2g; magnesium, 500mg in divided doses with meals; zinc, 5mg before bed; and regardless of height, five times the recommended daily allowance of a multi-B complex.*

Homeopathic

- *Homeopathic remedies should be considered before and after. For operations with no infection, use Arnica 30 four times a day starting three days before the operation. For infections that are deeply embedded or trapped in an abscess or the jaw bone, use Hepar sulphuris calcarium 30 four times a day starting as soon as the infection is noted. Immediately after the operation, commence on Calcarea fluorica 30, four times a day until healing is complete. These are basic and general recommendations that might be overridden by a homeopath, who would deal with specific symptoms.*

Orthodox

- *Find a dentist who is open to alternative and complementary medicine in an attempt to avoid the use of antibiotics. Do not go into an operation if you are 'under the weather' and consult with your complementary medical practitioner for a constitutional build-up prior to any operative procedure.*

THE LIPS
Care of the lips

The lips have several functions. They form the opening to the digestive tract and, together with the nostrils, the top part of the respiratory system. They act as a form of communication by forming many of our vocal sounds and are also an area that we use to attract the opposite sex, hence the use of lipstick! Once attracted, the lips are usually the first point of sexual contact.

The lips contain an intermediate form of cell between that of the skin and those of the mucous membranes. They have sweat or sebaceous glands and rely upon the moisture of the mouth (saliva) to keep their integrity. Internal moisture is therefore very important, as well as the constituents of saliva.

It is also worth remembering that the lips reflect the internal environment. For instance, dry, cracked lips mean dehydration; pale lips, anaemia; red lips, fever or internal inflammation.

RECOMMENDATIONS

General Advice

- *Dry or cracked lips require an increase in the hydration of the body.*
- *Avoid application of heat through hot drinks or smoking as much as possible.*
- *Spend as much time as possible without lipstick.*
- *Use sun block if in strong sunshine.*
- *If the lips are pale, see **Anaemia**.*

Homeopathic

- *A central crack in the lips is a guiding symptom for the homeopathic remedy Natrum muriaticum. Graphites, Calcarea carbonica and Sulphur are other remedies that should be reviewed in dry lips.*

Herbal/natural extracts

- *Calendula or Graphites creams should be applied. Avoid moisturizing creams that are geared towards temporary relief, thereby encouraging more use of the compound. Habitual users of chapsticks are habitual users because they use chapsticks.*

WISDOM TEETH

The backmost teeth at both sides of the upper and lower jaw make up the four molar teeth known as

WISDOM TEETH

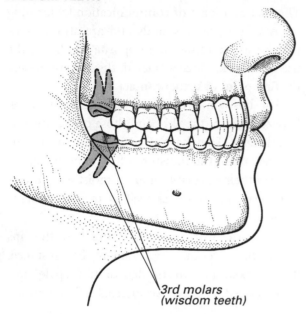

3rd molars
(wisdom teeth)

the wisdom teeth. They are so called because they finally push through the gum between the ages of 17 and 25 years (but usually around 21 years), a time when our childhood experiences supposedly convert into wisdom.

The emergence of the wisdom teeth should not cause a problem but in the West we are seeing increasing incidence of impaction (the wisdom teeth not coming out) and infections of the surrounding gum. This is probably caused by a decrease in the amount of chewy, fibrous food such as raw vegetables and fruit eaten and a higher amount of softer refined foods.

Pain may develop from impaction and infection, and teeth that only partially become exposed leave pockets of gum that allow bacteria to breed. Left unattended, erosion of the bone and loosening of these teeth and their neighbours can present a problem within a few years or later on.

RECOMMENDATIONS

General Advice
- *Pay special attention through brushing and flossing as soon as these teeth start to emerge.*

They are not easy to access and special brushes can be provided by your dentist.
- *Regular mouthwashes of a teaspoonful of salt and a teaspoonful of Arnica fluid extract in a cup of water is a useful daily treatment.*
- *Cranial osteopathy may be beneficial in impacted wisdom teeth.*

Orthodox
- *Many dentists are very quick to encourage the extraction of wisdom teeth and a second opinion from a less-invasive professional may be wise before this minor operative procedure is considered.*

THE CHEST

ASTHMA
See **Asthma** in chapter 3.
Asthma can be triggered at any age but quite often the teenage years are the starting point. Treatment from this age onwards is similar to that of a child.

RECOMMENDATIONS

General Advice
- *See* **Asthma** *in chapter 3.*
- *Acupressure may be used to help relieve an attack. Find the top of the chest bone (sternum) and move outwards along the collar bones on both sides. Move down the edge of the collar bone and find two sensitive spots on either side. Pull the shoulders back and gently apply pressure to the point of pain whilst inspiring for 3sec and expiring for 4sec.*
- *Relaxation and meditation. It is not easy to relax or meditate in the middle of an asthma attack. However, all asthmatics should practise a daily meditation routine and be able to utilize this technique during an attack.*

Supplemental

- At the first sign of an asthma attack take 10mg per foot of height of vitamin B_6 twice a day. Also, per foot of height: 500mg of vitamin C with each meal, 5mg of natural food-state zinc taken last thing at night, 500mg of magnesium twice a day, 1,000iu of vitamin A twice a day and 100mg of N-acetylcysteine twice a day.
- Beta-carotene 1000iu per foot of height.
- Chromium 10mcg per foot of height.

Homeopathic

- Homeopathy can be very effective but high potencies are required and a homeopathic consultation is recommended. Acute attacks can be helped by referring to a homeopathic manual with special reference to the remedies: Aconite, Arsenicum album, Calcarea carbonica, Ipecacuanha and Natrum sulphuricum. Do not stop using orthodox treatments such as inhalers without supervision by an experienced practitioner and even then only with your doctor's support.

Herbal/natural extracts

- Eucalyptus oil as a steam inhalation is very effective but it counteracts homeopathic remedies. Better to use a combination of lavender and chamomile oils (four drops of each in a bowl of steaming water).

Orthodox

- Do not give paracetamol (calpol) to asthmatics as it has been shown to worsen asthma.

BREATHING

If there is only one section of this entire book that I would ask everyone to read, it is this short note concerning breathing.

The Eastern philosophies of medicine all have breathing techniques as part of their health maintenance programmes. Evidence from all over the world shows that breathing techniques adjust the biochemistry of the body by influencing the amount of oxygen we take in and carbon dioxide that we breathe out. No part of the body functions without oxygen, and all active cells produce carbon dioxide that needs to be eliminated.

For many centuries it has been established that breathing techniques will aid meditation and relaxation as well as enhance athletic performance and activity.

There is no specific method of breathing that is best suited for all individuals because we are all unique, but basic rules hold steady.

We somehow manage to train ourselves out of good breathing as we age. Infants and children follow simple patterns.

- They breathe more frequently when they are active and reduce their respiratory rate at rest.
- When active, the depth of breathing increases; when asleep, the respiration is shallow.
- They exhale for a fraction longer than they inhale and when at rest they allow a moment before repeating the cycle.
- Children breathe 'into their navel'.

Western society seems obsessed with being slim, or appearing so, and much effort is spent by people as they age by holding in the abdomen. This causes stress which affects the flexibility of the diaphram – the large muscles that span the area below the lungs and which separate the chest from the abdomen. This leads to shallower breathing and less oxygenation into the lower and deeper aspects of the lung. Paradoxically, learning to breath abdominally tightens the abdominal muscles and flattens the stomach.

At the time of writing, a major debate is taking place concerning the use of breathing techniques in asthma and many other conditions. It has been thought for millennia that breathing techniques from yoga, Qi Gong and other exercise/relaxation techniques are the most beneficial for asthmatics. In many cases this is true. Recently there has been some contention brought forward by Western awareness of a Russian technique. Konstantin P Buteyko, a Russian medical scientist and practitioner, claims that the deep breathing techniques are compromising the brain and body's understanding of its own carbon dioxide levels that control many biochemical pathways in the body, including those that maintain normal airflow through the lungs. At the time of writing I understand that *The Lancet*, a most prestigious medical journal, is considering publishing an international trial supporting the breathing techniques of Dr Buteyko. The personal experience of some of my colleagues suggests that his is a technique worth learning if you are an asthmatic. This technique is not widely available yet, but search around.

RECOMMENDATIONS

General Advice

- *Ensure adequate rest and sleep when the body can govern its own respiratory pattern.*
- *Concentrate through the day on breathing abdominally. Place the hands over an area below the navel and breathe such that you move the hands at least one inch (2cm) forward.*
- *Spend time concentrating on opening the chest by stretching the top of the head upwards and pulling the shoulder back slightly.*
- *Avoid polluting the lungs with cigarettes, unnecessary perfumes and noxious fumes. If you are a city dweller, ensure as many trips into the countryside as possible.*
- *Learn a breathing technique from a meditation teacher. Deep breathing is not necessarily good breathing and a basic rule of thumb is to inhale for 3sec and passively (without forcing) exhale for 4sec. Allow 1sec before repeating the cycle. Practising even this technique a few times a day will help to retrain the body.*
- *Any conditions such as asthma and bronchitis that interfere with breathing may benefit from the Buteyko method.*
- *Consider learning techniques of Qi Gong, yoga and Tai Chi or a martial art, which will automatically teach you better breathing techniques.*
- *Consider using low oxygen therapy for any condition that affects breathing (see **Oxygen therapy**).*

ENDOCARDITIS

Endocarditis is inflammation of the inner lining of the heart, including the valves. It can be caused by viruses, bacteria and, in rare circumstances, autoimmune disease. Endocarditis most commonly follows infection from open wounds, such as teeth extraction or trauma.

It is characterized by cardiac symptoms such as irregular or rapid pulse, shortness of breath, general feeling of weakness and pain. It is a serious condition that should not be treated without expert medical advice.

Endocarditis can lead to persistent damage of the heart valves, as is often the case after rheumatic fever in childhood. The orthodox world recommends antibiotic cover whenever any major dental work is performed and, in the case of rheumatic fever, long-term antibiotic cover with penicillin is recommended to protect against further heart damage. Any decision to avoid antibiotic cover, whether acute or long-term, should be made only after discussion with a medically qualified complementary practitioner (*see* **Dental operations**).

RECOMMENDATIONS

General Advice

- *Any persisting symptoms in the chest should be reviewed by a physician.*
- *Complementary therapy should be administered by a medical practitioner or an alternative therapist only in conjunction with a cardiologist.*
- *Once the acute situation has settled, a complementary medical therapist may be consulted for long-term care and repair of damaged endocardial tissue.*
- *See **Atheroma**.*

THE LUNGS

Diseases and disorders of the lungs vary in type and severity and specific conditions are discussed throughout this book in different age groups. The lungs, more so than most other organs, deserve a few words because they are exposed to the outside world more than any other internal organ.

The lungs are the body's quickest method of taking in and expelling products.

Theoretically it may be possible to breathe through the skin (as an amphibian does) or even through the bowel, but the paper-thin qualities of the alveolar sacs within the lungs make this the fastest and most appropriate method. Excretion of the main waste product of metabolism – carbon dioxide – is performed through the lungs and the balance of acid/alkali within the body is governed by the lungs and kidneys working in harmony. Any damage to the lungs will prevent the fuel of life (oxygen) from getting in and the toxins from getting out.

I find it amazing that 5,000 years ago the Eastern philosophies were drawing the same conclusions. All Eastern medical beliefs stem from an understanding that the lungs are the main organ of energy input as well as being a major elimination centre. The scientific knowledge of how the lungs and kidneys control the acid/base balance is reflected by the connection in Eastern philosophies that the lungs pull energy into the body and the kidney energy is the store.

According to Eastern medicines the lungs are the organ that represent grief, loss and sorrow, which is perhaps why we sigh when saddened and why a few deep breaths can restore a sense of well-being.

The formation of the lungs takes up to 25 years and persisting infections or the self-assassinating habit of smoking are more damaging the younger we start. Like a house with poor foundations, any damage to the lungs at an early age will reflect throughout our lives not only in our breathing and tendency to recurrent infections but in every

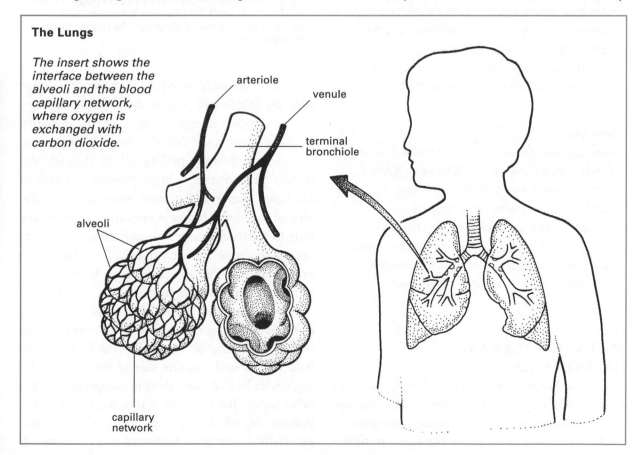

The Lungs

The insert shows the interface between the alveoli and the blood capillary network, where oxygen is exchanged with carbon dioxide.

arteriole

venule

terminal bronchiole

alveoli

capillary network

aspect of our energy flow. Pollution, including passive smoking by children in the homes of smoking adults, will be taking its toll. Asthma is on the increase and although no definite scientific evidence has been shown to incriminate air pollution I am dubious of the trials done to date.

RECOMMENDATIONS

General Advice

- *Above all other organs, pay the lungs respect from as early an age as possible.*
- *City dwellers should spend as much time as possible in the country even if it is simply a day trip to the seaside.*
- *Everyone should be taught and should practise a breathing technique and a yogic nasal washing procedure should be employed.*
- *Any lung problem, such as an inflammation or infection should be treated swiftly especially in those under the age of 25 years.*
- *Any grief or sadness should be dealt with through counselling as swiftly as possible because these emotions will drain the lung energy.*
- *An interesting study has shown that eating five or more apples a week may improve good lung function.*

Nutritional

- *Carrots, swedes, yam or sweet potato and deep-green leafy vegetables should be eaten regularly for the vitamin A content. Vitamin A has a profound effect on the lung membranes. Supplements should not be needed but can be used if the diet is poor. Take 1mg of beta-carotene per foot of height as a basic maintenance dose and treble this at times of lung infections.*

PNEUMOTHORAX AND HAEMOTHORAX

A pneumothorax is the presence of air in the space between the lungs and inner chest wall. A haemothorax is the presence of blood in the same space.

Air enters this space either through a puncture

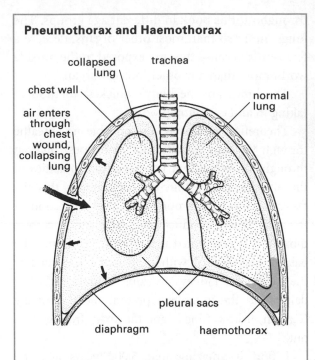

Pneumothorax and Haemothorax

The pneumothorax, shown on the left, is caused by air entering the pleural cavity through a hole in the chest wall. The haemothorax, on the right, is due to blood entering the cavity from broken vessels.

wound or through an injury that tears the lungs allowing inhaled air to pass through the damage. Air is inhaled into the lungs by the negative pressure created by the diaphragm contracting downwards, thereby pulling air in through the mouth and nostrils. A small puncture or tear in the lungs may mean it takes some time for the pleural sac to fill, but as it does the air causes the lung to collapse. A large hole may create an instant or spontaneous pneumothorax. A spontaneous pneumothorax can occur in apparently healthy individuals due to asymptomatic lung disease.

The symptoms are of a gradual or sudden onset of shortness of breath with or without pain on the affected side. Recognition is by failing to hear lung sounds on one side of the chest and a noticeable lack of movement in comparison to the other side. This is not easy to recognize. Confirmation is often required by a chest X-ray, especially if the pneumothorax is developing. A bilateral pneumothorax is, of course, extremely serious if not dealt with rapidly.

A haemothorax develops in the same way but is caused by a damaged blood vessel pouring blood instead of air into the pleural space. Treatment is a minor surgical procedure and should be performed at a local hospital.

If this is not available and the individual is moving into respiratory failure, follow the instructions below.

RECOMMENDATIONS

General Advice

• *An onset, sudden or otherwise, of a shortness of breath must be reviewed by a doctor.*

• *Keep the patient as still as possible and reassure them that the other lung will deal with breathing as long as they stay calm. This is true for most cases for a short period of time.*

• *If a doctor is not available or a bilateral pneumothorax is suspected, and the patient is in respiratory distress, losing consciousness or has passed out, an emergency 'chest drain' is recommended.*

Emergency insertion of a chest drain

• Do not start this procedure unless the following are available: a sharp blade or instrument; tube or piping at least one foot long; and a container and some fluid.

Emergency Chest Drain

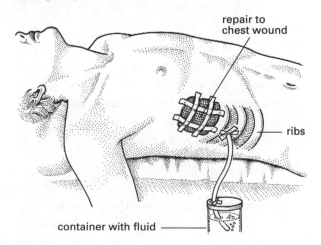

repair to chest wound

ribs

container with fluid

• With the patient on his/her back, find the lowest rib on the affected side in a line down from the front of the armpit. Count up two rib spaces.

• At this point insert the blade through the skin and, keeping it on the top of the lower rib, penetrate until any resistance appears to give. The tip of the blade is now in the pleural space.

• Insert the tube. Place the other end in the fluid in the container.

• Secure the tubing and seal, with whatever means possible, any obvious injury that is allowing air to penetrate.

As the patient breathes, the lung will expand and air in the pleural cavity will be pushed out through the fluid. The fluid will act as a valve and prevent air from re-entering and after a few breaths the lung will expand again. If the patient's breathing has arrested then please follow the instructions for artificial respiration (*see* **Artificial respiration**).

THE DIGESTIVE SYSTEM

BAD BREATH (HALITOSIS)

Most halitosis is caused by poor care of the gums, allowing small pockets of infection to breed bacteria that release noxious gases. The smell of fermenting food is combined with decaying flesh in bad cases.

Slow digestion may leave food in the warm acid of the stomach where bacterial action is unlikely but a certain amount of fermentation does take place. The gas produced may rise up the oesophagus and rarely cause halitosis. More commonly the lungs will eliminate noxious gases that have been absorbed into the bloodstream, as is apparent when garlic can be smelt on the breath many hours after ingesting the plant. The presence of bad bacteria or yeasts such as *Candida*, which produce gas as part of their metabolism, may reflect halitosis; enzymes may similarly be a reflection of halitosis.

General Advice

- *Ensure regular visits to the dentist and ask their opinion of your breath. Friends and loved ones may be too embarrassed to mention a problem. Respectfully, ask the dentist to consider the possibility of small pockets of infection and have a tri-annual cleanse by a dental hygienist.*
- *If bad breath comes and goes, reflect on the foods eaten up to 24hr previously and avoid any potential culprits.*
- *If none of the above techniques prove successful then consult a complementary medical practitioner to assess general health because a toxic system or poorly functioning liver may be the underlying cause.*

Supplemental

- *Take zinc 5mg per foot of height before bedtime.*
- *Obtain a pancreatic enzyme and hydrochloric acid supplement and good quality yoghurt bacteria extract and use at maximum dosage for three weeks.*

Herbal/natural extracts

- *Obtain an Arnica fluid extract, dilute it one teaspoonful to one cup of water and use as a mouthwash three times a day. Avoid antiseptic mouthwash because this kills good bugs as well as bad, thereby diminishing the competition for food and encouraging bad bacterial growth in the long run.*

COLITIS

Colitis literally refers to 'itis' (inflammation) of the colon (large intestine). Colitis is not an uncommon feature at any age and mild forms are created by eating a diet too high in acid or alkali, the ingestion of drugs, allergic foods and infections caused by bacteria, fungi and viruses.

Colitis usually presents as a mild pain and some diarrhoea and is self-limiting, lasting less than 24 hours. Medical books and some therapists erroneously confuse colitis with ulcerative colitis, which is a much more chronic and persisting condition requiring medical intervention.

General Advice

- *Any persistence of mild colitis should be seen by a healthcare professional.*
- *If there is a suggestion of ulcerative colitis (see* **Ulcerative colitis***).*

CROHN'S DISEASE

This condition, first described by Dr Crohn in the 1930s, is an inflammatory condition found anywhere from the mouth to the anus but most commonly in the small intestine, usually before the colon (large intestine) begins. The condition is characterized by pain, diarrhoea, bleeding and weight loss. Flatulence, fever and lethargy are all associated.

There are genetic predispositions and the problem usually shows itself between the ages of 15 and 30 years. There is a higher incidence in the Jewish race and slightly more in the female population.

The causes and treatments are the same as in ulcerative colitis (*see* **Ulcerative colitis**).

General Advice

- *Review the food eaten over the 24hr previous to the pain or discomfort and avoid these if there seems to be a correlation.*
- *Do not use colonic enemas in Crohn's disease unless the large intestine (colon) is particularly affected, and only under medical advice.*

Nutritional

- *More so than in ulcerative colitis, a link has been found between Crohn's disease and a bacterium* called Mycobacterium paratuberculosis, found in cow's milk and tap water. These two drinks and any cow's milk products should be avoided.

Supplemental

- Take a good form of Acidophilus with each meal for one week.

Orthodox

- If alternative treatments used for ulcerative colitis (see **Ulcerative colitis**) do not work, then the antibiotics rifabutin and clarithromycin have shown profound improvements. Complementary therapies to offset the side effects of these strong antibiotics are recommended.

DIARRHOEA

Diarrhoea is the passage of loose stool with more frequency than an individual passes stool normally. Therefore, one bout of loose stool is not, necessarily, diarrhoea. In most cases diarrhoea is not a serious problem and is merely the body or bowel clearing out a toxin. Diarrhoea is commonly associated with the ingestion of food that the body rejects or with mild viral or bacterial infections. More serious infection, such as *Salmonella*, will usually show up as diarrhoea, abdominal pains and associated vomiting and it needs to be treated under supervision. Less than severe cases – those improving over 48 hours or those with no other associated symptoms except perhaps mild abdominal discomfort – can be treated with the recommendations below.

Persisting diarrhoea (more than 72 hours) or diarrhoea associated with severe symptoms such as pain, vomiting, fever and debility should be reviewed by a GP and/or a complementary medical specialist. A change in bowel habit that is persistent may reflect a condition as sinister as a cancer and other problems such as ulcerative colitis (especially if there is blood and mucus associated with the stool), Crohn's disease and malabsorption syndromes. It is best to have a definite diagnosis before any self-help or complementary medical treatment is prescribed.

RECOMMENDATIONS

General Advice

- Diarrhoea that persists longer than 48hr or is non-responsive to the recommendations below should be reviewed by a GP.
- Once a definite diagnosis has been made, which may include stool sampling, a complementary medical view can be obtained.
- Avoid any medication or herbal treatment that 'stops' diarrhoea. It is better to obtain complementary medical advice when dealing with persisting diarrhoea than stopping the elimination.

Nutritional

- Ensure good rehydration because diarrhoea can very swiftly lead to dehydration. Replenish any fluid loss, pint for pint, by judging the amount lost. Take water every half-hour, alternating with diluted fruit juice, soups and slightly salted water, but avoid milk, caffeine, alcohol and any drinks containing refined sugar.
- Go with instinct and appetite. If you are hungry, aim at eating foods that 'mop up' poisons, such as wholegrain bread and pasta or rice. Avoid 'binding' foods such as eggs.

Supplemental

- Take a good-quality Lactobacillus acidophilus or equivalent, which must be encapsulated to avoid the acid in the stomach. Live yoghurt culture is useful but may not survive the acidity.

Homeopathic

- Consider from your preferred homeopathic manual the remedies Arsenicum album, Carbo vegetabilis, Mercurius, Nux vomica and Sulphur. Take the selected remedy at potency 6 every hour for three doses and then every 2hr until better.

Herbal/natural extracts

- Two teaspoons of chamomile tea with a teaspoonful of rosemary and a teaspoonful of sage per pint flavoured with honey is a soothing and potentially antibacterial drink that can be used as part of your fluid replenishment.

DYSENTERY

This condition of bloody diarrhoea, abdominal pain and associated debility is uncommon in areas of good sanitation and hygiene and is generally caused by a bacterium called *Shigella* or by an amoeba. It is an unpleasant condition and, if left untreated, may be serious or even fatal. Serious complications occur because of dehydration and electrolyte imbalance caused by persistent loss of body fluids.

RECOMMENDATIONS

General Advice

- *Any bleeding from any orifice that is persistent or recurrent needs to be reviewed by a doctor.*
- *Diagnosis is made by culture of the stool and unless the situation is very serious, antibiotics should be refused until a diagnosis of the causative organism has been made. The use of antibiotics against amoeba is at best pointless and at worst harmful to the body's natural flora, which are competing with the amoeba.*
- *Ensure constant rehydration with water and salt/sugar solutions.*
- *See* **Diarrhoea**.

Supplemental

- *Two billion units of Lactobacillus acidophilus should be taken every 4hr along with live yoghurt and polished rice. (This is one of the rare occasions where I encourage the use of a refined food over the harder-to-digest wholegrain foods.)*

Homeopathic

- *Dysentery should not be treated without expert help but the homeopathic remedies Phosphorus, Mercurius and Baptesia, all at potency 6 and taken every hour, can be considered until further medical or homeopathic advice can be gleaned.*

Herbal/natural extracts

- *Specific herbal preparations can be used against both bacterial and amoebic infections in the bowel but these should be taken under the guidance of a herbalist.*

FAECES

Faeces or stool are the correct and polite medical terms for the bowel's waste products. To the practitioner of medicine, the stool can be a mine of information and some basic knowledge can be great self-help in diagnosing problems at an early stage.

Blood in faeces

The presence of blood in the stool is abnormal and such a finding without a known cause must be investigated by a medical practitioner. The most common cause of blood in the stool is from a haemorrhoid or pile (*see* **Haemorrhoids**). Less common causes, but sadly more sinister, include cancer, ulcerative colitis, Crohn's disease and benign growths such as polyps. Blood may be mixed with the faeces or separate on the outside, in the pan or on the toilet paper, and these factors along with the colour (bright or dark) give the practitioner a clue as to the probable cause. The more the blood is mixed with the faeces, the higher up the gastrointestinal tract is the bleeding; the darker the blood, the longer it has been present.

Colour of faeces

The colour of faeces is dependent upon the diet. One should get used to looking at one's stool so that any variation from the norm may be noted.

A very black or tarry stool is known as melena and is caused by bleeding in the upper gastrointestinal tract, such as the stomach. The tarry effect is caused by blood being digested and is an indication of potentially serious gastritis or ulcer.

A white or yellow stool is indicative of the presence of undigested fat and may represent liver or gallbladder disease.

A persistent change in colour not related to dietetics should be mentioned to a complementary medical practitioner who should examine you from a broad, constitutional angle to ensure that there is no other digestive or systemic problem.

Frequency

Everybody should have their own bowel evacuation

frequency. In other words, we should all go a regular number of times per day. It is acceptable to open the bowels only once every other day provided that this is normal for you. Put simply, there is no correct number although once a day, in the morning, is preferable.

A change in frequency that persists and is not associated with an infection or a change in diet should be reviewed by a physician, who may choose to perform investigations. A change of frequency or bowel habit is an early and therefore invaluable sign of bowel cancer.

Mucus with stool

Mucus is a clear jelly-like compound that may be watery or gelatinous. The bowel produces mucus to protect itself from acids and alkalis but by the time the faeces reach the colon it should be mixed in and not noticeable as a separate entity. The presence of noticeable mucus is indicative of some inflammatory response and requires a medical opinion and investigations such as a colonoscopy or barium study.

Mucus may be associated with a temporary bowel infection but would therefore be associated with pain or diarrhoea. If this passes then no further action need be taken but a persistence of mucus production must be investigated.

Texture of faeces

See **Diarrhoea and constipation**
The texture of stool is dependent upon the diet and amount of dehydration. A dry crumbly stool is indicative of a lack of water whereas a loose stool may represent a diet lacking in fibre.

The presence of undigested food suggests that the diet or the digestive juices are not correct and a review with a nutritionist is advisable.

A change in the texture of stool, as with its frequency, that persists beyond two weeks and is not associated with a change in diet or recent infection might be an indication of something sinister and should be reviewed by a doctor.

IRRITABLE BOWEL SYNDROME (IBS)

Irritable bowel syndrome is a diagnosis only to be considered when all other reasons for the symptoms have been ruled out.

The characteristics of IBS are persistent and recurrent abdominal pains, usually gripping but sometimes with sharp or cutting episodes, bloating, irregular bowel habits with diarrhoea or constipation, flatulence and associated nausea, and lethargy. All or some of these symptoms may be present. Some authorities would also consider the passage of mucus as being a potential sign of irritable bowel but excess mucus and therefore the passage of it is, in my mind, an association of inflammation or other pathology and should not, therefore, be considered part of an irritable bowel syndrome. There is no inflammation in IBS.

There is no doubt that stress is a principal factor in IBS. Stress chemical or catecholamines, the most common of which is adrenaline, cause blood to move from non-essential organs to the heart, lung, brain and muscles in preparation for 'flight or fight'. The bowel loses some of its blood flow and in extreme cases a lack of oxygen will cause the bowel to contract and the individual will defecate. For those under a persistent level of stress, a small reduction in blood and therefore oxygen will lead to mild cramping as seen in IBS. Some consideration must be given to IBS being associated with a low-fibre diet because this prevents the bowel muscle from exercising and therefore it cramps more easily. Some studies have shown that increasing the fibre content may actually make IBS worse, so the jury is out on that possible cause.

A weakened hydrochloric acid production or pancreatic enzyme flow may also result in IBS by leaving undigested foods that may trigger some form of mild and transient inflammation.

More likely is a food allergy or intolerance, infestation of yeast, fungi or parasites and the inevitable disturbance of the normal bowel flora. The unwanted organisms cause the production of chemicals that trigger cramping, and a poor-quality normal bowel flora leading to an over-growth of these unwanted organisms.

RECOMMENDATIONS

General Advice

- Any persisting abdominal discomfort should be reviewed by a GP and serious pathology ruled out.
- All IBS sufferers must consider counselling and a relaxation technique. Yoga, Qi Gong, Tai Chi and meditation are all prerequisites to eliminating the underlying cause of the problem even if a physical reason is found. For those who disbelieve this, please have one session of hypnotherapy to ensure that there is no underlying and subconscious anxiety.
- Keep a journal and note bad days. Note accurately the foods and drinks you take in and the levels of stress you are under. See if there is any pattern, which may be delayed by 48hr, and try avoiding the possible triggers.
- Shiatsu and basic body massage may be very relieving by addressing the excess of adrenaline in the system and working on the lymphatic system and acupuncture meridians. Techniques of abdominal massage associated with manual lymphatic drainage can be instantly relieving and regular massage treatments can reduce the severity of symptoms.

Nutritional

- Avoid eating a lot of meat or dairy produce. Cut out greasy, spicy and sweet foods. During attacks of discomfort eat well-steamed vegetables, rice, potatoes and other soft foods such as bananas.
- If the diet is low in fibre increase this with fruit and vegetables at each meal but stop if the discomfort worsens.
- Consider a suitable blood test for food allergy or see a nutritionist who uses a bioresonance technique to isolate intolerances. Applied kinesiology is an alternative choice.

Supplemental

- If IBS is diagnosed, a course of capryllic acid (an extract from coconut) and grapefruit seed should be taken in combination. The maximum recommended dose on the product you buy is a guideline for prescribing.
- A high dose of a purified Acidophilus (yoghurt bacteria) should be taken at a maximum dose as recommended on the packaging.
- Try 500mg of bromelaine before meals three times a day.
- Consider a trial with a pancreatic extract or hydrochloric acid supplement, again as recommended on the product. Simple non-invasive hydrochloric acid and pancreatic enzyme-level tests are available.

Homeopathic

- Homeopathic remedies should be chosen on the basis of the symptoms. Pay attention to the homeopathic remedies Natrum carbonicum, Magnesia phosphorica, Carbo vegetabilis, Argentum nitricum and Ignatia.

Herbal/natural extracts

- Bach flower remedies Cerato, Gorse and Vervain can be taken.
- Herbal treatments such as those in Ayurvedic, Tibetan and Chinese medicine are all helpful when prescribed by a specialist.
- Enteric-coated peppermint oil (the oil is enclosed in a capsule that bypasses the strong acids and alkalis of the stomach and small

intestine, thus reaching the colon where the spasm most commonly occurs) can be used. This has a strong antispasmodic action and will act to relieve, although probably not cure, the problem.

- Two teaspoonsful of chamomile, one teaspoonful of rosemary and one of sage in an infusion taken every 2hr will also act as an excellent antispasmodic.
- Standardized Globe Artichoke (Cynara scolymus) can be beneficial in symptoms of dyspepsia, flatulence, nausea, cramping, constipation and diarrhoea. The active ingredient is cynarin and dosage depends upon the percentage extract and therefore should be taken according to the instructions on the package.

STOMACH ACHE

The lay use of 'stomach ache' is of course not medically accurate. The word stomach is used colloquially to cover the entire abdomen.

Abdominal pain needs to be treated depending upon the underlying cause. Most often the reason is clear and associated with the ingestion of some bad food or a nutrient to which an individual is intolerant. Stomach ache in association with other symptoms such as vomiting or diarrhoea will help the diagnosis.

RECOMMENDATIONS

General Advice

- Try to find an underlying cause and refer to that section in this book.
- If no reason is apparent, any severe pain or one that lasts longer than a few hours should be referred to a GP for a further diagnosis.
- There are two acupressure points that may be gently stimulated; they lie below the edge of the rib cage, the length of the individual's thumb away from the middle of the lower edge of the sternum (chest bone). They can be located easily because they will be slightly painful.

- Drink plenty of water, at least half a pint per foot of height during the day.
- In children and infants (see **Colic** and **Abdominal migraine**).

Homeopathic

- The homeopathic remedy Aconite can be used at the onset of any condition. Aconite may not only take away the discomfort but also bring forward other symptoms at a faster rate to help diagnose the underlying problem.

Herbal/natural extracts

- Chamomile (two teaspoonsful), rosemary and sage (one teaspoon of each) may be infused in one pint of boiling water and a cupful drunk every half an hour. This concoction has an earthy taste and may benefit from some honey.
- Ginger tea made by chopping up half an inch of fresh root ginger into a mug of hot water can be drunk and may be soothing.

ULCERATIVE COLITIS

Ulcerative colitis is an inflammatory condition of the large intestine (colon) that presents with sharp abdominal pains as well as cramps, diarrhoea, flatulence often associated with bloating, weight loss, symptoms of malabsorption and very often with blood in the stool or diarrhoea. Small cuts (fissures) are often found around the anus.

This can be an inherited tendency, although the hypothesis of the cause varies: food allergy, infection, autoimmune attack (when the body's immune system attacks itself), poor digestive enzymes, low levels of hydrochloric acid and psychological stress including anger, sadness and grief.

Diagnosis is made by barium meal or enema, X-rays and colonoscopy.

Ulcerative colitis and its small intestinal colleague, Crohn's disease, can spread through the bowel very rapidly. Do not underestimate these conditions. Full orthodox investigation and, in the first case, steroid treatment are often recommended to settle the acute situation before alternative therapies are employed. Do not stop orthodox treatment until resolution has occurred. Failure to control the inflammation can lead to surgical removal of the colon and/or other affected parts of the intestine in Crohn's disease.

RECOMMENDATIONS

General Advice

- *Any persisting bowel problem or show of blood from the bowels should be investigated by your GP with referral to a bowel specialist if required.*
- *Follow through with the orthodox treatment initially and then contact your complementary medical specialist. Self-help is not recommended but the following points should be brought up and discussed with your healthcare professional.*
- *A placebo study showed conclusively that many sufferers responded favourably to stress management. Relaxation, meditation techniques and gentle exercise are all mandatory in cases of colitis or Crohn's disease.*
- *Colonic enemas in the hands of specialists can be relieving in acute phases and beneficial in long-term care (not necessarily suitable in Crohn's disease).*

Nutritional

- *During an acute episode avoid raw or rough foods, preferably having soups and other easily digestible foods. Chew well.*
- *There is evidence that the following foods may be involved in inflammatory bowel conditions and they should be avoided, particularly when an attack is bad: refined sugars (white sugar), alcohol, caffeine, cow's milk products and any foods known not to be tolerated or to which you are allergic.*
- *Have a food allergy test.*

Supplemental

- *Ensure supplementation with zinc, magnesium, and vitamin C. During acute phases of ulcerative colitis and Crohn's disease malabsorption is common and therefore high levels of multimineral/vitamins, trace elements and protein supplements are all recommended. The amounts should be dictated by a nutritional or complementary therapist.*
- *Deglycyrrhizinated liquorice root and bioflavonoids such as quercetin may have healing properties.*

Herbal/natural extracts

- *Flaxseed, slippery elm and chamomile are all soothing.*

THE UROGENITAL SYSTEM

CHLAMYDIA

Chlamydia is a tenacious bacterium often found associated with vaginal irritation and discharge. It is blamed for inflammatory condition in the uterus and Fallopian tubes and can lead to blockages and therefore to infertility and should be treated swiftly and effectively.

It is important to treat an infected sexual partner and, as getting a partner to a clinic or doctor's surgery for a potentially uncomfortable, if not painful, swab is difficult, a first morning urine sample collected at home and sent or brought to a laboratory may suffice. It is also worth asking for *chlamydia* to be looked for on routine cervical smears since infection may be asymptomatic (without symptoms).

RECOMMENDATIONS

General Advice

- *See **Vaginitis**.*
- *Specifically make up a solution of zinc sulphate by adding 5ml of a two per cent solution to one pint of water and use this as a douche. Do not ingest.*

CYSTITIS

Cystitis is inflammation of the urinary bladder. It is usually caused by a bacterial infection but often overlooked is the possibility of viral or yeast infestation. The orthodox world is very swift to supply antibiotics, never considering the possibility that this might make things worse if a yeast is the problem. Also not considered is the possibility that the bladder is inflamed by toxins filtered from the bloodstream by the kidneys. Chemical compounds and specific food intolerances may also cause inflammation.

Infection is usually introduced via the urethra from outside the body. The urethra in the female is short and organisms do not have that far to travel. The male urethra is longer and has the added advantage of the protective effects of seminal fluid that collect in the prostate, which acts as a valve, before organisms can enter the bladder. Dehydration, being sedentary and sexual intercourse all predispose to urinary tract infections. Interestingly, women who do not achieve orgasm easily or frequently tend to have more cystitis, probably due to the fact that pelvic blood congestion occurs without the orgasmic release. (An orgasm is accompanied by blood flow from the pelvis.) One-fifth of women will have a urinary tract infection in any year and most will succumb to this uncomfortable condition at some time in their life. It is rare in men.

The symptoms are generally of pain in the vagina, penis or lower abdomen and this may be an ache or a sharp discomfort. Urination usually makes the pain worse. There is generally increased frequency and the urine may change colour becoming a deeper orange or even red if blood is present. A cloudy urine is not uncommon and particles (pus or bladder wall lining) may be visible.

Cystitis itself is not a pleasant condition but not particularly harmful unless the infection is allowed to travel up the ureters to the kidneys. This occurs in approximately 20 per cent of infections and is characterized by an ache, or worse, in the small of the back. The kidney area may be tender to touch. Renal involvement or recurrence, which may occur because of a general decrease in immunity, obstruction to the outflow or a bladder that has lost some of its sensitivity and therefore does not empty fully, needs to be treated by professionals. Pregnancy may apply pressure to the bladder outflow, as may a full rectum if the individual is constipated.

Asymptomatic bacteria

Four per cent of females carry bacteria in the urine with no symptoms. This is generally a sign of a good immune system. Asymptomatic bacteria increases markedly in pregnancy and anywhere up to 50 per cent of women may, at some time during the pregnancy, carry bacteria without symptoms. As the individual is symptom-free, the discovery of this condition is usually done on routine testing and no treatment need be preferred.

RECOMMENDATIONS

General Advice

- At the first sign of cystitis, increase water intake to at least one pint per foot of height in divided drinks throughout the day. In every second pint add two teaspoonfuls of sodium bicarbonate. These drinks should be at room temperature.
- Pass urine as frequently as is required and especially after intercourse.
- Unsweetened cranberry juice or juniper extract (one teaspoonful per glass of water) should be added if the sodium bicarbonate does not improve the problem within 12hr.
- Ensure good hygiene. Vaginal douching (see **Vaginal douching**) should be used if the problem is recurrent. Use Sandalwood or Calendula soap for the outer aspects of the vagina but only clean water for the vaginal vault. Do not use deodorants and remember to wipe up towards the abdomen after urination and towards the back after defecating. Use only cotton underwear to encourage absorption.
- Any cystitis that persists for more than 24hr

despite the above measures should be treated by a GP or an experienced naturopath.

- *Collect a mid-stream urine (MSU) sample by letting the first 2sec of urination flow into the pan, collect the urine until nearly completed and then let the rest go into the pan.*

- *Try to avoid antibiotics unless a culture and sensitivity test has been performed on the urine sample to ensure that the correct antibiotic is being used.*

Nutritional

- *Eat plenty of garlic with meals or take the maximum recommended dose of any good garlic supplement.*

- *Assess the possibility of any toxin if the condition is recurrent. Pay attention to foods eaten and if necessary consider food allergy testing. This is a must in any chronic or recurrent condition.*

Supplemental

- *The following supplements should be added into a predominantly vegetable and fruit diet. All should be taken in divided doses with meals in the following amounts per foot of height: beta-carotene, 1mg; vitamin C, 1g; and zinc, 5mg (if this creates any nausea, take the full dose before bedtime).*

Homeopathic

- *Refer to your preferred homeopathic manual and select a remedy based on the totality of symptoms. Pay special attention to Cantharis, Berberis and Apis. Staphysagria should be considered if symptoms occur predominantly in association with intercourse.*

Herbal/natural extracts

- *The herbs Uva ursi and Hydrastis can be considered by taking the maximum dose recommended of a proprietary preparation or after consultation with a complementary specialist.*

Orthodox

- *Persistent or recurrent infections that are not amenable to complementary specialist treatment may require a urologist's opinion. Treatment may*

include dilating any constricted or blocked urethra and in severe cases of cystitis (known as interstitial cystitis) may require partial or total removal of the bladder. This is an extremely rare occurrence and should be avoided.

DYSPAREUNIA

Dyspareunia is the medical term for painful sexual intercourse. Occasionally found in males, it is most commonly associated with females and diagnosis of the cause needs to be ascertained after consultation with a GP or, in the case of females, a gynaecologist.

Dyspareunia in men

This unusual situation is usually associated with mild inflammation or infection of the foreskin or penis (*see* **Balanitis**). Urethral inflammation such as caused by gonorrhoea or non-specific urethritis may also be a cause.

More rarely there are congenital deformities in the opening of the urethra (hypospadias), although this does not often cause pain.

RECOMMENDATIONS

General Advice

- *Establish a firm diagnosis by visiting a GP or specialist.*

- *Once a diagnosis is made, please refer to the relevant section in this book before embarking on any orthodox treatment, which may often include the use of antibiotics.*

Dyspareunia in women

Pain on the initiation of sexual intercourse is usually due to inflammation of the vaginal opening or the vagina itself. *Candida* and other infections may be the cause, as may trauma from previous vigorous intercourse or masturbation. Self-examination may isolate redness or white, cheesy patches (*see* **Candidiasis**).

Dyspareunia associated with penetrative sex may be caused by inflammation of the cervix, uterus, Fallopian tubes and ovaries. Occasionally, inflammation in the rectum or bowel may be incorrectly interpreted as dyspareunia. Infection, endometriosis and, very rarely, tumours may be associated and correct diagnosis is essential via a GP's or gynaecologist's examination, or other specialist and non-invasive techniques such as ultrasound. A vaginal examination is generally recommended.

It is worth going to your doctor armed with the knowledge of when, where and how the pain is brought on. Different sexual positions may relieve or exacerbate the problem and this information is helpful in forming a diagnosis.

The vaginal muscles may spasm involuntarily, creating a condition called vaginismus which can cause discomfort and pain if penetrative intercourse is attempted.

RECOMMENDATIONS

General Advice

- *Visit your GP, gynaecologist or specialist for an early and sound diagnosis.*
- *Try to avoid the use of antibiotics until complementary methods have been reviewed.*
- *Review the relevant section in this book for specific treatments once a diagnosis has been made.*

EJACULATION PROBLEMS

The most common problem with ejaculation in young adults is that of premature ejaculation (achieving orgasm and ejaculation with minimal or no physical contact). Strictly speaking this is not a problem of the urogenital tract, it is more to do with psychology. Other problems of ejaculation are due to the rare occasions when individuals may not produce semen or seminal fluid or if the sympathetic nervous system, part of the autonomic, uncontrolled, nervous system, is damaged. This may occur around the penis or throughout the spinal column. Injury to the penis

itself or infections that have caused scarring in the tubes from the testes upwards may all cause problems with ejaculation.

Premature ejaculation

If ejaculation is taking place too quickly there is rarely a need to bring a doctor into the equation but if ejaculation is absent then medical opinion should be sought.

Understand and believe that this is a very common problem faced by most males at some time of their life. It is often associated with early sexual experiments or erotic partners or situations and time usually heals the problem.

RECOMMENDATIONS

General Advice

- *If ejaculation is absent please see your doctor for referral to a specialist.*
- *If ejaculation is too swift (premature ejaculation), try the following routine:*

  (a) *Practise, either through masturbation or with your partner, intimacy without genital contact and conclude the intimacy before an orgasm or ejaculation occurs. Overenthusiasm may occur too often and it is important to put it down to experience and next time use even less stimulation until an acceptable level is reached that does not cause ejaculation.*

  (b) *If ejaculation seems imminent, stop the activity and squeeze firmly just below the head of the penis.*

  (c) *Slowly increase the sexual activity. An individual may find that although premature ejaculation occurs with initial contact, the 'second round' will be prolonged and more controlled.*

  (d) *Consult with a counsellor (most of whom will have had training in such matters) if the problem does not resolve within a few weeks. The longer premature ejaculation carries on, the more ingrained a problem it becomes.*

EPIDIDYMAL CYSTS

These are caused by a block in the epididymus (*see* opposite), which has many tubes collecting seminal fluid from the testes. They are noticed as painless lumps behind the testes, which are usually firm but indentable masses. Epididymal cysts are benign and rarely require treatment. They are generally caused by mild trauma, often unperceived.

RECOMMENDATIONS

General Advice

- *Any lump in the scrotum must be examined by a doctor.*
- *If an epididymal cyst is diagnosed, it should be left alone unless large enough to cause physical inconvenience.*

Homeopathic

- *The homeopathic remedies Apis and Graphites, potency 30, taken twice a day for two weeks have been seen to reduce testicular cysts.*

Orthodox

- *Surgical intervention should be considered only as a last resort because operations in this area may cause scarring that can block the seminal duct and lead to infertility.*

EPIDIDYMITIS

The tube that leads from the testes to the urethra is known as the seminal duct. The part that lies behind the testes through which the seminal fluid (the nutritious liquid in which the sperm flourishes) flows is known as the epididymis. Epididymitis is the inflammation of this coiled, lengthy tube.

Epididymitis, like testiculitis, is generally characterized by a sharp or dull pain, tenderness to the touch, possibly swelling and redness of the scrotal sac.

Inflammation may be caused by trauma, infection or, more rarely, an underlying tumour. It is because of this latter possibility that medical advice is essential but chronic inflammation from

Epididymitis

spermatic cord

epididymus

testis

When the coiled tube of the epididymus becomes inflamed this can be experienced as tenderness, pain or swelling.

infection or unrecognized damage from trauma also makes it preferable to obtain a medical opinion. Epididymitis is a very specific diagnosis and testicular pain may come from other causes such as torsion (twisting), which is a serious medical emergency (*see* **Testicular torsion**) or indeed may be referred pain from another part of the genital tract.

RECOMMENDATIONS

General Advice

- *Any testicular pain or swelling should be examined by a doctor.*
- *Apply a cold compress if it helps.*

Homeopathic

- *Use the homeopathic remedy Arnica 6 every half an hour until a firm diagnosis has been made. Once a diagnosis has been made, consider the following homeopathic remedies, depending on the cause and symptoms: Belladonna, Pulsatilla, Hamamelis – all at potency 6 every 4hr.*

Orthodox

- *If antibiotics are recommended and homeopathic treatment is not working, then consult your complementary medical practitioner without delay and consider using the antibiotics if an alternative treatment is not effective within 12hr. Incorrect or a lack of treatment may lead to sterility, especially if the cause is infection, which may spread to the testes.*

ERECTION FAILURE (IMPOTENCE)

Impotence is the medical term for an inability to raise or sustain an erection. It can be divided into physical and psychological causes. To understand the mechanism of this, it is necessary to illustrate how an erection works.

Under the stimulant of arousal, either physical touch or psychological eroticism, the nerves of the penis cause the arteries to expand and the veins to constrict. This allows more blood to fill the corpus cavernosa, which, like a fluid-filled tyre, will harden and erect the penis. Any interference with these mechanisms will lead to impotence. This reaction is caused by the autonomic (uncontrolled) nervous system.

Physical causes

- Trauma to the corpus cavernosa, arteries or nerves.
- Atheroma clogging the arteries.
- Disease (or trauma) of the central nervous system.
- Toxic effects.
- Certain drugs including alcohol, amphetamines and cocaine are a common cause of temporary impotence.
- Several orthodox drugs, including those used for cardiac and blood pressure problems, can cause temporary impotence.
- Postoperative trauma following prostate or bladder surgery can damage the nerves controlling erection.

Psychological causes

Over 90 per cent of erection failure that present to a holistic counsellor or GP are caused by psychological matters.

Evolution has made it very clear that the chemicals and hormones of stress must outweigh the effects of sex hormones. If we were busily procreating when a sabre-toothed tiger came into view then we would need to be more fearful than excited otherwise we would not, by preference, run away. Those of our prehistoric ancestors whose testosterone levels outweighed their adrenaline flow would stay to finish the job and were, presumably, killed. Nowadays we are rarely confronted by wild animals but the fear chemicals induced by bank managers, employment situations and domestic difficulties are just the same and override the hormones and neurological impulses involved with intercourse.

One most frequent cause is fatigue. Chemicals produced in response to tiredness inhibit erections. Anxiety, stress and phobias all produce large amounts of catecholamines, which directly affect the nervous system and specifically cause dilation in the penile veins, thereby preventing erections. The causes may be superficial, such as anxiety about performance, or they may be more deeply buried. Either way, a counselling session will help to illustrate the need of psychotherapeutic work.

Tiredness, stress and anxiety, fear and guilt are all, therefore, responsible for erection failure.

RECOMMENDATIONS

General Advice

- *Establish or rule out any physical cause by having a full examination from a GP or specialist if in doubt.*
- *Assess and remove bad habits and stress-creating situations wherever possible.*
- *Employ meditation and relaxation techniques through the practice of yoga, Qi Gong and meditation.*
- *Exercise. This reduces the amount of adrenaline in the system and enhances endorphins and encephalins, which are sexual stimulants and, paradoxically, stop the tiredness associated with stress.*
- *If the above measures are not easy to comply with, then techniques of counselling such as neurolinguistic programming are most often beneficial.*

Homeopathic

- *Consider the use of homeopathic remedies: Lycopodium if anticipating problems, Conium maculatum if erection occurs but does not last and Agnus castus if the erection is not firm enough. These remedies should be taken at potency 30 every night for two weeks. Further consultation with a homeopathic prescriber is well recommended as there are many remedies that are documented as being useful with erection problems.*

Herbal/natural extracts

- *Vitamins E and K, the botanical medicines Gingko biloba and Ginseng and a variety of Chinese, Tibetan and Ayurvedic herbs can be considered as adjuncts to the necessary treatment to deal with the underlying cause, but they should be prescribed by a complementary medical practitioner if taken above the doses recommended on the packaging that are necessary to elicit a response.*

Orthodox

- *Testosterone may be recommended by specialists if testosterone levels are found to be low. There are many side effects associated with this drug and I would recommend a visit to an Ayurvedic, Chinese or Tibetan physician who will prescribe herbal medicines appropriate to the case. Use testosterone as a last resort.*

- *Viagra, a popular drug for maintaining erection, has been around for several years and although it has a lot of associated side-effects, it is proving to be a safe enough drug.*

- *Orthodox specialists can teach an individual to inject a drug known as prostaglandin E1 into the base of the penis. This is only used in cases where other treatments have failed since penile pain and prolonged erection are just a couple of the more common side effects.*

GENITAL WARTS

Genital warts are caused by a group of viruses known as the human papillomavirus (HPV). There are over thirty types of HPV, of which two may be responsible for creating a cancerous condition in the cervix. Most are not serious from a medical point of view but are highly infectious, disfiguring and embarrassing.

They are recognized as small wart-like projections or raised areas found anywhere on the penis or within the vagina, most commonly on the moist surfaces.

As with most infections, the problem may not lie within the area infected but within the immune system as a whole. General health must be encouraged.

Warts very rarely undergo malignant change, but if one is bleeding, itching, growing rapidly or changing colour then an urgent dermatological opinion is recommended.

RECOMMENDATIONS

General Advice

- *The best treatment is avoidance, and self-inspection should be encouraged to reduce the risk of spread.*
- *Intercourse with a condom is extremely effective protection.*
- *Specific proprietary topical applications can be used with safety but pay attention to the warning not to place the compound on the surrounding healthy skin. Also, note that compounds used for warts on other parts of the body are not suitable for genital warts.*
- *See* **Warts and verrucas***.*
- *Viral warts are not an indication of poor hygiene or promiscuity. They may lie dormant from a sexual contact many years before. Be open about the problem and discuss the matter freely. Remember the safety of using a condom.*

Nutritional

- *Warts, like any viral infection, are dependent on a depressed immune system. Follow a detoxification programme for a few days and consider a consultation with a nutritionist to discuss diet and lifestyle.*

Homeopathic

• *Homeopathic remedies may be considered, depending on the type and place, but particular attention should be paid to Nitric acid and Thuja.*

Orthodox

• *Surgical intervention may be required if warts are disfiguring or spreading. Diathermy (burning), liquid nitrogen application (freezing) and, very rarely, surgical excision may be required.*

GONORRHOEA

This is a sexually transmitted bacterial infection that is characterized by a greenish creamy discharge, usually from the urethra but also from the vaginal vault in women. Similar discharge may appear in the pharynx, tonsils or anus as a consequence of oral or anal intercourse. Most often the discharge is associated with a sharp cutting pain and inflammation, although occasionally the discharge may be painless. It is this latter asymptomatic state that leads to inadvertent spread of this highly contagious condition.

Orthodox treatment ranges from a single large dose of a penicillin to longer courses of newer antibiotic generations – past injudicious use of antibiotics causing resistant and tougher strains of the gonococcal bacterium.

C S Hahnemann, the founder of homeopathy, paid special attention to gonorrhoea, which, until the 1940s (and even today if left untreated), was a debilitating, if not fatal, condition. Gonorrhoea can be responsible for urethral strictures leading to potential kidney damage, kidney infection, sterility, local abscesses and septicaemia, leading to infected organs including the brain. Hahnemann felt that a gonorrhoeal infection, like syphilis, may persist and be passed through generations. His fears may have less scientific foundation today, although congenital syphilis

has certainly been proven to exist and have devastating effects. Gonorrhoea, from an orthodox point of view, is not thought of in the same way, although arguments may be made on a hypothetical basis. Traditional homeopaths will invariably ask about sexually transmitted diseases and ideally would like to know whether these were contracted by parents and grandparents. Today, were he alive, Hahnemann may well have grouped together other venereal diseases such as *Trichomonas* or *Chlamydia* and registered these as having a deeper or greater significance to overall health than medicine does at the moment. The debate continues.

RECOMMENDATIONS

General Advice

• *Any discharge, discomfort or pain in the genitals should be seen by a GP immediately.*

• *Ensure that all sexual contacts are aware of the diagnosis and use condoms for intercourse until all symptoms and signs of infection have been absent for at least one week.*

Orthodox

• *Avoid antibiotic use until a clear diagnosis has been confirmed by a reputable medical laboratory. Swabs need to be taken. In severe cases an antibiotic may be started, provided that a sample is taken before.*

• *Herbal treatments are effective and, theoretically, homeopathic therapy may solve the problem but my recommendation is to use antibiotics and a suitable anti-antibiotic naturopathic therapy.*

HAEMATOSPERMIA – BLOOD IN SEMINAL FLUID

Blood in any body fluid or discharge is pathological and needs to be watched or investigated. The appearance of blood in the ejaculate is indicative of a bleed anywhere from the tip of the penis to the testes.

Trauma, infection or tumour are the most common causes.

General Advice

- *Any blood in the ejaculate should be investigated under the care of a physician or urogenital specialist unless an obvious cause such as trauma is acknowledged. Even then, if the bleeding persists beyond 24hr or is associated with pain, then have the problem checked out.*
- *Note when the blood appears: blood before seminal fluid suggests a problem in the urethra; blood at the end of the ejaculate is likely to be from the testes. Discolouration of the semen or a mix of blood and seminal fluid may indicate a prostate problem.*

Homeopathic

- *The homeopathic remedies Mercurius and Cantharis, potency 6, may be considered if infection is a likely cause. Take one dose every 3hr. (See* **Sexually transmitted disease***.)*

HERPES SIMPLEX

Herpes is a group of about 70 viruses, the most common of which are herpes simplex, varicella zoster (responsible for chickenpox and shingles) and the Epstein-Barré virus (EBV).

Each of these is discussed in its own section but in principle the treatments are as in this section.

Herpes genitalis (HSV-2), occurs most commonly around the entrance to the vagina, the vaginal vault, the cervix and occasionally up into the uterus. In men it is found on or around the head of the penis and foreskin. Herpes genitalis can, however, occur anywhere in the genital area and may even spread to the buttocks, lower back and upper thighs.

The symptoms range from small painless fluid-filled blisters, through mild stinging with associated redness, to excruciating pain, burning and marked inflammation. There may be associated fever and inflamed lymph nodes and most commonly a generalized malaise or lethargy that may be caused by the infection or be part of the depressed immune system that allows the virus to take a hold.

Up to 40 per cent of the population are liable to come into contact with herpes genitalis or labialis (HSV-1) (the type of herpes found around the mouth and called a cold sore). Eighty-five per cent of people who have an initial attack will deal with the problem and it will not recur. The other 15 per cent may have recurrent attacks and the top two per cent may have very severe and frequent symptoms. Bearing in mind that most of us will contract chickenpox in our youth, we all have had experience of fighting herpes and, in principle, a healthy body should not end up with recurrent herpetic attacks.

Transmission is by contact with the fluid associated with the viral lesions and is generally introduced to the next host through small cuts or abrasions (which are common and unnoticed during intercourse), and also depends on the new host having a depressed immune system at that time. By depression I am referring to being overworked, undernourished or with a mild infection such as a cold. Those who have recurrent attacks harbour the HSV in a nerve centre known as the ganglia. Herpes tends to lie dormant until an individual runs down with a cold, stress, periods, or allergic reactions to certain foods. Also, sunburn, overexercising and sexual activity can trigger the recurrence. The virus multiplies, travels back down the nerve, often to the original site of infection, and spreads through the dendrites or branches at the end of the nerve, causing a slightly larger area to be affected.

Combating herpes is carried out on two fronts. The first is to enhance the individual's own defence system and the second is to weaken the defence that the virus puts up by surrounding itself with an impregnable protein coat that the immune system cannot penetrate. The requirements to enhance the individual's immune system are rather dependent on the person. The recommendations below are specific for inhibiting the reproduction of the herpes virus and also weakening its defence.

General Advice

- *Recognize the cause of the immune suppression and try to avoid the situation (allergic foods, stress and lack of sleep).*

Nutritional

- *Increasing lysine and reducing argenine (both amino acids) in the diet is required. Foods to be discouraged through attacks are nuts, chocolate, seeds and pulses, all wholegrains, pork, sunflower oil and crustaceans such as crabs and shrimp. Foods to be encouraged through acute attacks are fish (especially halibut), chicken and turkey, yeast-containing foods such as raised white bread, potatoes, milk and lamb.*

Supplemental

- *Through an acute attack supplement each meal with the following: lysine 1g, vitamin C 2g, bioflavonoids (500mg), zinc (10mg, but if you feel any nausea then avoid this and take 30mg before you go to sleep) and a thymus extract as directed on the packaging.*
- *In the case of recurrent attacks the supplements mentioned above for acute attacks should be taken daily as recommended but only with one meal per day.*

Homeopathic

- *The homeopathic remedies Kali muriaticum, Rhus toxicodendron, Urtica urens and the nosode Herpes simplex can all be taken every hour for three doses in an acute attack, dropping to every 2hr. In chronic conditions a constitutional remedy is best selected by a homeopath.*

Herbal/natural extracts

- *The lesion can be treated with the following applications: apply moist coffee grounds four times a day; zinc (0.05 per cent) and vitamin E cream (0.1 per cent) may be used separately or combined four times a day; or vitamin E can be applied for 15min three times a day.*

- *For lesions that are resistant to the above recommendations, insomuch as attacks continue to be frequent and just as severe, discuss the use of liquorice or lithium succinate (8 per cent solution) with your complementary medical practitioners. Melissa officinalis (1 per cent solution) can be applied four times daily.*

Orthodox

- *Avoid the preparatory applications of the antiviral agent acyclovir because this only deals with the superficial infection and also has been shown to encourage the development of resistant strains of the virus that are much more difficult to deal with and can lead to much more serious complications, especially in the immunocompromised.*

It is unusual for treatment to be instantly effective and recovering is often shown by less frequent attacks of a shorter duration. Sometimes the more virulent viruses are not destroyed and a mild attack once or twice a year is the best that we can hope for – thus the concept that herpes, like diamonds, is forever. This is only the case in a very small percentage.

MENSTRUATION AND MENSTRUAL PROBLEMS

See **Uterus** *and* **Uterine problems**

Menstruation occurs in women on a cyclical basis. It is the clearing out of the inner lining of the uterus following a cycle where fertilization of an egg and pregnancy did not occur. The menstrual bleed, commonly known as a period, lasts from one to seven days, the average being a heavier flow of menstrual discharge on days 1–3 with a reduction in the amount thereafter.

The diagram overleaf shows the growth of the inner lining of the uterus, known as the endometrium, in relation to the hormones that control the cycle. The Eastern philosophies believe in a central energy that the Chinese call the vessel of conception (*see* **Vessel of conception**). The

Menstrual Cycle

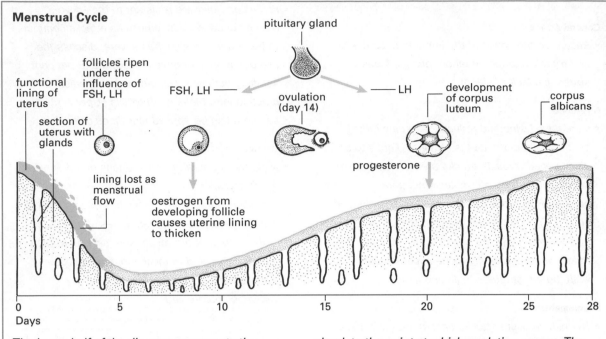

The lower half of the diagram represents the clearing out and regrowth of the uterine lining during the course of the female cycle. Above this we see the development of a follicle in the ovary, under influence from hormones secreted by the pituitary gland, to the point at which ovulation occurs. The empty follicle then develops into a corpus luteum which secretes the hormone progesterone causing the uterine lining to thicken. The corpus luteum then degenerates to become a corpus albicans.

energy connection between the pituitary gland, thyroid gland, pancreas and uterus has been well known for over 5,000 years and an imbalance in this energy can cause problems in any of these organs and is very often the underlying reason for irregularity in the menstrual cycle. Any stimulants that affect thyroid production, deficiencies, excess refined sugars or nerve-affecting drugs may alter the cycle.

Amenorrhoea

Amenorrhoea is the absence of periods. This can be primary – periods never started – or secondary – usually associated with hormone imbalances caused by stress, anorexia/bulimia and other causes of sudden weight loss. Amenorrhoea may also occur following childbirth, coming off contraception such as the coil or the pill and after diseases affecting other glandular (hormone producing) organs or severe illness leading to malnutrition.

The inner lining of the uterus builds up prior to ovulation and if pregnancy is not an occurrence then this lining is shed. A correct production of oestrogen and progesterone, as described in chapters 2 and 3, is required for a normal cycle to occur.

The Eastern medical philosophies include an energy line, the vessel of conception, that travels from the perineum (the area between the vagina and anus) up through the uterus, pancreas, thyroid and pituitary gland. This axis if deficient, can cause 'misbehaviour' in any of these organs, including amenorrhoea. (*See* **Menstruation and menstrual problems.**)

RECOMMENDATIONS

General Advice

• *Remember that the most common cause of amenorrhoea is pregnancy. Obtain a pregnancy kit if you have had intercourse, protected or unprotected, up to one month prior to missing a period.*

- *Review any weight loss or appetite changes. If any are present, then speak to a complementary medical practitioner.*
- *If no obvious reason is apparent from those mentioned above, consult a medical practitioner and your complementary therapist when you have missed three periods. Premature menopause and tumours of the pituitary gland are easy to diagnose and potentially treatable if caught early.*
- *Yoga, Shiatsu and acupuncture can all remove the energy blocks that can lead to amenorrhoea and they should be considered.*
- *Stress is a principal cause of amenorrhoea and if this is abundant or there is any evidence of anorexia or obsessive dieting, consider discussing matters with a counsellor.*
- *See **Delayed puberty** for discussion of primary amenorrhoea.*

Nutritional

- *Increase the protein in the diet. Ensure that iron, vitamin B_{12} and folic acid levels are normal (see **Anaemia**).*

Homeopathic

- *Homeopathic remedies can be most beneficial: Aconite and Arnica if the periods are associated with a shock; Natrum muriaticum or Ignatia if associated with grief or fear; and Sepia if emotionally indifferent or tearful. Consider Ferrum metallicum, Graphites and Pulsatilla when reviewing a good homeopathic book.*

Delayed, late or infrequent periods

The first two years of menstruation, which can start at any age from 11 years, may be irregular and a delayed or infrequent period should only be considered as abnormal if this is a new pattern differing from previously regular periods. A delayed or late period may have many causes and pregnancy must first be ruled out. The hormones that control the cycle are produced by the pituitary gland, which is a small walnut-sized piece of tissue that sits in the middle of the brain. This gland is very susceptible to changes in the neuro-transmitters or brain chemicals and therefore the cycle can easily be thrown by emotional disturbances. Problems with boyfriends, parents or impending exams may all trigger a suppression of the pituitary gland's production of follicle-stimulating hormone and luteinizing hormone, both of which are necessary for ovulation to take place and therefore for the period.

Once ovulation has taken place, a period generally follows 14 days later and most delays or long cycles are caused by an increase in the first part of the cycle known as the proliferative or follicular phase (*see* diagram opposite). The second part of the cycle is known as the secretory or luteal phase and this is followed, if pregnancy is not an occurrence, by the menstrual phase.

Delayed or late periods may result from overexercising or undereating. There is no firm scientific foundation for this occurrence but I suspect that it is to do with chemical suppression by exercise-induced hormones such as cortisol or endorphins. These are released when muscles are exercised or because of a lack of nutrients necessary to build up the inner lining of the uterus through the proliferative phase. Whatever the biochemical reason, energy is taken from, or not provided to, the uterus.

Certain metabolic conditions such as hypothyroidism and polycystic ovaries may be the cause of delayed or absent periods and this may need to be checked out.

RECOMMENDATIONS

General Advice

- *One or two late or delayed periods are generally not a problem. A missed period may represent a pregnancy and this needs to be tested for.*
- *Review psychological stresses and discuss the matter with a counsellor if no obvious cause is apparent.*
- *Avoid medication unless prescribed by a complementary medical practitioner experienced in this matter, because alteration of a body's normal*

cycle, delayed or otherwise, may be injurious.

- *Persistently late periods that are not altered after discussions with a nutritionist, counsellor or complementary practitioner should be viewed by a gynaecologist to rule out any underlying metabolic disorder.*

Nutritional

- *Ensure that the diet is regular and nutritious. Any alteration in the cycle in association with dieting suggests a deficiency and an incorrect dietetic plan. Remove excess sugars from the diet.*

Supplemental

- *Specific deficiencies in vitamins and trace elements may also cause a problem in the formation of the endometrium. Take a protein supplement, Vitamin B₆, Evening Primrose Oil and zinc at twice the recommended dose for one month.*

Homeopathic

- *Consult with a homeopath who will consider the symptoms in light of the individual as a whole and work from a constitutional standpoint.*

Orthodox

- *Avoid the use of the oral contraceptive pill as a technique of controlling the cycle except as a last resort.*

Dysmenorrhoea (painful periods)

Dysmenorrhoea is the medical term for painful menstruation. The start of menstruation, the menarche, occurs between the ages of 11 and 16 years in females. There is often a hereditary pattern and the start of a girl's periods may occur at the same age as her mother and grandmother. A textbook menstrual cycle is 28 days long with the bleed lasting 2–7 days (on average around 5 days). The first half of the cycle is under the control of oestrogens, which prepare the ovary to release an egg, and the second part of the cycle still has some oestrogen effect but is predominantly controlled by progesterone, which causes the build-up of the inner lining of the uterus in preparation for the implantation of a fertilized egg.

In the first part of the cycle the amount of oestrogen is controlled by the pituitary gland, which sits in the middle of the brain. In the second half of the cycle the progesterone and oestrogen production is produced by the corpus luteum, which is the 'shell' of the egg or ovum that has been released from the ovary.

If an egg or ovum is not fertilized, then the corpus luteum dies off and the progesterone and oestrogen levels diminish. These lower levels are a trigger to the pituitary gland to start the cycle all over again but before it does the unused inner lining of the uterus needs to be shed. This is done through menstruation (or a period). The process of removing this inner lining or endometrium is aided by mild contractions of the uterus. These contractions are painful and the amount of pain depends on:

- The force of the contraction.
- The amount of inner uterine lining.
- The pain perception of the individual.
- From an Eastern perspective, the amount of energy flowing through and supplying the uterus and female hormonal system. All Eastern philosophies believe in a mid-line energy flow which, interestingly, corresponds to the hormonal system. The top of the energy line is through or around the pituitary gland, which provides hormonal control for the thyroid and uterus in females. This energy line, called the vessel of conception (*see* **Vessel of conception**) in Chinese medicine, actually travels down through the thyroid and the pancreas on its way to the uterus. The pancreas is not directly under the control of the pituitary gland but insulin levels from the pancreas are related to sugar levels, which in turn are controlled, to a great extent, by the levels of adrenaline, growth hormone, thyroxine and natural body steroids, all of which are controlled by the pituitary gland.

It needs to be understood, therefore, that dysmenorrhoea, or painful periods, is not only to do with the uterus. It is important to establish an underlying cause, which may fall into any of the above categories.

RECOMMENDATIONS

General Advice

- Discuss the matter with your gynaecologist or GP and rule out any of the rare underlying conditions that may cause painful periods by having ultrasound, blood tests for hormonal imbalances and a full clinical check-up, including a cervical smear and internal examination.
- The perception of pain is exacerbated by stress. Good relaxation techniques and an evaluation of life's problems may be curative. Neurolinguistic programming and hypnotherapy, meditation, yoga and Qi Gong are all successful in helping to deal with painful periods.
- Acupuncture, chiropractic and osteopathy are all useful techniques and probably work on the strengthening of the underlying energy weaknesses or tensions that build up in the lower pelvis.

Supplemental

- Strength of contraction is dependent upon the body's levels of calcium, magnesium, sodium and potassium. It is also extremely important to be well hydrated and many cases of dysmenorrhoea are alleviated by taking a mineral supplement and ensuring an intake of 4–6 pints of water per day.
- The amount of endometrium (inner lining of the uterus) is associated with the uterine response to progesterone. Excess progesterone may be counteracted by the natural phyto-oestrogens found in soya milk and its products, celery, fennel, rhubarb and hops. An increase in these foods leading up to and during a period may be relieving. Conversely, stimulating the body's own progesterone production with the use of herbs such as Agnus castus or homeopathic derivatives at potency 200 or using natural progesterone through transcutaneous Mexican yam extracts may be of benefit. The amounts of these supplements and remedies should be decided in consultation with a complementary medical practitioner who has knowledge in these areas.
- The following supplements may be useful in divided doses: Evening Primrose oil (1g per foot of height) and Vitamin B_6 (10mg per foot of height) during the day and zinc (5mg per foot of height) at night.

Homeopathic

- Homeopathic remedies must be chosen on the type of pain, duration and associated factors, such as amount of bleeding and the presence of clots. Remedies that could be reviewed include: Magnesia phosphorica, Arnica, Belladonna, Calcarea carbonica and Cinchona officinalis. All should be taken at potency 6 every hour.

Herbal/natural extracts

- Chinese/Tibetan herbal medicine have much documented evidence of efficacy and a popular compound is Dong Quai (angelica), which, like most herbs, is best prescribed by a specialist.

Orthodox

- Before commencing any orthodox treatment discuss the matter with a complementary medical practitioner.
- If alternative techniques fail or the underlying cause is not amenable to change then the use of the oral contraceptive pill can be considered but, as always with any drug, weigh the potential risks with the benefits.
- Provided that there are no contra-indications, do not hesitate to use ordinary painkillers such as paracetemol. If this is not working well, mefanamic acid is prescribable by your GP and is a most popular pain reliever. Taken over the more painful couple of days, you are unlikely to do yourself any harm whilst you find the underlying cause.

Early periods (short cycle)

A short cycle may be considered as the arrival of an early period but is not a problem if this is the general pattern. A cycle of 20 days is not usually a disease process unless it is a departure from a longer cyclical pattern.

As for delayed periods, psychological matters can have a profound effect by the chemical influence of neurotransmitters from the pituitary gland.

An early menstrual phase is usually due to a shortened proliferative phase and is therefore commonly associated with a much lighter and shorter period.

Heavy periods – *see* Menorrhagia

Menorrhagia (heavy periods)

Menorrhagia is the medical term for an excessive menstrual flow. Many of the principles discussed in the section on dysmenorrhoea (*see* **Dysmenorrhoea**) are relevant to menorrhagia.

The amount of endometrial tissue discharged is proportionate to the amount that is laid down through the second part of the cycle. This is dependent upon the effects of progesterone on the endometrial growth, however this is not the only influence.

The uterus provides the female with another avenue to eliminate toxins from the body. Each month new tissue is laid down and provided with a rich blood supply. Toxins in the bloodstream will, therefore, automatically find themselves in abundance in this endometrial tissue. Toxins such as lead, from car exhaust fumes, are laid down and shed on a cyclical basis. Whether the body is actually intent on doing this is uncertain and one may argue that the body would protect against allowing toxins to settle in a part of the body where reproduction takes place, but the body is a phenomenally complex system. Assuming that toxins settle there with or without the body's blessing, menorrhagia may be a toxic excretion technique.

As with dysmenorrhoea, in Ayurvedic and yogic medicine a build-up of vital force or energy in the lower part of the vessel of conception (*see* **Dysmenorrhoea**) may be responsible for the overgrowth of endometrial tissue.

Energy must flow smoothly between all the chakras and an excess in any particular point will cause deficiency above or below. Therefore a block in the abdominal or solar plexus chakra may lead to an excess in the lower chakras which in turn can cause the overgrowth found in menorrhagia.

The Chakras

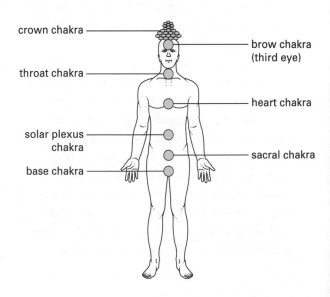

crown chakra
brow chakra (third eye)
throat chakra
heart chakra
solar plexus chakra
sacral chakra
base chakra

Certain deficiencies such as vitamin A, iron or hypothyroidism may all cause menorrhagia.

Menhorrhagia is rarely a symptom of a more serious condition. Fibroids, endometrial polyps and salpingitis (*see* **Salpingitis**) may present initially as menorrhagia, as may endometrial cancer.

RECOMMENDATIONS

General Advice

- *A full gynaecological examination including ultrasound and hormonal blood tests is a starting point. Having ruled out a serious condition, consider complementary techniques before orthodox ones.*
- *Assess the potential for stress because the pituitary gland, which indirectly controls the levels of progesterone, is centred towards the middle of the brain and is very much under the influence of the psyche. Techniques of relaxation and stress management should be embraced.*
- *The need to establish free energy flow through the chakras or vessel of conception requires consideration. Emotional, psychological, spiritual and physical causes may be at work and a review with an Eastern-thinking complementary practitioner is recommended. Yoga, Shiatsu and acupuncture may all be curative.*

Nutritional

- *Examine lifestyle and habits and eliminate any obvious toxins. Food intolerance testing through blood tests, Vega, bioresonance or applied kinesiology techniques are all recommended.*
- *Furthermore do not underestimate the toxic effects of caffeine, alcohol, tobacco and other recreational drugs.*

Supplemental

- *Menorrhagia may lead to deficiencies, particularly in iron and proteins, and supplements of amino acids and a multimineral including iron (which should always be associated with zinc and vitamin C) should be considered. A daily recommended dose of a natural food-state supplement should be taken until the problem is resolved and this level should be doubled throughout the actual bleeding period. Paradoxically, iron deficiency may cause menorrhagia.*
- *Supplement the diet with beta-carotene, 2mg per foot of height in divided doses with meals through the day.*

Homeopathic

- *Homeopathic remedies are, again, chosen on the symptom picture of the individual as a whole but those remedies mentioned in the section on dysmenorrhoea (see* **Dysmenorrhoea***) may be applicable. If anaemia is diagnosed or the individual is particularly pale then please consider the remedies Ferrum phosphoricum and Borax at potency 30 taken four times a day.*

Menorrhalgia (pain in pelvis)

This is the medical term for excessive pain in the pelvic area associated with menstruation but different from the individual's usual period pain.

All the suggestions and recommendations for dysmenorrhoea should be adhered to but your gynaecologist and complementary practitioner should consider the possibility of endometriosis (*see* **Endometriosis**).

Painful periods – *see* Dysmenorrhoea

NON-SPECIFIC URETHRITIS (NSU)

Non-specific urethritis (NSU) is a term initially provided for symptoms of cystitis (*see* **Cystitis**) that have no apparent cause. It was assumed that NSU was caused by viruses but in the last two decades the two organisms *Trichomonas* and *Chlamydia* have been thought to be the culprits. Most commonly these create vaginal infections that are often asymptomatic. At worst they may ascend into the uterus and cause salpingitis (inflammation of the Fallopian tube; *see* **Salpingitis**) but they frequently trigger urethritis.

Non-specific urethritis may also be a pseudonym for honeymoon cystitis created by the friction of intercourse. In my opinion the true definition is somewhat blurred.

RECOMMENDATIONS

General Advice
- *See Cystitis for specific symptomatic treatment.*

Herbal/natural extracts
- *If Trichomonas or Chlamydia are isolated, treatment of the vaginal vault is recommended. Single or combined treatments using pessaries of Tea Tree, Lavender, Hydrastis and Calendula may be beneficial if used morning and night.*

ORGASM

An orgasm is an intense, diffuse and pleasurable sensation experienced during sexual intercourse or masturbation. In the male it is associated with ejaculation (but please note that ejaculation may occur before and after orgasm) and in the female with uterine and pelvic muscular contractions, and a warm flooding sensation throughout the pelvis.

Orgasms may vary in intensity, depending very much upon the state of the nervous system both physically and psychologically. Persistent friction on the head of the penis, the clitoris or a small area just inside the upper aspect of the vagina (colloquially known as the 'G' spot) sends off nervous impulses to the central nervous system. An accumulation of these impulses triggers a profound neurotransmitter release that principally affects the pleasure centres but also blocks both pain and some neuromuscular channels. Co-ordination is particularly affected momentarily, heart rate, blood pressure and peripheral circulation can increase.

Achieving an orgasm requires a conscious effort but the actual nervous reflex is governed by the parasympathetic, autonomic (uncontrolled)

nervous system. Damage to these nerves can cause a decrease in intensity or a total loss of orgasm, whereas a hypersensitivity may cause an orgasm to arrive too quickly. Often associated with premature ejaculation, this oversensitivity can be created by natural hormones, excitement or stimulation and by the use of certain drugs. Other drugs may have a converse effect: alcohol, amphetamine, cocaine and ecstasy are commonly abused for this purpose (*see* **Ejaculation problems**).

The yogic philosophy believes that energy known as the *kundalini* is stored in the pelvis. Genital stimulation awakens this energy, which flashes up the spinal column and affects the brain. Masters of meditation can release this energy without physical stimulation and there are reports of telepathy being able to create orgasms in the partners of meditators. Certainly meditation will remove inhibitory chemicals and lead to easier attainment of orgasm.

Some physical disorders such as multiple sclerosis or other nerve diseases and problems with the prostate gland can interrupt the nerve supply and prevent orgasm. Damage to the central nervous system may also cause a loss. Anxiety, stress and phobias, often resulting from failed previous sexual experiences or guilt from religious teachings, can affect the ability to have an orgasm or might cause premature ejaculation. These are usually not serious conditions but may require some time and some special counselling.

RECOMMENDATIONS

General Advice
- *Delayed or absent orgasm may be a process of age but may also be caused by disease process and should be reviewed by a GP or specialist in the field.*
- *Meditation and counselling to alleviate anxieties or phobias may have a profound effect. Sexual counselling may be required.*
- *See Ejaculation problems.*

OVARIAN CYSTS

The ovaries are a complex of different types of tissue that harbour the female eggs. These are all produced at the foetal stage of an individual's development. Therefore a 40-year-old woman will have 40-year-old eggs. This is partially why the older a woman gets, the more chance there is of a genetic mishap in conception.

As an egg ripens it moves to the surface and is released, leaving behind a chemical-producing cell known as the corpus luteum. This produces chemicals, including human chorionic gonadotrophin (HCG), and other hormones, such as oestrogen and progesterone, until the placenta is formed and takes over this role after eight weeks of pregnancy. These corpus lutea are often the site at which fluid can accumulate, creating a cyst. A cyst may form in other parts of the ovary and may be triggered by infection that travels along the Fallopian tube. A common cause is when the mature egg fails to open or be released by the tougher outer fibrous coat of the ovary and this causes a follicular cyst.

Cysts in general may grow by an excess of fluid or damp in the system and the Chinese physicians consider cysts to be most commonly associated with an excess of Yin in the diet.

Most often cysts are symptoms and, without ultrasound techniques, may go unnoticed. Cysts are being found more commonly because of routine pelvic ultrasound, but I do not know of any study that has monitored whether these come and go as a regular occurrence. However, there is a belief that a cyst may be associated with cancer and the percentage chance of this being the case is equal to the age of the patient. Put more simply, a 20-year-old with a cyst has a 20 per cent chance of it being associated with cancer, but a 50-year-old has a 50 per cent chance.

A cyst may grow to the size of a football and cause pressure symptoms on the bladder, bowel or other internal organs. Usually bloating and a visible swelling would be noticed before any serious effects are created. An infected cyst may burst and lead to peritonitis, with severe pain and associated symptoms. Menstrual cycle changes may occur, although this is unusual, and the cyst may put pressure on nerves, leading to painful intercourse or back and leg aches.

An increasing number of women are presenting with multiple ovarian cysts not associated with the menstrual cycle and ovulation. Polycystic ovary syndrome has mild or considerable imbalances in the female/male hormonal structure often associated with excess follicle stimulating hormone (FSH) or testosterone. An absence of a normal cycle, hirsutism, lack of libido, are amongst the symptoms of this syndrome.

The orthodox world uses powerful oral contraceptive pills, many of which create unpleasant side effects, which may or may not be effective. Alternative therapies as mentioned below should be considered, especially the use of natural progesterone, before these are tried.

The apparent increase in the number of women with this condition suggests that there is some environmental hormonal effect, possibly from oestrogens in our food chain or even the use of the oral contraceptive pill. More study is needed, more research is not forthcoming.

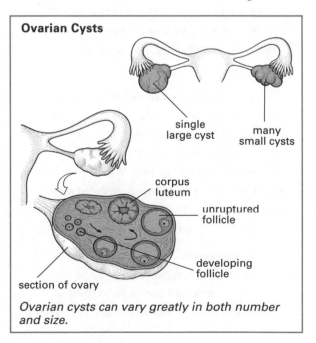

Ovarian Cysts

single large cyst

many small cysts

corpus luteum

unruptured follicle

developing follicle

section of ovary

Ovarian cysts can vary greatly in both number and size.

RECOMMENDATIONS

General Advice

- *Ovarian cysts are often picked up on routine gynaecological examination and will be confirmed by ultrasound. Do not be rushed into an operative procedure but consult a complementary medical practitioner.*
- *Some ovarian cancers release a particular chemical known as a marker into the bloodstream, which should be measured if there is any suggestion or risk of an ovarian cancer.*
- *Abdominal massage in experienced hands may remove a cyst.*

Nutritional

- *Remove sugar, alcohol, cow's milk products and caffeine from the diet.*
- *Fruit and watery vegetables should be reduced to a minimum and Yang foods should be increased (see **Yang foods**).*

Supplemental

- *The following supplements may reduce a cyst and should be taken as follows: vitamin E (200iu per foot of height in divided doses throughout the day with food) and gamma-linoleic acid (30mg per foot of height with breakfast). Beta-carotene (1mg per foot height in divided doses) should also be taken to counteract the effect that vitamin E has of draining the vitamin A.*

Homeopathic

- *Homeopathic remedies should be chosen depending upon the symptoms but the remedies Apis (right-sided cysts), Colocynthis (left-sided cysts), Oophorinum (cysts associated with menopause) and Kali bromatum (if there is any suggestion of the cyst being associated with a tumour) can all be used at potency 30 three times a day for three weeks.*

Herbal/natural extracts

- *The use of natural progesterone creams with or without the concurrent use of the herb Agnus castus can be administered and has been shown to remove ovarian cysts. The treatment must be under the control of an experienced practitioner or physician.*
- *Herbal treatments, especially Chinese, in association with acupuncture have proven successful.*

Orthodox

- *Surgical intervention may be required and is usually performed through a laparoscopy. A small tube is inserted through a 1cm incision just below the navel and passed into the abdominal cavity. Try to find a gynaecologist who is willing to remove the cyst rather than the ovary.*
- *Metformin, an antidiabetic drug, may be a resort to consider if naturopathic treatments and the use of orthodox drugs such as anti-androgens and the oral contraceptive pill do not work.*

OVARIAN CANCER

Ovarian cancer is an increasingly common diagnosis in the West. The reasons for this are uncertain, but an increase in the use of the oral contraceptive pill cannot be ruled out. Orthodox medicine has shown that there is an increased risk in those who use fertility-promoting drugs such as clomiphene or the group called gonadotrophins.

It is a difficult cancer to deal with since it can lie in the ovaries and spread to other parts of the body with very few symptoms until the disease is well advanced. Unlike breast cancer, it is not well screened although it is feasible to do so. Ovarian cancer tends to create a particular measurable component in the blood called CA125, and tumours or cysts can be visualized by ultrasound. A regular screen is advisable.

RECOMMENDATIONS

General Advice

- *See **Cancer**.*
- *Consider yearly screening if hyper-fertility drugs or long term oral contraceptive pills have been used.*

Orthodox

- *Operative treatment is recommended if there is no evidence of spread.*
- *Chemotherapy and radiotherapy may be beneficial.*

there will apply a painkilling gel (which is, unfortunately, only partially effective) and squeeze the head of the penis. It is worth taking a painkiller on your way to the hospital but advise the physician that you have done so.

PARAPHIMOSIS

Paraphimosis is the retraction and constriction of the foreskin behind the head of the penis. The event usually occurs after intercourse or masturbation and is more likely in those whose foreskin is tight, either as an anatomical anomaly or following infections of the foreskin (balanitis).

This retraction impedes the venous blood flow, causing swelling of the head of the penis. This tightens the foreskin even more and the engorgement causes intense pain.

RECOMMENDATIONS

General Advice

- *Prevention is the best cure. Make sure that the foreskin is pulled forward after intercourse and use a petroleum jelly or soap and water as soon as any difficulty in pulling the foreskin forward is noted. The problem is self-perpetuating and left to its own devices will worsen.*
- *If paraphimosis has occurred, place some ice cubes in soft material such as silk and surround the head of the penis. Apply gentle pressure and attempt to push the blood from the penile head up the shaft.*

Homeopathic

- *Use the homeopathic remedy Apis 6 every 5min and if the problem is solved, move onto Arnica 6 every 3hr until any residual ache subsides.*

Orthodox

- *If this technique fails it is sometimes necessary for an operation under general anaesthetic to incise the foreskin. This usually leads to a circumcision.*
- *If this technique fails, go to the nearest emergency unit as soon as possible. The doctor*

PELVIC INFLAMMATORY DISEASE (PID, SALPINGITIS)

Pelvic inflammatory disease (PID) is an infection of the uterus and Fallopian tubes typically caused by an infection with *Chlamydia* (*see* **Chlamydia**) or *Trichomonas*. Other infections – bacterial, viral or fungal – may cause PID, which may be recurrent or simply persist as a chronic infection.

The symptoms are of pain ranging from a dull ache to sharp and cutting. This may be felt from the vagina through to the back. A discharge is frequently associated and is most commonly unpleasant smelling but not always.

Pelvic inflammatory disease generally occurs following intercourse but any vaginal examination, uterine operation such as a dilatation and curettage (D & C) or a termination may introduce infection.

A severe or persistent infection may lead to damage of the narrow Fallopian tubes and is a major cause of infertility. Uterine and ovarian infection may lead to abscesses.

Any problem in the pelvis may represent a stagnation or lack of energy in the base chakra. There is a strong correlation between PID and sexual promiscuity and the reasons for this need to be confronted if the problem is a chronic or repetitive one.

RECOMMENDATIONS

General Advice

- *Any discomfort that persists or is severe must be examined by a GP.*
- *Ultrasound, vaginal swabs and full blood counts to test the level of white cells are recommended before any treatment course is started. In severe cases these may be done after initiating treatment.*

- *If PID is associated with promiscuity a truly holistic answer must include counselling to confront the need for multiple partners.*
- *Osteopathy and acupuncture are physical techniques to release blocked energy in the pelvis and encourage blood flow to wash out infections.*
- *Yoga, Tai Chi, Qi Gong and Polarity therapy techniques should be used in conjunction with other treatments.*
- *If intercourse was the initiating factor, the male partner needs to be examined using a penile swab and urine sample because many infections are asymptomatic. Urine samples, taken first thing in the morning may also isolate a causative bacteria.*
- *Chronic recurrent conditions should be assessed by a complementary medical practitioner with experience in this area.*

Homeopathic

- *Homeopathic treatments should be chosen from your preferred homeopathic manual depending upon the symptoms. Whilst deciding, use Aconite 6 every half an hour.*

Herbal/natural extracts

- *Herbal treatments can be used. Echinacea and Golden Seal are particularly useful for any infection and should be taken in the quantity recommended on a good quality product or via a naturopath.*

Orthodox

- *This is one of the few occasions when an antibiotic should be considered a first-line treatment. Failure to treat may lead to chronic, serious complications or infertility. Combination antibiotics for bacteria that breed well in non-oxygenated areas, as well as a broad-spectrum aerobic antibiotic, are usually used. Chlamydia and Trichomonas may require strong antibiotics and this treatment requires protection of the bowel and other body flora as described in the section on antibiotics (see* **Antibiotics***).*

PREMENSTRUAL SYNDROME/TENSION (PMS/PMT)

Most women will admit to some decrease in well-being in the 2–14 days prior to menstruation. This is predominantly caused by an increased sensitivity throughout the body because of raised oestrogen and progesterone levels. Deficiencies in vitamins and minerals, an excess of stress chemicals such as adrenaline and physical stress from food allergy may all make matters worse. Premenstrual syndrome is a troublesome and recurrent multi-symptom condition that can be anything from mildly disturbing to profoundly debilitating. The symptoms can be divided into categories.

Psychological symptoms

Anxiety, confusion, depression, memory deficit, irritability, mood swings, tearfulness, exacerbated tension and insomnia occur in 75 per cent of PMS sufferers.

Physical symptoms

Headache, lethargy, dizziness or fainting, fluid retention with associated weight gain, abdominal bloating and breast tenderness will be apparent in about 70 per cent of cases.

Studies have shown that the symptoms are directly related to hormonal imbalances. It is important to understand that on the way to making oestrogen and progesterone the body produces many similar chemicals all of which can have an effect on the system. Some symptoms are created by low levels whilst others by high levels. Other hormones such as androgens, aldosterones, prolactin, follicle-stimulating hormone (FSH) and thyroid levels can be affected.

Deficiencies in vitamin B_6 and magnesium can have a profound effect on the production of some of these hormones, as well as affecting brain neurotransmitters such as dopamine, which are responsible for the emotional changes. These two supplements also play a part in the production of a particular hormone known as prostaglandin E_1, the function of which is not well understood but is often found to be low in women struggling with PMS. Excessive fat intake or deficiencies in omega 6 and omega 3 fatty acids (which are included in extract of Evening Primrose Oil) can cause low levels of this compound. Mercury and lead poisoning may be associated with PMS, as may deficiencies in vitamins A, C and E and the minerals selenium, zinc and iron, in addition to those mentioned above.

RECOMMENDATIONS

General Advice

- *Premenstrual syndrome is not imagined. There is a lot of scientific evidence to support causes that can be treated without using the antidepressants that are the first-line treatment of the orthodox medical world.*
- *Hair mineral analysis should be considered if the above are not working.*
- *A study has shown that osteopathy can reduce the physical symptoms of PMS.*
- *Acupressure and acupuncture are beneficial.*
- *Reflexology with attention paid to the pituitary and adrenal glands will help.*
- *If all this fails, consider seeing a complementary medical practitioner because nearly everyone who practises medicine has some trick up their sleeve! The use of natural progesterone derived from the Mexican yam can be beneficial if the symptoms are created by low progesterone or unopposed oestrogen, but this needs to be prescribed by a practitioner with expertise in this area.*
- *Relaxation and meditation techniques through yoga or Qi Gong can be very beneficial.*

Nutritional

- *Avoid animal fats, fried foods and any hydrogenated oils (that includes many margarines) especially during the time leading up to the period. Reduce sugars and increase vegetable sources of proteins such as soya and legumes. Any compound that affects the liver, such as alcohol and caffeine,*

will reduce its ability to break down hormones and therefore exacerbate some cases of PMS.

Supplemental

- *Consider a trial of vitamin B₆ or magnesium, or preferably have these levels checked by a competent complementary medical practitioner.*
- *If deficient, for a trial period take vitamin B₆ and magnesium both at 50mg per foot of height in divided doses throughout the day starting on day 14 of the cycle and carrying on until the period starts (day 1 is the first day of a period).*
- *Obtain a fish oil or eicosapentaenoic acid (EPA) supplement and take three times the recommended daily allowance (RDA) from day 14 to the first day of the period. Vegetarians may use linseed oil – one teaspoonful per foot of height divided with meals through the day.*
- *Beta-carotene (2mg per foot of height) and vitamin E (5iu per foot of height) in divided doses during the day may be of some benefit.*
- *Gammalinoleic acid (GLA 50mg per foot of height) taken with breakfast may be beneficial. This can be found in Borage, Star Flower or Evening Primrose Oil capsules.*

Homeopathic

- *Homeopathic remedies that match the symptoms will be beneficial and specific attention should be paid to Calcarea carbonica, Sepia, Causticum, Pulsatilla, Ignatia and Kali carbonicum.*

Herbal/natural extracts

- *Liquorice taken as a tincture diluted 5:1 with water (1 teaspoonful per foot of height) in divided doses with meals.*
- *Alfalfa contains phyto-oestrogens (plant oestrogens), and should be considered but prescribed by a herbalist.*
- *Bromelain at twice the dose recommended of a good natural product may help.*
- *Extract from the plant Agnus castus (Vitex agnus castus) has been shown to have beneficial effects on irritability, mood alteration, anger, headache, breast fullness and bloating. Consider*

taking the maximum dosage recommended on the package.

Orthodox

- Resort to the oral contraceptive pill only if the above measures do not have an effect.

PRIAPISM

This is an abnormal, persistent, painful erection of the penis which, by definition, is unrelated to sexual desire. It is caused by certain blood disorders such as sickle cell anaemia which blocks the venous (blood flow outlet) system or by problems of the central nervous system that cause contraction of the corpora cavernosa, the blood spaces that fill and cause the hardening of the penis. If not dealt with impotence may result.

RECOMMENDATIONS

General Advice

- The problem must be dealt with by a urogenital specialist.
- Complementary treatment is dependent upon the underlying cause.

PUBIC LICE

Pubic lice are usually transmitted by sexual contact. These small parasites cause itching and appear as small freckles. Watched closely, especially in a bath, movement may be seen and the tell-tale sign of small white eggs will be found at the base of the pubic hairs stuck on with a remarkably tenacious glue. Raising a louse with tweezers will cause a very small pin-prick of blood.

RECOMMENDATIONS

General Advice

- (See **Lice**)
- Topical, orthodox preparations are effective and need to be applied to the affected area

including the lower abdomen, thighs and hairs around the anus, then covered by underwear and left on overnight. Repeat this process one week later.

SEXUALLY TRANSMITTED DISEASES (STD) AND VENEREAL DISEASE (VD)

A sexually transmitted disease is one that is passed from one sexual partner to another. It is most commonly associated with penetrative intercourse but may be passed through oral sex as well. Transmission can be divided into groups.

Viral infections

Acquired immuno-deficiency syndrome (AIDS) is transmitted by passing the human immunodeficiency virus (HIV). Herpes around the genitals is caused by herpes simplex type 2, and the human papillomavirus (HPV) causes warts. These are all discussed in their own sections.

Bacterial infections

The better-known bacterial infections are syphilis and gonorrhoea. These are stored in some part of the urogenital system and transmitted through associated fluid. Bacterial infections from other parts of the body, such as the bowel, may also be transmitted by the act of intercourse. Vaginal, uterine and bladder infections are commonly caused by a bacterium known as *Escherichia coli*, which thrives in the bowel and is part of the normal bowel flora. If this bacterium finds its way into another organ, it can be quite devastating and produces very unpleasant symptoms.

Other infections

Some organisms behave more like parasites, existing within cells in the same manner as viruses but also behaving like bacteria in their metabolism. *Chlamydia* and *Trichomonas* are commonly found in association with non-specific urethritis (NSU) and typically spread by sexual intercourse.

Pubic lice, or crabs as they are colloquially

known, are generally spread through sexual intercourse.

Candidal infection, most commonly known as thrush, is typically spread through sexual intercourse.

Safe sex

Safe sex is a phrase that has been coined since the rise of HIV/AIDS. It is an extremely accurate definition and it is becoming more relevant as Western societies become less critical of sexual promiscuity. This attitude is pervading the so-called Third World countries where unprotected sex is more common than not because of the lack of availability of condoms. Add to this an apparent increase in homosexual activity and the use of anal intercourse in poorer nations as a form of contraception and you have several reasons why the importance of practising safe sex is increasing.

There is some controversy as to whether oral sex is safe sex. Vigorous oral activity that produces small cuts or lesions will allow the transmission of infective agents. Bacterial infections such as gonorrhoea and syphilis are known to transfer from male ejaculate causing throat and tonsillar problems, as does *Candida* (thrush). It is unlikely that HIV will transfer in this way but the possibility cannot be excluded. The herpes simplex type 2 virus (genital herpes) prefers to live in tissue other than that found around the oral cavity. However, in rare instances transmission can occur and it is best to avoid unprotected oral sex if a herpetic lesion is visible.

RECOMMENDATIONS

General Advice
- *All of the above conditions are discussed in their relevant sections.*
- *All sexually transmitted disorders are best treated by avoidance. Sexual promiscuity should be reduced and safe sex practised.*
- *Maintaining hygiene and a personal high level of immune system activity will decrease the risk of*

transmission and encourage any infection to be destroyed effectively.
- *The use of drugs and alcohol reduces the immune system response and, in conjunction with sexual promiscuity, will increase the risk of an infection taking hold. Keep 'abuse' to a minimum.*
- *The use of a condom is effective against diseases which are vaginally transferred or carried in the semen.*
- *Anal intercourse and vigorous vaginal or oral sex will predispose to small (or large) lesions into which infected agents may travel directly into the bloodstream. Avoid these techniques or be gentle and use adequate amounts of lubrication.*
- *Wash the genitals before and after intercourse where possible.*
- *Urinate after intercourse when possible.*

THE TESTICLES

The testes descend from the abdomen and rest in the scrotal sac (scrotum) away from the body because their function and their maturity depend upon being below body temperature. Considering how sensitive they are, they have very little protection other than that the reflexes in that area which are very rapid and will draw the body around the midriff swiftly.

Sperm are produced at a rapid rate and each spermatozoon lives approximately five days. If no ejaculation has taken place the sperm break down and are re-absorbed. Sperm are stored in a collection of tubules known as the vas deferens before passing up into the urethra at the level of the prostate via the vas deferens.

It is here that the sperm mix with the seminal fluid from the prostate. This mildly viscous, sticky, milky compound completes the ejaculate and contains fructose in high quantities which provide the sperm with food on their journey.

Injury to the testes

Any trauma to the testes is extremely painful because of the high number of nerves in the area. The testes are associated with a complex of blood

The Testes and Penis

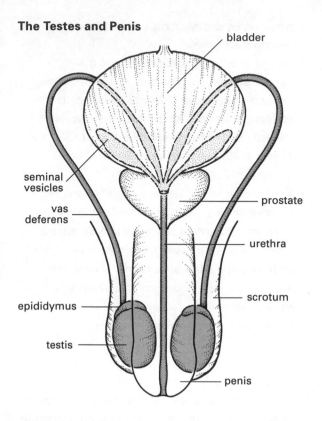

and lymphatic vessels and any trauma can rupture these, forming cysts (*see* **Hydrocele**). An injury to a blood vessel may bleed and cause a haematoma (bruise), which, while clotting, may cut off the blood supply and lead to testicular gangrene.

RECOMMENDATIONS

General Advice
- *Encase the scrotum in an ice-filled flannel to relieve the discomfort.*
- *Take deep breaths, pulling energy down into the lower abdomen.*
- *Any pain that is not easing within a couple of hours must be examined by a physician in case a more serious injury has occurred. Delay may run the risk of the loss of the testicle.*

Homeopathic
- *Take Arnica 6 every 10min until the discomfort is relieved and then every 2hr until the pain has gone completely.*

TESTICULAR TORSION

The testicle hangs in the scrotal sac to be kept away from the heat of the body (the testicle works best at 1°C lower than body temperature). This requires blood vessels and nerves to travel from the body along the spermatic cord from the testes up to the penis. The testicle is anchored into place through fibres that may be congenitally absent or damaged through trauma. If this is the case, the testes can twist causing occlusion of the blood vessels and an excruciatingly painful pressure on the nerves. If this twist or torsion is not corrected the testicle will die from a lack of oxygen and gangrene with its inherent dangers will set in. It is not possible to miss a torsion except in an infant since the pain is fierce.

RECOMMENDATIONS

General Advice
- *Please follow the advice for an injured testicle (see above).*
- *Any pain persisting without remission over 2hr must be reviewed by a doctor.*
- *Ice wrapped in a flannel and applied may reduce swelling but the slightest touch may make the pain worse and therefore even the ice is not desired.*

Homeopathic
- *The remedy Aconite 6 can be taken every 10min whilst awaiting treatment.*

Orthodox
- *Repair of a torsion that does not spontaneously untwist is surgical. In an emergency situation untwisting the testes may be possible provided that the turn is in the right direction. The pain is such that it is difficult to discern this as no relief will be immediately noticeable. This procedure must only be undertaken by somebody with experience who cannot operate immediately or if medical availability is too far away. In any case an operation is required because the testes need to be fixed to prevent recurrence.*

- *Please accept an anaesthetic or an intravenous tranquillizer such as valium, despite any alternative medical views of these drugs. The bravest of brave are unlikely to deal with the pain of examination, let alone treatment.*
- *See **Operations and surgery**.*

THRUSH

Thrush is the colloquial name for a *Candida* infection, commonly found in the vagina but also affecting other moist areas such as the anus and oral cavity. Men with foreskins may have an irritation there (*see* **Candida**).

TRICHOMONAS

Trichomonas is a protozoan (an organism that exhibits both bacterial and viral activity) that may be responsible for vaginitis and uterine infections.

RECOMMENDATION

General Advice
- *See **Chlamydia** as treatment is identical.*

URETHRA

The urethra is the tube passing from the bladder down the penis or to the upper aspect of the vagina. At the top end, just below the bladder, are consciously and unconsciously controlled valves (involved with the prostate in the male) that allow urine flow. Bacteria may travel up the urethra from the external skin surface but these are generally washed away by the flow of urine on a regular basis. The male urethra is a stretchable tube allowing for an erection but it is quite a long passage for bacteria to travel to infect the bladder. The urethra in women is much shorter, and markedly so in girls, increasing the chances of infection and cystitis.

RECOMMENDATIONS

General Advice
- *External hygiene is extremely important and washing the genitals is a must, especially at an early age or after intercourse.*
- *Good hydration leading to frequent urination is an important protective measure.*

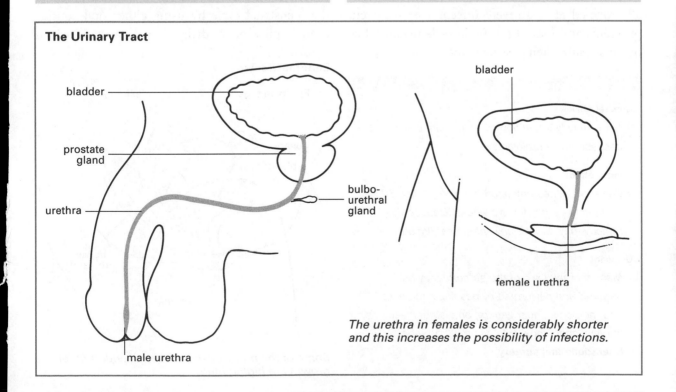

The Urinary Tract

bladder

prostate gland

urethra

bulbo-urethral gland

male urethra

bladder

female urethra

The urethra in females is considerably shorter and this increases the possibility of infections.

Urethral discharge

A discharge from the urethra is usually associated with bacterial infection although yeast infection such as *Candida* may be a culprit. The colour often gives away the causative agent. A yellow/green discharge is usually gonorrhoea, which is the most common cause.

RECOMMENDATIONS

General Advice

- *Immediately start treatment by water intake to flush the system.*
- *Collect a urine sample for the doctor's surgery.*
- *A urethral swab is recommended so that an accurate diagnosis can be made and the correct antibiotic used if required.*
- *See* **Cystitis** *for the treatment.*

Urethral stricture

A stricture is an obstruction, usually caused by scar tissue. Congenital malformations may account for a small percentage. Scar tissue is usually formed after a severe infection or recurrent problems and may, if severe, impede urinary flow or cause pain when passing urine.

RECOMMENDATIONS

General Advice

- *Any difficulty in the flow of urine must be assessed by a urologist.*

Homeopathic

- *Commence the homeopathic remedy Silica 30 three times a day for two weeks because this remedy may remove unwanted scar tissue.*

Orthodox

- *Manual breakdown of the stricture may be required and performed by passing a metal rod into the penis under general anaesthetic and surgical conditions. If this is required, see* **Operations and surgery**.

UTERUS AND UTERINE PROBLEMS
Endometriosis

This is a painful condition characterized by discomfort usually in the pelvis or abdominal areas and very often associated with cyclical changes of rising oestrogen levels just before and during the period.

The condition is caused by the presence of the inner lining of the uterus (the endometrium) existing in abnormal locations such as the outside of the uterus, Fallopian tubes or ovaries, or attached to the bowel, other organs such as the bladder or the bowel wall.

The pain occurs because this endometrial tissue behaves towards the oestrogen and progesterone levels as does the endometrium within the uterus. It engorges with blood and swells as if it were expecting a fertilized egg; this swelling causes inflammation and pain at the site.

Endometriosis, depending on its site and the amount of displaced tissue can lead to other problems such as painful intercourse, infertility and bowel and bladder problems.

The orthodox approach is to consider blocking the menstrual cycle by using either oral contraceptive pills or a drug called danazol, which

Endometriosis

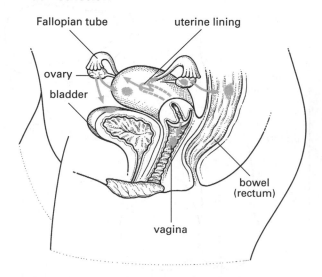

Some of the many possible sites of endometrial growth are highlighted.

blocks the pituitary gland (which controls the female cycle). Other drugs are being considered all the time. Surgery, either laparoscopic or open surgery, may have to be considered to remove aggressive or larger deposits.

Fibroids

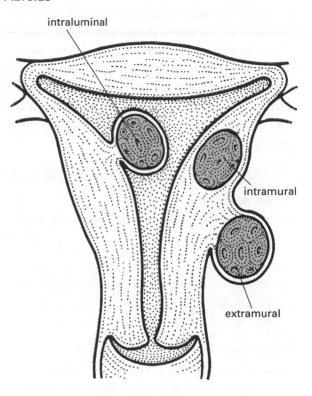

RECOMMENDATIONS

General Advice

- *Acupuncture can be useful both as a pain reliever and potentially as part of a curative protocol.*
- *Deep abdominal massage by a practitioner with knowledge in this area can break down adhesions.*

Homeopathic

- *Consult a homeopath. Depending on the symptoms, a variety of homeopathic remedies may be beneficial.*

Herbal/natural extracts

- *Consult a herbalist. Phyto-oestrols have a weak oestrogen effect, which may block the natural oestrogens and therefore lessen the amount of endometrial swelling. Herbs such as dong quai and glycyrrhiza, dandelion root and others may be considered.*

Fibroids

Fibroids are an overgrowth of uterine muscle that may develop as a type of polyp into the uterine space (intraluminal), within the uterine wall itself (intramural) or outside of the uterus (extramural). Depending on where they are, the symptoms of a fibroid may differ, although many fibroids are symptomless and will cause no problems. Their size is relevant to the level of discomfort they might cause by adding weight to the uterus which in turn will push on the sacral and possibly lumbar nerves causing discomfort and pain.

Intraluminal

Symptoms will include increased bleeding (menorrhagia), painful periods (dysmenorrhoea), painful intercourse (dyspareunia) and, much more rarely, discomfort.

Intraluminal fibroids are a cause of infertility and may be discovered when a couple investigate this distressing problem.

Intramural

Fibroids found in the wall of the uterus may create all the problems associated with intraluminal fibroids and are actually far more common.

Extramural

These fibroids do not carry the same number of complications, although painful intercourse and pressure-induced discomfort are the principal clues to discovery.

The orthodox world is uncertain as to the cause of fibroids but the consensus of opinion in the holistic medical world is that an excess of energy builds up in the pelvis, uterus or lower chakra (*see* **Menorrhagia** *and* **Dysmenorrhoea**).

Fibroids are much more under the control of oestrogen than endometrial tissue build-up, which is under the control of progesterone. Bear this in mind when referring to the section on menorrhagia below. Fibroids often diminish through the menopause (when the oestrogen levels drop dramatically) and therefore progesterone treatment may be considered when dealing with fibroids.

RECOMMENDATIONS

General Advice

- *Please refer to the recommendations in the next section on menorrhagia.*

Homeopathic

- *Homeopathic remedies should be considered at high potency and in particular Calcarea iod and Thuja should be reviewed.*

Herbal/natural extracts

- *Natural progesterone absorbed into the body through the skin can have very beneficial effects but often needs to be taken over a 2-year period. This needs to be monitored by a doctor or complementary medical practitioner with experience in this field. Please note that natural progesterone is currently available by extraction from the Mexican yam (no other wild yam has the same proven efficacy) but it cannot pass through the acid in the stomach and is therefore not available in pill form.*

Orthodox

- *Orthodox treatment is restricted to operative procedures, either dilatation and curettage (D & C) or modern techniques using laser. It is becoming less common but hysterectomy is still too frequently recommended.*

THE VAGINA
Care of the vagina

The vagina is a remarkably tough area of the body. It is the hallway to the cervix and uterus and the exit of the urinary system. Urine is constantly passed through it and the vagina is approximately one inch away from the anus. Intercourse constantly introduces foreign matter and the act of sex itself can be quite bruising. The vagina has to act as a barrier and protector of the womb whilst undergoing pressure from all of these external influences.

The vaginal vault has its own protective secretions in which there live normal body bacteria that attack and compete with invading organisms. The vaginal secretions contain many immuno-globulins and white blood cells in preparation for this activity. The secretions must also be lubricating enough to allow intercourse and receptive enough not to attack and kill sperm and thereby reduce the chances of fertilization.

The vagina manages all this through a very careful regulating system that keeps the acid/alkaline levels balanced and is very much under the control of the body's hormonal system especially oestrogen and progesterone. Different times of the cycle will produce different levels of these female hormones, which in turn affect the

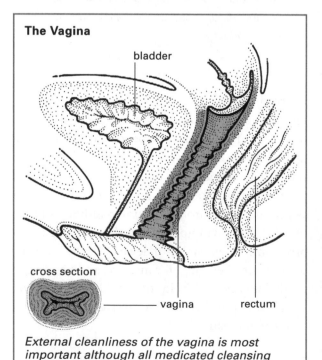

The Vagina

bladder

cross section

vagina

rectum

External cleanliness of the vagina is most important although all medicated cleansing products should be avoided.

cellular production of these secretions. These tend to thicken and take on a characteristic viscous feel around the time of ovulation, which is of great benefit to the survival chances of the sperm.

External cleanliness is important and the wiping of the urethral exit away from the vagina is as important a learned trait as wiping the anus backwards and upwards. Medicated soaps and toiletries should be avoided because these will interfere with the normal bacterial flora and natural soaps and fresh water should be the only cleansing agents. Vaginal perfumes are not to be encouraged. Any unpleasant odour is generally due to dietetic problems, hormonal imbalances or infections and should be treated appropriately. Cleanliness is especially important throughout menstruation. Old blood is a perfect medium for bacterial growth. External pads are theoretically more hygienic than internal tampons, but not so popular and may give a greater rise to discomfort and odours. Both should be changed frequently in any case.

Vaginal douching

There is no need for a vaginal douche as a regular cleansing mechanism. The healthy body will produce ample lubrication and immune response to protect the vagina and a douche should only be used to support this basic cleansing mechanism. Douching should not be performed during a period because the cervix may be slightly more open and may allow easier access for infection. However, this is generally counteracted by the blood flow and therefore douching may be desirable if the vagina is uncomfortable or odorous or in preparation for sexual intercourse.

RECOMMENDATIONS

General Advice

- *Douche only when necessary.*
- *Douche bags are available from chemists or ask your GP for a 50ml syringe.*

- *Preferably use boiled water in the preparation of a douche.*
- *A basic cleansing solution may be obtained by adding one tablespoonful of cider vinegar to one pint of water or one tablespoonful of live yoghurt to one pint of water. These quantities may be doubled in the case of a vaginal discharge or infection. Douching with these solutions may be done up to every 4hr and may be very beneficial in infections if used on an alternating basis.*
- *Boric acid (500mg in half a pint) of water can be used, but not more than once a week.*
- *All of the above can be used up to four times a day in acute infections but if there is no improvement after five days then bring the problem to the attention of your doctor or gynaecologist.*

Herbal/natural extracts

- *Douching solutions can be made from Hydrastis, tea tree oil and zinc sulphate (one tablespoonful of a 2 per cent solution to one pint of water), but generally only use these for treatment rather than regular hygiene.*
- *Arnica or Calendula lotion may be used at a dilution of one tablespoon per pint of boiled water.*

Vaginal discharge

A vaginal discharge is either due to excessive secretion or the action of the vaginal defence mechanism. The former is usually associated with sexual excitement or hormonal or neurological stimulation. The latter is a general reaction in an attempt to flush out any foreign object or organisms that may be causing irritation.

Candida tends to produce a thick whitish discharge with a typical yeasty smell, soreness and itching. Green/yellow discharge is indicative of bacterial infection – *Streptococcus* or *Trichomonas* are the most frequent. A grey discharge is often associated with *Gardnerella*, and *Chlamydia* often produces a clear, runny discharge.

Foreign objects

A foreign object may well be found in a vagina in children or infants who show a discharge. Adults are less likely to be unaware of the contents of the vagina but all too frequently internal tampons may be forgotten. Bacteria have a predilection for living in a blood-soaked tampon and a syndrome known as Toxic Shock Syndrome (TSS) is a surprisingly common occurrence. In this condition bacteria grow at a rapid rate in a forgotten tampon, release toxins and cause severe poisoning, not infrequently resulting in death.

Irritated or itching vagina

Itching of the vagina is most commonly found on the outer lips (vulva) but can be anywhere. It is generally caused by minor infections or contact dermatitis from irritating creams and deodorants. In older ladies the menopause leads to a diminution in normal secretions, which automatically encourages dryness and potentially infection. Different stages of the normal menstrual cycle may alter the level of secretion, protection and normal vaginal flora, and this may lead to an irritation.

The quality of the vaginal secretions is dependent upon nutrition, and deficiencies in nutrients and excesses of sugar and toxins, such as from smoking and alcohol can lead to irritants being expressed through secretions. Poor hygiene will lead to mild infected irritation, and fungal infections by skin fungi can affect the vagina in the same way as athlete's foot.

Infections of the vagina

Vaginal infections may be asymptomatic (without symptoms), or present as a discharge which may be coloured or clear, an irritation or a pain, or may only be discovered during intercourse.

The vaginal vault has a considerable amount of its own normal bacteria which compete with bad bugs for food, thereby keeping unwanted bacteria at bay. Provided regular hygiene is maintained, vaginal infections are infrequent.

A persisting problem requires a medical examination whereby a swab may be sent to a laboratory for culture to see if anything is growing. Antibiotics are the orthodox world's first line of treatment but should only be used as a last resort.

RECOMMENDATIONS

General Advice

- *Depending on the symptoms, see* **Vaginal discharge** *and* **Vaginitis**.

Herbal/natural extracts

- *Tea tree oil, lavender, Hydrastis or Calendula pessaries or any combination should be considered for use as directed by the practitioner who prescribes them.*

Orthodox

- *Chlamydia or Trichomonas infections may warrant an antibiotic as a first-line treatment. See the relevant sections in this book on these infections.*

Odour

Odour is generally created by a bacterium or yeast infection that has settled into the vaginal vault despite the body's normal vaginal flora. The normal flora will have a characteristic smell but should not be offensive.

Vaginal secretions, like any discharge from the body, will reflect the contents of the bloodstream, and diet will have a strong influence on the smell.

RECOMMENDATIONS

General Advice

- *Consider diet and mild infections as being relevant. Correct the nutrition and visit a doctor for a swab to isolate any causative organism.*
- *Please refer to the relevant section if an infection is present.*
- *See* **Vaginal douching** *and use the technique after a sample or swab has been taken.*

- *Do not use vaginal deodorants directly because this will interfere with the normal vaginal flora. Instead, if necessary, deodorize the groin area of the outermost clothes.*

Vaginal dryness

Lubrication is produced by special cells that line the vaginal walls and are under the influence of oestrogen and progesterone. These cells themselves are governed by the autonomic (involuntary) nervous system and both the hormones and these nerves stimulate the production of lubricant in response to sexual stimulus.

General dryness may be due to neurological problems but most frequently are the result of diminished hormonal activity or production. Menopause is notorious for creating vaginal dryness.

The lack of secretions leads to a diminution in the protection of the vaginal vault due to a loss of the immunoglobulins and white blood cells that attack invading organisms. The normal vaginal flora also need a moist environment, and this too will diminish. Intercourse becomes painful or irritating.

RECOMMENDATIONS

General Advice

- *Vaginal dryness for no apparent reason, but often due to age, needs to be reviewed by a complementary medical practitioner and doctor.*
- *Ensure that dehydration is not an aspect by drinking half a pint of water per foot of height.*
- *If hormonal imbalances are ruled out and no neurological conditions are found, consider using non-medicated lubricants. KY Jelly is the best known, although vitamin E creams or olive oil may be used.*
- *Ensure adequate foreplay before intercourse. This is particularly important after menopause when lubrication is physiologically diminished but still capable of being produced given enough stimulus.*

Homeopathic

- *The homeopathic remedies Belladonna, Lycopodium and Natrum muriaticum should be reviewed and the most suitable remedy for the individual constitution should be chosen.*

Vaginismus

Vaginismus is a painful spasm of the vagina created by constriction of the muscles within the vaginal wall. It is a nervous condition usually associated with a trepidation of intercourse. Most frequently found in teenage girls, this condition may persist and can be painful and embarrassing.

RECOMMENDATIONS

General Advice

- *Vaginismus is not a disease and is treatable but it requires psychological intervention. Please seek a counsellor with experience in sexual dysfunction.*
- *Do not try to force intercourse, but digital insertion may remove some of the anticipation.*

Vaginal warts – *see* Genital warts

Vaginal pain

Pain in the vagina is usually associated with trauma following violent or aggressive intercourse or the traumatic insertion of foreign objects. Inflammation from any cause of vaginitis, especially infection, may cause vaginal pain.

Often overlooked is a lower spinal nerve entrapment that causes a referred pain; and food allergy has been cited as creating a variation to the normal vaginal secretions, causing irritation and discomfort.

Pain of the vaginal lips (vulvodynia) is occasionally present with no known cause. This condition is thought to be neurologically based rather than a local problem.

RECOMMENDATIONS

General Advice

- *Any pain in the vagina that is without obvious cause, severe or persistent must be reviewed by a GP or gynaecologist.*
- *If associated with back pain or is persistent, regardless of treatments for specific problems, it may be relieved by osteopathy especially with the use of ambulatory traction as offered by a lightweight contraption fitted for a few minutes by osteopathic specialists.*

Nutritional

- *Surprisingly, consider food allergy for unexplained and unremitting vaginal discomfort.*

Orthodox

- *The tranquillizer amitriptyline may be of benefit in unrelenting vulvodynia.*

Vaginitis

Symptoms of itching, even pain, discharge, burning, redness and pain on intercourse can all be symptoms of vaginitis.

The vagina is a resoundingly tough part of the anatomy considering the battering it gets from intercourse and foreign compounds such as sperm, douches, deodorants, tampons and condoms etc. The vagina also houses many bacteria, most of which are useful and attack bad bacteria but also, amidst the colonies, there lurk small amounts of 'bad guys' who are no trouble at all until the normal healthy vaginal flora are disturbed by the use of antibiotics and other drugs and chemicals such as perfumes and proprietary-made douches. Hormonal imbalance, often created by oral contraception and the eating of non-organic meats (which contain oestrogens), can all create vaginitis. Excess white sugar and specific allergic foods can also encourage bad bacterial/fungal growth.

RECOMMENDATIONS

General Advice

- *Maintain good hygiene with daily baths and cleaning the vagina after intercourse with water or a natural douche (see **Vaginal douching**). Ensure that the area between the anus and vagina (the perineum) is cleaned by washing with strokes away from the vaginal opening.*
- *If forced into using an antibiotic or chemical douche, ensure protection through complementary medical means, including natural douches and ingestion of high doses of Lactobacillus acidophilus or an equivalent.*
- *Any persistence of a problem despite treatment after five days should be reviewed by your GP or gynaecologist. If any discomfort appears to be travelling to the uterus or lower abdomen visit your specialist straightaway.*

Nutritional

- *Avoid refined sugars (white sugar) and foods containing them through any acute episode.*

Herbal/natural extracts

- *Vaginal pessaries containing one or a combination of the following as instructed on the container or by a complementary practitioner are beneficial: tea tree oil, Hydrastis, Calendula, Pau d'arco.*

WET DREAMS

Wet dreams are an essential part of the normality of growing up. There is no pathological cause of ejaculating in the sleeping state. There is no 'normal' frequency and there may be times when wet dreams will occur several times in one week.

STRUCTURAL MATTERS

ACHES AND PAINS

Aches and pains in a young adult that are not associated with exercise must be reviewed by both a medical practitioner and a complementary body worker such as an osteopath or chiropractor. Diseases of the muscles and joints in young adults are unusual and may require treatment.

RECOMMENDATIONS

General Advice

- *Ensure that you are well-stretched out before and after exercise.*
- *Ensure that you are well hydrated. Half a pint of water per foot of height drunk through the day, and an extra amount of water for any extra sweating or the intake of alcohol, caffeine or excessively sweet foods. All of these are dehydrating.*
- *Persisting pains with no obvious reason must be brought to the attention of a medical practitioner, orthodox or complementary to begin with.*

Nutritional

- *Ensure that you have a high intake of vegetables of all varieties because mineral deficiencies can lead to persisting cramps, etc.*

ACHILLES TENDON

The Achilles tendon is the lower part of the calf muscle that attaches through a dovetail-like insertion into the heel bone. This tendon is commonly strained, especially in young adults, due to poor stretching before vigorous exercise. It is most commonly strained when playing hardcourt games such as squash or tennis and can be extremely painful.

The Achilles tendon can split due to excessive contraction of the calf muscle. This most commonly occurs if the tendon is not stretched before activity, if the body is dehydrated or if the calf muscle is swollen.

RECOMMENDATIONS

General Advice

- *Always stretch out before and after exercise.*

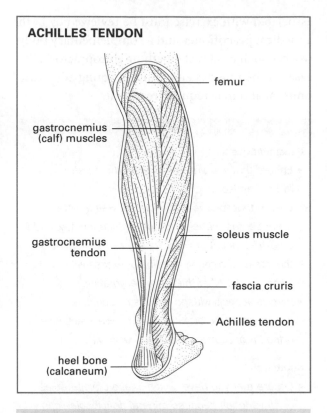

ACHILLES TENDON

- femur
- gastrocnemius (calf) muscles
- gastrocnemius tendon
- soleus muscle
- fascia cruris
- Achilles tendon
- heel bone (calcaneum)

- *Alternate hot and cold applications via a bucket of iced and hot water.*
- *Persisting discomfort should be reviewed by an osteopath or body worker with knowledge of posture. Incorrectly fitting shoes can be very detrimental.*

Homeopathic
- *The remedies Arnica, Rhus toxicodendron and Ruta should be reviewed.*

Herbal/natural extracts
- *Apply an Arnica cream to the tendon and calf if ever there is soreness in that area.*

Orthodox
- *An Achilles tendon rupture (commonly sounds like a gun shot) must be surgically treated.*

BRAS
It may be surprising to come across a section on the brassiere in a medical book. However, more so than any other garment, the brassiere can lead to or harbour problems.

Correct fitting is essential. A tight-fitting brassiere can rub on the skin over a period of time and may lead to slight abrasions that can allow mild infection or *Candida* to set in. Persistent rubbing can lead to skin cancers, and moles that lie underneath the tight-fitting lining of a brassiere have a higher tendency to develop cancerous changes.

Support is essential, especially for larger breasts in athletic women. Unfettered bouncing can lead to stretching of the ligaments that support the breasts and this can cause unnecessary sagging in later life.

RECOMMENDATIONS

General Advice
- *Ensure correct fitting brassieres. Bear in mind that breasts may change depending on the time of the month and it may be necessary to have different-sized brassieres. Avoid forcing the breasts into cups that are too small.*
- *Spend as much time braless as possible.*
- *Pay special attention to any abrasions or moles that might come into contact with the harder parts of the brassiere.*
- *Change brassieres frequently. Despite washing, certain fungi and yeasts can live in brassiere straps and cause minor irritations.*

BREASTS
Full discussion on care of the breasts is in chapter 5 because more problems arise in that age group.

RECOMMENDATION

General Advice
- *Read thoroughly the section on breasts in chapter 5 because the sooner you learn how to examine and what to look for, the better.*

COCCYDYNIA
I have yet to meet a non-medical practitioner who has heard of this condition although nearly every patient I have ever questioned has suffered from

it! Coccydynia or coccygodynia is simply pain in the region of the coccyx, which is the bone at the base of the spine or at the top of the buttock cleft. Most of us will have fallen on it at some point and this is a major cause of discomfort although pain can emanate from that area without trauma due to compression of nerves and muscular spasm.

DISLOCATIONS

Normally a joint is made up of two or more bone surfaces opposing each other. They are covered by layers of cartilage and surrounded and separated by an oily fluid called synovial fluid. The joint is held together by strong fibres known as ligaments, and muscles connect within a few centimetres either side of the joint via tendons. A dislocation occurs when the two surfaces become unopposed.

A joint may separate and stay unopposed or it may slip back once having dislocated. This is described as persistent or replaced. If a joint partially dislocates it is known as a subluxation – these usually spontaneously replace themselves.

Dislocation and subluxation usually occur through injury although certain conditions weakening the ligaments that hold the joints in place or musculature that give added protection to the stability of joints may be relevant. Dislocations may cause damage to blood vessels, lymphatic system and nerve tissues that are associated with the joint, and the pain of a dislocation may cover damage to cartilage or even a fractured bone. It is for this reason that medical attention must be sought whenever a dislocation occurs.

Recognizing a dislocation is often difficult, especially if it has replaced or was a subluxation. A persistent dislocation will show an irregularity of that joint, immobility and considerable pain. A replaced or subluxed joint may not be quite so apparent. The shoulder joint is the most commonly dislocated

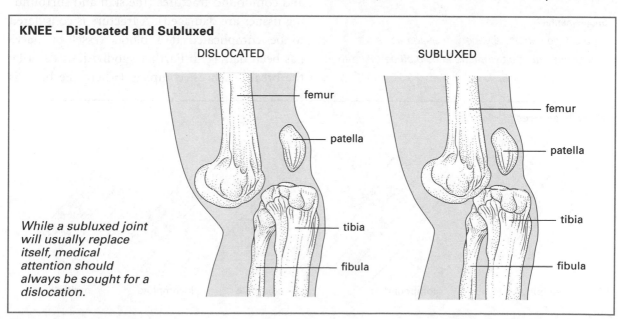

KNEE – Dislocated and Subluxed

DISLOCATED

SUBLUXED

femur

patella

tibia

fibula

femur

patella

tibia

fibula

While a subluxed joint will usually replace itself, medical attention should always be sought for a dislocation.

main joint of the body and is discussed in its own section. (*See* **Dislocation of the shoulder.**)

General Advice

- *Any suggestion of a dislocation of any sort should be treated as an emergency. Check the part of the body furthest away from the suspected dislocation for blood flow by checking for a pulse and constantly monitoring the area for coldness or blueness. Obtain medical attention as soon as possible.*

- *Persisting discomfort will be relieved by acupuncture.*

- *Depending on the joint, a period of time will be advised by the expert dealing with the injury when immobilization is essential. Do not reduce the time of immobility because this will lead to recurrent dislocation because the tissues will not have had time to repair.*

- *Osteopathic or chiropractic assessment is recommended because an injury to a joint will inevitably cause extra pressure on the corresponding joint of the body and also the joints above and below the injury. Backache is not uncommon following any body injury because of an imbalance in the body's natural fulcrum and structure.*

Supplemental

- *Ruta fluid extract, a variety of amino acids, minerals and multivitamins should all be taken to help speed up the repair process. The amounts vary depending on the individual and the extent of injury. A naturopathic practitioner will advise.*

Homeopathic

- *Use the homeopathic remedy Arnica up to potency 30 every half-hour until the joint has been re-established and splinted. Thereafter use Arnica 30 and Ruta 30 alternately every 4hr for five days.*

Herbal/natural extracts

- *Application of Arnica and Calendula creams will draw blood into the area and help healing.*

Orthodox

- *Radiography (X-rays) should be considered.*

- *Feel free to use analgesia, especially if the joint has to be replaced.*

- *Orthopaedic specialist opinion is warranted with any such injury but if the problem is recurrent then a surgical procedure may be required.*

FRACTURES OR BROKEN BONES

In medical parlance a broken bone is referred to as a fracture regardless of its severity. Fractures are divided into simple (the skin is not broken) and compound fractures (the skin and surrounding tissues are damaged). A fracture is considered to be complicated if a blood vessel or nerve has been damaged. Further subdivisions describe the break, such as: complete (where the bone is

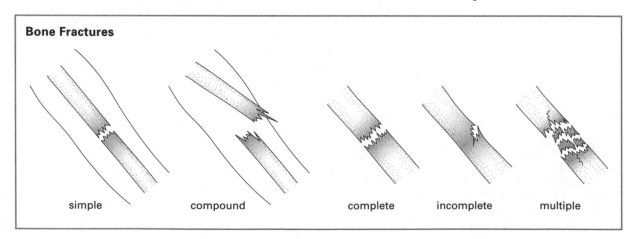

Bone Fractures

simple   compound   complete   incomplete   multiple

separated), incomplete (there is just a crack) and multiple (several fragments are visible on X-ray). The term 'greenstick' fracture is now used less frequently but refers to a crack in the bone.

If there has been displacement there is usually deformity visible but this is not always the case. Diagnosis of a fracture is difficult without an X-ray but one must suspect a fracture and seek medical attention in any injury that has:

- Swelling
- Immobility
- Pain
- Discolouration from bruising
- An inability to bear weight.

Immediate first aid

RECOMMENDATIONS

General Advice

- *If a break is suspected, organize medical attention.*
- *Whilst awaiting medical expertise, immobilize the suspected broken bone by splintering to a piece of wood or similar material or, in the case of the lower limb, the other leg. Fingers and toes can be used similarly.*

Nutritional

- *Increase your protein intake. The calcium in bones is attached to a protein network and both are required for rapid bone healing.*

Supplemental

- *Calcium and magnesium supplements should be taken at a maximum dose as recommended on packaging.*

Homeopathic

- *Homeopathically the following routines should be administered: Aconite 6 or 12, four pills every 10min, or Aconite 30 every half-hour for 1hr; then Arnica 30 alternating with Symphytum 30 until the pain has diminished.*

After medical treatment

Medical treatment will include assessment, pain relief and immobilization. If there is much swelling in the area, a plaster of Paris 'back slab' will be used. This is only a partial circumference plaster that prevents the swelling from being compressed. After keeping the damaged area raised above the heart (to help decrease the swelling) for 24–72 hours, a full plaster of Paris or fibre-glass plaster will immobilize the bone for, on average, six weeks. More aggressive fractures may require much longer in plaster.

Whilst in plaster the muscles will lose approximately 15–20 per cent of their mass, which is usually rebuilt within a few weeks following the correct exercises.

RECOMMENDATIONS

General Advice

- *Follow your orthopaedic consultant's advice. It never pays to shorten the expected healing time, especially if a break is around a joint because this will lead to an increased risk of arthritis.*
- *Attend a physiotherapist. The techniques of muscle exercise and ultrasound and electromagnetic therapy can speed up repair.*
- *Ensure that you exercise the joints and muscles that are not restricted by the plaster.*
- *Any injured part will be compensated by its opposite side. This generally leads to an imbalance in the structure and a visit to an osteopath, Polarity therapist, Shiatsu practitioner or Alexander Technician is advised as soon as the injury has been secured.*
- *Acupuncture can be very beneficial in speeding up long-term injuries. Electro-acupuncture is most beneficial.*

Homeopathic

- *The homeopathic remedy Symphytum 30 should be taken three times a day for at least half the length of time you are expecting to be in plaster and if, following further X-rays, the healing is slow, also use the remedy Calcarea phosphorica 30, twice a day for the remainder of time in the plaster.*

Herbal/natural extracts
- *The herbal remedy comfrey can be taken as tea but not more than one mugful every two days because it may have a toxic effect on the liver if taken in large quantity.*

FROSTBITE

Frostbite is the non-medical term for an area that, having been exposed to extreme cold, loses its circulation. Characteristically the area will be cold, firm, pale or streaked and, contrary to popular belief, painless. There is initial pain as the cold sets in but the nerves are numbed by the cold and pain only returns as the area is warmed. Left untreated, the tissues will die and gangrene will set in.

Individuals with poor circulation are more prone to frostbite, which may occur at higher temperatures than for the rest of the population. Smokers, those with diabetes and individuals using certain drugs such as beta-blockers may all have a greater predisposition.

RECOMMENDATIONS

General Advice
- *Do not warm the area rapidly. Apply the affected area to a warm body part, ie place the hand in the groin or armpit only.*
- *Common sense prevails: cover the individual with blankets or coats and find shelter.*
- *Administer warm but not hot drinks.*

Homeopathic
- *Apis 30 every 15–30 min whilst part reheats.*
- *Damaged skin and tissues may respond to the remedy Agaricus muscarius 30 four times a day for five days.*

Herbal/natural extracts
- *Apply Arnica cream to the area of the injury and above to encourage circulation.*

Orthodox
- *Use painkillers if available.*

SHIN SPLINTS

Shin splints is a colloquial term for the medical condition 'anterior tibial compartment syndrome'. The tibia is the shin bone and on the outer aspect, on the front of the leg, lie the muscles that cause the foot to flex upwards. These muscles are encased in a tough fibrous sheath known as the anterior tibial compartment. Pressure and inflammation within this compartment is the cause of a characteristic dull ache with periods of sharp pain most commonly associated or worsened by movement.

The term shin splints actually has nothing to do with the shin bone but is caused by small tears in the muscles within this compartment that cause fluid to leak into the tissues, which in turn cause a build-up of pressure in this tightly compacted area. The pressure leads to a diminution in blood flow, causing ischaemia (lack of oxygen), which the nerves register and leads them to send pain impulses to the brain.

RECOMMENDATIONS

General Advice
- *At the first sign of this condition, rest is essential. Continuing to exercise the area will worsen the condition and make treatment more difficult. A period of inactivity of up to six weeks may be necessary if the condition is bad.*
- *Whilst warmth may be more soothing, icing the area will reduce the inflammation by decreasing the blood flow.*
- *Very gentle massage moving the encased fluid up the leg may help the symptoms. If the massage is too aggressive, the bruising will worsen. Massage is important once the condition has settled because it will prevent recurrence.*
- *Ultrasound or deep heat treatment is occasionally given by those who do not understand the underlying physiology. This will*

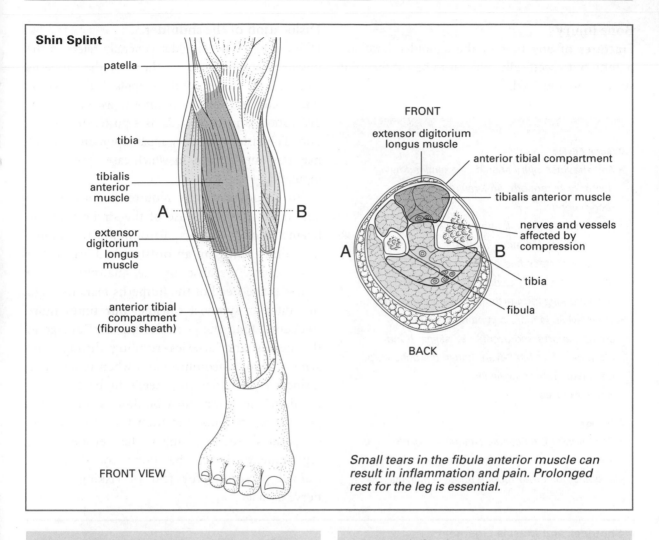

Shin Splint

patella

tibia

tibialis anterior muscle

extensor digitorium longus muscle

anterior tibial compartment (fibrous sheath)

FRONT VIEW

A ···· B

FRONT

extensor digitorium longus muscle

anterior tibial compartment

tibialis anterior muscle

nerves and vessels affected by compression

tibia

fibula

A B

BACK

Small tears in the fibula anterior muscle can result in inflammation and pain. Prolonged rest for the leg is essential.

---

encourage blood flow and prolong the condition.
- *Acupuncture may be instantly relieving.*
- *Osteopathy should be considered because manipulative techniques may help the lymphatic drainage, thereby clearing the excess fluid, and also the malalignment that is common because of the other side of the body taking more strain.*
- *When returning to exercise, start slowly and avoid exercise on hard surfaces, such as road running, basketball and tennis.*

Homeopathic
- *The homeopathic remedies Arnica, Bryonia, Rhus toxicodendron and Ruta should all be considered through examination of your preferred manual. Take potency 6 every 3hr when the condition starts and after three days increase the potency to 30 but reduce the frequency to twice a day until the condition has resolved.*

Herbal/natural extracts
- *Rub in Arnica-based creams several times a day.*

THE SHOULDER

This region, where the arm joins the trunk of the body, is formed by the meeting of three bones – the clavicle, scapula and humerus – that create several joints, all and any of which can cause shoulder pain and varying degrees of immobility.

The shoulder is a complex area and its ball-and-socket joint between the upper arm bone (humerus) and the scapula is the most flexible in the body.

Bone injury

Fractures of any part of the shoulder joint are painful but specifically difficult to heal if the joint surfaces are involved.

RECOMMENDATIONS

General Advice

- *Any shoulder injury should be examined by a doctor or osteopath. An X-ray is usually recommended.*
- *Immobility for a minimum of six weeks is recommended in most fractures, or longer if the articular surface has been compromised. Do not shirk on this or try to do too much too soon because long-term arthritis is the usual outcome.*
- *The clavicle is more commonly fractured in contact sports and events like skiing. It may often be left to heal even though the bones may be considerably malaligned.*
- *See* **Fractures**.

Orthodox

- *Fractures of the scapula cannot be splinted and severe breaks in this area or anywhere in the shoulder joint may require surgical pinning.*

Dislocation of the shoulder

Dislocation of the shoulder generally refers to the misalignment between the head of the humerus and the socket aspect of the scapula. If the dislocation occurs forward it is known as an anterior dislocation, and backwards as a posterior dislocation. The dislocation may repair spontaneously or may stay out of place, in which case it needs manipulating.

To dislocate usually requires a considerable amount of force because of the strength of the ligaments and muscles surrounding the shoulder joint. Falling on an outstretched arm is the usual cause. Because of the anatomy of the shoulder the head of the humerus tears through the anterior synovial capsule four times more frequently than the posterior aspect. Damage to the nerves and arteries running through the armpit is not uncommon and when replacing a dislocated shoulder this needs to be borne in mind. A relocation must be done swiftly if the pulse is compromised at the wrist. If numbness or paralysis of the fingers has ensued then replacement should be done by medically-trained personnel for fear of risking further nerve damage.

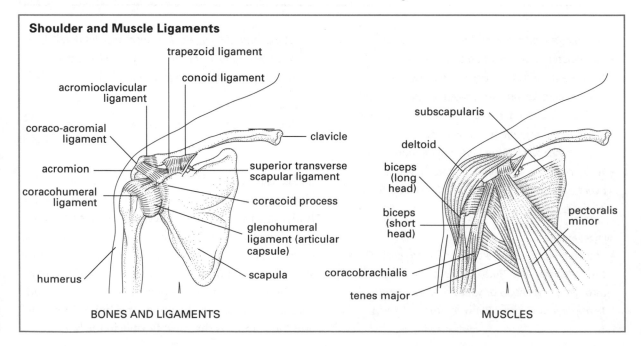

Shoulder and Muscle Ligaments

trapezoid ligament

conoid ligament

acromioclavicular ligament

coraco-acromial ligament

acromion

coracohumeral ligament

clavicle

superior transverse scapular ligament

coracoid process

glenohumeral ligament (articular capsule)

humerus

scapula

BONES AND LIGAMENTS

subscapularis

deltoid

biceps (long head)

biceps (short head)

pectoralis minor

coracobrachialis

tenes major

MUSCLES

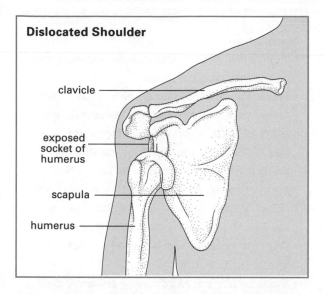

Dislocated Shoulder

clavicle

exposed
socket of
humerus

scapula

humerus

General Advice

- *See **Dislocations**.*

- *Emergency replacement or relocation of the humerus when no complications are observed should proceed as follows, but only if the joint cannot be stabilized until a professional can do the job:*

  (a) The arm will be flexed at the elbow because of the shortening of the biceps tendons and will automatically be across the chest in an anterior dislocation. Hold the forearm as close to the elbow as possible and apply gentle downward traction.

  (b) Move the hand of the dislocated arm outwards, continuing to apply strong but gentle traction downwards at the elbow as in (a) above.

  (c) If the shoulder has not re-aligned, gently pull the elbow towards the other shoulder whilst continuing the downward traction and keeping the hand rotated away from the body.

  (d) This is a painful process and should preferably only be done if analgesia is available.

Frozen shoulder

A frozen shoulder is a chronic or longstanding inflammation of the tendons and synovial capsule around the shoulder joint. It is characterized by pain that gets worse on moving the shoulder. Any motion is limited by this pain.

This lay-term has passed into medical parlance and represents a painful tightening of the muscles around the shoulder joint. It is most commonly created by an initial pain causing a lack of movement on a persistent basis, leading to a profound stiffness and worsening of the pain in these muscles.

The causes are generally unknown but there is increased vascularity, degeneration and scarring of the fibres within the tendons and synovial capsule. Arthritic conditions and trauma are often associated.

Several meridians or energy channels travel across the shoulder joint or are indirectly connected. These include the large and small intestine, heart, lung and reproductive organs. The triple heater (arguably the energy line that controls the heat of the body via its influence on the adrenal and thyroid glands) is very much associated with shoulder problems. The triple heater is often weakened in stress situations. Problems such as frozen shoulder that have no obvious causative factor need to be reviewed from this point of view.

General Advice

- *Osteopathic or chiropractic assessment is necessary for a firm diagnosis.*

- *Manipulative treatment, including work on the neck and spine, is mandatory.*

- *Acupuncture may be instantly relieving and should be used in combination with osteopathy.*

- *Shiatsu may take the place of both of the above.*

- *The application of heat may pull blood to the surface, reducing inflammation; or holding an ice bag over the area for a period of time may cool the area down. Both techniques may be soothing but neither are particularly relevant in long-term care.*

- *Ensure good hydration because persistent*

cramps may be indicative of dehydration: three pints of water on top of current intake (up to a maximum of six pints per day) is necessary.

- *Avoid orthodox practitioners because the treatments of choice are anti-inflammatory drugs and steroid injections, which may give temporary relief and a full sense of well-being that will allow further movement but longer-term injury and recurrence are not uncommon.*

Supplemental

- *Ensure that calcium and magnesium supplements are being taken at three times the daily recommended dose on a chelated product.*

Homeopathic

- *Homeopathic remedies should be reviewed in your preferred manual and specific attention paid to Arnica, Rhus toxicodendron and Ruta.*
- *Arnica 6 can be used every hour if pain and limitation of movement is being noticed.*

SPINAL INJURY

An injury to the spine is a serious and potentially grave injury. At best it may represent a rupture of ligaments or a crack in the vertebrae, but at worst it may mean injury or severance of the spinal nerve cord. The possibility of an injury progressing due to instability of the vertebrae means that all spinal injuries need to be treated the same and with the utmost care and urgency until a firm diagnosis is made by a qualified medical practitioner or casualty team.

If the casualty is not correctly handled, the spinal cord may be permanently damaged, with paralysis or death resulting.

Spinal injury generally occurs as a result of a direct force, a fall or hyperflexion or extension such as in a whiplash injury.

A fracture of the vertebrae will not be known until an X-ray is taken, but a dislodged vertebrae may be palpable. If the patient is conscious the pain must be taken into account but pain is generally a better sign than no pain.

General Advice

- *If the patient is conscious then remind and insist that he/she does not move.*
- *Assess by asking questions, which should include: 'Where does it hurt?', 'Can you feel your fingers and toes?', 'Can you move your fingers and toes?'. The point of asking these questions is simply to reassure and to have an idea of the gravity of the situation. Whatever the answers, the individual must not move until medical expertise has arrived. Brief the medic on his/her arrival.*
- *Cover the individual with a blanket or whatever it takes to keep him/her warm.*
- *If medical aid is not forthcoming or unavailable, only then should transportation of the individual be considered.*
- *Enlist as much help as possible and keep the individual's shoulders and pelvis firmly held in the position that the casualty was found. Place pads of soft material between the thighs, knees and ankles.*
- *Tie the ankles and feet together with a figure-of-eight bandage and tie bandages around the thighs and knees. Make do with whatever material is available.*
- *The casualty is best transported in the face-upwards position but only if that was the position in which he/she was found. Do not turn the neck to accommodate this.*
- *An unconscious casualty must be supported with blankets, pillows or any material to avoid movement.*
- *A stretcher must be a stiff board. Consider a door if nothing else is available.*
- *Once the casualty is on the board and supported, strap down around the forehead, shoulders, pelvis and knees and then place in the smoothest vehicle available.*
- *Avoid giving anything by mouth.*
- *At all times throughout this procedure ensure that the airways, breathing and circulation (ABC) are intact. Commence cardiopulmonary resuscitation (CPR) at any stage, attempting to keep the patient in the correct position.*

STRESS FRACTURE

A stress fracture is a small crack or break in a bone that occurs because of excess pressure or overuse of a part of the body. It is most commonly found in soldiers who march or athletes whose footwear has not protected them from the hard surface they may be exercising on. Basketball players who constantly land on a hard-covered wooden playing area are very prone to stress fractures of the feet.

RECOMMENDATIONS

General Advice

• *Rest is unfortunately an essential part of healing a stress fracture.*

• *See **Fractures**.*
• *The use of ultrasound may speed up the process in bone stress fractures beyond that of most other bone injuries.*
• *Reflexology will speed up healing in most injuries.*

SWELLING

For swelling that is generalized throughout the body or the swelling of both ankles or legs, *see* **Oedema** *and* **Fluid Retention**. The swelling of one part of the body, such as a leg, arm, hand or foot, may be due to lymphatic obstruction caused by a trauma, inflamed or infected lymph glands or tumours blocking lymphatic flow. All of these

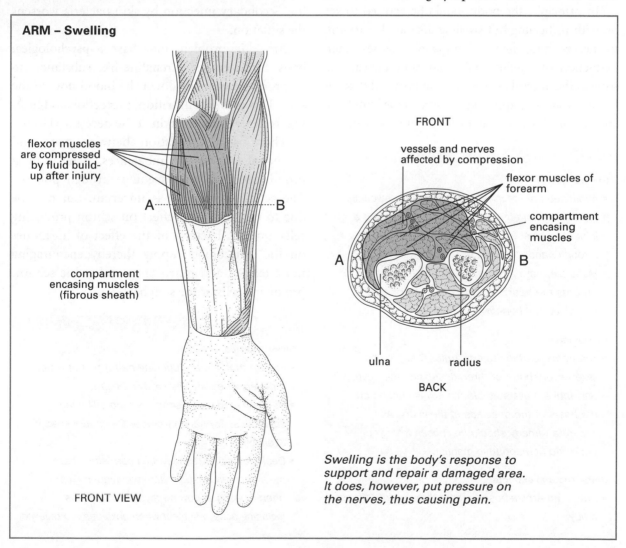

ARM – Swelling

flexor muscles are compressed by fluid build-up after injury

compartment encasing muscles (fibrous sheath)

A ········· B

FRONT VIEW

FRONT

vessels and nerves affected by compression

flexor muscles of forearm

compartment encasing muscles

A   B

ulna   radius

BACK

Swelling is the body's response to support and repair a damaged area. It does, however, put pressure on the nerves, thus causing pain.

conditions need to be reviewed independently once a cause is established.

A swelling caused by an injury or infection represents the body's attempt to splint, immobilize and repair the area. The site of a swelling is also a warning to the conscious mind that protection is necessary and a similar injury-causing event should be avoided.

Damaged tissue sends a nervous reflex to the spinal column that returns instructions to the surrounding blood vessels to open up and flood the area with more nutrition, oxygen, white blood cells and scar-forming cells. Blood vessels are also encouraged to open by the release of certain chemicals from injured cells.

In principle, the body should be allowed to get on with its healing but swelling does apply pressure to nerves and, like inflammation, causes pain. Reduction of swelling will occur automatically as soon as the injured area is given support and this can be encouraged by applying pressure to the lymphatic and venous flow, thus taking fluid from the area.

RECOMMENDATIONS

General Advice

- *Application of ice in a cloth may relieve swelling.*
- *Ensure that the injured area is immobilized if a joint is involved, has pressure applied to it through bandaging and is rested.*
- *Massage, paying special attention to moving fluid towards the heart; any physical therapy technique will benefit.*

Homeopathic

- *The homeopathic remedy Arnica 6 should be taken every hour for three doses and then every 3hr until a more suitable remedy is chosen on the basis of the specifics of the injury. An accurate remedy should be chosen from your preferred homeopathic manual.*

Herbal/natural extracts

- *Rub in an Arnica-based cream three or four times a day.*

THE SKIN

ACNE

Acne is caused by an excess production of sebum, the waxy substance that our skin produces. The overproduction clogs the skin's pores, leading to blackheads, pimples and pustules. Nearly everyone at some time will have this problem but unhappily it can be very severe in a few of us.

There is some correlation between poor diet or hygiene and acne, and a certain amount of improvement can be made by changes of habit. Very often the difficulty lies in the sebum being too viscous, and dehydration may be a major factor. Secondary infection by skin bacteria worsens the situation.

Any skin problem may have a psychological basis. Stress causes adrenaline-like substances to be produced that cut down the blood flow to the skin. This prevents nutrition, protection and healing from reaching the skin at the necessary levels.

There is a correlation between acne and hormonal changes or imbalances. Acne is most prominent in teenagers going through puberty. The actual mechanism is uncertain but may be due to the hormonal effect on sebum-producing cells, on skin bacteria or the effect of hormones on the skin blood supply thereby encouraging more oxygen and nutrition to either the sebum-producing cells or the skin bacteria.

RECOMMENDATIONS

General Advice

- *Ensure that you are drinking half a pint of water for every one foot of your own height.*
- *Use non-medicated soaps and no oil-based cosmetics. Try sandalwood or Calendula soap if available.*
- *Deal with your stress levels. Learn some basic meditation and visualization techniques. I am often amazed at how swiftly skin conditions, including acne, will clear when anxieties are relieved.*

- *Consider hypnotherapy if basic relaxation has no impact.*

Nutritional

- *Some people will benefit by reducing fried foods, spicy foods, citrus and all refined (white) sugars.*

Supplemental

- *Try Evening Primrose Oil (1g three times a day), zinc (15mg before sleep) and copper (2mg with breakfast).*

Homeopathic

- *Homeopathy can work wonders. Look up the remedies Sulphur, Kali bromatum, and Antimonium tartaricum. A homeopath's opinion is well warranted.*

Herbal/natural extracts

- *Tea tree oil (one drop to five drops of olive oil) applied to the skin after cleaning can be curative. Dilute further if this stings.*
- *In moderate to severe cases use a teaspoonful of chickpea flour with a teaspoonful of almond powder mixed in goat's milk. Apply for a few minutes twice a day.*
- *Under the supervision of a complementary medical practitioner, try a natural oestrogen extract and if this does not work try a natural progesterone treatment. The herb Agnus castus can be very beneficial.*

Orthodox

- *Benzoyl peroxide can be applied to the face twice a day after prescription from a doctor. This compound, like hydrogen peroxide, releases oxygen that kills the proprionibactium acnes that cause the problem.*

AEROSOLS

Do not use them. They are environmentally unfriendly and contain innumerable chemicals that are, to some extent, absorbed through the skin. Use natural fragrances in basic oils rubbed onto the skin instead.

BLISTERS

Blisters are caused by fluid leaving damaged blood vessels, generally after a pinch, friction or excess heat. This fluid contains many of the nutrients that help the repair process and should be allowed to stay in the area. If the blister becomes too full it can start to cause pressure on the stretch-sensitive nerves and produce pain. This is the only indication to burst a blister and it should be done under medical supervision only.

RECOMMENDATIONS

General Advice

- *Do not burst a blister.*
- *See **Burns**.*
- *Applying gentle pressure to the blister may take away some of the discomfort.*
- *Recurrent blisters or blisters that occur after no apparent injury may represent an underlying condition that requires medical diagnosis and this should be assessed by your GP.*

Homeopathic

- *Review the homeopathic remedies Cantharis and Rhus toxicodendron for small blisters.*

Herbal/natural extracts

- *Apply Arnica creams or lotions. If the blister is on the fingers or toes, use Hypericum creams or lotions.*

BOILS (FURUNCLES)

A boil is a localized infection of the skin and sub-cutaneous tissue. It usually starts around a hair follicle and develops into a solitary abscess. An abscess is defined as a collection of pus (the body's dead white blood cells) that drains to the nearest surface through a single tract. This may be external to the skin or internal to the bowel, lungs, etc.

They are differentiated from pimples by an arbitrary decision on the size.

RECOMMENDATIONS

General Advice

- *Recurrent, numerous or persistent boils should*

be addressed by a complementary medical practitioner.

- *Application of hot and then cold compresses can draw a boil out.*
- *Soaked oats and wholegrain bread poultices may be most beneficial.*
- *Boils should only be lanced under medical supervision.*
- *Any boil around the anus must be treated by a medically qualified complementary practitioner immediately. They have a higher tendency to drain inwards, allowing a tract for the faeces and related bacteria to travel into the boil/abscess.*

Homeopathic
- *The homeopathic remedy Hepar sulphuris calcarium 6, four pills every hour, is one of the rare master remedies for a general condition.*

Herbal/natural extracts
- *Application of Arnica creams is encouraged.*

BRUISES

A bruise is caused by damage to capillaries and larger blood vessels, allowing blood to drain into the tissues. The variety of colours that appear in the skin are due to the amount of blood and the contents of the blood cells moving to the surface. Superficial bruises are rarely complicated, deeper bruises can cause extreme pain by cramping muscles and a bruise underneath the tough lining of bones is excruciating.

If bruising occurs with minor knocks or for no apparent reason this may indicate fragile capillaries or an underlying deficiency in the body's clotting mechanism.

RECOMMENDATIONS

General Advice
- *Hot and cold applications can be very relieving.*
- *Fragile capillaries can be improved through nutritional and herbal treatments but these require a consultation with a complementary medical practitioner.*

Supplemental
- *If there is no underlying illness for recurrent bruises, then one can administer the following in divided doses with each meal: vitamin C (1g per foot of height per day), vitamin E (100iu per foot of height per day) and vitamin A (1,000iu per foot of height per day).*

Homeopathic
- *The homeopathic remedies Arnica and Bellis perennis can be used at potency 6, four pills every 4hr.*

Herbal/natural extracts
- *Apply Arnica and Urtica creams on a regular basis throughout the day.*
- *Large bruises can be dissipated quicker by the use of massage and an unusual aromatherapy oil called Helichrysum. Hyssop or lavender are more easily available and can be equally effective. Place a few drops into five tablespoonsful of extra virgin olive oil and apply.*

Orthodox
- *If a bruise is persisting or is extremely painful, obtain an examination from a doctor or osteopath/chiropractor to ensure that no underlying damage is being concealed. A specialist in haematology should be consulted if bruises are occurring too easily.*

CARBUNCLES – *see* Boils

CELLULITIS

The medical term for inflammation is 'itis'. Cellulitis is, therefore, inflammation of cells. It presents as a red area, usually around or spreading from an injury or lesion. Cellulitis can occur at any age but is most commonly found following accidents, allowing bacteria to get underneath the skin and cause infection. The body's response is to send blood into the area carrying white blood cells and this increase in blood flow causes redness, swelling and pain.

Cellulitis is often associated with 'tracking', which is seen as streaks of red travelling away from the area of inflammation through lympathic ducts towards the nearest group of lymph nodes.

Cellulitis can spread very rapidly, especially if the infection is a virulent staphylococcal bacteria. Often associated with conditions that reduce the immune system, such as diabetes, use of steroids, AIDS and nutritional deficiencies, the problem should not be underestimated.

RECOMMENDATIONS

General Advice

- *If the cellulitis is mild then complementary medical care can be used provided that the condition does not worsen.*

Homeopathic

- *The homeopathic remedies Apis, Urtica, Belladonna, Calendula and Hypericum can all be reviewed in your homeopathic manual.*

Herbal/natural extracts

- *Apply hot and cold compresses to the area and clean any associated wound with Arnica, Calendula or Hypericum solution.*
- *Take some white bread, steep in Arnica, Calendula or Hypericum solution, apply to the area and gently wrap with a suitable cloth or bandage.*

Orthodox

- *Any cellulitis that is spreading rapidly should be seen by a GP and antibiotics should be utilized along with complementary medicine to help protect against the unwanted side effects from the antibiotics.*

CHLOASMA

This patchy hyperpigmentation is most often seen on the face, nipples and down the middle of the abdomen, although it can show up anywhere. The patches may be of varying size and often become marked during pregnancy, menstruation, and with disorders of the ovaries or uterus and occasionally in association with tumours.

Very often the condition has no obvious cause

Chloasma

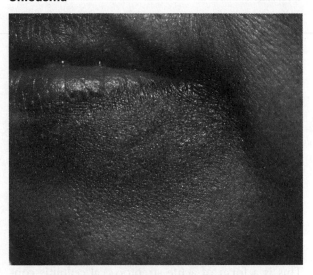

but may be due to the action of sunshine on areas of the skin affected by perfumes and cosmetics, as well as certain hormonal problems.

RECOMMENDATIONS

General Advice

- *A full assessment from a medical practitioner to rule out anything nasty is the first step.*
- *Avoid buying any medicated compounds, cosmetics or perfumes for use on the areas affected.*
- *Obtain a complementary medical view from a homeopath and/or herbalist because these two branches of medicine claim to have the highest success rates.*
- *As with all skin conditions, subconscious or underlying psychological conditions must be determined either through counselling or hypnotherapy.*
- *Ensure the continued use of a good sunscreen, regardless of the strength of the sun.*

Orthodox

- *Consider stopping the oral contraceptive pill.*
- *Consider bleaching using hydroquinone cream, applied twice daily this can be used with acid facial peels.*
- *Laser pigment lightening treatments are available.*

CRABS

This most unfortunate term is given to an infestation of small parasites that do, under the microscope, resemble the shape of beach crabs. Generally considered to be a sexually transmitted parasite, although transmission can occur through any contact (not only sexual) these small parasites tend to live in the pubic hair.

RECOMMENDATION

General Advice
- *See* **Lice**.

ERYSIPELAS

This is a form of acute streptococcal cellulitis confined to the skin and having a slightly raised red area with a well-demarcated advancing border. There are many types, depending on associated symptoms and the presence of pustules or vesicles. The condition may be very aggressive and spread rapidly or persist over a period of time. Diagnosis is made by a GP.

RECOMMENDATIONS

General Advice
- *A slow or persistent area of erysipelas may be treated constitutionally by a complementary medical practitioner.*
- *See* **Cellulitis**.

Orthodox
- *When a diagnosis of erysipelas is made, treatment should depend upon the speed of spread. If fast and aggressive, then antibiotics must be considered.*

FUNGAL INFECTIONS

Fungus is a low form of plant life most commonly thought of as mushrooms and growths on the side of trees. Similar but different organisms live on and under the human skin and may even colonize our intestine. Many of these fungi are harmless and may compete with more aggressive or pathogenic fungi, thereby being protective. This is an important factor when treating fungal conditions because we do not wish to wipe out our own beneficial flora.

Most fungal infections are noticed because of red, itchy, inflamed areas on the skin. Athlete's foot (*see* **Athlete's foot**) is the most frequent but fungi will grow in any darkened or moist area such as the groin, under the breasts, armpits and skin folds, especially in those who are overweight.

Fungi will predominate in those who are immunocompromised and, whilst not dangerous, can be an indication of a depressed immune system.

Medically speaking nails are an extension of the skin and therefore fungal infections of the nails should also respond to the following recommendations. Fungal infections of the nails are characterized by a discolouration (usually yellowing) and thickening of the nail without any discomfort. The fungus is embedded in the growing part of the nail (the nail bed) and is difficult to get at. Orthodox treatment recommends oral antifungal agents that will, unfortunately, not only destroy the harmful fungus over a six-month period but will also potentially damage the healthy fungus that we have on our skin and in our bowel. This treatment is not recommended by holistic practitioners, who are more concerned with the underlying deficiency in the immune system that has allowed the fungus to settle.

RECOMMENDATIONS

General Advice
- *Aerate the affected areas as much as possible.*
- *There may be an association with yeast infection in the system and persisting fungal infections should be treated systematically (by looking at the whole body) by a complementary medical practitioner.*

Nutritional
- *Reduce refined sugars and sweet foods.*

Herbal/natural extracts
- *Twice daily applications of vinegar, selenium-containing solutions or grape seed extracts can be applied.*

- *Garlic can be applied, although the smell may be unsociable. Fungal infections under the nail respond well to twice daily applications of garlic under the nail and around the nail bed.*
- *Tea tree oil applied in a solution as concentrated as the skin will allow (there should be no discomfort) is effective.*

Orthodox

- *If the above techniques fail then antifungal drug treatments from the chemist can be used but avoid oral antifungal drug treatment by seeking complementary advice.*

MOLES

A mole is a fleshy, pigmented lesion known in medical parlance as a naevus. These lesions contain increased amounts of melanocytes, which give the skin its pigmentation. In themselves moles are harmless but disfiguring and if very obvious or very numerous can cause social embarrassment and feelings of inadequacy.

A mole carries a slight chance of becoming a melanoma (*see* **Melanoma**) and it is therefore important to watch out, for the following signs:

- An increase in size
- A change or variation in colour

Melanoma and Solar keratosis

Melanomas should be distinguished from solar keratosis – a pre-cancerous condition caused by over-exposure to the sun.

- Bleeding
- Itching.

Moles may appear on meridians or energy lines and be reflective of underlying weakness in an organ. Multiple moles probably have no relevancy but a single mole, especially if there at birth or developing in the first few years of life, could be assessed by a Chinese or Tibetan practitioner who may compare its position with weaknesses in the pulses.

RECOMMENDATIONS

General Advice

- *Most moles are harmless but any of the changes mentioned above should raise suspicion and a GP or dermatologist should be consulted.*

Homeopathic

- *The homeopathic remedy Thuja can be taken at potency 200, one dose daily for three days every three months, as a possible protective measure in individuals with many moles.*

Orthodox

- *Removal and microscopic examination of the mole is the only sure way of establishing the innocence of a mole.*
- *See* **Operations and surgery** *if necessary.*

PIMPLES

A pimple is a small pustule or circumscribed elevation of the skin that, by definition, is less than 1cm in diameter. Any bigger than that and it is considered a boil or abscess.

Pimples can be found at any age but are particularly prominent through the teenage years in response to hormonal activity and increased intake of refined sugar.

RECOMMENDATION

General Advice

See **Acne** *and* **Boils**.

PITYRIASIS

Pityriasis is a fine scaly condition of the skin. There are many different types, defined by the position on the body or shape of the lesion. There may be an association with vesicles and pustules and the condition may even be in the body, such as on the tongue.

Pityriasis rosea

This is a common self-limiting skin disease of the trunk that usually clears up within three months. It is characterized by a pale red patch with a fawn-coloured centre. There may be one or many patches, which usually appear on the trunk and upper arms and thighs.

RECOMMENDATIONS

General Advice
- *See Rashes.*
- *Examination of where the lesions are by an acupuncturist or specialist with a knowledge of acupuncture points may be beneficial to discover any underlying weakness in the system that has allowed this condition, of unknown origin, to occur.*

Homeopathic
- *Specific homeopathic treatment should be selected on the symptoms and the person as a whole by a homeopath, but Natrum muriaticum 6 taken four times a day may clear the problem.*

Herbal/natural extracts
- *Application of Calendula or Urtica-based creams are useful.*

PRURITUS

Pruritus is an itching or uncomfortable sensation due to irritation of the peripheral sensory nerves, usually caused by inflammatory chemicals being produced from surrounding cells due to infection or external irritation.

Most commonly, pruritus ani (an itchy anus) is seen in childhood and is discussed in chapter 3 (*see Pruritus ani*). Other common causes include a cold climate, particularly the dry, cold conditions caused by air conditioning. Pruritus senilis is triggered in the elderly by a lack of sebum (the body's skin oil). Pruritus vulvae is an intense or mild itching of the vulva and vagina.

The causes may be chemical irritation, mild infections such as thrush (*Candida*) or a contact dermatitis. If left unattended, secondary infection from bacteria may evolve, which will lead to damage of the skin and, in the case of the vulva, possible malignancy.

RECOMMENDATIONS

General Advice
- *Treatment is dependent upon the cause being removed.*
- *See Itching skin and Itching vagina.*

Nutritional
- *Pruritus senilis may benefit from increased levels of EPA or fish oils and the levels should be determined by consultation with a nutritionist because digestive processes may be troubled in some cases.*

Herbal/natural extracts
- *Application of a Calendula or Urtica cream may be curative in pruritus ani or vulvae.*

PSORIASIS

Psoriasis is a skin disease that is characterized by the development of red patches that are covered over with silvery-white scales. The disease affects the scalp and extensor surfaces of the elbows and knees mostly but can appear anywhere on the body.

The skin grows from a basal cell at the bottom of several layers of cells. These basal cells multiply in psoriasis up to 1,000 times faster than they should. The resulting higher layers cannot shed off quickly enough and the characteristic appearance results. There are two chemical complexes called cAMP and cGMP that inhibit or encourage cell proliferation, respectively. An imbalance caused by a decrease of cAMP or an increase of cGMP results in excessive cell growth.

There are many factors that can imbalance these chemicals. Certain proteins and toxic compounds from bacterial and yeast metabolism in the bowel are known to inhibit cAMP, or increase cGMP respectively. The proteins and toxins responsible are derived from unbalanced bowel flora or digestive incapabilities and are an essential factor in treating psoriasis.

Toxins are normally broken down by the liver and any deficiency in liver function will cause or encourage psoriasis. Alcohol and smoking are particularly straining on the liver, as are most drugs. Several studies have shown the damaging effect of alcohol and cigarettes on psoriasis cases.

Deficiencies in certain oils, amino acids and zinc have all been shown to cause psoriasis. Increased levels of insulin and glucose also seem to have an effect.

There is evidence that stressful events may trigger psoriasis and certainly stress is an important factor in most skin conditions because adrenaline and other catecholamine levels affect the amount of blood flow to the skin.

There may be some connection to an autoimmune syndrome (the body attacking itself) because an arthritic condition may be associated with psoriasis. Nails may become characteristically pitted due to fluctuations in the growth rate of the nail bed.

RECOMMENDATIONS

General Advice
- *Regular bowel motions are necessary to keep the colon cleansed and increased fibre and water intake is essential.*
- *Learn a meditation technique and increase exercise to a substantial level.*
- *Ultraviolet light from sunshine is beneficial. Ultraviolet B is a preferred treatment although ultraviolet A (PUVA therapy) is offered by orthodox treatment centres. The PUVA therapy*

may be associated with side effects.
- *Localized heat through electric pads or ultrasound may be effective.*

Nutritional
- *The association with bowel toxicity is well documented. It is necessary to remove animal fats, refined sugars and sweetness in general and yeasty or fungal foods such as bread and mushrooms.*
- *Weight-reducing diets automatically cut out refined foods and may be beneficial.*
- *Oily fish such as salmon, herring and mackerel should also be added into the diet along with one teaspoonful of linseed oil per foot of height.*
- *A high percentage of psoriasis sufferers will benefit from a gluten free diet. A three-month period without gluten is essential and if an improvement is apparent try eating gluten again. If the condition returns then consider techniques of desensitization against gluten.*

Supplemental
- *The following supplements should be taken in divided doses with food per foot of height: folic acid (100µg), beta-carotene (2mg), vitamin E (100iu), selenium (40µg), eicosapentoenoic acid (1g) and zinc (5mg before bed). All of these should be administered daily for one month and if improvement is noted remove one supplement each ten days, starting with the vitamin E. If any deterioration is noted, add back that compound and see if you can isolate the particularly active supplement. Discuss with a nutritionist the foods that may be absent in your diet that contain any culprit.*

Herbal/natural extracts
- *Vitamin D, liquorice, comfrey and chamomile-based creams or lotions have been shown to be beneficial. Try one at a time and note any benefits.*
- *The herb Sarsaparilla taken as a dried root should be used (1g per foot of height in divided doses throughout the day).*

• Milk thistle could be taken. Take twice the advised dose on any product recommended by your local healthfood store or herbalist.

SHAVING RASH (BARBER'S RASH)

This red, itching and irritating rash is associated with shaved areas. It is caused by the normal skin bacteria (*Staphylococcus*) accessing the lower levels of the skin due to small abrasions following shaving.

RECOMMENDATIONS

General Advice

• Avoid shaving an infected area until the problem has cleared.

• The use of aftershave causes a reflex closure of opened pores and also acts as a mild antiseptic against skin bacteria for a short while. Its use, especially on skins with a tendency to shaving rash, may be painful but lessens the risk of infection.

• Choose an aftershave that is as non-medicated as possible and use small amounts because the chemicals used in proprietary types may cause local or toxic problems.

• See **Itching skin**.

SUNBURN

A burn from the sun may be as mild or serious as a burn from any other source of heat. First-, second- and third-degree burns are all conceivable. Sunburn may be more damaging than other burns because generally more of the skin is damaged. Sunburn frequently occurs in a relaxed situation where sun-tanning was intended or the effect of the sun went unnoticed or was underestimated, perhaps because of being in a swimming pool or the sea, with its cooling effects.

Sunburn is often associated with heat-stroke and because the damage may be caused by ultra-violet light, not heat alone, a sunburn can penetrate below skin level.

Sun screens

There is an increased use being made of ultra-violet light-blocking chemicals in preparations known as sun screens. These are expensive and tend to be improperly used. Their principal function is as a barrier and if significant amounts are not actually placed on the skin then the effect is minimal. Most users will rub the lotion in, as opposed to leaving it on the surface.

What is more disturbing is the suggestion in a recent study that those who use sun screens to achieve a tan run an increased risk of melanoma and possibly other skin cancers. This may be because the sun screen gives a false security that prolonged exposure is safe or the chemicals are imparting some form of cancer-causing effect.

RECOMMENDATIONS

General Advice

• If a burn has occurred, see **Burns**.

• Prevention is the best form of treatment. Avoid exposure and when this is unavoidable or time is spent in the sun with large areas of the skin exposed, use sun-screen compounds efficiently.

• Strictly avoid any antiseptic soaps or lotions because the loss of skin bacteria will predispose to the secondary infection of a burn.

• See **Melanoma** and **Moles**.

Nutritional

• Ensure that at least five portions of fruit and vegetable are eaten to encourage higher levels of antioxidants.

Supplemental

• If exposure is inevitable or intended, take the following supplements per foot of height in divided doses with food throughout the day: beta-carotene (2.5mg), vitamin E (100iu) and selenium (40µg).

Homeopathic

• Homeopathic remedy Sol can be taken at

potency 30 three times a day, starting three days before the holiday or sun exposure and continuing until your return.

Herbal/natural extracts
- *Aloe vera and lemon juice or gels can be soothing.*
- *Calendula or aloe vera gels will be soothing and potentially healing for any sunburn.*

Orthodox
- *Many orthodox drugs, especially tranquillizers, antihistamines and anti-nausea drugs, all of which are commonly used in holiday situations, may increase the sensitivity of the skin to the sun.*

Sunbeds

As a general rule of thumb, avoid them. If this is not possible, stay well within the recommended time-dose because many beds are faulty or poorly serviced and the amount of ultraviolet light emitted is not necessarily accurate.

Please follow the general advice for sunburn above if a sunbed is going to be used.

SUN STROKE – *see* Dehydration *and* Sunburn

SWEATING (PERSPIRATION)

We all perspire to some degree. Sweating is an essential bodily function and should only be considered a problem if absent or in excess.

The primary function of sweat is as a cooling mechanism. For instance, one minute of running produces 10Kcal of heat. This heat has to be removed from the body and this is done by cooling down the skin's surface. Sweat passes from sweat pores, settles on the skin, evaporates using heat to do so and thereby cools the skin's surface. This in turn cools the body and maintains a steady internal temperature. Sweat that drips off the body is not cooling. The sweat glands are under the control of the nervous system and sweating is the main physiological adjustment to an increased heat load. The control comes from specific centres in the brain that recognize and increase heat in the bloodstream.

A second, less well thought of, reason for sweating is based on the fact that sweat is similar in composition to urine. Urea, a nitrogenous waste product from protein metabolism, does not come out in the sweat, but most other compounds can. The body may use sweating to eliminate toxins or to regulate electrolyte balance by removing salt and other elements.

Anything that heats the body, such as exercise, alcohol, caffeine, smoking and spicy foods, will increase sweating. Outside air temperature causes a body temperature rise and a reflex sweat. High humidity will prevent evaporation and prevent the cooling mechanism. The body sweats more in a vain attempt to encourage evaporation, but may fail to do so. Overheating may occur in a humid climate and dehydration is also a risk.

The sweat glands are under the control of the

Sweat glands

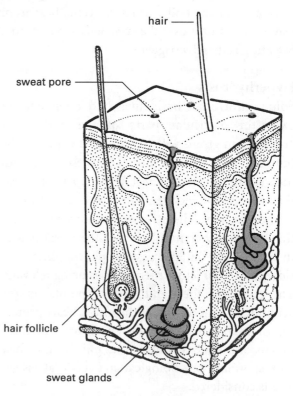

hair

sweat pore

hair follicle

sweat glands

nervous system, which in turn responds to stress chemicals such as adrenaline. Nervousness or anxiety can trigger sweating. This is an evolutionary reaction in principle to prepare the body's cooling mechanism if a fight or flight reaction is required.

An absence of sweating may be found in individuals who have a genetic pre-disposition to a warmer core body temperature and, therefore, cooling is not required. A lack of sweat is most commonly associated with dehydration and needs to be corrected.

Excessive sweating is also a genetic predisposition and may not be a sign of ill-health. Generally, however, sweating is a sign of a raised body temperature, usually due to infection or an overproduction of thyroxine or adrenaline. Any situation that creates fear or anxiety can promote sweating and, interestingly, there is an internal fear mechanism associated with heart conditions and sweating may be an early sign of heart disease.

Obesity (being overweight) puts an insulating layer around the body, which prevents heat from leaving and thus raises the core body temperature. Sweating is thereby triggered.

Hyperhydrosis

Some unfortunate individuals have a tendency to sweat in particular parts of the body. Our armpits and groins will appear moist with exercise but some will sweat profusely in these areas with little strain. The hands, feet and scalp are all areas that may sweat independently of body temperature or anxiety. There is no orthodox reason for this nervous overstimulation of the sweat glands in these areas but the Eastern philosophies consider the acupuncture meridians as being relevant. The palms of the hand contain points on the acupuncture meridians of the lungs, heart protector or sexual function and the heart. All these organs and systems must be examined and their corresponding psychological and spiritual associations considered.

RECOMMENDATIONS

General Advice

- *Try to establish a cause and remove it. It may be necessary to lose weight, remove the heat-creating foods mentioned above from the diet or learn a relaxation/meditation technique to take nervous anxiety away.*

- *Absorbent material such as cotton should be worn, especially in humid conditions, to mop up sweat and aid the evaporative process. It may seem illogical to wear something if you are hot, but in fact a cotton vest is cooling for this reason.*

- *Remember that fever is a friend and that sweating in association with infection or disease should not necessarily be inhibited (see* **Fever***).*

- *If excessive sweating is creating an unpleasant smell (see* **Body odour***).*

Homeopathic

- *A genetic predisposition to sweat may be difficult to alter but homeopathic remedies at potency 200 or higher may alter fundamental tendencies. Prescribing is best done by a homeopath but special attention should be paid to Calcarea carbonica, Hepar sulphuris calcaria, Lycopodium, Psorinum, Silica and Veretrum album. The place, time of day or night, smell and other variables will lead to the best choice.*

Orthodox

- *Excessively sweaty palms may interfere markedly with an individual's social life and if the above measures do not resolve the problem, surgical intervention to cut the nerves that control sweating can be considered. This is a technically difficult operation for fear of damaging other neurological controls. It is therefore not a particularly successful procedure and is best avoided.*

- *A general practitioner may offer topical applications of aluminium chloride or refer you to a physiotherapist who uses the electrical current therapy, Iontophoresis, although this is only useful for hands and feet. An injection of a neurotoxin known as Botulinum A can be used for excessive sweating in the axilla (the armpits) or the forehead. There is high level of efficacy but the effect may not last much longer than five months. Surgical sympathectomy is the cutting of the nerves governing sweating. This is now done through endoscopic procedures and is far less traumatic than the old techniques.*

THE NERVOUS SYSTEM

CONCUSSION AND UNCONSCIOUSNESS (LOSS OF CONSCIOUSNESS)

From a medical point of view concussion is actually the state of being shaken or the result of such a jarring. The term has, however, passed into both lay and medical colloquialism, referring only to brain concussion and so is now used to describe an immediate loss of consciousness, transient in nature due to a violent shaking or agitation of the brain within the cranium (skull). Concussion may be associated with a penetrating injury but usually it is due to a blunt blow and is caused by a change in the momentum of the head. What this means is that a blow causes the skull to go in one direction but the brain, because it is floating in cerebrospinal fluid, stays stationary and gets 'hit' by the skull.

Most often such an injury results in a headache and nothing more, but if a loss of consciousness is associated then the term concussion is used to describe the situation.

Concussion may also be used for a partial loss of consciousness where an individual is clearly unaware of where they are or aspects of reality that relate to that current time.

Associated with concussion may be a shallowness of breathing, a massive adrenaline response leading to pale, cold and clammy skin, a tachycardia (rapid heart rate) and a drop in blood pressure noted by a weak pulse. Recovery may also be connected with nausea and vomiting, and loss of bowel and bladder control. Upon recovery, a loss of memory is not uncommon.

It is important to remember that concussion is a temporary state and if it persists then the term used is unconsciousness. Further symptoms occur in unconsciousness which are generally not associated with concussion. These include twitching of the limbs or convulsions, a flushed face rather than pallor and, as the patient recovers consciousness, weakness or paralysis may be noted in any part of the body and the awareness or alertness of the individual may be deficient.

A warning sign that the brain has been damaged and that an intracranial bleed may be occurring is an inequality in pupil size, a bilateral dilation of the pupils, or pupils that are not reactive to light (*see* **Intracranial bleeds**).

RECOMMENDATIONS

General Advice

- *Whether concussion or unconsciousness is the ultimate definition, emergency first aid is relevant and the ABC (airways, breathing, circulation) routine or cardio-pulmonary resuscitation (CPR) is the first step.*
- *Once the ABC of resuscitation is performed, establish the probable cause of concussion. If there is any suggestion of spinal injury, ensure that no movement takes place and follow the instructions for spinal injury (see* **Spinal injury***).*
- *If movement is permissible (no spinal injury is likely and all injuries are splinted), move the patient into the recovery position (described overleaf).*
- *Cover with a blanket and, if possible, also place one underneath the casualty.*
- *Check the patient's wallet and pockets for any medical notification, such as a diabetic card, steroid card, anti-coagulant card or medical-alert bracelet that may be worn.*

The recovery position

Any unconscious patient should be placed in the recovery position to avoid the possibility of vomiting, which may be inhaled and cause asphyxiation. The positioning of a casualty into the correct position, which used to be known as the coma position, must be preceded by clearly establishing that there is no neck or spinal injury. Moving a patient with such damage may lead to paralysis or death by putting pressure on or severing the spinal cord.

Moving a body safely

If there is no possibility of neck or spinal injury use the following procedure as illustrated below:

- Place both arms of the casualty close to the body.
- Turn the casualty on to his/her side. This is done most conveniently by grasping clothing at the hip (1).
- Pull up the upper arm until it makes a right angle with the body and then bend the elbow (2).

- Draw up the upper leg of the same side until the thigh makes a right angle with the body and then bend the knee (2).
- Pull out the other arm, which is generally underneath the body at this stage, and extend it slightly behind the back (3).
- Bend the undermost knee slightly.

This position places the body in such a way that it will be stable and prevent asphyxia (4). The heavier the body, the more difficult this procedure and it is often easier to do all of the above in a kneeling position beside the casualty.

MULTIPLE SCLEROSIS (MS)

Multiple sclerosis is the medical term given to a condition that strips the nervous system of the sheath that surrounds the neurone, which is the part of the nerve that transmits the impulses. The sheath is called myelin and, therefore, MS is a 'demyelinating' disorder.

The orthodox world has postulated a variety of

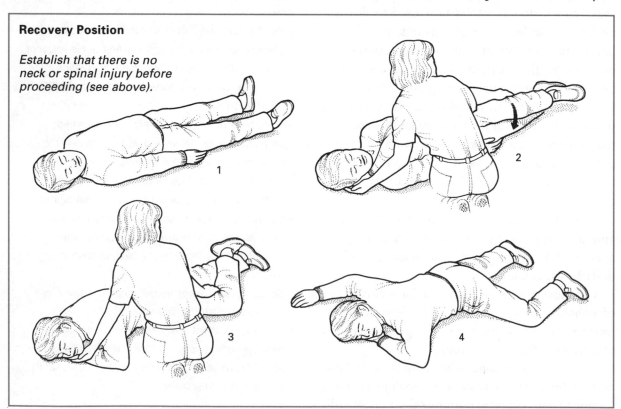

Recovery Position

Establish that there is no neck or spinal injury before proceeding (see above).

1

2

3

4

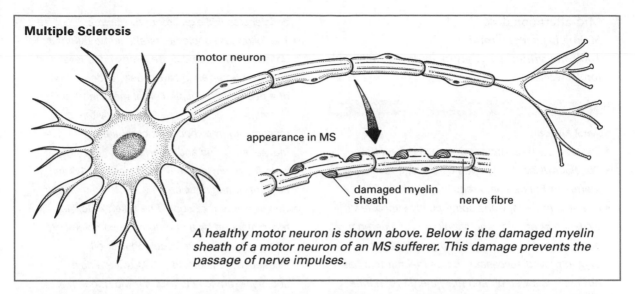

Multiple Sclerosis

motor neuron

appearance in MS

damaged myelin sheath

nerve fibre

A healthy motor neuron is shown above. Below is the damaged myelin sheath of a motor neuron of an MS sufferer. This damage prevents the passage of nerve impulses.

causes for MS, including viral, autoimmune disease (the body's immune system attacking the nervous system), dietary causes and specific chemical reactions in the nervous system, probably caused by genetic errors. The complementary medical world views the cause as being all of the above plus the possibility of heavy metal toxicity, food allergy, vaccine reaction and, arguably, psychological factors.

My experience suggests that anger produces chemicals within the nervous system that have a direct effect on the body's ability to protect the nervous system's myelin sheaths. The anger is usually repressed and stems from childhood and most often is associated with problems between the child and a parent.

Symptoms of multiple sclerosis are many and variable. They can be divided into sensory symptoms, such as visual disturbance, tingling and numbness and movement symptoms, such as loss of balance, loss of bladder or bowel control, weakness and paralysis. Problems usually occur in one part of the body, although they can rarely be bilateral and may come along for a matter of minutes or last for years. Repeated episodes of neurological disturbance need to be assessed by specialists before a diagnosis can be made. Multiple sclerosis is well known for going into remission. This means that people with neurological condi-

tions may resolve them and not have problems again until many years later. It is this principle of remission that alternative practitioners work on because it shows that the body is capable of overriding the condition. After all, a permanent remission is the same as a cure.

Diagnosis is made by excluding other causes and is confirmed by specific visual tests called visual evoked response (if the patient has visual disturbances), magnetic resonance imaging and, on occasions, biopsy.

A Multiple Sclerosis sufferer by the name of Cari Loder discovered that her problem was alleviated with the use of tricyclic antidepressant in combination with an amino acid and with regular intake of vitamin B_{12}. There has been no study published to date but anecdotal evidence and support from people who have used her course of treatment is hopeful. Whilst we await results of studies, I see no reason why people should not try the course. Because it involves a drug, a doctor needs to prescribe the antidepressant and it would be best to have the doctor keep an eye on the situation.

Adrinex – The Cari Loder suggested treatment
Morning dose
70mg lofepramine
500mg L-phenylalanine

Mid-afternoon dose
500mg L-phenylalanine
1000 mg vitamin B_{12} given by injection weekly for 10 weeks.

RECOMMENDATIONS

General Advice

- *Exercise such as yoga or Qi Gong is essential.*
- *Consider using the Ayurvedic massage technique Marma or Shiatsu on a regular basis.*
- *Bee-venom therapy has some poorly supported evidence of efficacy and should be considered if other treatments are not helping. Hyperbaric oxygen proved successful in one trial but this has not been followed up and may, therefore, not be an effective treatment.*
- *Lastly but most importantly address any anger – conscious or subconscious, present or past, known or unknown – via regular counselling and meditation/relaxation techniques.*

Nutritional

- *Establish and remove any food allergies. Specifically, have a very low animal fat intake (less than 10g/day) and reduce even vegetable fats to less than 50g of polyunsaturated oils. No cow's milk products, although sheep's and goat's products can be used in small quantities. Absolutely no caffeine or tannin, which therefore means no coffee, tea or cola drinks. Cocoa needs to be avoided as well, which includes chocolate.*
- *Vegetable proteins such as soya, lentils and grains should be increased to compensate and fish should be eaten at least every other day. Salmon, herring and mackerel are the best.*
- *Polyunsaturated fatty acids need to be assessed, preferably by an essential fatty acid blood test, and any deficiencies corrected through diet or supplements.*

Supplemental

- *Have your essential amino acid, copper, calcium, magnesium and zinc levels checked out because deficiencies will exacerbate symptoms.*
- *The following supplements should be taken at doses of twice the daily recommended level and can even be given intravenously, under the care of a doctor with supplemental medicine training: Vitamins B_1, B_5 and B_{12}, folic acid, vitamin C, magnesium, molybdenum, chromium, manganese, zinc and selenium.*
- *Take D,L-phenylalanine, approximately 100mg per foot of height twice a day.*
- *Supplements that should be taken at levels recommended by a nutritional or complementary medical specialist include cod liver oil, eicosapentaenoic acid (500g twice a day), docosahexanoic acid (300mg with meals), N-acetylcysteine (500mg with meals every other day), zinc, copper, selenium and vitamin E.*

Herbal/natural extracts

- *Discuss the use of the herb Ginkgo biloba.*
- *Consult a Tibetan physician and ask about Padma 28, a combination of different herbs which has shown to be an effective treatment in a scientific study.*

Orthodox

- *Self-help for MS should take the form of advising your health practitioner of the following recommendations but you should be under the care of an orthodox neurologist.*
- *Orthodox treatments such as adrenocorticotrophic hormone (ACTH) or steroids may be recommended and should be considered if the following alternative treatments are not effective. The use of beta-interferon is distinctly a last resort.*

PARALYSIS

Paralysis is the loss of muscle function with or without loss or diminution of sensation. It is classified in many ways, depending on: the body part involved; the cause; the tone of the muscle – a paralysis can be described as flaccid or spastic; and the distribution, such as monoplegic (one limb) or hemiplegic (one side of the body).

Certain types of paralysis are sometimes called palsies (*see* **Cerebral palsy**).

A partial paralysis is known as paresis. The variety of types and causes of paralysis require different treatments and it is best to refer to that section in this book concerning the underlying cause. There are, however, certain treatments and techniques that can be used for all those with paralysis.

Paralysis occurs because of damage to the nervous system. This can occur anywhere from the brain to the local nerves controlling the area or part paralysed. Paralysis may be of a digital limb or may affect the muscles of breathing in which case the damage is extremely serious and potentially fatal. Paralysis of a part of the body may be caused by a progressive disease and the cause must be found as soon as possible.

The orthodox medical world will point out that nerve damage is irreparable. This is true to a great extent although naturopathic techniques may encourage some repair and they work predominantly to encourage other nerves to take over the sending of instructions to muscles that have been lost by the damage to the original nerve. I consider the possibility of repairing a paralysed area as being similar to teaching a right-handed person to use their left hand. It requires another part of the nervous system to learn functions that it has not used, but there is a strong possibility that this may occur. A lot depends on the extent of the damage.

RECOMMENDATIONS

General Advice

- *Identification of the cause of paralysis is paramount because it will help to decide which treatments are of benefit.*
- *Establish good communication with a physiotherapist and use the techniques recommended as often as possible. It will make a big difference in most cases.*

- *Ensure full support from 'home services'. Take advantage of all household gadgets that can make life easier.*
- *Ensure that clothes, footware, wheelchairs and other accessories are comfortable.*
- *Try to find a practitioner of Marma massage or neurotherapy, which are physicotherapy techniques derived from Ayurvedic medicine.*
- *If Marma or neurotherapy is not available then consider osteopathy, chiropractic, Polarity therapy, yoga or the Alexander Technique. Any of these structural or energetic treatments may be of benefit.*
- *Definitely utilize acupuncture.*
- *Bioresonance techniques and healing hypnotherapy are useful.*
- *Cranial osteopathy or craniosacral therapy should be tried for at least six to ten sessions because marked benefit may occur.*
- *Please undertake some training in a meditative technique in association with counselling. Great benefit will be derived if an inner peace and understanding of what has happened can be reached. For those with a strong religious faith then time spent with your spititual advisor will also prove invaluable.*

Herbal/natural extracts

- *Tibetan medicine encompasses bodywork, nutrition, acupuncture and herbal treatments and is probably the best all-round medical treatment if available. If not, an Ayurvedic or Chinese assessment is essential.*
- *Herbal and homeopathic treatments may be of benefit. In traumatic paralysis Arnica potency 6 or 30, given every 15min may make a difference in the long term. A homeopath or herbalist would be required for more specific prescribing according to the symptoms.*

SEIZURES – *see* **Epilepsy** *and* **Convulsions**

PSYCHOLOGICAL MATTERS

ADDICTION

It is arguable that all of us are addicts. Problems only arise when the addiction is detrimental to health. It is also arguable that the 'abuse' of a healthy action or substance in an addictive manner may in fact be beneficial. Frequent visits to a church, temple or mosque could be considered an addiction, especially if it changes one's life. Provided that religious fanaticism does not set in, this could be considered a non-destructive addiction. Can we extrapolate this to the use of alcohol? Do two or three gin and tonics each evening to shrug off the day and engender a relaxed feeling for the evening constitute addiction? One may argue that if it is felt to be beneficial then it may be an addiction but is not one that is harmful. On the other hand, would we do better without the toxins, but then the issue becomes to 'do better' or to be more content?

You can see that the discussion is tricky, with tangent after tangent proffering itself for philosophical discussion. I feel that treatment for addiction depends very much on establishing whether one is addicted or not. If the answer is 'yes' to any of the following questions, then my recommendations should be studied.

- Is there anything that you do or take that you wish you did not?
- Is there anything that you do or take that others wish you did not?
- Is your life negatively affected by something you do or take?
- Is somebody else's life negatively affected by something you do or take?
- Is your health or fitness affected by something you do or take?
- Have you had to debate any of the above questions to reach the conclusion 'no'?

If you have answered 'yes' to any of the above, then you are probably an addict and would benefit from changing.

RECOMMENDATIONS

General Advice

- *There is no simple answer to breaking an addiction, and fighting the battle by yourself is slow and often ineffective.*
- *Establish a rapport with a counsellor you like. There are no 'good or bad' points to look for when choosing a psychologist. If you get on with the professional you have your initial starting point.*

Homeopathic

- *Use the following homeopathic remedies depending upon your addiction: for alcohol addiction – use Lycopodium 200 nightly for one week; for tobacco addiction – use Tabacum 200 nightly for two weeks. For the following addictive substances obtain homeopathic potency 200 of the recommended remedy and use nightly for seven nights. Further recommendations must come from a homeopath: cannabis addiction, take Cannabis indicus; cocaine addiction, take Coca; heroin addiction, take Morphinum; addiction to ecstasy, LSD and other manufactured drugs requires a high potency of the corresponding remedy, available through homeopaths or homeopathic pharmacies.*

Herbal/natural extracts

- *Consult a Bach flower remedy manual to establish the best remedy to keep in your pocket at all times.*

Eastern philosophies regard reincarnation to be an important aspect of health. With regard to addiction, the philosophy is the same. To reach Nirvana one must free one's spirit of all shackles. Addiction is a tie to the mental and physical plane and must be dealt with to be 'free' or enlightened. This is not a religious concept, more a spiritual one, but even strong religious dogmas such as Christianity will place an abuser in 'Hell', suggesting as usual a strong tie-in between Eastern and Western theology.

RECOMMENDATIONS

General Advice
- *Do not fight addiction alone. Get help from a specialist, a support group (including Alcoholics Anonymous and Narcotics Anonymous), and a complementary medical practitioner.*
- *When dealing with addiction, learn a meditation technique that is suitable for you. This may be transcendental, a personal technique taught to you or an active form such as yoga, Tai Chi or Qi Gong. Dealing with the mental and physiological aspects is only two-thirds of being released from addiction.*

Dealing with an addict

Living with an addict, being related to an addict, befriending or loving an addict is a situation that requires help in itself. Addiction is not just about the addict. There are one million registered alcoholics and drug addicts in the UK. If each one has a parent, a lover, a child, a brother or sister and a best friend, we can estimate that five million people are directly influenced by an addict. If you consider that only one in five people register or realize they are an addict we have anywhere from 5 million to 25 million (nearly half the population) influenced by addiction. You can multiply these figures in the USA by five!

An addict without a will to change and the support structure to do so will continue to be socially disruptive by being deceitful, untrustworthy, violent, changeable, vindictive and hateful. The addict will lie, cheat and steal, all beyond their control and all with a self-hatred that overpowers the care and love that those affected can offer.

RECOMMENDATIONS

General Advice
- *Do not try to solve this yourself. Professionals fail, so you probably will.*

- *Seek help for the addict if they wish but, importantly, contact a support group for yourself via your GP or complementary clinical therapist.*

ASSERTIVENESS

A lack of assertiveness must be differentiated from shyness and timidity, both of which are character traits. A lack of assertiveness is sociologically unacceptable, leading to difficulties with social or professional life.

RECOMMENDATIONS

General Advice
- *Self-help is difficult and a consultation with a psychologist is most beneficial to differentiate between acceptable and unacceptable levels of poor assertiveness.*
- *Martial arts training is excellent at increasing assertiveness, especially Qi Gong.*

Homeopathic
- *Homeopathic remedies can have a profound effect on areas of psychology and special interest should be paid to the remedies Baryta carbonica, Pulsatilla, Gelsemium and Petroleum.*

CLAUSTROPHOBIA

This condition is characterized by acute anxiety in enclosed spaces or in areas where immediate escape is not evident, such as in a crowd.

The symptoms may range from a mild discomfort to profound anxiety including panic, uncontrolled tears or screaming, sweating, palpitations and fainting.

RECOMMENDATIONS

General Advice
- *If the condition is affecting well-being, then neurolinguistic programming, hypnotherapy or*

---

other behavioural modification techniques are usually beneficial.

- *Eye movement desensitization, a new branch of psychotherapy, may be very effective.*

Homeopathic

- *The homeopathic remedy Aconite 6 should be kept in the pocket and used every 10min if a situation that may encourage claustrophobia is liable to occur. Argentum nitricum 6 may also be tried.*

EATING DISORDERS

The term 'eating disorder' is extremely broad. It may represent a food phobia leading to deficiencies and illness, excessive eating leading to obesity or the conditions of anorexia or bulimia.

Any of the eating disorders may be mild, moderate or severe and move from one category to another. Severe and prolonged eating disorders will lead to ill-health and be potentially fatal. With anorexia, which strikes most usually in young females (20 girls to 1 boy) below the age of 25 years, 1 in 10 will be admitted to hospital and 1 in 10 of these will die.

Eating disorders are rarely caused by physical conditions, although any eating disorder can lead to pathology. It is unusual for a food allergy to create anorexia or bulimia but it may well create a phobia towards a food or to overeating leading to obesity.

More commonly, eating disorders are in fact an imbalance of energy or a matter of psychological concern. The Eastern philosophies consider the stomach to be the energy meridian responsible for the intake and absorption of food. The small intestine and heart meridians are involved in absorption and distribution and the liver meridian is concerned with energy for the processing. Imbalance in any of these meridians can lead to the apparent condition of an eating disorder.

The orthodox world will most often cite emotional disturbance as the cause. Suppressed or unrecognized anger, depression, low self-esteem or psychosexual crises are all found in association with eating disorders.

In my practice I have noted a tendency for those with eating disorders to fall into a category that I define as the 'pretty-person syndrome'. At some point in a child's development, usually at a psychologically susceptible age (often around puberty), the child has found him/herself in a situation where physical appearance or beauty has taken on a profound sociological meaning. Very often this stems from overadoring parents or finding oneself in a social group that places too much emphasis on prettiness or ideal body measurements. The correlation between being sociably acceptable and being thin is very much a Western development, as indeed are eating disorders. The association, therefore, between the perfect body and not eating is clearly seen.

At some point in our development we consider our own inner self-worth. If our society (parental or social) focuses on our outward appearance then the inner self or soul questions whether it is loved for itself or the shell in which it is encased. By shutting off that part of our consciousness that truly sees the shape of the body and by focusing on the 'unattractiveness' of fat, the subconscious can feel confident that if someone likes the individual then it is because of them and not because of the way they look. There are many holes in this argument as being the underlying cause of eating disorders and in particularly anorexia, but it may account for why the disfigurement of anorexia is not seen by the individual and why a large number of sufferers are often young and attractive and can be found in the modelling, acting or singing professions.

Identifying an eating disorder

The sooner that a problem can be identified the sooner it can be treated. Individuals may be blind to a problem and may need help in spotting the difficulty. Also, individuals with an eating disorder may be in denial or be unable to establish whether they really do have a problem or not. St George's Hospital Medical School, London, have suggested five simple questions that can be asked. If two or more are positive then consider the possibility of an eating disorder. They have termed the assessment the **SCOFF** questionnaire:

1 Do you make yourself **S**ick because you feel uncomfortably full?
2 Do you worry you have lost **C**ontrol over how much you eat?
3 Have you recently lost more than **O**ne stone (14 lbs – 6 kilos) in less than a three month period?
4 Do you believe yourself to be **F**at when others say you are too thin?
5 Would you say that **F**ood dominates your life?

RECOMMENDATIONS

General Advice
- *Establishing an eating disorder requires not only the individual's perception but also the input from those around because the patient may not be aware.*
- *Ten to twenty per cent of body weight loss must be apparent in association with dieting or irregular eating patterns before an eating disorder should be considered as a diagnosis.*
- *Self-help is usually inadequate and counselling from psychotherapists and nutritionists is advisable: the former to deal with the cause and the latter to deal with the inevitable imbalances that occur.*
- *Biochemical changes such as depression and cessation of periods are often associated with dehydration. Try to ensure that 4–6 pints of water are taken per day regardless of any other intake.*
- *Mineral deficiencies, particularly zinc, are associated, whether as a cause or an effect is uncertain.*

Anorexia nervosa

Anorexia is the medical term for a loss of appetite. Anorexia nervosa is a severe condition where individuals starve themselves because they incorrectly view their body as overweight. This psychological pathology occurs 20 times more frequently in girls than in boys and can range from mild obsession to being a fatal condition.

RECOMMENDATIONS

General Advice
- *If you or someone close recognizes that your dieting is encroaching into your lifestyle, sit down with a counsellor and discuss the matter. There may be an early sign of anorexia nervosa.*
- *If you disagree with other people's image of your body, go to see a counsellor.*
- *Do not assume that this problem will go away by itself. Go to see a counsellor.*
- *A good study has shown that anxious mothers could cause anorexia in their children. Such maternal anxiety should be treated and mothers should receive counselling.*

Nutritional
- *Having seen a counsellor, you may consider sitting with a nutritional expert to establish whether any supplementation is necessary to replace deficiencies.*

Homeopathic
- *See a homeopath to obtain a constitutional remedy.*

Bulimia

This is a non-medical term for an insatiable appetite with excessive food intake. It is in common use for the correct medical term Bulimarexia, where an individual will alternate bingeing or gorging with self-emptying by enforced vomiting, prolonged fasting or self-induced diarrhoea, usually under the influence of laxatives.

Bulimics are not as obvious as anorexics because their body features may not change. Bulimia, unlike anorexia, does not focus itself in young adults only and has quite an even distribution of ages.

Bulimia is less inclined to lead to physical pathology although vomiting can tear the oesophagus and cause biochemical imbalances and is considered much more of a psychological problem occurring in young, affluent women who have low self-esteem, a history of rejection or a fear of failure.

RECOMMENDATION

Homeopathic

- *Constitutional prescribing by a qualified homeopath is highly recommended.*

FRIGHT AND FEAR

Fright is an essential emotion for survival. Those of our prehistoric ancestors who did not respond to a fearful situation with fright generally did not run away or fight and their gene line will have stopped abruptly. Adrenaline and other similar hormones called catecholamines are produced in response to frightening situations and prepare the body for action by moving blood into areas such as the heart, lungs, muscles and brain and removing it from non-essential areas such as the skin, bladder and bowel.

A severe fright or shock can produce such a surge of adrenaline that the sudden change in the position of blood in the body can cause a faint or temporary paralysis. This faint mechanism was another survival technique, namely 'playing dead'.

Fright, like fear, is not a disease process and does not need specific treatment unless it is persistent and socially disruptive. In this case the condition is known as a phobia (*see* **Phobia**).

RECOMMENDATIONS

General Advice

- *Learn a relaxation–breathing technique if you have a tendency to be fearful.*

Homeopathic

- *Keep the remedy Aconite 6 at hand and use up to every 15min in the case of a sudden shock.*

Herbal/natural extracts

- *Keep a rescue remedy (a Bach flower remedy) at hand and use two drops every 15min if required.*

FRIGIDITY

Frigidity refers to an unwillingness to have sexual relations and one needs to consider carefully whether or not this is a pathological situation. It is neither right nor wrong to have a high or low sex drive and discussion is essential to establish whether or not frigidity is actually a problem. Social pressure nowadays encourages young adults to have sexual relations at an ever-decreasing age. Nature did not intend us to have an interest nor indulge in sexual intercourse until we were in our mid- to late teens and therefore it is important to differentiate between the absence of our natural sexual drive and frigidity.

RECOMMENDATIONS

General Advice

- *Discuss the matter openly with parents or friends to establish whether the emotional block is within normal parameters. If you feel uncomfortable with this, then a counsellor should be able to give guidance.*
- *If a problem is identified then counselling is an essential aspect of treatment, starting as soon as possible and continuing in weekly sessions for as long as is necessary.*
- *Do not confuse frigidity with a difficulty in intercourse, such as vaginismus (see* **Vaginismus***). A physical discomfort (dyspareunia) that creates a dislike of sexual intercourse is not frigidity.*

Homeopathic

- *Constitutional homeopathic remedies can be chosen by a homeopath with experience.*

HYSTERIA

Hysteria is commonly envisaged as 'that screaming woman' in a Hitchcock movie. Whilst this is an extreme example of sensory hysteria, it is important to understand that one can also have motor hysteria. Sensory hysteria is an inability to control an emotion, most usually fear. Usually associated with stress, hysteria can present as a continuous babbling in association with a loss of awareness of what is being said around them. Motor hysteria refers to a loss of function of the body, the most dramatic of which is hysterical paralysis.

Whatever the type of hysteria, the effect is caused by an overload of adrenaline and catacholamine chemicals into the nervous system. The brain loses its normal neurotransmitter control and nervous system failure ensues.

Hysteria is usually short lived, resulting in a self-limiting event such as a faint, or it can take some time to pass, as is often the case in hysterical paralysis. In very rare events hysteria can persist and lead to a deep psychotic event or persisting paralysis.

RECOMMENDATIONS

General Advice

- If in attendance of a hysterical individual, use a calming voice and any necessary common sense advice to placate the panic.
- A slap on the face is potentially injurious and a safer technique is to apply pressure to the tissue at the base of the thumb and first finger. Try it now and you will appreciate how painful that point can be.
- A recurrent hysteria needs to be treated by a counsellor with knowledge in specific relaxation and breathing techniques.

Homeopathic

- Hyperventilation often associates with hysteria and is often the cause of worsening panic (a respiratory alkalosis affecting the brain – see **Hyperventilation**) and paralysis (due to alkalosis preventing muscular action). The homeopathic remedy Aconite, potency 6 or higher, can be given every 5min until the situation is completely under control. One dose is often enough to placate the individual.

NERVOUSNESS

Nervousness is not so much a medical term but in common parlance covers milder forms of anxiety and fearfulness. Nervousness is divided into two levels: acute and chronic.

Acute nervousness

Acute nervousness or anxiety is generally brought on by events that are real or imaginary. Public speaking, pre-exam nerves or pre-event anxiety are all common and will be faced by most of us.

Symptoms include a rapid heart beat (tachycardia), 'butterflies' in the abdomen, a desire to defecate – even as diarrhoea, a desire to urinate, trembling and muscular tension that can lead to headaches. Nausea and vomiting may also be present. These are all acceptable symptoms provided that they are controlled and pass once the event has started or concluded.

RECOMMENDATIONS

General Advice

- If the following tips do not help or the symptoms are severe enough to be disruptive, then a complementary medical opinion should be sought.
- Ensure a good breathing technique, preferably by learning one in association with a relaxation technique through yoga, Qi Gong, Tai Chi, etc.
- Ensure at least six hours of sleep per night, avoid caffeine and other stimulants (the brain does not memorize as well under such adrenaline-like affects) and exercise daily for at least half an hour to reduce the build-up of adrenaline compounds.

Nutritional

- Regardless of appetite, ensure that the diet includes at least four portions of fresh fruit or vegetables and complex carbohydrates (wholegrain foods) for at least three days prior to the event.

Supplemental

- Take three times the recommended daily dose of a vitamin B complex starting three days before any event that may be causing the 'nerves'.
- Use D, L-phenylalanine (100mg per foot of height) with each meal starting three days before the event.

Homeopathic

- *The following homeopathic remedies can be taken at potency 30 four times a day starting three days before the event and at potency 6 every hour on the day of the event: Argentum nitricum if you are unable to concentrate or memorize and suffering from abdominal upsets such as nausea, vomiting, diarrhoea or abdominal pains; Lycopodium is ideal for a nervous individual who is full of bravado and has a tendency to do well regardless of the strong anticipation of failure; and Gelsemium is a master stage-fright remedy for when the body becomes weak, bordering on paralysis and the mind goes blank.*

Herbal/natural extracts

- *Before you advance to this level of drug treatment, consider using a teaspoonful of Passiflora or Valerian fluid extract diluted in a cup of water four times a day.*

Orthodox

- *In uncontrolled cases your GP may recommend beta-blockers, which will temporarily deal with physical symptoms.*

Chronic nervousness

Persistent anxiety or fearfulness can be most disruptive and at its extreme can be considered a phobia. This is the case if the nervousness focuses on a particular theme or object, such as not wishing to go outside or a fear of spiders.

Longstanding nervousness arguably stems from early childhood experiences, psychological trauma such as accidents or relationship problems and may simply be a character trait that does not require treatment. If, however, the nervousness is affecting lifestyle or well-being, advice should be sought.

Nervous dispositions may be created by improper intake. Drugs (both prescribed and those of abuse), alcohol and tobacco (which are all potentially depressive) and nutritional deficiencies such as zinc, the amino acids tryptophan, tyrosine and phenylalanine and vitamin B complex may all cause nervousness.

RECOMMENDATIONS

General Advice

- *Counselling should be sought for an initial discussion on the options available. Hypnotherapy and neurolinguistic programming may be of benefit in isolating underlying causes at a faster rate than psychotherapeutic or psychoanalytical techniques.*
- *Embark upon a course of meditation. The release of endorphins (the body's natural painkillers and calmants), let alone the connection with your higher spiritual being, may be curative on its own.*
- *Avoid tranquillizers like the plague. They cover the symptoms, encourage dependence and, from the onset, are not curative. Herbal preparations are available but should only be taken on the advice of an experienced herbalist.*

Nutritional

- *Establish any nutritional deficiencies through a consultation with a nutritionist or specific blood and/or bioenergetic tests.*

Homeopathic

- *A homeopathic consultation to establish a constitutional remedy treatment is essential.*

SCHIZOPHRENIA

Schizophrenia is actually a group of problems and not a single psychotic disorder. It often starts in the teenage years and is characterized by an alteration in the ability to form concepts, with misinterpretation of reality. This affects behaviour and the intellect in varying degrees. The most common disorders are a tendency to withdraw, ambivalence, inappropriate responses and irregular moods, difficulty in maintaining a stream of thought and, in severe cases, hallucination and delusion.

This condition is not necessarily easy to establish if symptoms are mild so the term 'borderline' schizophrenia is often used when symptoms are mild but nevertheless noticeable. Symptoms of schizophrenia in childhood are termed autism (see **Autism**) but a shy, withdrawn, overly nervous adolescent may be all of those things or borderline schizophrenic. As the individual grows up, these tendencies may be assumed to be normal and the underlying psychiatric disorder not noticed and therefore not treated.

Terms such as *hebephrenic* (childish behaviour and markedly disorganized thoughts), *paranoid* (a conviction of persecution) and *catatonic* (completely cut off from the outside world, often associated with rocking in the foetal position) are all types of schizophrenia. The underlying cause is, from an orthodox point of view, an imbalance of brain chemicals. Holistically it is well established that certain nutritional deficiencies, environmental hazards and heavy metal poisoning are associated on the physical plane. There is always a fine line between 'genius and madness' and there may be a strong spiritual link to those labelled schizophrenic and those a step closer to God. The Eastern philosophies would assume that a chemical imbalance in the brain could be created by an excess energy flow in the higher chakras and therefore spiritual or emotional effects, especially in childhood, may be at work.

Diagnosis is generally made by a psychiatrist using a variety of tests. Other tests include checking for deficiencies in all the B group vitamins, checking the mineral levels and assessing from other physical symptoms the possibility of deficiencies in essential fatty acids. Amino acids may be deficient and investigation of any specific absence may be relevant. Schizophrenia has been associated with coeliac disease, which is an oversensitivity of the bowel to gluten and other gliadins and glutenins found in wheat, rye, corn and, to some extent, in all other grains and starches. Most naturopaths with experience in this area would support the view that other food components may also trigger psychiatric problems.

Schizophrenics are more likely to harm themselves than others, but their presence can be extremely disruptive both to family life and society. Correct professional treatment is necessary.

RECOMMENDATIONS

General Advice
- *Family therapy is essential for both the individual and home life. Any illness within the household will affect all members. Individual psychotherapeutic sessions are a must for children or adolescents because early recognition and counselling can have a profound effect in the long run.*

Nutritional
- *Perform nutritional deficiency tests under the care of a complementary medical specialist with experience in this area.*
- *Test for food allergy and eliminate any allergens.*

Homeopathic
- *Consult with a homeopath. There are many remedies when used at potencies above 200 that will have a profound effect on the psyche. Self-prescribing can be considered in acute schizophrenic episodes when the remedy Stramonium 6 can be given every 10min. Paranoia may be helped by Hyoscyamus 30 given every 10min and should be kept or carried by an individual or their families or partner especially if travelling away from home.*

Orthodox
- *Assessment by a psychiatrist for a definitive diagnosis is essential before any treatment is undergone.*
- *Test for heavy metal poisoning and, regardless of the results, remove mercury from the mouth and aluminium from the kitchen. Specifically, look for copper levels (via red blood cells, not hair only).*
- *Chelation therapy is recommended if toxicity is found.*

CHAPTER 5

ADULT

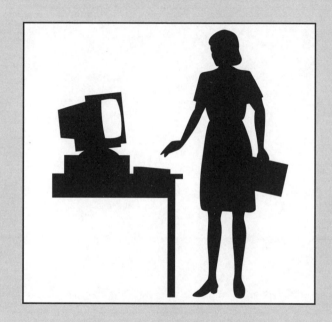

CHAPTER 5
ADULT

GENERAL

ANAPHYLAXIS

Anaphylaxis is the term used to describe an over-allergic reaction. The body becomes flushed and sweaty, the patient feels strong palpitations, becoming short of breath because of narrowing of the airways. The mouth, tongue and lips can swell and there is usually considerable fear associated with the symptoms.

Anaphylaxis can occur from bee/wasp stings, ingestion of certain foods (especially peanuts and eggs) and the use of drugs (both prescription and those of abuse). *See* **Cardiopulmonary resuscitation**, and learn the technique.

RECOMMENDATIONS

General Advice

- *Any suggestion of a shortness of breath or chest pains – call an ambulance.*
- *Apply pressure to acupuncture points one inch below the middle of the clavicle (collar bone) on both sides.*
- *If the patient loses consciousness, check for breathing and pulse and if necessary commence cardiopulmonary resuscitation.*

Homeopathic

- *Whilst waiting for the ambulance, administer Aconite 6 or Apis 6, four pills every 10min.*

Herbal/natural extracts

- *Place a few drops of Olbas or lavender oil in steaming water and encourage the patient to do some inhalations.*

ARTERIOSCLEROSIS OR ATHEROSCLEROSIS (ATHEROMA)

This short section of the book is the most important.

Arteriosclerosis (AS) is the highest cause of death in the Western world, claiming one in three lives. It is the underlying cause of heart disease, strokes and high blood pressure.

Arteriosclerosis is the clogging of the body's arterial system. It is part of the natural ageing process and arterial wall changes have been noted in babies as young as one year old.

The inner lining of all the arteries in the body should be smooth. Anything that causes damage to this delicate layer predisposes to AS. Infections, drugs, radiation and free radicals formed from the ingestion of toxins such as pesticides, insecticides, smoking and alcohol all actively damage the arterial wall. The body automatically tries to repair this by releasing chemicals that attract platelets (a specialized type of red blood cell), scar tissue-forming cells and nutrients. Nearly every cell in the body has cholesterol as part of its cell structure and this is one of the main nutrients pulled into the damaged area. All these different components knot together to create an irregular patch in the

Arteriosclerotic artery

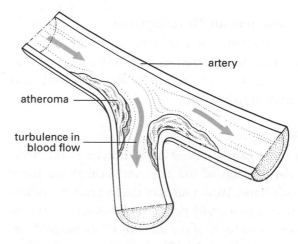

artery

atheroma

turbulence in blood flow

Arteriosclerotic artery, showing the build up of atheroma on the inner lining.

arterial wall, which then grows by trapping other passing molecules such as cholesterol and platelets.

Arteriosclerosis is a silent condition that will not show up until occlusion of the artery creates a problem for the tissues being supplied. The build-up of debris within the artery is known as a plaque. This will finally obstruct the blood flow, cutting off oxygen and nutrients. The plaque may also become loose and travel to a more narrow part of the artery, causing the blockage at a distant point. This moving plaque is known as an embolus (*see* **Embolism**). The occlusion of arteries to organs such as the brain or heart can have an instant and potentially fatal effect. Occlusion to one kidney may not be fatal because the other will take over and, as another example, the blockage of part of the liver blood supply will still leave plenty of liver cells elsewhere to carry on normal function. The plaque also hardens the arteries, making them less responsive to the neurological control that governs their diameter. This 'hardening' of the arteries causes the blood pressure to rise, which in turn leads to a further risk of strokes and cardiovascular disease.

It is feasible that most disease conditions associated with age are caused, or contributed heavily to, by AS. A decrease in oxygen or nutrition will lead to disease and is the main cause of 'ageing' and its characteristics.

Assessment and investigation

Arteriosclerosis is a difficult condition to assess without being invasive. The following observations may be made to assess the level and potential risk of AS.

Pulses

A pulse can be felt easily in arteries at the neck, wrist, on top of the foot and behind the inner ankle bone. Weak pulses in the feet may be indicative of a genetically poor blood flow and cannot be used to assess AS if the individual has had cold feet for most of their life. However, anyone with 'poor circulation', as exhibited by cold feet and hands,

must be especially careful not to encourage AS.

Practitioners may often 'roll' their fingers backwards and forwards over the pulse in the wrist (the radial pulse) to feel the texture and tension within this superficial artery. An individual may do the same on their own pulse but a comparison is needed and because AS develops slowly this is a difficult technique to use. The harder the artery the more likely AS is involved.

Listening to blood flow (auscultation)

A practitioner may place the stethoscope over the carotid arteries (beside the Adam's apple) or over the femoral arteries (in the groin) to listen for a gentle buzz. This is known as a 'bruit' (French for noise) and is caused by turbulence within the artery, in turn caused by blood flowing over the roughened artery. This is similar to the gentle rumble of rapids. The louder the bruit the greater the damage.

Fundal examination

The back of the eye is known as the fundus. A practitioner can look with an ophthalmoscope through

Ear Crease

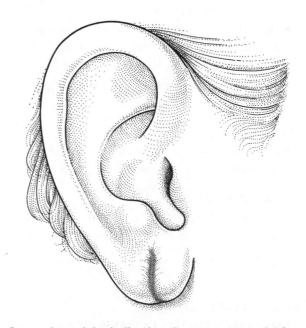

Crease in earlobe indicating the occurrence of AS. The deeper the crease, the worse the AS.

the front of the eye and examine the blood vessels at the back of the eye. Arteriosclerosis reflects the light more brightly and damaged arterial walls will show up like two shining railway tracks either side of a central core of blood flow.

Earlobe crease

Perhaps the easiest technique of assessing AS is by examining the earlobe. Many studies have shown and correlated the development of a crease running down the earlobe. The deeper the crease, the worse the AS. The development is created by clogging of the arteries to the ear. Anybody with a crease needs to take preventive action to avoid the almost inevitable development of AS.

Blood tests

A blood sample can be sent to the laboratory for assessment of total cholesterol, high-density lipoprotein (HDL) and low-density lipoprotein (LDL) levels. These can be correlated as mentioned below in the section on cholesterol, and a risk level obtained.

Doppler examination

The Doppler test is a non-invasive, sound-related investigation that tells the patency of arteries (*see* chapter 9).

Arteriograms

This invasive procedure carries a small risk and should only be used as a last resort; it is also important to bear in mind that the accuracy of this investigation has been questioned. *See* **Radiography** in chapter 8.

Risk factors

Cholesterol

Cholesterol levels are the highest risk. There are different types of cholesterol and their functions are discussed in chapter 7 (*see* **Cholesterol**). It is extremely important to read that part of the book.

Several factors are very relevant in AS with regard to maintaining lowered cholesterol levels. Refined sugars and all fried foods and saturated fats (*see* **Fats**) raise the LDL 'bad' cholesterol. Deficiencies in calcium, copper and chromium, as well as an excessive level of zinc in the bloodstream, can all create too much LDL and decrease the good HDL.

Remember that cholesterol will be drawn into any area of damage and the lower the levels of the LDL cholesterol the less likely that plaques will form. Although I discuss this in the cholesterol section, it is worth reiterating the importance of knowing whether one has good or bad cholesterol in abundance. The best measure of this is the total cholesterol: HDL ratio. This should be below 5 in males and below 4·4 in females. A high cholesterol level does not necessarily mean that an individual will have a problem.

Toxins

Any compound that may cause damage to the arterial wall must be considered a toxin and removed from the diet or lifestyle. The biggest risks are smoking and free radicals. Cigarettes contain over 3,000 chemicals, any of which may be responsible for damaging the inner lining of the arterial wall. Smoking also creates free radicals along with high fat, sugar and red meat diets. Anything that stresses the liver will prevent the breakdown of toxic substances so alcohol and drugs (prescribed and those of abuse) are all liable to predispose to AS.

A special mention needs to be made of coffee. Coffee has a direct effect on the liver as well as on the cholesterol levels. It is worth noting that tea does not have the same detrimental effect and therefore it is not only the caffeine but other compounds within coffee that cause the problem. Caffeine itself may not act directly but its effect on blood pressure may exacerbate the effects of AS.

The platelets

These specialized red blood cells are an important part of the blood clotting mechanism (*see* **Blood clots**). They have a structure that allows them to adhere to damaged tissue and they also release chemicals to attract 'healing' compounds such as white blood cells, scar tissue-forming cells and nutrients. Platelet stickiness is increased by a lack of vitamins B_6 and E, excess saturated fats or a lack of omega 3 and omega 6 oils, deficiency in the amino acid methionine (found predominantly in vegetable proteins) and deficiencies in the minerals magnesium and selenium.

Aspirin is known to decrease platelet stickiness and is therefore the orthodox world's choice of basic prevention of AS-related diseases such as stroke and heart attacks. The use of correct diet and naturopathic supplements are, probably, more effective than aspirin and carry a low risk of side effects (*see* **Diet** below).

Arterial muscle condition

The arteries have muscles within their walls that contract or relax depending upon neurological and hormonal instructions. Magnesium or calcium deficiencies will lead to poor muscular control thereby making the clogging of arteries more dangerous.

Exercise

Exercise increases HDL, encourages arterial dilation and thereby increases arterial patency (openness). A good exercise programme is extremely important in reducing the risks of AS.

Stress control

Many studies have shown that the endorphins released through meditation and relaxation techniques reduce cholesterol levels and increase arterial patency. A good meditation and relaxation program is essential for all of us but more so with AS.

Diet

The diet controls the amount of nutrients we absorb and, as can be seen from reading the above, many components can have a direct effect on AS.

The ideal diet for those at risk of AS or those who would like to avoid this condition developing is simply a vegetarian diet with oily fish such as herring, salmon, tuna and mackerel eaten four times a week. Vegetables carry fibre which binds with cholesterol in the gut, and also contain vegetable proteins that are known to lower cholesterol levels. Methionine is the best example. A compound called carnitine, manufactured in the liver, is made up from lysine found in lamb and poultry but is more prominent in vegetable proteins. Vitamin B_6, co-enzyme Q_{10}, beta-carotene (synthesized into vitamin A), chromium and selenium are all found along with calcium, copper and magnesium in most vegetables.

Onions, garlic and especially ginger act by decreasing platelet stickiness. The protein lecithin from soya beans binds with cholesterol in the gut and bloodstream. It is worth pointing out that eggs are often criticized for having high cholesterol levels. There is a rule in nature that insists upon balance and the white of an egg contains lecithin that binds with much of the cholesterol in the yolk, rendering eggs less dangerous than advertised. An occasional egg for anyone at risk from AS is not a big problem.

The oily fish contain the 'good' oils omega 3 and 6, as well as eicosapentrenoic acid. Vegetarians can find these in linseed and cold-pressed olive oil.

Water is the best fluid for reducing AS risks by diluting toxins but specific treatment may be obtained from the oriental green tea. A small amount of alcohol on a daily basis may be beneficial. Do not drink particularly sweet drinks and even fruit juices may be harmful if taken in excess. One pint of juice a day is an acceptable level but should be diluted down and taken in divided doses.

RECOMMENDATIONS

FOR AVOIDANCE OF AS
General Advice
• *Consider being assessed by a complementary medical practitioner on a yearly basis.*

- *Avoid all risk lifestyle factors such as smoking, heavy drinking, drug use and coffee.*
- *Establish a good exercise programme.*
- *Learn and practise a good meditation and relaxation technique.*

Nutritional

- *Consider the Ornish or Pritikin diets (see chapter 7).*
- *If at risk (or otherwise), consider a vegetarian diet supplemented with some oily fish and fowl. Avoid fried foods and red meat.*
- *Consider using the macrobiotic diet (see chapter 7).*

RECOMMENDATIONS

FOR THOSE WITH AS

General Advice

- *Follow the recommendations of avoidance above.*
- *Discuss the matter with an experienced complementary medical practitioner.*

Supplemental

- *Take the following in addition to a good diet. The doses prescribed are per foot of height and should be taken in divided doses throughout the day with food.*

Beta-carotene	2mg
Vitamin C	500mg
Vitamin E	100iu
Vitamin B_6	10mg
Methionine	200mg
Carnitine	200mg
Linseed oil	1 teaspoonful
Eicosapentaenoic acid	1g
Ginkgo Biloba	200mg
Lecithin	500mg
Cysteine or N-acetyl cysteine	50mg
Zinc	5mg
	(taken before bed)
Copper	0·5mg

These dosages should be considered for six months following an AS-related event such as a heart attack or stroke and then reduced to half the amount thereafter. I would encourage lifelong use.

Homeopathic

- *With the guidance of a practitioner, consider the homeopathic remedy Cratageus.*

Orthodox

- *Chelation therapy. This is described in chapter 9.*

ARTERITIS

Arteritis is the inflammation of an artery. It most commonly occurs in the temporal arteries at the side of the forehead and is an extremely dangerous condition.

Temporal arteritis can occur as a sudden pain or one of gradual onset. It is very severe, unrelenting and rarely affected by mild painkillers. The temples may or may not be sensitive to touch. This condition is associated with arterial supply to the eyes and brain and if not suppressed can lead to blindness or death.

RECOMMENDATIONS

General Advice

- *Any suggestion of symptoms as described above, go immediately to an emergency department. They may recommend steroids – take them.*
- *Once the condition is under the care of an orthodox physician refer yourself to a cranial osteopath and naturopathic physician.*

AUTOIMMUNE DISEASE

Autoimmune disease is the term used when the immune system turns on the body itself. Through complex and poorly understood biochemical mechanisms, the immune system recognizes its own body parts. When foreign matter enters the system the immune system recognizes it as being alien and destroys it. The reasons why this recognition system fails are not well understood. The Eastern philosophy considers the immune system to be overburdened by defending against infections, food allergies and pollutants, and certain body tissues get caught up in the battle.

Principally the immune system recognizes its own and foreign proteins and the introduction of these into the system can trigger a self-attack response. Viruses, bacteria, drugs and pollutants all fall into this category. The most common autoimmune diseases are rheumatoid arthritis and systemic lupus erythematosus (SLE).

Autoimmune disorder is a complex matter and signifies the failure of the immune system after prolonged ill-health, even if it has been symptom free. Autoimmune disease can be very serious and even fatal. Most cases, however, are treatable with complementary and orthodox therapies and many are self-limiting, lasting only a few years.

RECOMMENDATIONS

General Advice

- *Consult a complementary medical practitioner with a knowledge in homeopathy, herbal medicine and nutrition. All these areas must be reviewed.*
- *Any lifestyle habits such as smoking that are clearly polluting the body should be avoided.*
- *Please refer to any specific condition in this book.*

Nutritional

- *Any foods that are known to cause reactions should be eliminated and food allergy testing can be of great benefit.*

Systemic lupus erythematosus (SLE)

This condition, commonly termed Lupus, is a surprisingly common autoimmune disease. The orthodox world is uncertain of its cause but most complementary practitioners with experience in this field would consider it to be an aggressive over-sensitivity by the body's immune system as a whole, and the underlying reasons that cause it may be multiple.

One study has linked the Epstein-Barr virus to the condition.

Systemic lupus erythematosus is characterized by inflammation of any tissue in the body and is often referred to as a 'mimicker'. The condition must be suspected in any persisting joint pain, fever and general malaise but is often associated with a 'butterfly' rash, which shows as a red lesion covering the forehead and cheeks (the wings of a butterfly). The rash may cover the entire body and may be associated with any number of symptoms.

Diagnosis is generally made after other conditions are excluded, and there are specific blood tests that show positive in over 90 per cent of cases.

Orthodox treatment is steroids, pain relief and drugs aimed at any of the multitide of symptoms that may appear. The complementary medical world must look at any autoimmune disease, as discussed in the section above, but special attention must be paid to diet, food intolerance/allergy, stress levels and environmental toxins, all of which can trigger an overreactive immune system.

RECOMMENDATIONS

General Advice

- *This is a condition that should be treated by an experienced complementary medical therapist, who should coordinate treatment with a homeopath, herbalist and nutritionist.*
- *Stress management through counselling or meditation teaching is a prerequisite.*
- *Do not smoke.*
- *Rule out a leaky gut using an intestinal permeability test.*
- *See **Arthritis** for relief of pain if relevant.*

Nutritional

- *Avoid vegetables in the nightshade (solanum) family, such as tomatoes, potatoes and peppers.*

Supplemental

- *Pain associated with SLE may be due to a magnesium deficiency. This should be checked by a blood test for intracellular magnesium, and replenished if the test is positive.*

- Take 1gm of omega 3 essential oils with each meal.
- Consider using DHEA at the maximum dose recommended on the packet.

Herbal/natural extracts
- The Ayurvedic technique of drinking the first morning urine may be of benefit, although techniques of extracting the sediment from the urine and taking this in drop form (somewhat more appealing) may be available through an experienced complementary medical practitioner.
- The roots and stem of a plant called Tripterygium wilfordi at a dose of 10–15g three times a day was shown to be effective in a study reported in China. The side effects of abdominal discomfort, nausea and loss of menstruation in women all disappeared after a few days of treatment or within six months of stopping.

BLEEDING
See Haemorrhage

Bleeding from trauma
Loss of blood is pathological in all instances. Bleeding from cuts and trauma needs to be controlled as soon as possible. The arteries have an inbuilt spasm mechanism should an artery be cut. Interestingly, the cleaner the cut (ie the less trauma to the vessel), the less the constrictive response. The more traumatic the injury, the more spasm is likely. This accounts for the fact that a swift cut with a knife will bleed more than an amputation.

RECOMMENDATIONS

General Advice
- If an injury does not stop bleeding in 10–15min then seek medical attention. This should be sought sooner if blood loss is heavy or in children as they have less blood in the body.
- Apply compression to the wound and only consider constriction of a bleeding vessel above the site of the injury if medical attention is close at hand and compression itself is not working. Occlusion of an artery can cause permanent damage to a limb within half an hour.
- Do not attempt to stitch a wound without medical supervision except in extreme circumstances.

Homeopathic
- Arnica 6, four pills every 10min is a master remedy.

Bleeding from areas other than the skin
Bleeding from an orifice such as the anus, penis, vagina or from sensory organs such as the eyes, ears and nose is *always* pathological except for a female's period.

RECOMMENDATIONS

General Advice
- Such bleeding must be investigated by a medically qualified professional.

Homeopathic
- Sudden onset of bleeding can be treated with Aconite 6, four pills every 10min, slower but persistent bleeding noticed over 24hr can be treated with Phosphorus 30 every hour until medical advice is sought.

Internal bleeding
Injuries such as road traffic accidents or trauma with a blunt instrument can cause bleeding inside the body. Diagnosis can only be made by experienced medical personnel but the signs to look for are:

- Dizziness, visual disturbance and headaches for head injuries.
- Pain, dizziness and difficulty in breathing for chest injuries.
- Pain, nausea and vomiting and bloating for abdominal trauma.

Anybody who faints after receiving a blow from a blunt instrument must be rushed to an emergency room.

BONE MARROW DISORDERS

The bone marrow found predominantly in the long bones (arms and legs) and the sternum (chest bone) is responsible for the production of the blood cells. Those that we all know about, the red blood cells (erythrocytes) and the white blood cells (leucocytes), are manufactured along with others including the platelets – a modified type of red blood cell very important in the mechanism of blood clotting.

The bone marrow function can fail in one of two ways. It may cease to produce any of these cells or it may produce too many of them. Specific conditions such as polycythemia rubra vera (increase in red blood cells and, usually, white blood cells) and thrombocythemia or thrombocytosis are conditions marked by an absolute increase in the number of platelets (throbocytes is the medical name for platelets). Thrombocytopenia is a lack of platelets.

Excessive production of white blood cells in the bone marrow form myeloid leukaemias which are covered in their own section.

Certain drugs, radiation and viral infections are all associated with bone marrow disorders but who will succumb to this group of disorders is not known. There may be some genetic predisposition, but these problems tend not to run in families.

I have a theory. Stress releases adrenaline and cortisol which are the stress chemicals (*see* **Stress**). To counteract this, the body will try to make calming chemicals such as serotonin. The platelets are cells that contain and release serotonin when the body is under stress. I hypothesize that at certain levels of stress the platelet–serotonin release function may increase and the body may be tempted to make more platelets due to some chemical response. If the stress is persistent this mechanism may trigger a permanent effect leading to thrombocytosis. If the stress persists, perhaps the controlling chemical may run out, therefore the stimulation to make platelets may be reduced leading to thrombocytopenia. These are rare conditions and I have only treated a few cases, but in each there has been a noticeable stress-related time period prior to the condition forming.

The condition is often found only on routine blood test but may also be discovered because of symptoms related to clotting difficulties. Unexplained bruising and bleeding or conditions such as stroke may occur because of excessive clotting.

drugs, radiation or surgical treatments. Look at the alternatives which may reduce the amount or the level of intervention.

CANCER

Before I discuss cancer and its treatment from a holistic point of view, I would like to discuss exactly what it is and some of the salient facts.

Cancer cells have three characteristics:

- They are cells in the body that have lost their growth regulatory system. Each cell of the body contains chromosomes, which divide to form other cells. Part of these chromosomes are known as telomeres. Each time a cell divides, some of these telomeres are cleaved off and once their number falls below a certain level the cell can no longer multiply. In cancer cells these telomeres are not cleaved.
- Cancer cells infiltrate adjacent tissue and this differentiates them from benign tumours.
- Cancer cells can spread through the lymphatic or blood system. These are known as metastases.

The causes of cancer

The orthodox world has few treatable causes of cancer but does accept that the following are relevant:

- Poor nutrition and excess calorific intake in childhood.
- Genetic factors.
- Infections – probably by viruses. Those known to cause problems are the human papilloma virus, hepatitis B virus, certain herpes viruses and HIV.
- Chemical compounds – such as asbestos, metals, hydrocarbons, chemicals known as olefins in solvents, *N*-nitroso compounds in tobacco smoke, certain natural substances such as aflatoxins (mould that grows on foods, especially stale grains).

- Deficiencies – specifically vitamins A, C and E, the mineral selenium and dietary fibre.
- Radiation – ultraviolet, gamma and X-ray.
- Persistent irritation.
- Defects in the immune system.
- Age – due to a natural failing of cell division.
- Psychological causes. It is known, for example, that women are more likely to develop breast cancer if they have had a serious shock, such as a bereavement or divorce within the previous two years.

The Holistic world accepts all of the above causes but also considers the possibility of parasitic infection, persistent food allergy/intolerance, the possible carcinogenic affects of food preservatives, additives and organophosphates used as crop sprays, and certain amino acid deficiencies, in particular methionine and cysteine. Whilst psychological shocks have been established, the complementary medical world looks at longstanding suppression of emotion or stress to be potentially capable of causing cancer.

Staging of cancer

The medical world has tried to simplify passing information from one physician to another by creating a clinical classification of tumours. The most commonly used classification is the TNM system.

T (stands for tumour size)
T – primary tumour
Tis – carcinoma *in situ* (confined to an area)
T0 – no evidence of a primary tumour
T1–4 – an arbitrary description of the local size
Tx – location and size unknown

N stands for lymph node involvement
N – regional lymph nodes involved
N0 – no evidence of regional lymph node involvement
N1–4 – arbitrary differentiation of the number of lymph nodes involved
Nx – cannot be assessed

M stands for metastases

M – distant metastases

M0 – no evidence of distant metastases

M1 – distant metastases present

Mx – cannot be assessed

Certain tumours have their own terminology, such as stage or grade, that generally can be thought to substitute for T and N as described above.

Prognosis

One of the big questions that anybody is faced with when dealing with a cancer is the chance of cure or surviving the disease. It is difficult nowadays to assess the outcome of patients who are not treated because anybody with a cancer is generally subject to orthodox treatment. What is more, the orthodox world does not seem to differentiate for the lay-person the difference between 'cure' and five-year survival rate. The table below shows this survival rate as published by the American Cancer Society. I was unable to locate comparable figures for cases before modern intervention came into play but statistics suggest that in the last 30 years there has been little if any change in the overall cure rate despite aggressive intervention.

Site of malignancy	5-year survival rate
Pancreas	3%
Bronchi (lung tubes)	13%
Leukaemia (all sorts)	34%
Ovary	48%
Ear, nose and throat	52%
Colon and rectum	52%
Cervix	67%
Prostate	70%
Breast	75%
Urinary bladder	75%
Melanoma	80%
Uterus	85%
Testes	87%

The orthodox world does not ask why certain people do less well than others but I am convinced that it is to do with the individual and their immune system rather than the cancer itself.

Cancer is a chronic condition that arises because of a multitude of factors ranging, as I have mentioned above, from genetic to environmental. Orthodox treatment against cancer takes strides forward every day but the majority of cases still end up with poorer results than they should because complementary treatments are not considered.

There are thousands of reports of spontaneous regression and alternative cures for cancer. Many of these have scientific validation and are not in common or orthodox use simply, but sadly, because trials are not completed due to financial and political considerations. Also, the necessity to stand up to double-blind placebo-controlled studies is not, and will never be, an acceptable method of testing for alternative treatments. This does not mean that they are not effective or in common use – as the art of surgery shows. No surgical technique has ever been proven double-blind in a study.

Treatment

Working against cancer requires the consideration of six different areas:

- Establishing and removing the cause
- The use of orthodox treatment
- The activation of the immune system
- Psychological and spiritual aspects
- Dietetics and nutrition
- Alternative anticancer treatments

Establishing and removing the cause

Some cancers have a clear cause. Lung cancer and smoking, bowel cancer and low-fibre diets and skin cancers with excessive exposure to the sun are examples. Many cancers are being shown to have a genetic predisposition and I am sure that over the next decade genetic reasons and answers will be found to fight cancer. At the moment a hereditary trait puts most cancers beyond our control.

The use of complementary diagnostic techniques (*see* chapter 8) in association with orthodox screening techniques should be used to clarify an individual's health on a regular basis, and also to establish the origin of the tumour. The cause of cancer can range from psychological and stress-related causes to food intolerance and environmental pollutants. The need to look at an individual holistically and consider their mind, body and soul is clearly as relevant in this disease as in all chronic illnesses. The orthodox world is advancing at an enormous speed as far as diagnostic capabilities go. The advent of computers with X-rays, magnetic resonance imaging (MRI) and other visualizing techniques can pinpoint down to a millilitre the location of a tumour buried deep in the body. Unfortunately, none of the billions of dollars that is spent on diagnostic research appears to go towards predicting or forecasting the development of cancer. The smallest of masses may be isolated once formed, but we seem unable to predict where or when this might happen. However, there is hope.

Over the last 50 years research has gone into proving that the body contains energy channels that can be measured using sensitive electromagnetic transmitters and receivers. These basic machines have now been developed into sophisticated computers known as bioresonance computers. These machines are capable of measuring the normal flow of energy through an individual and can differentiate any irregularity in the system. Cancer cells have a particular resonance that will differ from normal tissue and this can be measured.

A simple blood test, known currently as the Humoral Pathological Laboratory Test, examines a dried drop under a high-powered microscope and compares what is seen with samples of known conditions or samples taken from people who have gone on to develop certain conditions. Blood changes rapidly and is extremely sensitive to deficiencies and toxins and can therefore, theoretically, predict the presence of a cancerous tendency. For example, red and white blood cells behave in a particular way in the presence of free radicals: negative ions that can trigger cancerous changes in the nuclei (the brain centre) of cells.

It is becoming clear that chemicals within our food chain, often placed there through crop spraying or actively injecting livestock, can cause cancer within our system. A recent study showed over 12 cancer-causing compounds in a basic three-course – prawn cocktail, meat and two veg and pudding – meal provided in a popular chain restaurant. Removing these chemicals from the body may not be easy but homeopathic principles may work alongside detoxification diets.

There is some evidence that food allergy may be relevant to certain tumours and possibly, by inference, all cancer. Establishing food allergy response is essential in all chronic conditions but especially in cancer because correct dietetics may be curative (*see* **Dietetics and nutrition** *overleaf*).

All the above investigations are becoming more available and are discussed more fully in the chapter on 'Alternative Therapies' (chapter 9).

The use of orthodox techniques

Orthodox medicine has come a long way in the treatment of cancer and should rarely be discounted in a holistic treatment course. The surgeon's knife is curative and chemotherapy and radiation treatments are improving constantly. The side effects of these treatments continue to be a problem and orthodox treatments are often toxic to the system. Full and frank discussions in consultation with medically qualified orthodox practitioners and thereafter alternative practitioners with experience or specialization in the treatment of cancer are essential. Very often an attempted cure may be pointless or even worse than the disease. It is arguable that a slow-growing tumour in someone elderly should be left alone because the body will wear out before the cancer can affect it. Complementary treatments to prepare the body for these procedures, treatments to speed healing after surgical and radiation damage and the correct alternative therapies to protect the

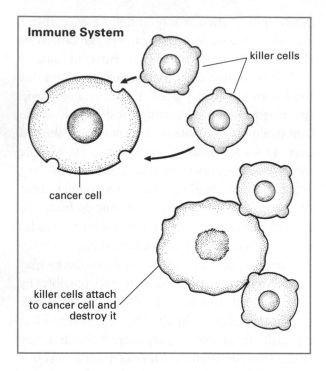

Immune System

killer cells

cancer cell

killer cells attach
to cancer cell and
destroy it

body from the toxic effects are all essential.

The orthodox world is experimenting to find a vaccine for cancer and whilst the possibility is not close at hand, I believe this to be a very important area of research.

Activation of the immune system

Cancer may be created and certainly proliferates due to a failure of the individual immune system. The body has specific anticancer cells named 'killer' cells and produces chemicals that act as antioxidants to remove the free radicals that cause or promote cancer cell growth. Cancer is the proliferation of a particular type of cell. This means that the normal multiplication rate has been lost and the cell is replicating too fast. There are certain genes called telomeres that are cleaved off each time a cell multiplies. When all these have been removed the cell can no longer multiply and eventually dies. In cancer this cleavage does not occur. The reasons for this, I am sure, will soon be illuminated by science. Whatever the cause, the fundamental energy that keeps these cells healthy is absent and part of the body's defence mechanism has gone wrong. This too

needs to be corrected and working on this energy plane is as important a part of supporting the immune system as promoting the effects of the killer cells.

Psychological and spiritual aspects

The field of psychoneuroimmunology has recently come to prominence. The ability of the psyche to affect the neurones (the nerve cells), which in turn send out chemicals to the entire central nervous system, is well established. This affects all parts of the body, including the immune system, and stimulates other areas that are essential for dealing with illness or maintaining health. Breast cancer has now been correlated with sudden emotional shocks and the holistic consensus of opinion is that tension, stress and anxiety over a long term can also create cancer.

There are many examples of prayer curing cancer and whether a religious or purely a spiritual attitude is concentrated upon, this is an area that must not be overlooked in dealing with the fight. The use of antistress techniques, counselling, hypnotherapy, visualization and meditation techniques must all have a place in the treatment of cancer.

Dietetics and nutrition

There is much evidence to support the use of strict dietetics in both preventing and hampering the growth of tumours. Some researchers have shown, although not to double-blind scientific levels, that diet may cure cancer. I believe that dietetics have an important role to play alongside most other forms of treatment. The best known anticancer regimes are based on the works of the physician Max Gerson in the early part of the twentieth century and the philosophy of the macrobiotic diet. A review of individual nutrition is mandatory in the treatment of cancer.

Alternative anticancer treatments

There are a myriad of claims and much anecdotal evidence supporting alternative medical treatments. I have read books, spoken to their authors, worked with healers and been involved with patients, all of whom have an answer to cancer. There are many potential cures out there presently being destroyed by the advance of humankind into tropical rainforests with the associated destruction of dozens of curative plants each day. Of treatments that are available and discussed, the following should be reviewed by the individual with a complementary specialist and should not be taken without a full understanding of their 'unproven' effects. They are, however, not toxic if taken as recommended, which cannot be said for orthodox regimes.

High-dose antioxidant therapy (AOT)

There is much high-level scientific research and study done on the effects of antioxidants on cancer. Antioxidants are vitamin-based molecules that neutralize negatively charged particles found in the bloodstream known as free radicals. These free radicals cause changes in normal cells to allow cancer to develop. There is scientific proof that antioxidants can prevent the development of cancer and research is ongoing to confirm studies that suggest that AOT is potentially curative.

In advanced cases, those patients undergoing radiation or chemotherapy, those patients due for or recovering from surgery and any patients who are found to have high levels of free radicals will possibly be recommended to have initial treatment by intravenous administration of antioxidants.

The complementary medical world expects negative press that is encouraged, if not funded, by the pharmaceutical industry regarding the use of antioxidant therapy in cancer. An example was a well-publicized study suggesting that vitamins A and E made smoking-related lung cancer worse. It is easy to pick holes in the study but perhaps smokers with lung cancer should avoid vitamins A and E for the moment. Watch this space. Personally, I suspect that beta-carotene (as opposed to vitamin A) and D-alphatocopherol (natural vitamin E) as opposed to DL-alphatocopherol (synthetic vitamin E), as was used in the study, would show different results.

IP-6 (Inositol hexaphosphate)

This is a vitamin-like derivative best taken in concentrated form. It is extracted from brown rice, which is high in the B group vitamin inositol. IP-6 stops cellular reproduction. The dosage is around 80mg per kg of body weight taken in divided doses three times a day.

Native legend tea (Essiac)

Essiac is a combination of herbs used as a basic 'tea' by the Ojibway Indians in North America. Doctors noted that the number of cancer cases in the tribe were far below those expected and did some basic studies on the Essiac tea. No acceptable scientific studies have been performed on Essiac and the evidence is purely anecdotal at this time. It is worth noting, however, that a highly esteemed and established physician who looked after the Kennedy family has written a letter endorsing this product based on the evidence to date.

MGN-3 (arabinoxlan)

Research carried out in Japan on a reportedly large number of patients with a variety of cancers has highlighted the possible benefits of this rice bran extract. Its action is to stimulate specific parts of the immune system, especially the killer cells (T-cells) that attack tumour cells.

Mushrooms

There is considerable evidence that mushrooms originating from Chinese medicine, such as Maitaki, Cordyceps sinensis and Coriolus, have efficacy in dealing with the stimulation of the immune system and should be considered as part of a holistic/integrated treatment once interreaction with other therapies has been excluded. More research is required but some of the scientific evidence is very encouraging.

Naltrexone

This drug has been approved for use at doses of 50mg for maintaining withdrawal of addicts to heroin or opium, but it may be beneficial in this and other conditions at doses of 3mg nightly. This unlicensed treatment has undergone initial studies and may be a treatment in tumours such as lymphoma, lymphocytic leukaemia, Hodgkin's disease and cancers of the prostate, rectum and pancreas. Its method of action is uncertain although it is known that it increases the body's natural opiates, endorphins, by briefly blocking endorphin receptors giving the body the impression that it is deficient. Endorphins increase immune system function. Other than some sleeping difficulties, side effects have not been noted. This compound should not be taken through pregnancy or if the individual is using morphine or codeine as a painkiller.

Iscador

Iscador is a mistletoe extract and this has had a lot of research performed on it, with some considerable success, via the Cancer Research Society in Switzerland. It is administered by injection, sometimes as frequently as daily, depending on each individual case. Iscador may be taken orally but this is not as effective.

Ukrain

Ukrain is an extract from the celandine plant. It has been shown over the last 15 years to have an anticancer effect. Attempts to organize trials have been ongoing for 15 years under a medical professor in Vienna, Austria. Scientific evidence is strong and case histories have been very promising.

Ukrain is administered intravenously (it can be given intramuscularly but is painful) at least twice a week. This may be inconvenient, although your GP or a local physician could be asked to administer the compound but very often orthodox practitioners are resistant to unlicensed therapy even though they are entitled to administer it. The cost of Ukrain is also prohibitive.

Hydrazine sulphate

This is an extract from rocket fuel that was initially found (goodness knows how!) to be beneficial for patients who were cachectic (losing weight). Cachexia is a prominent feature in many cancer cases and through experimentation on cachectic-cancer cases there has been a suggestion that hydrazine sulphate may have an anticancer effect. The compound comes in easy-to-take capsules and is considered in any case where weight loss is relevant.

Shark cartilage

There are at least three proteins found in shark cartilage, all of which have weak anticancer effects due to the inhibition of the development of new blood capillaries needed to feed a fast-growing tumour. When put together, the effects seem to be enhanced and multi-centre trials are currently under way. The Federal Drugs Administration (FDA) have approved shark cartilage for second-level trials, which is a considerable achievement for any naturopathic compound. Early trials have been very encouraging. On average, a patient needs to take around 1g of this powdery, fish-tasting compound per kg of their own body weight. Treatment is divided into three doses per day. This is not easy to take, which is a slight disadvantage.

Chelation, hydrogen peroxide, ozone and chelox therapy

There is some evidence to support the use of a compound called ethylene diaminetetraacetic acid (EDTA) and the use of hydrogen peroxide or ozone in treating cancer.

Chelox is a combination of EDTA, oxygen therapy and high-dose vitamin/antioxidant therapy administered intravenously.

Bioresonance techniques

Forty years of practitioner experience has shown that passing small electromagnetic waves transmitted by healthy cells into cancerous tissue can prevent cancer growth and even act in breaking the cancer cells down. There is poorly documented scientific evidence but impressive amounts of anecdotal evidence. This treatment requires a visit to a bioresonance practitioner on a weekly basis and is non-invasive and easy to apply.

Other treatments

There are several other potential treatments, the most well-known being an extract from almond called Laetrile, which showed remarkable results in the hands of the alternative practitioners who initially used it over 40 years ago. The governments and pharmaceutical industries removed this as well as other potential products from the market. The reason was not the poor efficacy or the dangers of the compound, but the lack of substantial evidence through scientific trials. These were only unavailable because governments and the pharmaceutical industry would not pour the necessary millions of dollars into the research as the compounds are natural and therefore cannot be patented. The finding of a simple, naturopathic cure for cancer or, for that matter, any disease process would cost the pharmaceutical industry billions of dollars. These billions, that are received and circulated through universities, laboratories, government departments and pharmaceutical employees make it largely undesirable for a cure to be found. When confronted by:

- a pharmaceutically backed clinical laboratory asking for funds for research;
- a trial on a manufactured compound that has much evidence to support its efficacy; or
- a single physician who has worked on a compound in his garden shed;

where would you distribute the millions of dollars collected from the well-caring public? We are, at this point, at an impasse when dealing with the funding of cancer research.

CARDIOPULMONARY RESUSCITATION (CPR, ARTIFICIAL RESPIRATION)

All adults should know the technique of CPR. Thousands of lives a year could be saved if oxygen is fed into the blood and the heart is kept

Artificial Respiration

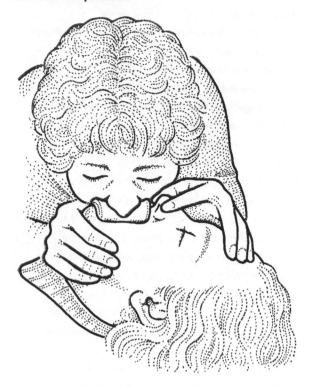

The first aspect is to remember ABC – Airway, Breathing, Circulation.

General Advice

- *Ensure that the airway is clear. Pushing with one hand on the jaw muscles will open the mouth. With your other hand push one finger to the back of the throat and ensure that there are no obstructions. Look as well. Remove false teeth.*
- *Place the patient flat on the ground. Tip the chin upwards, which will automatically open the mouth and straighten the trachea (the airway tube).*
- *Place a handkerchief or piece of material over the patient's mouth. Clamp your mouth over the patient's mouth through the material.*
- *Take a deep breath and breathe into the patient's mouth, holding the chin up with one hand and with your other hand on their forehead.*
- *Look at the chest to see that it is rising. If it is not, double check that there is no obstruction in the upper airway.*
- *Perform this twice before commencing cardiac massage.*
- *Cardiac massage. Place yourself on your knees next to the patient. Place one hand on the sternum (breast bone) and the other hand on top of the first. Rocking forward and applying firm downward pressure, imagine compressing the sternum onto the heart lying below. Successful cardiac massage may result in broken ribs. This is not a pleasant sensation or sound but is an indication that the massage is efficient. Judgement is required because you do not want to push too hard for fear of pushing a rib into the lungs.*
- *Repeat this five times before repeating the breathing technique.*
- *Carry on until the emergency services arrive or the patient starts to breathe spontaneously.*
- *It is important to stop occasionally to check for a carotid pulse or chest movements. Cardiopulmonary resuscitation is not beneficial if the heart is beating and breathing is occurring.*

pumping whilst awaiting emergency services.

It is important not to move anyone who has been involved in an accident because of possible damage to the spine and neck. However, if there is no pulse or respiratory movement the patient will need to be moved. The first step, therefore, is to establish whether breathing is occurring and the heart is beating.

- Watch the chest. If there is no movement, place your ear by the nose and mouth and listen. The mirror test (placing a mirror or glass by the nose and mouth to see if it mists) is an ancient but effective technique.
- To establish if the heart is beating place two fingers, index and third, on the patient's Adam's apple and push gently but firmly to one or the other side. The carotid artery is easily felt pulsating below your fingers. You can also try the pulse in the wrist which is found less easily one inch (2cm) up the arm from the wrist on the side of the thumb.

I recommend that everybody take a first-aid course and practise this technique on a dummy. Do not practise this technique on patients who do not have an arrested heart or breathing.

CHOLESTEROL, HIGH – *see* Cholesterol

DEEP VEIN THROMBOSIS (DVT)

Deep vein thrombosis is most commonly associated with the formation of a blood clot in the lower legs and is characterized by pain in the calf. Simply put, deep vein thrombosis can occur in any deep-lying vein. Most commonly found in the calf, they also appear elsewhere in the legs, pelvis and abdomen.

Deep vein thrombosis is a dangerous condition due to the not infrequent movement of the clot from the site of origin through the larger blood vessels to the heart. From the heart, these clots are pumped into the lungs causing a blockage and a pulmonary embolism.

The characteristics of DVT are localized pain, swelling and discomfort caused by an inability of blood to pass the blockage and associated redness. These symptoms must be taken to your doctor and treated as an emergency if there is any suggestion of a chest pain or shortness of breath.

Deep vein thrombosis is often associated with superficial varicose veins although clots in this area are not dangerous because they are unlikely to travel into the larger veins leading to the heart. Any conditions thickening the blood (including dehydration) and any condition that may block the venous blood flow such as pregnancy, injury, obesity or oestrogen drugs (found in the oral contraceptive pill and HRT) may predispose to DVT. Individuals who are restricted by sedentary jobs, driving, air travel or those confined to wheel-chairs may also compromise the blood flow from the legs and therefore be predisposed to DVT. Anyone in this group should be wary of any characteristic symptoms and bring them to the attention of a doctor immediately.

RECOMMENDATIONS

General Advice

- *The possibility of a DVT should be treated as a medical emergency, reviewed by a doctor and if necessary treated in the acute phase with anticoagulants such as heparin or warfarin.*
- *Establish the most probable cause and discuss this with a complementary medical practitioner with experience in this condition. Homeopathy, herbal medicine and dietetics are all beneficial.*
- *Establish a good exercise regime to encourage blood flow generally.*
- *Consider regular massage or Shiatsu as part of your lifestyle.*
- *Ensure that you drink 4–6 pints of water per day.*

Homeopathic

- *In an acute situation, whilst awaiting the doctor's opinion, use the homeopathic remedy Lachesis 6 every 15min.*

DIZZINESS, GIDDINESS AND VERTIGO

In common parlance these three words are often taken to be synonymous but medically speaking the difference in symptoms between the three definitions following is very useful to the practitioner trying to isolate the cause.

- Giddiness is an unpleasant situation of losing one's relationship to surrounding objects.
- Vertigo actually reflects the sensation that the world is revolving about oneself (objective vertigo) or that one is moving in space, although one knows that one is stationary (subjective vertigo).
- Dizziness is a mixture both of combining a difficulty in relating to objects, as well as feelings of rotation or whirling. Very often weakness, faintness and unsteadiness is associated.

Depending on your symptoms, an experienced practitioner or doctor will be able to isolate whether the problem is occurring because of sensory input (vision or problems with the pressure receptors in the feet if standing) or motor control (loss of control of the body through nervous or muscular uncoordination). The other reason that dizziness, etc may occur is because of problems in perception actually within the central nervous system or brain. The causes can be as serious as brain tumours and other space-occupying lesions, or less serious such as low blood sugar not providing the brain with enough energy.

Dizziness, giddiness and vertigo may be initial symptoms of the presentation of atherosclerosis causing clogging of the arteries and therefore reducing the blood supply and oxygen to parts of the brain. The intake of any drugs or specific food allergens may also affect the perception of the brain, sensory input or motor control of the body. Except when an obvious cause has created dizziness, such symptoms should be reviewed by a doctor.

Eastern philosophies consider dizziness to be a deficiency in being 'earthed' or an excess of space/air. Treatment is therefore based on centring or earthing the body and, according to the Chinese, nourishing or working on the stomach meridian is useful.

RECOMMENDATIONS

General Advice

- *For any persistence of dizziness please visit a doctor. The practitioner will need to check your sugar levels through your blood and urine and if examination does not reveal anything may suggest further investigations such as computed axial tomography (CAT or CT scans) of the brain to rule out anything nasty. Follow through with these investigations as treatment is dependent upon accurate diagnosis.*
- *Once a diagnosis has been established, review the situation with a complementary medical practitioner.*
- *In an acute situation try drinking a small glass of fruit juice, water and some non-refined*

carbohydrate such as a slice of wholegrain bread. (This will raise blood sugar and feed the stomach meridian.)

- *Pressure can be applied to stomach meridian points; the most well used is stomach 36, situated four fingers widths below the knee cap in a small dent found on the shin bone. Apply gentle pressure for about 2min at least.*
- *When the cause of the sensations has been isolated, such as hypoglycaemia and arteriosclerosis, please refer to the relevant section in this book.*

Nutritional

- *Avoid alcohol, caffeine or refined sugars.*

Homeopathic

- *The following homeopathic remedies may be of benefit if taken at potency 6 every 15min until the problem relieves itself or medical attention is sought. Kali carbonicum if worse for movement or concentrating on something or if the individual is better in the open air or by an open window; Conium maculatum – if symptoms are worse for lying down; Gelsemium – if the dizziness is associated with weakness and feeling shaky.*

EMBOLISM

Embolism is the medical term for the occlusion of a blood vessel by matter that is foreign to the bloodstream, such as a blood clot, air, tumour, fat, bacteria or a foreign body that may have entered the bloodstream through an injury.

Symptoms of an embolism depend upon the size and position of the artery that has been occluded. The body forms small clots constantly which are destroyed by the anticlotting mechanism in the bloodstream and specific white blood cells that attack any foreign matter. Occlusion of small vessels will, therefore, go completely unnoticed.

An embolism that obstructs a major artery can lead to a stroke if it is in the brain, a heart attack if a cardiac artery is obstructed or neurological symptoms such as pins and needles, numbness and coldness if the artery that is blocked is supplying a limb or digit. Occlusion of a bowel artery or other internal organ may give sudden and severe symptoms.

One of the main causes of embolism comes from deep vein thrombosis (*see* **Deep vein thrombosis**) and dislocation of a clot from the deep leg veins can lead to the more serious complication described below.

Pulmonary embolism

A commonly heard term is that of pulmonary embolism, where a clot, very often following an operation in the lower part of the body, such as a hip replacement, dislodges and blocks the artery to the lung. This blockage prevents blood from reaching the lung tissue, resulting in poor oxygenation and a major stress on the heart. Symptoms of sudden breathlessness and chest pain, a bloody cough and faintness or fear following an operative procedure or trauma that has affected the lower part of the body should all warn of the possibility of a pulmonary embolism.

RECOMMENDATIONS

General Advice

- *Any symptoms resembling an embolism must be treated as a medical emergency and reviewed at the nearest hospital.*
- *Decoagulation with drugs and possibly even operative procedures may be required and these should be followed through without hesitation.*
- *Vitamin E, certain herbal preparations and relevant dietetic changes, especially increasing water intake, should all be discussed with a complementary medical practitioner as soon as any emergency has passed.*

Homeopathic

- *The homeopathic snake remedies Bothrops and Lachesis, potency 6, can be taken every 15min en route to the hospital.*

FLUID RETENTION

Fluid retention (oedema) describes an excess of fluid in the tissues caused by an incorrect leakage from the blood vessels, especially the capillaries. Fluid in the body exists in three compartments. In the cells (intracellular), in the tissues (interstitial) and in the blood vessels. There is constant interchange between these three compartments and they are all 'fed' by fluid taken in from the bowel.

The balance is maintained by osmosis (where water molecules follow larger molecules through blood vessel and cell walls) and by chemical messengers that increase or decrease the size of the pores in the blood vessels and cell walls.

There are many reasons why fluid will build up in the interstitial compartment but in principle this is either because protein leaks from the capillaries pulling water with it or the fluid cannot enter the cells because of a protective fat/protein layer that is laid down around the cells. Specific areas of the body may become oedematous because of a blockage in the drainage system (the lymph system), which can occur through infections causing elephantiasis, trauma or tumour.

Many conditions affect capillary permeability but hormone imbalance is one of the most common. Low thyroid levels and imbalance between oestrogen and progesterone and hormones produced by the kidneys and nervous system all affect the size of blood vessels and their permeability. Water is attracted into tissues by osmosis. Osmosis is a physiological reaction caused by molecular electromagnetic attraction that, put simply, pulls water through a membrane until there are equal numbers of water molecules either side. A similar situation will occur if there is a lack of sodium or potassium and other electrolytes and minerals within the bloodstream. Excess salt or sugar in the tissues will pull water into them, as will toxins. This latter process is an attempt by the body to dilute down the potentially poisonous effects.

Simple back-pressure caused by obstruction to venous flow or heart failure will literally force fluid through the capillary pores. Symptoms of oedema or water retention are dependent upon where the fluid has settled. The biggest complaint is about water that settles in the ankles and lower legs, hands and fingers, around the face and jaw and the midriff. The more serious places for oedema to occur are within the vital organs such as the brain and lungs. The latter two are associated with medical complications and need urgent attention.

Fluid in the lower limbs is often associated with venous obstruction and is commonly found in pregnancy and obesity. More serious conditions such as heart failure and diseases of the liver (through which the main vein of the body – the vena cava – passes) causes back-pressure and forces fluids into the tissues.

More generalized oedema is often noted with hormonal fluctuation and pre-menstrual syndrome is notorious for having this as one of its most awkward symptoms. Shoes become tight to wear, and rings obstruct circulation to the fingers.

Dietary deficiencies will lead to poor electrolyte, amino acid and mineral content, allowing water to move cosmetically into the tissues and a food allergy may create a toxic state within the tissues that causes water to be pulled in for dilution. Other toxins such as alcohol and its breakdown product aldehyde, cigarette by-products and other drugs of abuse may all cause a toxic state requiring dilution as well as creating a chemical effect directly on the permeability of the capillaries. Orthodox drugs may well induce oedema for the same reason.

One of the major causes of water retention that is commonly overlooked is, paradoxically, dehydration (*see* **Dehydration**). Although it is not immediately obvious why not drinking enough water may cause an excess of water in the tissues, the mechanism is simple. If not enough water is ingested, the individual cells in the body recognize dehydration. They attract fluid into themselves and when replete will surround their outer walls with a waterproof lipid/protein protection. This cover is generally a cholesterol-based compound manufactured in the liver and is a cause for raised cholesterol levels in the bloodstream.

Despite the cells being hydrated and therefore normal metabolic function progressing without illness forming, the body will recognize the dehydration and give instructions to hold water in the system because there is not enough. The bloodstream will provide fluid to the body tissues, particularly to the fat stores, thereby creating oedema and the midriff effect so commonly associated with PMS. This leaves the bloodstream concentrated, triggering further reflex water retention.

Another less respected cause of water retention is the build-up of toxins in the system. The body will often hold water to dilute poisons that may be found in the interstitial and cellular compartments, thereby rendering the concentration less dangerous. The characteristic bloating often found after drinking or abusing drugs is caused by a combination of dehydration and toxic build-up.

RECOMMENDATIONS

General Advice

- *It is important to rule out underlying hormonal or biochemical changes that may be due to conditions such as hypothyroidism and diabetes. Diseases of the heart, liver and kidney, the former two leading to venous back-pressure and the latter to electrolyte disturbance, all need to be ruled out.*
- *Review any drug prescription via the doctor who prescribed in case one of its side effects is water retention. This may need to be changed or removed.*
- *Drink plenty of water. As described above, the mechanism is paradoxical but the more water that is drunk, the less the retention is maintained. Normal input should be half a pint per foot of height at the least but in cases of water retention this should be doubled. Water intake may need to be restricted in cases of fluid retention caused by heart, liver or kidney problems. Discuss this with your practitioner.*
- *Any retentive disorder (one that forms lumps, bumps or cysts) including water retention may be a bodily reflection of a mental or spiritual attitude.*

Water retention associated with depression or an inability to express is literally 'holding it in' and it is necessary to confront these emotions. Counselling is invaluable in water retention that does not seem to have an underlying physical illness associated with it or does not respond to the naturopathic recommendations above.

Nutritional

- *Review the diet. Restrict salt and processed foods, which are inevitably high in sodium content.*
- *Consider testing for food allergies. Whether this is required may be established by using a Detox diet or fast for three days, ensuring adequate water intake. If an improvement occurs, food allergy is probable.*

Supplemental

- *Water retention associated with the hormonal cycle may benefit from vitamin B_6 (20mg per foot of height divided into two doses) taken with breakfast and supper.*

Homeopathic

- *The homeopathic remedy Natrum muriaticum 30 taken four times a day for five days may shift the problem and can be repeated up to twice a month.*

Herbal/natural extracts

- *Herbal treatments such as Uva ursi, Herberus and Juniper can be utilized but should be considered as a drug or a diuretic and should be prescribed by a herbalist rather than taken off the shelf.*

GEOPATHIC STRESS

The earth carries magnetic and electrical fields and lines that travel in different directions depending on an area's relation to the North and South poles. The movement of water, the position of the sun and the moon and 'man-made' electrical power stations all affect this natural electromagnetic status.

The human body is known to have electro-magnetic energy travelling through its system from both an orthodox point of view as well as that of Eastern philosophies, which conclude that all health is created through these meridians or channels.

The subject of geopathic stress is enormous and is poorly documented, although there is much evidence of disease and illness being created through interfering with these lines.

RECOMMENDATIONS

General Advice
- *See* **Feng Shui.**
- *See* **Radiation.**

GIGANTISM (ACROMEGALY)

This is a chronic disease due to excessive secretion of growth hormone by the pituitary gland. It causes overgrowth of bone and tissues but has a particular effect on the hands, feet, face and head. It is a rare condition and does not particularly jeopardize longevity although specific problems caused by moving an excessively large frame around may be apparent as muscular strains, including that on the heart muscle.

RECOMMENDATIONS

General Advice
- *The reason for excess production needs to be eliminated. Consult an endocrinologist.*
- *Complementary treatment is dependent upon any particular problems associated with acromegaly.*

THE GLANDS
(The Endocrine System)

Glands are a special type of tissue that produce chemicals that travel through the bloodstream and affect cells in other parts of the body. These chemicals are called hormones and they are extremely potent, being produced in very small amounts but having profound effects. The true meaning of gland is 'tissue that secretes hormones' but the term is also used for tissues that secrete products that travel locally.

ADRENAL GLANDS

These sit on top of the kidneys and are divided into two parts: the outer cortex, which makes steroids, and the inner medulla, which produces adrenaline in response to nervous control from the central nervous system. Some consider the adrenal glands to be governed by an energy meridian called, in Chinese medicine, the 'triple heater', and the adrenal glands in turn govern the *pitta* or fire energy in Ayurvedic beliefs.

Stress, both physical and psychological, will drain the adrenal glands of energy, leading to biochemical–chemical imbalances caused by poor steroid production as well as general malaise and tiredness from the lack of adrenaline. Tumours may arise in all glands but the most common in the adrenal glands is phaeochromocytoma, which is a tumour of the adrenal medulla that causes an excess of adrenaline, which in turn can cause rapid heart rate, a rise in blood pressure, weight loss and sweating. This is a serious condition that mimics hypothyroidism and requires immediate medical attention and probably surgery.

BARTHOLIN'S GLANDS

These are not truly glands because they do not secrete a hormone. They are small amounts of tissue found in the labia on either side of the vagina that secrete a lubricating and cleansing fluid. A blockage in the duct from these so-called glands leads to Bartholin's cysts (*see* **Bartholin's Cysts**).

LYMPHATIC GLANDS

In the truest sense of the word, these are not strictly glands. They are a mesh of protein found in the lymphatic system. After the goodness from blood has left the blood vessels and fed the tissues, it is collected with waste product in the lymphatic system and drained, through a complex of vessels that match the arteries and veins for quantity and length, before going back to the bloodstream in the chest. Along the way the lymph, which will be carrying bacteria, viruses and any other foreign matter, will pass through lymph glands. Caught in the meshwork are white blood cells, which devour the foreign matter and break it down before releasing it back into the lymph flow.

These glands can swell in the presence of infection and this is generally a good sign, showing that the body's defence mechanism is active. Unfortunately if the body is overreacting or out of control, such as in leukaemia or lymphoma, the numbers of white blood cells increase, get trapped in the lymph glands and these swell excessively.

Cancer can also drain from its primary site into lymph glands, which then harbour the cancer cells which help to prevent their spread around the body. Temporary swelling in the lymph glands in association with an obvious infection can, and should, be left alone but any persistence or pain within glands should be reviewed by a health practitioner.

PARATHYROID GLANDS

These small glands are found in the middle of the thyroid tissue in the neck. They are responsible for the balance of calcium and thereby magnesium in the body tissues.

Problems with the parathyroid glands are a potentially serious medical condition and are often found by routine blood screening showing incorrect levels of calcium. Any persistent swelling in the neck should be reviewed by a physician (*see* **Thyroid**).

PAROTID GLAND

This gland is found at the side of the face in front of the ears and overlying the jaw joint. It is a salivary gland with a tube passing down the side of the cheeks to a small opening. The parotid gland produces saliva, helping digestion and cleanliness of the mouth.

The parotid gland is surrounded by a tight

Endocrine System

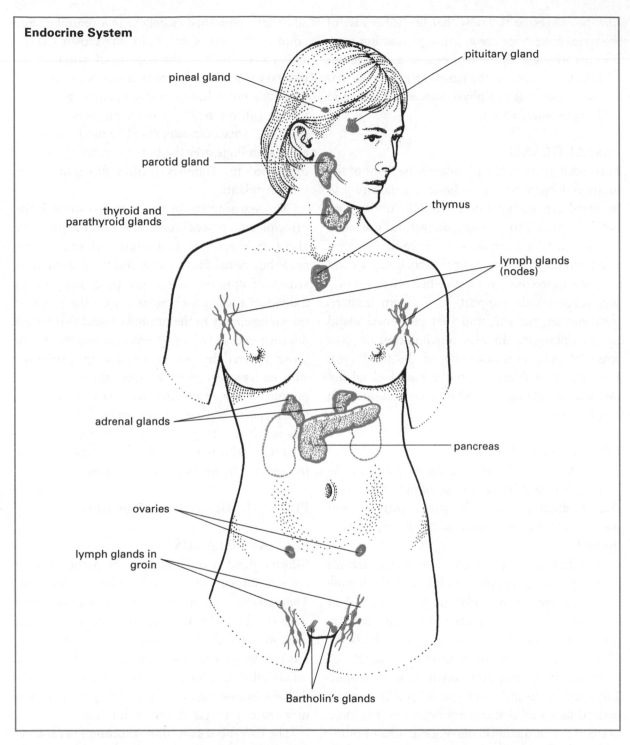

pineal gland

pituitary gland

parotid gland

thyroid and parathyroid glands

thymus

lymph glands (nodes)

adrenal glands

pancreas

ovaries

lymph glands in groin

Bartholin's glands

capsule and infection or inflammation that causes swelling can be very painful and should be treated urgently. Tumours in the parotid gland are not uncommon and may be dangerous if left unattended. Stones may form in the parotid duct,

leading to a blockage and swelling. This too needs to be attended to swiftly.

If anyone has occasionally noticed a sharp but transient pain in the side of the cheeks when putting anything sour or tart in the mouth, they may be interested to know that this is because of the immediate response of saliva production from the parotid gland, which causes a restriction within the muscles of the parotid gland tubes that is like a cramp. It is a physiological response and nothing to worry about.

PINEAL GLAND

This small gland is found towards the front of the brain and corresponds in Eastern philosophy to the third eye. Its function is not fully understood but it is known to produce the natural hormone melatonin, which controls our circadian rhythm and sleep pattern. There is probably some control over our mood and, as I notice that science slowly but surely finds support for ancient Eastern philosophies, we will find that the pineal gland has something to do with our intuition or sixth sense (thereby corresponding to the third eye). Diseases or problems with the pineal gland are rare and usually only found on investigations such as CT scans.

PITUITARY GLAND

This is probably the most complex gland in the body. It is found in the middle of the brain tissue and is divided into two parts, anterior and posterior, that control most of the other glands in the body.

The hormones produced control the thyroid gland, growth (especially in children), the female hormonal cycle and ovulation, water content in the body, steroid production from the adrenal glands and other functions throughout the body. This walnut-sized gland may cause a variety of problems if it does not function as it should. Tumours of the pituitary gland initially may be noticed as visual disturbance because it sits close to the route of the optic nerve. Diagnosis of pituitary malfunction requires a physician's expertise, although many minor problems may be associated with the pituitary gland and its relevance to Eastern medical philosophy.

I find it fascinating and not coincidental that all Eastern philosophies believe in a central energy point at the top of the head, the crown chakra. This corresponds to the superficial point of the pituitary gland. It is interesting that for over 5,000 years this point has been documented as being a master control point of the entire system. This belief has since been supported by modern science and its findings over the last 100 years as we have unravelled the complex control function of the pituitary gland.

Not well accepted by the orthodox world is the principle of a psychological effect on the pituitary gland. It is accepted that stress and anxiety can cause hormonal fluctuations and the holistic consensus of opinion is that the psychology of an individual produces chemicals from the brain or transmits energy to the pituitary gland that have a negative effect. The most obvious symptoms are those suffered by young females, in particular, who under pressure may throw their cycle. The pituitary has a connection to a part of the brain that registers and recognizes smell and it may be this sensitivity to pheromones (airborne chemicals) that induces a coinciding of hormonal cycles in women who live in close proximity.

PROSTATE GLAND – *see* Prostatitis

SALIVARY GLANDS

Salivary glands (which include the parotid gland) are distributed around and under the jaw line. They produce saliva, which contains enzymes to start the breakdown of food, fluid to moisten what we eat and different types of immunoglobulins to help protect and clean the mouth. Saliva is mildly alkaline which accounts for its extra production in association with gastric problems that may cause an excess of acid production.

The control of salivation is through neurological reflexes and some neurological problems, such as motorneurone disease and tumours of the salivary gland, can produce excess salivation. It is necessary to bring to the attention of a physician any persistent excess salivation or pain in the soft

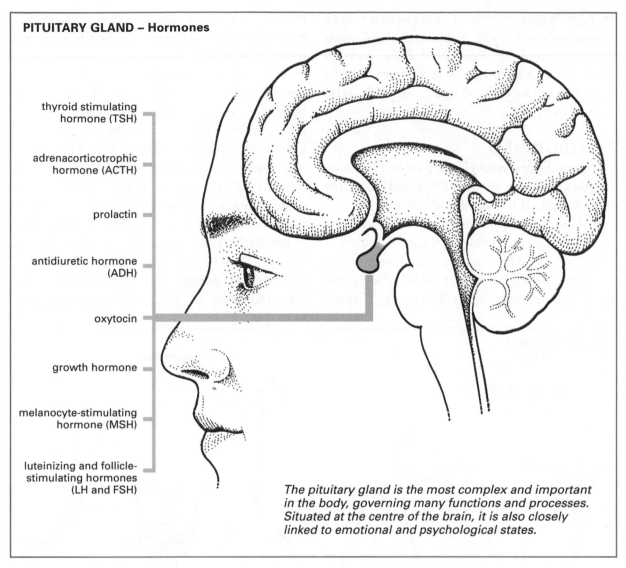

PITUITARY GLAND – Hormones

thyroid stimulating hormone (TSH)

adrenacorticotrophic hormone (ACTH)

prolactin

antidiuretic hormone (ADH)

oxytocin

growth hormone

melanocyte-stimulating hormone (MSH)

luteinizing and follicle-stimulating hormones (LH and FSH)

The pituitary gland is the most complex and important in the body, governing many functions and processes. Situated at the centre of the brain, it is also closely linked to emotional and psychological states.

tissues underneath the jaw line. A dry mouth may be caused by disease of these glands or a stone in the duct (*see* **Saliva**).

SEBACEOUS GLANDS

Sebaceous glands are found in the skin and produce sebum, which is the characteristic moistening and protective compound necessary for healthy skin. Excess sebum production leads to oily skin, and blockages in the ducts from these microscopic glands can be the cause of pimples, acne and sebaceous cysts (*see* the relevant sections).

There are rare genetic conditions that prevent the sebaceous glands from functioning, leading to

persistent dry skin open to infection. Dehydration may affect the constituency of sebum and the function of sebaceous glands and this needs to be corrected by increased intake of water (*see* **Skin**).

THYMUS GLAND

This small amount of tissue is found behind the sternum (breast bone) and is responsible for the production of T-cells. These T-cells are a vital part of the body's white blood cell immune system.

Problems with the thymus gland are rare although it corresponds with the heart chakra and therefore is influenced by the emotional state of an individual. A recent hypothesis suggests that the thymus gland may store parasites that may be released on contact with petrochemical pollutants in the atmosphere. Release of these parasites causes destruction of the T-cells, which may be instrumental in the ill-health of HIV/AIDS patients (*see* **AIDS**).

THYROID GLAND

The thyroid gland is an H-shaped structure about the size of a palm situated along and under the Adam's apple. It is made up of cells that are concerned with the synthesis of thyroid hormones, the most prominent being thyroxine (T_4) and Tri-iodothyronine (T_3). These are both made up from iodine and the amino acid, tyrosine. (The thyroid gland also contains a small amount of tissue known as the parathyroid, which produces a hormone called calcitonin that controls calcium levels in the body.)

The thyroid hormones are responsible for regulating the metabolism of cells throughout the body. The amounts in the body are controlled by a chemical released from the pituitary gland known as thyroid-stimulating hormone (TSH). This itself is controlled by another hormone called TSH-Releasing Hormone (TRH), which comes from a part of the brain known as the hypothalamus. This is a prime example of a biofeedback mechanism. An increase in the level of thyroid hormones depresses the production of TRH, which is not available to stimulate the production of TSH, which, thereby, does

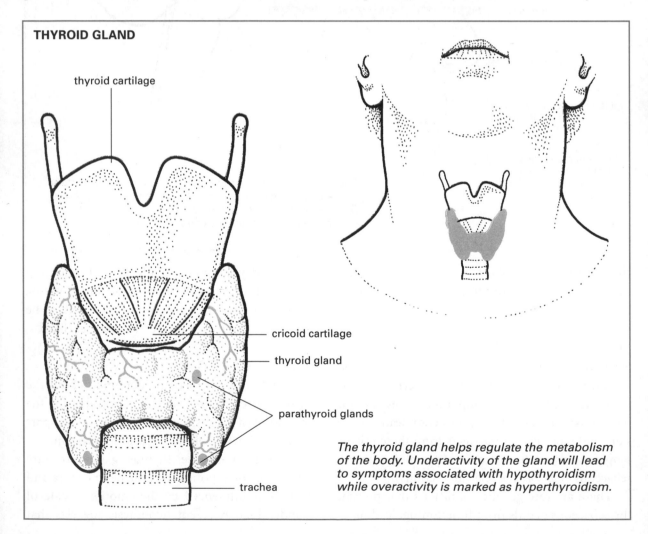

THYROID GLAND

thyroid cartilage

cricoid cartilage

thyroid gland

parathyroid glands

trachea

The thyroid gland helps regulate the metabolism of the body. Underactivity of the gland will lead to symptoms associated with hypothyroidism while overactivity is marked as hyperthyroidism.

not stimulate the thyroid gland unless T_3 and T_4 are made. This cycle attempts to maintain a constant level of circulating hormone within a suitable range.

Blood tests are now freely available but the normal ranges are only guidelines. For example one laboratory has a normal range of 44–143nmol/l. Somebody with a figure of 50nmol/l would therefore be considered normal. If that individual should, however, have a level around 120 then they are, in reality, hypothyroid.

High or low figures should not be considered by themselves. It is better to evaluate thyroid status by measuring the basal body temperature (BBT), which gives us some indication of the metabolic rate of the cells of the system. This, in combination with the blood tests and symptoms of hypo- or hyperthyroidism, provides a much better guideline. Individuals may have T_3 or T_4 levels in the low part of the normal range and be considered 'euthyroid' (normal for thyroid function), but in reality their levels should be, say, 120. The orthodox medical world would consider the thyroid to be functioning normally but in fact the person is considerably hypothyroid.

Basal body temperature (BBT)

To measure the BBT, place a thermometer beside your bed before sleeping and then, first thing on awakening, place the thermometer under the tongue whilst remaining in bed for at least 5 minutes. It is best to repeat this test on ten successive days and take the average temperature. Normal body temperature is between 97.6°F (36.4°C) and 98.2°F (36.7°C).

A BBT below the norm in association with thyroxine levels in the lower half of the normal range is much more indicative of a hypothyroid state than just a blood figure. Numbers at the other end of the scale may indicate hyperthyroidism.

I have described elsewhere in this book the principle of the vessel of conception described by Chinese acupuncturists. If you refer to that section (see **Vessel of conception**) you will see that the thyroid may well be controlled not only by hormones from the pituitary and hypothalamus but also by a direct energy flow. Problems, either biochemical or energetic, with these parts of the brain may therefore strongly influence the entire body by affecting the thyroid.

GOITRE

A goitre is the term used for *any* enlargement of the thyroid gland.

Goitre is therefore the definition of a symptom similar to jaundice rather than a condition itself. A cancer or inflamed thyroid may show up as a goitre. Bacterial infections causing an acute thyroiditis are very uncommon but a viral infection such as mumps is a little more frequent. These are known as subacute thyroiditis and generally present as a tender thyroid with severe pains throughout the neck.

A goitre can be described as non-toxic or toxic. A toxic goitre is a swelling associated with hyperthroidism, discussed in that section.

A non-toxic goitre is caused by the thyroid gland enlarging in an attempt to trap more iodine to make more thyroxine. This occurs in people who are not taking enough iodine into their system through diet or who have a glandular defect (see **Hypothyroidism**).

The goitre in hypothyroidism, therefore, tends to be diffuse with an equal growth throughout the gland. Hyperthyroidism may exhibit a diffuse growth but also appears in a uninodular or multinodular pattern. Frequently a rumble may be heard if the gland is listened to through a stethoscope because of the increased vascularity.

Most goitres are asymptomatic (without symptoms) but, if they grow too much, local pressure effects may be noted, particularly a tightness around the neck, a persistent irritation of the throat or a change in voice due to pressure on the vocal cords.

Physiological goitres may occur at puberty and pregnancy. This is due to the influence of oestrogen and progesterone.

General Advice

- *Any swelling in the neck should be reviewed by a physician for a firm diagnosis. This may include investigations via ultrasound and blood tests.*
- *Please refer to the relevant sections on hypo- or hyperthyroidism depending upon the cause or effect of the goitre.*

GRAVES' DISEASE

Named after an Irish physician in the early 19th century, this disease is characterized by a diffuse swelling of the thyroid gland, known as a goitre, and a bulging of the eyes, known as exophthalmos. The cause of the disease is unknown, although it tends to be hereditary and most commonly affects women. The thyroid gland is overactive and symptoms of hyperthyroidism are prominent; the condition has a specific symptom of circumscribed lesions under the skin over the shinbone (this is known as pretibial myxoedema).

General Advice

- *Any suggestion of a swelling in the neck or development of bulging eyes with or without symptoms of sweating, palpitations, weight loss, insomnia or overactivity should be reviewed by a doctor to check that hyperthyroidism is not the diagnosis.*
- *See* **Hyperthyroidism**.

HYPERTHYROIDISM

The symptoms of hyperthyroidism are principally:

Weight loss	Heat intolerance
Increased sweating	Warm and moist skin
Shortness of breath	Palpitations
Tachycardia	Flushing
Increased blood pressure	Irregular heart beat
Weakness	Tiredness
Anxiety	Irritability
Insomnia	Occasional psychosis
Tremor	Diarrhoea
Irregular periods	Miscarriages

Left untreated, a characteristic bulging of the eyes known as exophthalmos develops and is known as Graves' disease (*see* **Graves' disease**). The causes of hyperthyroidism are little understood. The thyroid gland becomes overprotective throughout the tissue, through multiple nodules or occasionally a single 'hot' nodule. Frequently a chemical known as long-acting thyroid stimulator (LATS) is found in the system. This is an immunoglobulin and is being produced somewhere, for some reason, by the body's immune system. It may well be in response to some other factor and its effect on the thyroid is purely a side effect. A group of antibodies known as the thyroid-stimulating antibodies (TSAbs) can be demonstrated in the serum of thyroid-toxic patients and these seem to attack the receptors in the thyroid for THS, thereby stimulating the activity and causing the thyroid to produce too much T_3 and T_4. There is some suggestion that there is an autoimmune (the body attacks itself) stimulus, but holistic physicians look more at toxicity, potentially parasitic or fungal infection of the thyroid, food allergy and vital force imbalance then at the vessel of conception or mid-line chakra points.

Naturopathic treatment is remarkably ineffective against hyperthyroidism in my experience. Severe hyperthyroidism is a potentially swift lethal condition and needs to be treated with the appropriate respect. Mild hyperthyroidism may respond to naturopathic treatment but all cases must be monitored carefully.

General Advice

- *Establish a baseline of thyroxine levels in comparison to the BBT. If very high, do not hesitate to follow orthodox treatment; if only just outside the normal scale, monitor the situation frequently and pay attention to the worsening of any symptoms.*

Nutritional

- *Add goitrogens (foods that inhibit thyroxine production) to the diet by increasing the intake of broccoli, cabbage, turnips, spinach and collard greens, Brussels sprouts, soya products, peanuts, pine nuts and millet.*

Homeopathic

- *The homeopathic remedy Thyroidinium 200, one dose nightly for one week.*
- *Specific symptoms may be relieved by a correctly selected homeopathic remedy. A homeopath should be consulted.*

Herbal/natural extracts

- *Try the following herbal tinctures in divided doses three times a day: lycopus, five drops per foot of height; cactus, five drops per foot of height.*

HYPOTHYROIDISM

The thyroid hormones affect all the being. The symptoms of hypothyroidism may be seen in any part of the body and should be considered if one of the following symptoms appears, persists and in combination with any two or more others.

Depression	Insomnia
Anxiety	Poor concentration
Loss of memory	Numbness or tingling
Dizzy spells	Carpal tunnel
Poor vision,	syndrome
especially at night	Weight gain
Fatigue	Sensitivity to the cold
Water retention	Hoarse voice
Slow speech	Abnormal rhythms
Slow heart beat	Increased number of
Palpitations	cold symptoms
Constipation	Decreased appetite

Irregular periods	Infertility or
Absent periods	miscarriages
Dry skin	Muscle cramps
Hair loss (notably	Brittle hair
eyebrows)	Ridged nails
Irritability	

There are also other less common symptoms.

If left uncontrolled, the above symptoms will continue and a condition known as myxoedema may develop. This term is derived from the deposition of a fatty material around the body that causes an oedema-like swelling all over the body. If myxoedema is profound then a coma may be the outcome, associated with very low body temperature and damage to other organs through low oxygen supplies.

Hypothyroidism may be divided into primary or secondary.

Primary hypothyroidism

In primary hypothyroidism there is a failure of the thyroid to develop and if severe or not spotted will lead to a marked inability known as cretinism. There are many causes.

- Iodine deficiency – which occurs in specific parts of the world where iodine is not in the food chain to any great extent. Seafood in particular is high in iodine and mountainous areas that may not consider fish as part of their regular diet are more prone to iodine deficiency. Damage to the thyroid by foods known as goitrogens, which contain substances that prevent the utilization of iodine, is another cause. This list includes soya bean, peanuts, millet, turnips, cabbage and mustard. It is worth noting that cooking usually inactivates goitrogens.
- The stress hormone, cortisol, is known to block the production of T_3.
- Rarely, thyroid levels may be normal (or even raised) but symptoms of hypothyroidism continue. This may be due to the cells of the body not recognizing thyroid hormone. Metal

toxicity may be relevant in this condition.

- Destruction of normal thyroid glandular tissue by tumours, operations or radioiodine. The latter two are more frequent because these are common treatments for hyperthyroidism.
- Autoimmune thyroiditis (Hashimoto's disease) most commonly affects middle-aged women and is due to antibodies being formed against different constituents of the thyroid gland. Simply, the body attacks its own thyroid.
- Drug-induced hypothyroidism may be caused by certain prescribed drugs including those used for heart arrhythmias, some tranquillizers, anti-epileptic drugs and others.

Secondary hypothyroidism

Secondary hypothyroidism is created by reduced TRH or TSH caused by afflictions of the pituitary gland by the hypothalamus.

The treatment for hypothyroidism is generally replacement with thyroxine, which replenishes the blood levels but does not attempt to isolate or treat the cause. Holistic practitioners may try to restimulate the thyroid once they have removed any possible underlying causes of hypothyroidism but may have to resort to thyroxine replacement because restimulation is frequently not achieved. The following recommendations should be tried for a short time and thyroid function tests and symptom assessment should be made very objectively. Many patients are reluctant to consider having to use a 'drug' for the rest of their lives but need to be reminded that it is simply a replacement of what the body naturally produces. Complete natural thyroid is available although the pharmaceutical form is much purer and a physician knows exactly how much is being given.

RECOMMENDATIONS

General Advice

- *Rule out any changeable cause of hypothyroidism such as iodine deficiency or drug-induced deficiency.*
- *Practise a relaxation or meditation technique*

regularly and sit with a counsellor to discuss and attempt to resolve underlying stress-creating conditions.
- *Check mercury, lead and other chemical contamination through blood and hair samples and treat accordingly (see **Poisoning**).*
- *Acupuncture can be used to try to stimulate the thyroid.*
- *Yoga or Qi Gong should be used because exercise may stimulate thyroid production and the techniques move the energy through the chakras thereby potentially relieving blocks or deficiencies in the throat chakra, that overlies the thyroid.*

Nutritional

- *Remove the goitrogens mentioned above from the diet.*
- *Check for nutritional deficiencies, specifically tyrosine (the amino acid), iodine, zinc, copper, iron and selenium, all of which are necessary for thyroid function.*

Supplemental

- *Add the following nutrients into your diet regardless of blood results because the system may simply need more thyroxine to function normally. The following should be taken with breakfast at the recommended dosage per foot of height: iodine (50µg), selenium (50µg), copper (500µg) and tyrosine (100mg); and zinc (5mg per foot of height) should be taken before bed.*

Orthodox

- *Thyroxine replacement through orthodox preparations should be used if symptoms of hypothyroidism are troublesome. The above recommendations may still stimulate the thyroid and brain centres regardless of the presence of thyroxine in the bloodstream. Taking thyroxine will diminish symptoms swiftly.*
- *Desiccated natural thyroid can be used, although I see no advantage. Whichever is taken, ensure that blood levels and BBT are taken every three weeks until normality is achieved and symptoms have regressed.*

TUMOUR AND CANCERS OF THE THYROID

Single or multiple benign growths in the thyroid are common and frequent in areas where iodine intake is low. These are harmless and have no greater tendency to become cancerous than normal thyroid tissue.

Cancer of the thyroid should be suspected in any thyroid with a single nodule. Initial testing is done by scanning the gland after administration of radioactive iodine. Overactive thyroid tissue will pick this up and is termed a 'hot' nodule. This may be an indication simply of an overactive area of the thyroid and nothing more than a hyperthyroid state, but it can also indicate cancer. Benign nodules do not pick up the radioiodine to any great extent and are known as 'cold' nodules.

RECOMMENDATIONS

General Advice

- *Any swelling in the throat must be examined by a physician.*
- *Do not avoid investigation of thyroid nodules because early detection increases the chances of a better outcome.*
- *Treatment of a goitre is dependent upon the cause and the associated symptoms.*
- *Do not shirk from investigation for fear of a bad result because most goitres are innocent and easily proven so.*

Orthodox

- *A 'hot' nodule may need a biopsy or even a lumpectomy and this should be undertaken, usually under general anaesthetic, with your permission to remove the thyroid if cancer is found.*

HAEMORRHAGE – *see* Bleeding

The term haemorrhage is generally reserved for a serious bleed and not the inevitable scratches and cuts obtained in the garden and kitchen.

Haemorrhages that occur through trauma may be external or internal, the latter being more serious as symptoms may not appear immediately. A fractured femur (thigh bone) can cause severe blood loss and yet show no signs of swelling because of the powerful sheath around the leg muscles. A ruptured spleen or liver can bleed into the abdominal cavity which will be painful if the patient is conscious but may not show if the patient is not.

Bleeding from specific areas such as the nose, ears or bladder should be reviewed in the specific sections in this book.

RECOMMENDATIONS

General Advice

- *Any trauma or injury, especially of the head, must be reviewed by a doctor to rule out the possibility of internal bleeding.*
- *External bleeding should have firm compression over the area that is bleeding. Do not tie a ligature around a limb unless compression is not preventing the bleeding or an amputation has occurred. Even then ensure that the ligature is loosened every 15min to allow profusion of the tissues above the serious injury. Send someone for or obtain medical assistance as soon as possible.*

Homeopathic

- *Homeopathic remedies Arnica 6 and Phosphorus 6 should be alternated every 10min until medical advice is obtained.*

HAIR

Hair is an evolutionary remnant of our ape ancestry. Intended to keep us warm and protected from the elements, the use of protective clothes encouraged natural selection to remove our fur. Hair has remained on our heads, our armpits and groins in greater abundance. That on the scalp I can understand as a protective factor, but armpits and groins … ? If anybody knows, do please write in with the answer!

Hair is principally made of keratin, which is a protein, and may accurately be described as a 'dead' material. However, the follicle from which

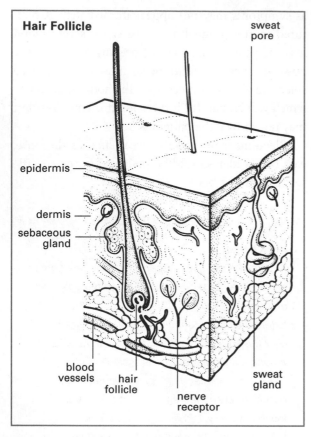

Hair Follicle

sweat pore

epidermis

dermis

sebaceous gland

blood vessels

hair follicle

nerve receptor

sweat gland

the hair grows is very much alive and is considered by complementary practitioners to be a useful eliminatory cell and the hair itself to be a reflection of health. Many conditions, such as hypothyroidism, will be reflected by dry, brittle hair and hyperthyroidism may actually cause hair to fall. Some less well-proven food allergies/intolerance tests examine the hair for molecules of food that have become enmeshed with the keratin structure in the belief that the follicle will remove toxins or compounds less well tolerated by the body, which can therefore be measured.

Most cultures consider the hair to be an adornment worthy of spending much time keeping it attractive. This is an important factor in 'mate' selection and care of the hair should be looked upon as a necessity, not a vanity.

Care of the hair and the scalp

Medicated hair products detract from the ability of the scalp to maintain its hair in good condition.

If you look at the hair of healthy children you will see that very little needs to be done if the individual is in good health.

The hair follicles and sweat glands act as elimination organs and the more toxins in the system the more the hair will contain debris and the more the sweat will coat the hair with poisons. Dehydration, excess fats, refined foods, additives and preservatives will all take the shine and gloss out of the hair.

The hair itself is dependent upon the production of a protein called keratin which demands an amino acid supply in the diet. The easier the protein is to digest and break down the easier it is for hair to be formed. Therefore amino acids from vegetable proteins and light meat (fish, chicken) will be better for the hair.

Remember that the skin absorbs compounds, albeit at a slow rate, and the highly vascular scalp is an effective route of entry for compounds into the body. Certain plant extracts are less toxic than chemicals and will adhere to the hair just as efficiently. The more natural the hair product, the less likely it is to create a toxic environment in the system. The scalp in which the hair follicles live is a very active part of the skin surface. Sweat, sebum and hair are constantly produced and diseases of the scalp, which include dandruff and alopecia, are best prevented rather than treated. Stress will affect the condition of the hair. When under pressure or stressed, the body produces more adrenaline, which cuts down the blood supply to the skin in order to provide more oxygen and nutrients to essential organs for a fight-or-flight reaction. This 10 per cent reduction in blood flow may not be noticeable but will cut down the nutrient and oxygen supply to the hair follicle, sweat and sebum glands and thereby diminish the amount of essential nutrients reaching the hair follicle.

RECOMMENDATIONS

General Advice

• *Do not wash the hair more frequently than is*

necessary. If your hair is losing its lustre or appearing dirty every day, then reflect on your diet, not your hair products. Daily washing removes the natural oils, which in turn diminishes the quality and condition of the hair.

- *Do not use medicated shampoos. Shampoos with plant extract such of jojoba are perfectly safe and just as beneficial as most chemical additives.*
- *Hair that is dry may benefit from a weekly application of olive oil and lemon juice. Mix one tablespoon of olive oil with one teaspoon of lemon juice and apply until all the hair is covered. Leave this on for 15min and then wash off with a natural shampoo. Dry hair generally suggests dehydration (see **Dehydration**).*
- *Avoid medicated conditioners, again using natural products instead.*
- *Scalp massage either by oneself, a professional or a partner will encourage blood flow and, potentially, promote healthy hair.*
- *Meditation or relaxation techniques are an essential aspect of healthy-looking hair in those who are stressed or under pressure.*
- *Persisting lacklustre hair may be a reflection of poor diet or underlying ill-health. A trichologist and/or a complementary medical practitioner should be consulted.*

Supplemental

- *A multimineral supplement may be beneficial if hair growth is slow.*

Grey hair

There are several hypotheses for the physiological reaction that allows hair to grey, but in principle the colour of hair is genetically predisposed and is to do with the way light reflects off the protein structure in the hair rather than any additive to the hair matrix. Grey hair is often found to run in families although the Eastern philosophies believe that grey hair is an indication of a lack of fundamental energy, especially when associated with youth (premature greying). There is no doubt that shock (an excess of adrenaline) can cause the hair to grey and persistent pressure or stress (persistent production of adrenaline) will encourage greying. The mechanism is described in the section above on care of hair.

RECOMMENDATIONS

General Advice

- *Be proud of your hair colour rather than fighting it.*
- *Reduce stress and alter lifestyle to avoid persistent pressure.*
- *Correct diet and mineral supplementation may affect hair colour.*
- *Hair dyes should not be used because the products will be absorbed to some extent by the scalp, but if the use is considered necessary then try to obtain as natural a product as possible.*

Hair dyes

Changing the colour of the hair stems from an evolutionary need to camouflage or attract attention, either for courting purposes or making the appearance more aggressive before going into battle. The latter use is not so much required any more although the brightly coloured hair of some younger people may be making a form of social statement!

Dyes will be absorbed to some extent by the highly vascular scalp and may create a toxic reaction, major or minor, within the system.

RECOMMENDATIONS

General Advice

- *Use only the most natural of hair colourants because the body will deal with natural herbs much better than artificial chemicals.*
- *Medically speaking, avoid hair dyes. Be comfortable with yourself and possibly consider sitting with a counsellor if you have a strong need to appear as that which you are not.*

Hair loss

About one in three women report hair loss. We all lose some hair naturally each day and the amount varies from person to person, depending on the type of hair, external heat and nutritional factors. It becomes relevant when an individual notices more loss than previously or when they or their hairdresser recognizes thinning. There are 100,000–350,000 hair follicles on the human scalp and they tend to grow hair for about three years before resting for about three months. Some people have a short growing phase of about 600 days while others can be longer than 1,000 days. Most people follow the average but this can vary. This is why a regular haircut is sometimes needed but at other times can be delayed for a couple of weeks.

Evenly distributed hair loss is known as 'chronic telogen effluvium' and it usually affects women between the ages of 18 and 50. Men are also affected by hair loss but they tend to have genetic hair loss or androgen-dependant alopecia.

Losing hair may be a physiological or a pathological response. A certain amount of hair loss will occur when the weather becomes warmer, through pregnancy and lactation, and with ageing. Pathological causes may vary from overwashing, medicated or poor quality shampoos, persistent use of hair dryers, especially in association with the current hair design or cutting and possibly from overuse of hairsprays or gels. More serious conditions can cause hair loss, such as hypothyroidism and other metabolic diseases. Skin fungus, most often responsible for dandruff, may cause hair loss and toxins such as excess alcohol, drugs of abuse, steroids and anticancer drugs can all cause the hair to fall.

Nutritional deficiencies of minerals (especially sulphur), proteins and vitamins may all cause hair to thin; and stress, as discussed in the section above on the care of hair, will also have an effect.

RECOMMENDATIONS

General Advice
- *Feel assured that if hair loss is associated with physiological causes the hair will regrow.*
- *Persistent hair loss with no obvious cause*

requires a studious examination of hair care and the products used, or a consultation with a complementary medical practitioner or, preferably, a trichologist initially.
- *Persistent hair loss should be considered by a GP with possible referral to an endocrinologist.*

Nutritional
- *Whether physiological or pathological, increase vitamin and mineral intake through fresh fruit and vegetables (at least five portions a day).*

Supplemental
- *Take the following:*
  - *L-lysine 300mg per foot of height in divided doses per day.*
  - *Iron (preferably not in sulphate form) at maximum recommended dosage on packaging.*
  - *Multi-vitamin B complex which must include vitamin B_{12} minimally at 3mcg daily.*
  - *Vitamin C 300mg per foot of height in divided doses with meals.*
  - *Folic acid 50mcg per foot of height in divided doses daily.*
  - *A multi-mineral supplement.*

Excess hair

Excess hair is usually only considered a problem if it is facial. Excessive growth is usually an ethnic or genetic predisposition although certain rare metabolic conditions and drugs may encourage hair growth. Hormone imbalance, particularly excess testosterone and other male hormones (androgens), is a cause in women.

RECOMMENDATIONS

General Advice
- *If no ethnic or genetic reason is apparent, then a consultation with a trichologist and a GP will be in order.*
- *Discuss naturopathic oestrogen and*

progesterone treatments before using orthodox drug approaches to blocking androgen effects.

- *If no metabolic or drug problems are the cause, then hair removal can be considered. Both chemical and electrical techniques can be used, although the latter is less likely to create a toxic response.*

HAY FEVER

Hay fever or allergic rhinitis is characterized by itchy nose, throat and palate, congestion and/or runny discharge from the nasal passages, itching or stinging eyes. These symptoms are often associated with tiredness, lethargy and sinus-type headaches. Hay fever is caused by the body producing chemicals, including histamine, in response to pollens from plants attaching themselves to membranes in the nose and throat.

The orthodox treatment is the use of antihistamines, which temporarily blocks the effects of histamine. Other types of decongestant can be used concurrently. These treatments do not offer cure, only temporary relief, and it is worth trying alternative treatments, which can be very effective.

Complementary practitioners may look at hay fever as being an inappropriate response to pollens or other inhaled particles due to an over-sensitivity created within the body by food allergy or intolerance. Treatment for hay fever is therefore a complex, all-body concern and not one that demands a topical therapy.

RECOMMENDATIONS

General Advice

- *See **Allergies**.*
- *Nasal washing techniques. The easiest to use is a yogic technique called Jala Lota, which employs a salt solution and a little watering can. One passes the solution from nostril to nostril by holding the head in a downward position; the solution washes off the pollens and the salt solution helps the congestion. Pots are available through many healthfood outlets but it is best to be trained by a yoga practitioner.*

Nutritional

- *Avoid alcohol, caffeine, refined sugars and cow's milk products, all of which encourage mucus production and make congestion worse.*
- *The holistic consensus of opinion is that hay fever sufferers have, generally, an overaggressive immune system, attacking things like pollen that should not cause a problem. This is often caused by persistently eating or drinking foods to which the individual is allergic. Food allergy testing is recommended through blood tests or bioresonance techniques.*

Supplemental

- *Vitamins C and A and zinc have all been shown to desensitize membranes and relieve hay fever. These supplements should be taken in the following amounts per foot of height in divided doses with food throughout the day: vitamin A (1,000iu), vitamin C (1g) and zinc (5mg just before bedtime).*
- *Quercetin 100mg per foot of height per day may help reduce allergic response.*
- *Pantothenic acid 200mg per foot of height per day can reduce allergic response.*

Homeopathic

- *Gencido ointment and injections are a Swiss-made pollen-based homeopathic preparation that can be applied to the nostrils or, in more serious conditions, injected. This needs to be prescribed by a doctor with knowledge of the compound.*
- *The homeopathic remedies Allium cepa, Pollen and Arundo can be taken at potency 6, four times a day, as can the various hay fever homeopathic combinations.*
- *Desensitization with specific homeopathic remedies for that type of pollen can be beneficial. It is possible to check the bloodstream for immunoglobulins for airborne pollens in order to isolate which ones are the culprits.*

Herbal/natural extracts

- *Extract of nettle has been shown to reduce the symptoms of allergic rhinitis.*
- *Garlic, horseradish and ginger in tincture form*

help to ease breathing difficulties, reduce nasal congestion and boost the immune system.

Orthodox
• Enzyme potentiated desensitization (EPD) is a specific desensitization technique being studied by the John Radcliffe Hospital in Oxford, England. Only a few doctors around the world have the equipment to use this new but effective treatment in severe cases.

HEAT STROKE – *see* Dehydration *and* Sunburn

HICCOUGHS

A hiccough is caused by the spasmodic contraction of the diaphragm. This causes a jolt of the upper body and is in itself quite harmless. A hiccough can only be considered a problem if it is persistent.

Hiccoughs occur because of an irritation or inflammation of the diaphragm. Psychological stress can cause a mild cramp and ingestion of a compound that may irritate or inflame the oesophagus or stomach which in turn touches the diaphragm can also cause the problem. Rarely, the irritation of the phrenic nerve in the neck can cause problems because this controls the diaphragm.

RECOMMENDATIONS

General Advice
• Try a couple of old wives' tales: drinking a glass of water with the head between the knees, or dropping a cold object down the back of the collar and holding the breath. Each of these techniques causes the diaphragm to spasm which can take away the irritation.
• A persistence of hiccoughing may indicate an underlying sinister cause of an irritation to the diaphragm such as a tumour or abdominal cavity abscess and needs to be investigated by a GP initially.

Supplemental
• Ginseng taken with meals at twice the dose recommended on any bought product may be beneficial.

Homeopathic
• The homeopathic remedies Ratanhia and Sulphuric acid are first-line remedies but they are unusual; you may find Nux vomica in your medical chest and this can be tried initially. Take potency 6 every 10min.

HIGH BLOOD PRESSURE (HYPERTENSION)

Any tube with a fluid in it will exert a pressure. Like the garden hose, the amount of water being pushed through it and the flexibility of the tube will affect the pressure in the same way as a thumb held over the end. The more of the opening that is obscured the faster the water spurts out of the end. This is an indication of increased pressure. The arteries in the body act on exactly the same principles.

The heart pumps blood out into the aorta, exerting a pressure known as the systolic blood pressure. The aorta and other major arteries expand because more blood is pushed into them and the contractile muscles around the artery constrict for the same reason as a stretched rubber band will contract. The pressure exerted by these constricting arteries is known as the diastolic pressure. When your blood pressure is taken, reference

Blood Pressure Chart

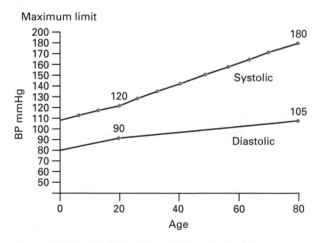

The typical systolic and diastolic blood pressures rise as the age of the individual increases.

will be made to two figures. For example, 120/80 represents a pressure of 120mmHg due to the systolic push of the heart and a pressure of 80mmHg due to the diastolic constriction of the arteries.

A rule of thumb for normality is an individual's age plus 100 (give or take 20mmHg) for a systolic pressure and a figure below 90mmHg for a diastolic pressure.

High blood pressure may be variable. 'White coat' blood pressure is well established and describes the rise in blood pressure that occurs when an individual is subjected to a visit to the doctor's surgery. Persistently high blood pressure on repeated visits needs treating but any fluctuation can be checked by a 24 hour ambulatory blood pressure monitor, which may show that the blood pressure only rises in situations of stress. This is extremely relevant to ensure that unnecessary treatment is not undertaken.

High blood pressure occurs for several reasons:

- The development of atheroma in ageing arteries, those who smoke or who have high cholesterol levels leads to inflexibility in the arteries, which decreases the arteries' ability to expand and also narrows the lumen. Liken this to placing half of your thumb over the end of a hose pipe and see how much further the water will squirt.
- Increased weight requires the heart to beat with more strength to get the blood around the increased amount of tissue. The fat also constricts major arteries and causes the muscles to have to work harder, which requires more oxygen, again encouraging the heart to beat harder to pump more blood through. Carrying too much weight also increases the amount of insulin produced, which in turn increases sodium which is known to increase blood pressure.
- A lack of exercise or sedentary lifestyle will cause a blood pressure rise. Exercise reduces adrenaline, oxygenates the body and works in several other biochemical ways to reduce blood pressure.
- Adrenaline, thyroid hormones and the body's

natural steroids all control blood pressure and both dietary and stress factors that increase these will raise the blood pressure.

- Dietetic factors such as salt, alcohol and caffeine all raise the blood pressure and a reduction or cessation of the use of these can bring the blood pressure down to normal limits.
- Toxins or poisons such as cadmium and lead are known to raise the blood pressure, probably by a direct action on the centre in the brain that monitors and tries to control blood pressure, by increasing or decreasing the heart rate and opening or closing blood vessels around the body. Food allergies have been researched and shown to cause hypertension.

Recognizing high blood pressure

High blood pressure may cause symptoms ranging from headaches, dizzy spells, nose bleeds, throbbing in the ears or tinnitus, or it may be asymptomatic (no symptoms at all). Many people who do not check their blood pressure regularly may exist with high blood pressure and have no problems at all and have no increased risk of heart failure, heart attacks or strokes. A high blood pressure may indicate that the heart is working too hard, therefore heart failure or a heart attack may ensue; a raised pressure may fracture small or damaged arteries to cause bleeds, which, if occurring in the brain, will result in a stroke but other factors need to be present also.

It is important to put high blood pressure risks into perspective. You will read that high blood pressure increases the risk of a cardiovascular accident by anywhere from two to six times. This sounds like a great risk. However, if the chances of a heart attack or a stroke at a young age are 1 in 1,000 and high blood pressure may increase that to 6 in 1,000, then the odds are still low. In my opinion, and this will be hotly argued by most doctors and pharmaceutical companies, high blood pressure, whilst potentially dangerous, should not be made into the evil that it currently is. Basic naturopathic treatments can and usually do make a profound difference and drug medicine should be used only as a last resort. Long-term studies have shown that individuals with hypertension who control the pressure but do not take orthodox blood pressure lowering medicine do much better than those who take prescription drugs. I am sure this is because blood pressure is, like most signs or symptoms in the body, a warning about some aspect of lifestyle. Even those who have a genetic predisposition to high blood pressure may be found to have a specific trigger that needs to be eliminated. Simply dealing with the high numbers is not dealing with a cure. What a surprise to find that no orthodox drug for high blood pressure is intended to cause a cure but merely lowers the figures, ignoring any underlying factor. The intricate control that the body shows in controlling blood pressure through centres in the brain, the delicate balance of sodium and other electrolytes in the kidney, the strength of the heart and the nervous control of the vessels suggests that the body may know what it is doing when adjusting blood pressure. It may be that an individual needs to have a raised blood pressure for specific functions and it is only the persistently very high or sudden hypertensive (a condition known as malignant hypertension) that need to be treated.

Secondary hypertension

'Secondary' hypertension is found in approximately six per cent of all high blood pressure cases and is due to some underlying disease process such as a tumour, which produces adrenaline or thyroxine, or kidney tumours, which affect specific chemicals from the kidney that act to control blood pressure. Certain metabolic conditions, pregnancy and drugs such as the oral contraceptive may raise the blood pressure. Theoretically, but I think somewhat outside the definition of secondary hypertension, one might consider alcohol and tobacco to be a cause of secondary hypertension because these compounds do cause the problem. The volume of blood within the

arteries will also be relevant to the blood pressure reading. The higher the salt content, the more water will be present through the process of osmosis.

Primary hypertension

Most high blood pressure has no orthodox disease causing it. It is called primary or essential hypertension and is generally treated immediately by GPs with an orthodox drug. Such drugs are diuretics (which remove water from the bloodstream and thereby, like turning down the tap on the hose pipe, lower the blood pressure but they do nothing to answer the question why the blood pressure was raised in the first place), beta-blockers (which slow the heart rate or prevent arterial contraction), calcium channel blockers (which stop arterial muscle contracting) or anti-angiotensins (drugs that block controlling hormones that come from the kidney). Other drugs are slowly but surely being prepared but they all aim at lowering the figures without dealing with underlying causes.

High blood pressure does run in families but as I mentioned above there is probably some form of environmental or lifestyle trigger. It is important to note that geographical studies show that high blood pressure is far more prevalent in Western societies than in others. A prime example is the Negro race who have far higher blood pressure than Caucasians when living in the USA but in Africa high blood pressure is negligible. Studies have shown conclusively that the Western diet, high in refined sugars, caffeine and alcohol, is directly responsible.

Generally speaking, complementary or alternative methods of treating this condition can bring the diastolic pressure (the one that is most often raised and the figure that is most often monitored to see if treatment is helping) down by 10–15 points.

RECOMMENDATIONS

General Advice

• *Lose any excess weight through a slow, steady dietetic plan.*

- Stop smoking, drinking alcohol or caffeine until the blood pressure is normal and then reintroduce slowly, keeping a close eye on the pressure rise.
- Increase exercise. Yoga has been shown to help control hypertension and is a must, regardless of any other aerobic exercise taken.
- Investigate the possibility of cadmium or lead poisoning through specific blood or hair analysis.
- Stress reduction through biofeedback, hypnosis and counselling will all help to lower blood pressure.
- The integrity of the arterial vessels may determine the danger of hypertension and the recommendations in the section on arteriosclerosis should be reviewed (see **Arteriosclerosis**).

Nutritional

- Remove salt completely from the diet.
- Check for food allergies using a bioresonance technique or accurate blood test.

Supplemental

- Calcium and magnesium taken in divided doses throughout the day as follows may help: calcium (200mg per foot of height) and magnesium (150mg per foot of height). These should be taken in the form of citrates or aspartame.

Herbal/natural extracts

- If blood pressure is proving resistant, consider herbal treatment in the hands of a specialist. Crategus and Viscum album should be discussed.

Orthodox

- Antihypertensive drug treatment should be considered only when the above measures have failed, and only if blood pressure is shown through 24hr monitoring to be persistently high, especially if the individual has a family history of stroke or cardiovascular disease, smokes, remains overweight or is taking the oral contraceptive pill.

HOT FLUSHES

Hot flushes usually occur in women who are going through the menopause. The sensation occurs because the peripheral blood vessels expand and allow more warm blood from the centre of the body to reach the peripheral nerve endings, thus creating a sensation of heat. The dilation of the blood vessels occurs because of a diminution of ovarian oestrogen and the fluctuating amounts made to compensate this loss by the adrenal glands. Oestrogen has exerted some control over the contraction of blood vessels since the start of the indivudual woman's periods.

Hot flushes that occur away from the menopause are most commonly associated with anxiety. Nervous conditions, diseases of the liver and problems associated with an excess production of thyroxine or adrenaline may also be associated.

RECOMMENDATIONS

General Advice

- Hot flushes not associated with the menopause or anxiety should be investigated by your GP.
- Wear only natural fibres next to the skin.

Nutritional

- Avoid caffeine, alcohol, spicy foods and smoking, all of which can cause hot flushes in themselves and will certainly exacerbate the situation.
- Increase the following foods in the diet: fennel, celery, rhubarb and any soya product (this may be contraindicated if the individual has a thyroid deficiency – please consult your complementary medical practitioner).

Supplemental

- Try the following supplements at the recommended doses per foot of height in divided doses throughout the day with food: vitamin B_6 (20 mg), zinc (5mg; if this makes you feel nauseous, take the recommended dose in one go before sleeping at night) and Evening Primrose Oil (500mg).

Homeopathic

- *The following homeopathic remedies may be suitable and any one of these can be taken at potency 30 every 3hr for one week. If there is no improvement, please try the next remedy. If an effect is found, then reduce the dose of that remedy until the flushes return, step up in frequency and maintain on that level for one month: Belladonna, Agnus castus, Amyl nitrate, Lachesis, Pulsatilla and Sulphuric acid.*

Herbal/natural extracts

- *The herb Agnus castus can be used by following the maximum dose recommended on a good brand. Phyto-oestrogens (plant-derived oestrogens) that have a mild oestrogenic effect can be used with safety except in those who are known to have an oestrogen-dependent cancer, and even then it is best to discuss this with a practitioner.*

Orthodox

- *Persisting flushes may require the consideration of hormone replacement therapy.*
- *Before orthodox drugs are used, try natural progesterone in combination with natural oestrogen. This needs to be prescribed by a practitioner with experience in this area.*

HYPERLIPIDAEMIA

Hyperlipidaemia is the medical term for an excess of fats in the bloodstream. There are many types but basically the two that are measured are cholesterol and triglycerides. These two compounds are essential for the integrity of cell membranes and are involved in many biochemical processes.

An excess of triglycerides without a rise in cholesterol levels is generally associated with the eating of a fatty meal and should not be considered a particular risk.

INFLUENZA (THE FLU)

Influenza is most commonly abbreviated to the word 'Flu'. There are a variety of symptoms,

ranging from mild to severe, all created by specific viruses.

The symptoms range from head and eye aches, sore throats, coughs (dry or productive), glandular swelling and pains that can often create abdominal pains in children, aching limbs, lethargy, malaise and depression. Secondary infection from a bacteria is not uncommon and is often the cause of serious complications especially in the elderly, very young or those who are immuno-compromised.

The flu generally lasts 4–5 days, as opposed to a cold that can linger for 10 days or more. This often surprises people, who think that flu is longer lasting.

RECOMMENDATIONS

General Advice

- *Please refer to the relevant section in this book with regard to the specific symptoms being suffered.*
- *Rest, preferably in bed.*
- *Any underlying illness may be worsened by an influenza virus and your health practitioner should be contacted if you are asthmatic, diabetic or carrying the human immunodeficiency virus (HIV).*
- *Acupuncture and Shiatsu can be useful if breathing is compromised or congestion is prominent.*

Supplemental

- *The following supplements should be started for each foot of height in divided doses: beta-carotene (2mg), vitamin B complex (10mg) taken with breakfast only and vitamin C (1g).*
- *Glutathione, a naturally occurring potent antioxidant, has been shown to protect against influenza infections if used either as a lozenge or as a mouth and nasal spray.*

Homeopathic

- *Please refer to your preferred homeopathic manual for a suitable remedy depending on your symptoms. Consider Bryonia, Gelsemium and Arsenicum album initially.*

IRON DEFICIENCY

A deficiency in iron is often associated and thought of as anaemia. Indeed a deficiency in iron can be one of the many causes of anaemia but iron is required for many functions in the body and problems such as dermatitis, neurological problems, general lethargy and tiredness and muscular weakness can all be caused by iron deficiency. Problems in the uterus such as fibroids or polyps may be associated with low iron levels.

As ever, the orthodox world suggests that there is a normal level within the blood and tests can be beneficial. It is always worth remembering that blood levels do not necessarily correspond to the levels in the tissues and that iron deficiency may be a problem despite normal levels. It is better to correlate blood analysis with the Humoral Pathological Laboratory Test (*see* chapter 8) or if this is not available, hair analysis.

Vegetarians and vegans are more likely to become iron deficient because of the lack of red meat in their diet. Vegetable sources include green-leafy vegetables, with particular interest to be paid to spinach and collard greens. Parsley is a good source but large amounts need to be eaten regularly, as do dried peaches, nuts, beans, asparagus, molasses and oatmeal. Heavy periods are a most common cause of iron deficiency and, paradoxically, anaemia can actually encourage heavy and painful periods.

A French study has shown that 15 per cent of children are iron deficient. This is due to poor iron intake through breast milk, formula milks and the type of foods given early in life. This may be the cause of tiredness and lethargy with persistent coughs and colds in children under the age of five.

RECOMMENDATIONS

General Advice

• *Iron deficiency should be recognized by specific cellular iron levels and not simply by blood levels.*
• *Persisting iron deficiency or iron deficiency without an obvious cause should be reviewed by a doctor because it may indicate unrecognized bleeding, malabsorption syndromes or even more serious conditions such as cancer.*

Nutritional

• *Ensure an increase in the sources listed above.*
• *Elemental iron should not cause constipation but if this occurs pay special attention to increasing the fibre in the diet or temporarily adding bran or psyllium husks throughout the day.*

Supplemental

• *Replenishment should be made using iron in chelated combination with gluconate, citrate, fumerate or peptonate at a level of approximately 50mg per foot of height in divided doses with meals. Do not use ferrous sulphate. This should be carried on until symptoms alleviate and then the dose should be halved for two weeks.*
• *Vitamin C at approximately 250mg per foot of height in divided doses with meals should be taken to enhance iron absorption.*

Herbal/natural extracts

• *The plant extract of broom can be used under direction from a herbalist if iron levels are not rising or if constipation is not avoidable.*

JAUNDICE

Jaundice or, as it used to be known, icterus, is a yellowing of the skin, mucous membranes and secretion due to hyperbilirubinaemia – an excess of bilirubin in the blood. Bilirubin is a breakdown product of old blood cells that is formed in the liver and should be excreted in the bile. If there is any obstruction to the bile flow, an absence of enzymes in the liver or the liver cells are diseased or inflamed, bilirubin cannot be processed correctly and backs up and flows into the bloodstream instead of the bowel. Once travelling in the blood, the yellow pigmentation will settle all over the body, thus causing the yellow appearance.

So you can see that jaundice is actually a symptom and not a disease. It can occur at any age and is commonly seen in the newborn within the first five days of life (*see* **Jaundice of the newborn**). The causes of jaundice are numerous, with hepatitis, gallstones and tumours of the head or the pancreas (which surrounds the lower part of the bile duct) being potentially serious conditions.

A false jaundice may be noticed by those who have an excessive amount of beta-carotene. Carrot juice in excess is a very typical cause of a mild yellowing of the skin.

RECOMMENDATIONS

General Advice
- *Any sign of jaundice must be reviewed by a GP and a firm diagnosis made.*
- *Please refer to the relevant section in this book once the underlying cause is isolated.*

LEGIONNAIRE'S DISEASE

This is a pneumonia that is caused by a bacterium called Legionnaire's bacillus. It is so called because it was first recognized at a convention of the American Legion in 1976. It is a dangerous pneumonia because it affects the kidneys, the bowel, the liver and the nervous system.

The Legionnaire's bacillus lives comfortably in air conditioning units and is spread through airborne transmission.

RECOMMENDATIONS

General Advice
- *See* **Pneumonia**.
- *Ensure that all filters in air conditioning units are changed frequently.*

LEUCOPLAKIA

This is an abnormal thickening and whitening of the lining of an internal body cavity. The mouth and vagina are the most common. It is uncertain what creates this thickening of the epithelium of mucous membrane, although smoking and persistent friction (as from a pipe) may be responsible for leucoplakia in the mouth. An ill-fitting dental bridge may also be a cause. Viral infection is another probable cause. Leucoplakia may indicate a precancerous condition.

Leucoplakia on the tongue may be isolated to particular areas and be representative of disease in part of the body, according to Eastern philosophies of tongue reading. The condition arising in the vagina is probably a viral creation but effectively lies on the vessel of conception meridian and an individual needs to look at their relationship to their parents and loved ones.

RECOMMENDATIONS

General Advice
- *Any white patches need to be reviewed by a physician.*
- *Stop smoking and remove any item that may be causing friction.*
- *See a complementary medical practitioner for a review of lifestyle and general health because there may be a precancerous tendency or condition lurking.*

LEUKAEMIA

Leukaemia is a definition of any disease of the blood or bone marrow that is characterized by an uncontrolled multiplication of white blood cells. The term 'uncontrolled proliferation' is the same as cancer. Leukaemia is classified on the basis of the speed with which the white cells will multiply, specifically being known as acute, subacute or chronic. Further differentiation is made by naming the type of white blood cell that is out of control and lastly by the difference in the cells themselves. The more varied the white blood cells, the more dangerous the cancer.

White blood cells are initially made in the bone marrow with further production and modification in the lymphatic system. White blood cell proliferation in the lymphatic system is known as lymphatic leukaemia, whereas that in the bone marrow is known as myeloid leukaemia. The latter condition can overwhelm the bone marrow and the production of normal cells becomes diminished, leading to symptoms of anaemia. An acute situation can come on within a matter of weeks and be triggered by viruses, radiation and, possibly, agrochemicals/pesticides. The chronic forms may not be noticed for months, if not years, but if left untreated the outcome will be the same.

Symptoms depend on the type of leukaemia. Those affecting the bone marrow will lead to lethargy, paleness, lack of appetite, shortness of breath and a rapid heartbeat, whereas the lymphatic leukaemia will lead to enlarged lymph glands, liver and spleen; in both acute and chronic leukaemia eventually there is a marked decrease in immune function. Leukaemia can strike at any age, the acute lymphatic leukaemia most commonly affecting children.

RECOMMENDATIONS

General Advice

- *See Cancer and Anaemia.*
- *Chronic more so than acute, and lymphatic more so than myeloid, appear to be susceptible to chemotherapy, radiotherapy, blood and bone marrow transfusions. Do not necessarily refuse these but use complementary medicine alongside.*

LIBIDO (SEXUAL DRIVE)

Sexual drive is governed by the sex hormones: testosterone in males and oestrogen/progesterone in females. Testosterone has an added aspect of aggression. Both men and women have levels of all three major sex hormones, and, as always in nature, it is about balance.

It is rare for a physician to come into contact with patients who complain of too high a sex drive. Nymphomania, which is defined as an excessive sexual desire on the part of a woman (it is interesting that there is no male counterpart!) is more often a psychological problem rather than a chemical one. Excessive sexual desire on the part of a male is hard to define because men do not have an oestrus cycle and are, therefore, 'on heat' all the time. Women are primarily, from an evolutionary point of view, geared towards procreation and therefore reach sexual peaks under the influence of luteinizing hormone (LH) and follicle-stimulating hormone (FSH), which are produced around the time of ovulation when the woman is at her most fertile. The definition of a sexually aggressive male is generally used inaccurately. Sexual abuse and rape have very little to do with sex and mostly to do with sociopathic aggressive behaviour.

Most complaints about libido are to do with a low sex drive and the most common causes are linked with stress. Evolution made it very clear as to whether adrenaline (the fear chemical) or the sexual hormones should be more dominant. A couple copulating and faced with a sabre-toothed tiger needed to feel fear above sexual excitement to stand a chance of surviving. Those of our ancestors who found sex more titillating than fear would attempt to finish the act and were in all probability killed. Natural selection did the rest. Whilst we are rarely confronted by wild animals, we do have to put up with other stressful situations. Adrenaline is produced in response to these with the same suppressing effect on our sex drive.

Longer-standing and deeper-seated anxieties stemming from our childhood, relationship with parents and siblings and our early sexual encounters are all relevant to the amount of adrenaline and other stress chemicals that we produce and can therefore have a detrimental effect on our sexuality.

I find it interesting that the Eastern philosophies

consider sexuality to be a source of energy. On reflection, it is understandable that because life is created from intercourse, sex is really the fountain of vital force. Indeed, the more tired we are, the less sexually active we feel. The yogics believe in *kundalini*, which can be thought of as a coiled snake lying in the pelvis. Sexual arousal is the same as the uncoiling of the snake and an orgasm can be thought of as the rapid strike of the cobra. The serpent launches itself up the spinal column and spreads its cheeks to embrace the brain. A strikingly accurate analysis, considering that 5,000 years ago the understanding of neuroanatomy and physiology was non-existent. The Chinese and Tibetans, whilst using a different language, reflect sexuality in much the same way. A weakened libido is therefore a combined physical and psychological problem stemming from present and past conditions and needs to be reviewed holistically by considering physical, mental and spiritual well-being.

The use of stimulants is only of temporary benefit and will inevitably lead to a longer lasting and more difficult problem to deal with. Alcohol, cocaine and marijuana all act by lowering inhibitions and heightening the senses. At the time this is not a problem and on occasion is fine and should be considered a treat. The difficulty arises when the mind and soul lose contact and the memory of the pleasures of sex for sex's sake. A French fry with a sprinkling of salt may not be a healthy enjoyment but a pleasure all the same. Once that chip has been dipped in ketchup many people find it hard to go back to having their minor sin without the red sauce embellishing the product. Sex 'under the influence' can very rapidly lead to a dependency upon a drug without which the act is no longer enjoyable.

It is also important to remember that a decrease or lack of libido may simply be an ageing process. As we age, we move away from the more material needs and our spiritual and mental requirements become more important. Nature does not particularly want us to sire or mare offspring at an older age when we are less likely to be able to protect them. The universe prefers that as we age we use our experience to teach the younger generation and our usefulness becomes more cerebral and spiritual. It is not illness to be lacking or to enjoy a level of sexuality at any age but one must be careful not to try to conform to what society expects but instead to look inside and ensure that we perform at a level that is satisfactory to ourselves.

RECOMMENDATIONS

General Advice

- *Remove any stressful stimuli such as alcohol, caffeine and other drugs of abuse. Smoking is a notorious neurological depressant and often overlooked in weakened sexuality.*
- *Remove stress chemicals such as adrenaline by increasing physical exercise and reducing levels of anxiety.*
- *Meditation minimally, through counselling and then to active spiritual practices such as Tantric yoga (a branch of yoga using specific sexual positions and practices), should be considered, learned or studied.*
- *Time spent toning the body will release the body's natural opiates (which are natural aphrodisiacs), reduce adrenaline and simply make us look better and therefore feel more attractive, and is a simple process of raising the libido.*
- *Ensure that you are getting enough sleep. Introduce variety into the sexual act. Monotony is a notorious damper of libido.*

Herbal/natural extracts

- *Homeopathic and herbal treatments, especially Chinese, Ayurvedic and Tibetan, can be utilized to increase both masculine and feminine energies.*

LOW BLOOD PRESSURE (HYPOTENSION)

Some authorities would consider low blood pressure to be a problem that requires treating.

Doctors in Germany are quite active in raising blood pressure although there is little, if any, evidence to suggest that this is necessary. A low blood pressure should only be treated if symptoms of fainting, dizziness, depression or persisting lethargy are associated with a blood pressure that has a systolic level below 80 or a diastolic level below 50. (Systolic pressure is that of the heart beating and diastolic is the pressure exerted by the arteries, *see* **Hypotension**.) So nonplussed appear the authorities that I was unable to find any reference to treatment for non-emergency hypertension in the English language.

Low blood pressure will occur when the heart fails to pump correctly, there is marked blood loss or the blood vessels dilate, usually in response to some toxin, most probably a hypertension drug such as a beta-blocker. Hypotension that occurs suddenly should therefore be considered a medical emergency and be treated accordingly.

RECOMMENDATIONS

General Advice

- *A sudden drop in blood pressure must be assessed by a doctor and treated accordingly. Ensure that any blood pressure-lowering drugs are not being taken in excess. Different people have different sensitivities.*
- *Low blood pressure without symptoms should be left alone.*
- *If symptoms are present, try increasing water and protein intake to enhance the volume of blood.*

LUMPS AND BUMPS

Lumps and bumps come and go and those that persist need a diagnosis because rarely they may turn out to be something nasty.

Most lumps are completely innocent, being formed by trauma, which can cause cysts or scar tissue, or hormonally related such as breast lumps, which could be encouraged by oestrogen or progesterone production.

Putting it simply, there are three different body types, just as there are 12 astrological signs. The description is more fully embellished in the introduction chapter but basically the body should be a balance of elimination, reaction and retention. Lumps and bumps are a tendency to be too retentive, suggesting some form of lifestyle inbalance. Frequent formation of lumps and bumps tends to suggest that a consultation with a complementary practitioner to review lifestyle, diet and exercise would be beneficial.

RECOMMENDATIONS

General Advice

- *Any lump that arises anywhere without cause, or a lump that persists despite a known causative event, should be seen by a doctor.*
- *Please refer to the relevant section in this book once the underlying diagnosis of lump has been made.*

Orthodox

- *Consider ultrasound and magnetic resonance imaging (MRI) before radiological investigation (X-rays), but do not shy away from investigations.*
- *Surgical lumpectomies should be a last resort but, again, not ignored as an option of diagnosis especially if the lump is associated with the breasts or genitalia.*

LYME DISEASE

This is an acute, transient form of arthritis that is accompanied by a fever and skin lesions, transmitted by the bite of a deer tick. It is so named because it was first observed near a town called Lyme in Connecticut in 1974. The condition is now spreading and, although rare, is found throughout Europe and the British Isles.

The symptoms, whilst debilitating, are not particularly dangerous but the parasite is now known to attack major organs, especially the nervous system. The condition should be suspected if an individual has been in an area where deer are found. Any sort of insect bite that has a clear centre and red circles of inflammation surrounding it must raise suspicions. The tick may not be felt and a close inspection of the body after a ramble through deer country is important because if the tick is removed within 36 hours the chances of contracting Lyme disease is reduced. Symptoms such as fever, stiff neck and painful joints usually appear within four weeks.

RECOMMENDATIONS

General Advice

- If you think that you have been bitten by a tick, please see a doctor with knowledge of the subject. Prophylactic antibiotic treatment may be offered and is probably a wise precaution, especially if the tick has been on the body for more than 24hr. A blood test for Lyme disease can be performed but not for around three weeks after the bite, by which time early interventional antibiotic treatment is still possible but may not be as effective.
- See **Antibiotics**.
- See **Arthritis** if the disease process has taken a hold.

Homeopathic

- The homeopathic remedy Ledum 30 should be taken twice a day for one month whilst undergoing any orthodox treatments. If possible potency 6 should be taken every 15min if a tick bite has been noticed, for five doses.

Orthodox

- The use of antibiotics is necessary because alternative treatments may not be effective and any delay in destroying this bacterium can have long-term effects.

MALARIA

Malaria is one of the world's most frequently fatal diseases. It is endemic (meaning part of the natural system) in Africa, the southern half of Asia and South America. The entire population of sub-Saharan Africa will contract malaria and suffer to some degree. Those with strong constitutions and good immune systems may suffer from infrequent mild fevers and chills with general malaise whilst those who are weaker may have severe symptoms and, at worse, suffer severe anaemia, immune collapse and renal failure.

The malarial parasite, of which there are many types, has a group name of *Plasmodium*. *Plasmodium falciparum* is the most aggressive and has probably developed to become so dangerous because of resistance to antimalarial drugs that have been used over the last 20 years. *Plasmodium falciparum* can infect the nervous system, giving rise to severe neurological symptoms, including paralysis and coma.

Antimalarial agents have recently been given a bad name because one particular compound, mefloquine, was reported as causing neurological symptoms. Whilst this is true, most people who used this aggressive drug had no problems and were protected against *P. falciparum*. There is always resistance to having to take a drug but if one weighs the risks of malaria against the risk of a serious side effect, the ratio is negligible. Alternative anti-malarial medicines derived from herbs have been used both in treatment and prevention for thousands of years, derived from plants from all parts of the world where malaria is found. In principle these are fine to take, but they probably act in the same way as the manufactured drugs. The advantage of a pharmaceutical preparation is that doctors know exactly how much of what they are giving. Herbal preparations vary greatly in their constituents and we may be under- or over-dosing.

The drug treatments are very effective prophylactically and less so as a treatment but nevertheless have made a profound difference on the prognosis. Ideally the scientific community needs to concentrate their efforts on controlling the *Anopheles* mosquito that transmits the malaria parasite. Much work is being done in this field but, as always, nature is very tenacious and mosquitoes resistant to insecticides are developing at the same speed as the malaria parasites are becoming immune to antimalaria drugs.

Preventing being bitten is probably the best treatment. The use of drug repellents runs the risk of absorbing these chemicals, which may have a detrimental effect on general health, but at this time, again, the risk of malaria is greater than the hypothetical dangers of insecticide poisoning. Natural repellents are undoubtedly safer but, in my experience, tend not to work so well. Individuals have a greater or lesser predisposition for attracting mosquitoes and, other than levels of vitamin B_6 in the bloodstream, there is no evidence to suggest why this is.

RECOMMENDATIONS

General Advice
- If you are pregnant or unwell, avoid travelling to malaria-endemic areas. If this is inevitable, discuss the matter with your doctor.
- The best treatment is prevention. Use mosquito repellent sparingly but effectively.

Supplemental
- The use of vitamin B_6 at a level of 10mg per foot of height taken with breakfast and before dusk can have a profound antimosquito effect.

Homeopathic
- Some unsubstantiated homeopathic sources suggest that the homeopathic remedy Natrum muriaticum can be taken, potency 6, three times a day and has a protective effect against malaria. An individual is taking a risk if relying on this alone.
- If malaria is contracted, review the homeopathic preparations of Cinchona, known as China, or two of its derivatives, Cinchona arsenicum or Cinchona sulph. These should be taken as potency 6 every 2hr through the fever and every 4hr between bouts.

Herbal/natural extracts
- Only if you react badly to the drugs should you consider the use of Peruvian bark (Cinchona succirubra): either one teaspoonful of the bark per cup of boiling water that has simmered for 30min, drunk three times a day; or 1–2ml of the tincture three times a day.
- Burberry (Berberis vulgaris): put one teaspoonful of bark in a cup of cold water, bring to the boil, leave for 15min and drink three times a day; or take 2–4ml of the tincture three times a day.
- The above concoctions may be used as a treatment if orthodox drugs are failing, or at the same time.

Orthodox
- Unless a specific intolerance or symptoms develop to antimalaria drugs, these should be used as directed by the World Health Organization (WHO), who advise all pharmacists of the best drugs for the area to be visited.
- Mefloquine should be avoided wherever possible because of its neurological side effects.
- Antimalarial drugs should be started at least one week before travelling and continued for at least three weeks after leaving the malaria-endemic area, because the parasite may lay its eggs in the red blood cells, which may not hatch for at least two to three weeks. The drugs are ineffective unless the parasite is swimming freely in the bloodstream outside of the red blood cells.
- If prevention fails and the fevers, shakes, sweating, fatigue and headache of malaria are suspected, then a blood test for diagnosis is usually available and needs to be taken at the peak of the fever if possible. Orthodox drug treatment with quinine derivatives is usually initiated immediately and should be taken alongside alternative treatments.

MEDITATION

Throughout this book I will advise people to learn a technique of meditation for physical, psychological and spiritual benefits. With respect and with the assumed consent from the few teachers I have come across, I will paraphrase their teachings.

What is meditation?

Meditation is many things to many people. To some it is a concept as alien as a holiday on Mars and conjures up visions of portly Indians levitating cross-legged in orange robes and sandals. Fair enough. Meditation may be like that but in the broader sense meditation is whatever it takes to allow an individual to recognize his part in the big scheme of things.

The Eastern philosophies believe that every molecule within our body is connected with all others, both within the self and the surrounding environment and universe by an, as yet, unmeasurable energy. Attempting to achieve a connection with this energy source is what meditation is about.

Most of us achieve some contact either through prayer or formal meditative techniques, and all of us achieve a glimpse of meditation when we drift into sleep. At that time most of us, provided that we have not taken any extreme anxieties to bed, and even then, find that those moments before sleep are blissful.

A more orthodox view suggests that meditation is a technique that stimulates relaxing chemicals within the brain, which takes us to a happier place. In reality both the orthodox and alternative views are accurate and, actually, the same.

Maharishi Mahesh Yogi has probably done the most to bring meditation to the Western consciousness. His association with the superstars of the 1960s attracted much media space and time and made a distinct change in Western consciousness. However, the Maharishi simply spread to the West those techniques that had been formalized thousands of years ago but have probably been practised since our higher mental state developed. 'Since' might actually be unfair to primates, who, for all we know, meditate at a very high level.

Meditation positions

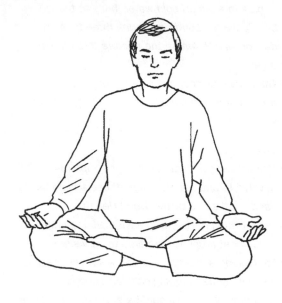

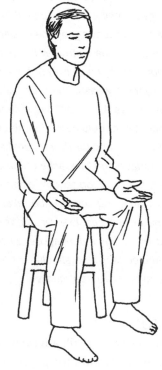

There is no 'right' meditation position. While the two shown above are popular, experiment and see what works for you.

Why meditate?

There is no reason why anybody has to meditate. But then again there is no reason why anybody should exercise or eat correctly. It is simply how an individual's consciousness may choose to exist. Healthily or unhealthily, that is the option. Meditation can be looked upon as the aerobics of the mind and whether one takes the orthodox approach to the production of calming chemicals or the Eastern philosophy of connecting with the 'whole', the benefit is better than not meditating at all.

How to meditate

Meditation may be a silent, passive event or found in prayer, chant or non-aerobic exercise. The body's energy (Qi) or neurochemistry can be influenced by all and any technique. The important thing is to find the avenue that you feel most comfortable with.

Personally, I have had the privilege of befriending or being in the presence of some of the world's greatest meditators. I have never felt comfortable in a passive, stationary meditative technique. I have found it easy enough to learn but difficult to continue at my current level of spiritual development. I think I need and hope to get to a point where passive meditation is accessible to me but for now the use of Qi Gong seems perfect. The breathing techniques, stretches and positions in association with the conscious practice of finding the time can lead me into a state of relaxation within 10–15 minutes.

Twenty minutes twice a day is an acceptable minimum in order to benefit from meditation, but 5 minutes a day is better than none. I suggest that a human being is geared towards 8 hours of sleep, 8 hours of work, 6 hours of play and 2 hours of meditation within a 24-hour cycle to balance the body's energies. It is difficult to imagine contriving a lifestyle that allows this but I believe that we should all have this goal.

I considered describing a basic meditative technique that I have found benefits most people but somehow I felt that it would defeat the object of this short section by creating a finite technique. An individual may find that it is perfect but most may demand an alternative and be put off by attempting the wrong concept – a bit like trying to learn tennis, not enjoying it and therefore considering all racket sports an anathema.

RECOMMENDATIONS

General Advice

- Ask around and see if any of your friends or acquaintances practise an art of meditation. Very often those within your social circle may share your preferences.
- Do not give up if one particular type of meditation does not suit. Try others. See if yoga, Qi Gong, Tai Chi or a martial art attract your attention rather than a more passive form.
- If you find one that you enjoy but get bored, persevere and keep returning to the practice even if it is only for a few minutes, days or weeks apart. The body, mind and soul will appreciate even a few moments of meditation. Can you think of anything that you have achieved that you have not had to work at? Meditation is the same.

OPERATIONS AND SURGERY

Surgery carries risks but is, at the end of the day, the most curative aspect of modern medicine. This is a debatable point because removing a lump may, indeed, rid the individual of the symptom but will not necessarily answer the cause. However, a cancer that is taken out may not spread and therefore, it is arguably true to say that the problem is cured.

Any holistic approach to health must include surgery as part of its whole. Ayurvedic, Tibetan and Chinese medicine all have surgical techniques – some of them extremely sophisticated considering the lack of technical knowledge – entrenched in their roots. Modern medicine, by using incredibly sophisticated scientific techniques, has made surgery much safer than even ten years ago. Techniques include the use of laser instead of scalpels, 'keyhole' endoscopic surgery instead of open surgery and robotic techniques. Surgeons can work using X-rays and magnetic resonance imaging (MRI) without actually visualizing the organ upon which they are operating. All in all, the techniques are fascinating and not to be discouraged when required.

Plastic surgery

A special mention, I feel, should be made of elective (optional) operations and most of these fall into the category of cosmetic surgery or, as it used to be known, plastic surgery.

While surgical techniques have much improved, there is still a 1 in 500 chance of having a severe adverse reaction to an anaesthetic. A bad reaction may even include death. Surgery itself may entrap nerves or create scar tissue that irritates and hurts well past the healing of the wound and I feel that all of this must be taken into account. I also feel that much cosmetic surgery is done for the wrong reasons; principally, as we age we should not try to compete with those younger than us but accept that wrinkles and wisdom – being saggy and sage and eroding whilst gaining experience – are inextricably linked.

RECOMMENDATIONS

General Advice

- *Always ask the questions, 'Does this procedure need to be done?' 'Does this procedure have a medicinal alternative?'*
- *A physician should decide if a surgical procedure should take place. Surgeons cut, that is what as a profession they do, therefore that is what they will recommend.*

Pre- and post-operative care

Sometimes, when the body fails to heal itself, it is necessary to resort to mechanical repair, in other words, surgery.

Pre-operative preparation

Leading up to an operation is invariably an anxious time whether it is sprung upon you through an emergency or planned, elective surgery. As soon as anxiety starts we produce adrenaline, which speeds up the body's metabolism and certain compounds may run into deficiencies. Combine this with the inevitable 'nil by mouth' instructions at least 6 hours before an operation and it generally means

that an individual is going into a damaging process with poor nutrition. Preparation to avoid this should start two weeks before an operation by building up stores of vitamins, minerals, trace elements and water.

Suggestions for medication prior to an operation are given in the recommendations below.

The operation

When having an operation it is necessary to view the patient from four angles:

- Psychological
- Repair of operated area
- Liver toxicity
- Nervous system shock

Psychological aspects

Going in for an operation can be a very harrowing experience and a full explanation by a physician, a surgeon and if necessary a counsellor should be provided. This explanation of the procedure and its side effects must be clear to the patient. People who are particularly anxious should be introduced to techniques of relaxation and meditation, thereby often negating the need for a premed (a drug given to keep you calm on your way to the operating theatre) and thus reducing the drug effect on your body.

Many operations can leave individuals disfigured and psychological support for operations leaving visible signs such as amputations or mastectomies is often very necessary.

Repair of the operated area

When operating, the skin or membrane is cut, the underlying tissues are damaged and the surrounding blood vessels and deep tissue all need repairing. The repair process requires scar tissue formation as well as many other biochemical reparative processes, all of which use proteins, vitamins, trace elements and other nutrients. Before an operative procedure, therefore, a check-up with your health professional is recommended and supplemental advice should be offered to ensure that the body has a pool of required nutrients, etc to enable the body to heal without hindrance. Supplementation can be given orally or, preferably, intravenously and this should be discussed with your health professional.

Liver toxicity

An anaesthetic is a powerful drug. As with any medication the liver is instrumental in its breakdown and removal from the body. The effects on the liver are mild in nearly all cases but the liver is nevertheless poisoned and requires support. Supplements, herbal medicines and homeopathic remedies should be utilized to strengthen the liver.

Nervous system shock

An anaesthetic works by preventing the vibration of electrons within nerve tissue. Whilst this very rarely damages the nerves permanently, it gives the central nervous system quite a shock. As far as the brain is concerned, unconsciousness has occurred for no reason. The chemicals within the nervous system that activate us are instructed to awaken us and there is quite considerable activity on that level as the anaesthetic effect wears off. As with the liver, the nervous system needs to have its building blocks in abundance to allow it to repair itself rapidly and supplementation and homeopathic remedies are useful in this area.

Post-operative oxygen

Of patients who undergo a surgical procedure, 5 per cent will develop a surgical site infection. This can add 4–12 days to a hospital stay and, as hospitals tend to carry much tougher infections, this increases risks to general health. A good medical study showed that administering oxygen through a mask can benefit patients considerably.

RECOMMENDATIONS

General Advice

- *Advise your complementary medical practitioner of any operation, major or minor, involving a*

general or a local anaesthetic, preferably two weeks before the procedure. The following recommendations should be administered by a professional preferably. Operations should not be undertaken unless as good a standard of health as is feasible, considering that a surgical operation is required, is achieved. Do not go under anaesthetic with a upper respiratory or chest infection.

- *Be absolutely certain that you are comfortable about having the operation and understand the need and probable outcome. Do not hesitate to consult your doctor, surgeon or a counsellor if you have any doubts or insecurities.*
- *Ensure that the risks and side effects are clear.*
- *Ensure that you are taught a technique for relaxation and thereby reducing the need for a 'pre-med'.*
- *Good hydration is essential because no water will be allowed for several hours prior to, during and whilst recovering from an operation. The day or so before an operation, drink at least three-quarters of a pint per foot of height throughout the day and start drinking water as soon as it is permissible after the operation. This is important to dilute down the anaesthetic toxins and encourage the biochemistry of healing.*
- *Request post-operative oxygen by mask or nasal applicator for 24–48 hours after an operation. If the surgeons have not come across this study or trial, suggest that they contact BOC Gases in Guildford, Surrey, England.*

Nutritional

- *Avoid any junk food at least one week before an operation. Ensure that five portions of fresh fruits or vegetables are taken every day for that period and at least ten days after. These will not be provided by hospitals and should be organized from outside.*

Supplemental

- *Three days before the operation take the following supplements as directed below and* carry this on until healing is complete: vitamin C, 1g per foot of height in divided doses with meals; zinc, 5mg per foot of height taken before bed; argenine (an amino acid), 5g with each meal. Argenine may not be tolerated and may cause digestive upset, in which case halve the dose and see if this can be tolerated. If not, take the minimum amount to avoid problems. Please note that argenine may trigger viral herpes attacks and carriers should not attempt to use this supplement.

Homeopathic

* Nux vomica, potency 30, should be taken four times a day starting the day before an operative procedure and carried on at hourly intervals on the day of operation. After the anaesthetic use Arnica, potency 200 three times a day for three days and then potency 30 four times a day until repair is complete.

Herbal/natural extracts

* A herbal liver cleanser available in most healthfood stores should be taken at twice the daily recommended dose. If this is not available then milk thistle at twice the recommended dosage can be used. Either should continue for one week postoperatively.

PARASITES, COMMENSALS AND SYMBIONTS

Organisms that live off the cells or fluids to the detriment of another organism are known as parasites. Those that feed off or within a host but do not do harm are known as commensals. Some commensals actually benefit their host and are known as symbionts.

A common example of a symbiont is the bowel bacteria, a commensal is *Candida* and a parasite is malaria. The human being benefits so much from bowel flora that without them we would actually die. We provide food and shelter, they provide essential nutrients and digestive processes. *Candida* is a yeast that generally lives in small colonies

Blood Parasites

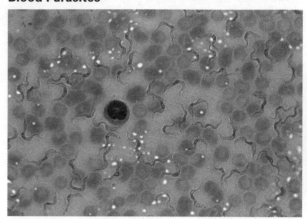

This blood sample contains the blood parasite that causes the serious tropical disease sleeping sickness which is spread by the bite of the tsetse fly.

in many of us, doing little good, but relatively little harm. An excessive growth of *Candida* will lead to a problem and this is often the case in those who are immunocompromised through conditions such as AIDS, or in people who are forced to use steroids. Parasites actually do harm. Theoretically they may kill. Generally, parasites are single-celled organisms that have a lifecycle, such as malaria and amoeba, but they may also be complex organisms such as a tapeworm which may grow up to several feet in the intestine of those infected.

Parasitic infections may be asymptomatic or create reactions in the area that is affected. Bowel infections frequently create diarrhoea, liver infestation may cause jaundice, but most will cause malaise and fatigue. A tapeworm may eat vital nutrients and leave an individual deficient.

As an interesting philosophical discussion point, try to place a foetus during pregnancy into one of these categories!

RECOMMENDATIONS

General Advice

* Diagnosis of a parasite, commensal or symbiont is by discovery following investigations for any number of symptoms.

Herbal/natural extracts

- *For those who are reluctant to use orthodox medicine, herbalists with experience in this field may be able to offer a treatment. There are hundreds of years of reported success of treatment through botanical means.*

Orthodox

- *High magnification blood analysis, known as the Humoral Pathological Laboratory Test, may show up parasitic infestations within the system either by isolating an organism in the bloodstream or by showing changes that are reflected by the blood cells caused by the chemicals produced by the parasite. This is not a fully accepted orthodox test but it is available and, in my opinion, accurate.*
- *Parasitic infection is best dealt with by a suitable orthodox drug with concurrent protective alternative treatments prescribed by a complementary practitioner.*
- *Orthodox treatment for parasites in the gut is generally effective and rarely produces side effects. Treatment against parasites in the bloodstream or organs, such as malaria or amoeba, often requires courses of antibiotics (see* **Antibiotics***).*

POISONING

Poison is a substance that kills or impairs health if introduced into the body. Some substances are instantly toxic, whereas others may require large or protracted ingestion before they cause a problem. I classify poisoning as either accidental, intentional, doctor-induced (iatrogenic) or environmental.

This emotive term reminds us of the serial killers such as Crippin in the early 20th century in England, but unfortunately poisoning is taking place most of the time either unintentionally or by governments and industry turning a blind eye. There is very little that an individual can do to avoid environmental poisoning but

supporting the charities and bodies that lobby on our behalf against such pollution is, I think, everybody's duty.

We hear about the ozone layer and the pollution of our atmosphere, the disposal of toxic products into our rivers and streams, thereby polluting our rivers and seas, but we do little to recognize the toxification of our livestock and the application of pesticides and agrochemical is not criticized or closely monitored.

Many homes have lead in their pipes, aluminium in their cooking pans and we are subjected to fluoride in our water, and chlorine and its derivatives in most of our detergents, which are left on table tops. We have a suggestion that fumes from our babies' mattresses may be involved in cot deaths, there is radiation from our televisions, microwaves and computers and very little is said to the masses who smoke in their houses leaving cancer-causing residues in the carpets, curtains, clothes and bedding that our children are fully exposed to.

It is a wonder that we survive and no wonder that most chronic disease processes are increasing. We survive them better because of the miracles of emergency medicine but we need to do something to protect ourselves individually and *en masse*. Different sections in this book deal with individual toxic problems and how best to remove them from the system.

Environmental poisons

Metal poisoning

There are many types of metal found in our environment, all of which can cause a poisonous effect. Those I have listed below are the most common.

Iron

The clinical features of iron poisoning are vomiting and bloody diarrhoea within a couple of hours of ingestion; 6–8 hours later dizziness, confusion, fainting and even coma may ensue. The pulse will be rapid and weak and if blood pressure is measurable it will be very low. This is due to iron having a direct effect on the cardiovascular system causing peripheral dilation. The individual may appear flushed at some point. If left untreated or if the levels are not high enough to cause the above collapse, then liver necrosis, renal failure and gut spasms can all occur.

RECOMMENDATIONS

Homeopathic
- *The homeopathic remedy Ferrum metallicum should be given, potency 30, every 20min if poisoning has taken place at a single incident or twice daily if the poisoning has been over a period of time.*

Orthodox
- *Acute ingestion is a medical emergency and hospital treatment is required. This will include gastric aspiration and lavage (washing) and the use of a compound called desferrioxamine, which will bind with the iron in the gut, thus preventing absorption. This compound may be used intravenously if blood levels are found to be high.*

Lead

This is difficult to diagnose because the ingestion of lead is usually via cooking in lead pots or by those working in smelting and refining factories. Absorption used to be common through lead-based paints, either by painters and decorators or children who would chew on lead-painted toys. Rarely, lead can be ingested by drinking home-brewed wine or beers that were made and stored in earthenware pots, and an unsuspecting vagrant may drink lead in an anti-knock compound.

Lead poisoning can cause fits, anaemia, colic and constipation. Lead has recently been shown to be responsible for bad behaviour in children. Specific toxicity of the nervous system can cause weakness, specifically a weak wrist. This causes a characteristic sign called wrist drop. Another specific sign for lead poisoning is a blue line forming on the gums.

RECOMMENDATIONS

General Advice
- *Investigate lead levels in the blood for a firm diagnosis.*

Homeopathic
- *The homeopathic remedy Plumbum metallicum can be given, potency 30, every hour in an acute poisoning or twice a day over three weeks if the toxicity has been over a longer period.*

Orthodox
- *An intravenous administration of a compound called EDTA binds with most heavy metals.*

Mercury

Most commonly ingested by a child who chews on a mercury-filled thermometer, this metal used to be the cause of 'Hatter's shakes' because hat makers would paint mercury nitrate onto felt – thus the term 'Mad as a hatter'. The features include anxiety/depression, an imbalanced walk, tremors that affect the face and limbs, blushing and excessive salivation.

More recently, concern about mercury poisoning has come about following the use of thiomersal as an anti-microbial agent in vaccinations. The symptoms mentioned above may occur, but the orthodox medical world remains unconvinced. We await more studies and the results of a recent retrospective analysis by the US Center for Disease Control and Prevention. Holistic dentists are also concerned about the leakage of mercury from dental fillings over a prolonged period of time.

RECOMMENDATIONS

General Advice
- *See **Fillings**.*
- *Test for mercury levels through hair analysis and white blood cell sensitivity tests.*
- *Check mercury levels through blood and urine samples and re-measure after an eight-week course.*

Agricultural chemical poisoning (pesticides)

There are approximately 5,000 different frequently used pesticides and other agrochemicals that affect all the foods provided to us that are not strictly organically grown. The intention of these is to stop the growth of fungi, yeasts, bacteria and viruses. They do an effective and excellent job and will continue to do so in our system unless we are able to wash them off. Unfortunately we need our fungal, yeast, bacterial and viral populations to maintain our health. This is not so easy because many of the chemicals are actually designed to penetrate into the food substance. This is especially the case when agrochemicals are used in animal produce such as beef, lamb, pork, chicken and fish.

We are also exposing ourselves to chemicals through the use of insect repellents, weedkillers, lawn fertilizers, pet sprays and household cleaning agents.

In the UK, in 1999 the working party on pesticide residues found pesticide residues in 27 per cent of the range of food samples tested which included children's foods. The levels exceeded the legal limits in 1.6 per cent of the samples.

The orthodox medical world claims that the levels that we ingest are negligible and cannot cause problems but these are also the same scientists who tell us that they have no idea why we have increasing asthma, eczema, irritable bowel syndrome, cancer ... shall I go on? There is no doubt that these compounds do cause serious conditions such as cancer because numerous studies have shown that individuals who are exposed to these compounds, especially from youth, are more prone to have serious problems. It is possible that pesticides can actually cause genetic damage and therefore are particularly able to create illness in pregnancies and children. The effect of phosphate-based chemicals on the brain of children is known to create aggression, emotional problems and even schizophrenia. We also know that these chemicals can attack the nervous system, causing multiple sclerosis, muscular dystrophy and Guillain-Barré-like syndromes. There are hypotheses that chronic fatigue syndrome and allergic responses may also be worsened, if not caused, by these compounds.

This may not be a problem for the human race in the long run because there is a strong correlation between declining sperm counts and agrochemical poisoning. There has been a marked and noticeable decline in sperm counts in the Western world over the last 20 years which coincides with a far greater increase in the use of these chemicals. If we carry on we shall become an infertile race and, pesticides or no pesticides, health books or no health books, the problem will become academic!

Nutritional

• *Wherever possible only eat organically grown foods.*

Homeopathic

• *The use of homeopathic remedies derived from any specific poisons should be administered at potency 30 twice a day for at least three weeks.*

Environmental chemicals

Depending on what you read, we are constantly assaulted by anything between 5 and 20,000 chemicals from our environment. Some have been mentioned above but many others are inadvertently inhaled or absorbed through the bowel or skin. Over the millennia, the body has developed techniques to break down natural compounds. However, man-made chemicals are often more difficult to remove and may remain in our systems for a lifetime.

Typical examples are fluorocarbons present in aerosol propellants, resins and printer toners. These may cause considerable discomfort or even dangerous symptoms such as cardiac arrhythmia, swelling of the throat, nasal congestion, skin irritation and abdominal discomfort.

If burnt, polychlorinated biphenols, which occur as part of the insulating material around some electrical wires, can produce a neurological toxin. Paraffin oil (kerosene) is related to asthma and the food dye/additive tartrazine can cause autoimmune disease.

Wood treatments, such as lindane, can cause skin, neurological, eye and immune problems, and so-called 'volatile organic compounds' are released from computers and have been associated with emotional and behavioural changes, decreased immunity and respiratory problems.

RECOMMENDATIONS

General Advice

• *Obviously, try to avoid all contamination where possible.*

• *Breathe away from aerosol sprays if using them.*

• *Use a mask whenever confronted by a potentially toxic, inhalable compound.*

• *Consider having a Bioresonance test – an unscientifically validated method of assessing chemical toxins. Doctors may know of certain laboratories that can test for chemical toxins. Consider introducing your doctor to the Biolab (see 'Useful Addresses')*

Supplemental

• *Ensure double dosage of high potency antioxidants if having to work with noxious chemicals (see Antioxidants).*

Homeopathic

• *If a toxin is known to have been absorbed, consider taking the homeopathic equivalent at potency 30 three times a day for two weeks.*

Iatrogenic (doctor-induced) poisoning

One hopes that it is never the intention of a doctor to poison a patient but, unfortunately, this does occur all too often. Rarely is this due to a doctor's mistake, more commonly it occurs because an individual does not tolerate a particular drug or the prescription label is misprinted or misread. Many drugs are taken as over-the-counter preparations and therefore are not actually doctor-prescribed but doctor-encouraged. I believe I read in a non-medical journal that over 2,000 deaths in 1994 were attributable to over-the-counter prescriptions being taken incorrectly.

The effect of poisoning may vary from a mild nausea to diarrhoea, vomiting and sweating. Persisting lethargy, tiredness, malaise or any physical symptom that does not clear up may be a gradual onset of poisoning. In any case, whether the symptoms are mild or marked, or the medicine was taken intentionally or unintentionally (say, by a child), any symptoms that may be associated with drug ingestion should be dealt with immediately.

Complementary medical practitioners are not blameless. Incorrect or overdosed prescribing of herbal medicines or, very rarely, supplements may also be toxic to the system.

RADIATION

When most of us consider radiation we think of medical investigations like X-rays and those 'our government would never let us take a risk' stories about leakages from nuclear power stations. These situations are very true to life and I, personally, have no faith either in the medical technological industry or the governments advising us of safe levels. We are also constantly exposed to radiation by:

- The sun – and the diminished protective ozone layer.
- Air travel – being closer to the sun increases our exposure to X-rays.
- Microwaves and car phones – leak emissions and these appliances emit low-level microwaves that have been shown to affect our DNA (genetic material). Asthma, neurological symptoms and skin problems have all been reported and much more serious diseases may be being triggered by the DNA effect.
- Computers and visual display units (VDUs) – these create minor symptoms such as tiredness,

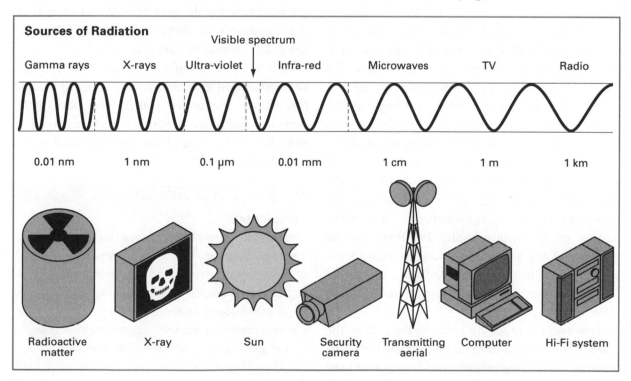

Sources of Radiation

Visible spectrum

| Gamma rays | X-rays | Ultra-violet | Infra-red | Microwaves | TV | Radio |

| 0.01 nm | 1 nm | 0.1 µm | 0.01 mm | 1 cm | 1 m | 1 km |

Radioactive matter — X-ray — Sun — Security camera — Transmitting aerial — Computer — Hi-Fi system

headaches and skin and eye problems but also have been shown, conclusively, to increase the risk of miscarrying and may even create birth malformations.

- Pulsed and static fields – created by our every-day appliances and the wiring within houses, thus changing the electrical and magnetic fields within our environment. These emissions may have the same effect as electromagnetic radiation.

- Electromagnetic waves (EMR) from power lines – strong correlation with leukaemia. (Televisions emit EMR.)

- Radioactive material – this is being dumped into our rivers from hospital waste, especially as radioactive iodine.

- Ultrasound radiation – considered absolutely safe until we found that scans in pregnancy more frequent than 11 within the gestation period created small-for-dates babies. Does that make ten scans safe?

Not all radiations are necessarily bad and the body is very capable of dealing with exposure most of the time. Indeed, radiation keeps us alive. Without sunlight we would not exist. The ethereal energy that we term vital force or Qi is also radiation. Used correctly it may block the harmful effects of the 'man-made' energies. I wonder if our attempts and dabblings in the realms of physics are some deep or subconscious attempt to attain a better understanding of the vital force energy that we understand and utilize so little? Radiation is being used to 'purify' our food and in the process of killing the unwanted bacteria is, hypothetically, altering the natural energy within molecules. Food has an energy and the way it is prepared is vital to the availability of this life force. Radiation acts at the core level of an atom and must be having some effect, surely.

However the radiation gets into the system, the areas that it is most likely to damage are the chromosomes (affecting processes such as cancer) the nervous system and the more delicate organs such as the back of the eye (retina). Investigations such as X-rays and radiotherapy are meant to target certain areas of the body. The accuracy is now marked, especially with computerization, but what the orthodox world seems to overlook is the blood in the area when the X-ray exposure is conducted. The blood cells become irradiated and 'carry' radiation to other areas of the body. This is partially why even pinpoint radio therapy may create radiation sickness and feelings of tiredness and malaise.

This is an incredibly difficult and sensitive subject. We need some very clear studies and a move away from the greed culture that promotes money-making above the potential for health damage. I do not see this happening in my lifetime. We receive the same assurances that the scientists gave in the 1950s when using radiation to perform tonsillectomies and allowing our soldiers to stand a few unprotected miles away from atomic bomb experiments. We did not know the damage we were causing then and, giving the authorities the benefit of the doubt, perhaps we do not know the dangers now. We need to heed the warnings that many trials are showing that any radiation may be harmful.

It is not easy to avoid radiation in the Western or Westernized environments that are spreading throughout the entire planet, but both small measures and major lifestyle changes may be possible for all of us and the options need to be considered.

RECOMMENDATIONS

General Advice

- Keep household electrical appliances to a minimum.
- Avoid sitting within ten feet of a television. This is extremely important in the case of children. Furniture should be situated away from any electrical source wherever possible.
- Avoid microwave emissions by limiting or avoiding the use of microwaves, and mobile phones

should be used hands-free wherever possible. The proximity to the brain may be detrimental.

- Use protective screens with VDUs and computers, remembering that emissions from the side and from behind are often greater than from the screen. Pregnant women should be even more wary.

- Avoid keeping electrical appliances in the bedroom as you may spend one third of your life there.

- It is possible to have the electrical fields in your home measured. You may hire or buy a magnetometer and, apparently, your local power company may offer to come out and test. They won't do this at night but a daytime reading is attainable. The difficulty is believing the current guidelines on safety levels, but if your environment is overcharged, take action to reduce it.

- It is not ridiculous to avoid or refuse housing near 'risk' sites. Nuclear power stations and electricity substations may make a profound difference to your health, and especially those of your children, and one must never counteract health with convenience. Pay attention to overhead power lines and move away from them if possible. More difficult to assess is the possibility of power lines under the house, but your local electricity company should be able to tell you.

- Diviners, with their now very sophisticated instruments, and practitioners of radionics, who often use pendulums to assess radiation fields, may be able to isolate areas within the house that are energetically incorrect. Beds, and once again, especially our children's beds, should not be close to these areas.

- If radiation is unavoidable within the home environment, powerful magnets placed around the areas that are liable to be injurious may create a specific field that will block other radiation. The question is: might these be harmful; at this stage I can find no evidence either way. We watch and wait for further evaluation.

- Lastly, but probably most importantly, consider the possibility that the vital force or Qi is the most potent form of radiation, although little

understood. Meditation techniques and active Qi control through Qi Gong, Tai Chi and yoga are principally the best defences we have. Daily use, especially in those who are confronted by radiation professionally, is essential.

Supplemental

- Radiation may have an effect on the body by producing free radicals and daily use of antioxidants can only be beneficial. Increase your intake of natural organic fruit and vegetables.

- Take the following in addition to a good diet. The doses prescribed are per foot of height and should be taken in divided doses throughout the day with food:

  ○ Beta-carotene 2mg

  ○ Vitamin C 500mg

  ○ Vitamin E (D-alphatocopherol) 100IU

  ○ CoQ 10–20mg

  ○ Selenium 20mcg.

- Take zinc 5mg per foot of height (before bed) and a multi-B complex daily as directed on the label.

- Soluble oxygen solutions are to be found in health food stores. These should be taken at the maximum dose recommended on the bottle, usually a teaspoonful to a tablespoonful per litre of water drunk through the day.

Homeopathic

- A dose of the homeopathic remedy X-ray 200 every three months may protect and should be considered by any frequent flyer on a monthly basis.

SALMONELLA (INCLUDING TYPHOID FEVER)

Salmonella is a group of bacteria of which there are hundreds of types. They cause generalized fevers and illnesses, acute gastroenteritis and, if severe, can multiply in the bloodstream causing septicaemia, which may affect every part of the system.

One of the most dangerous types is *Salmonella typhae* (or *typhosa*), commonly contracted in hot climates and characterized by fever, headache, a cough, rose-like spots on the skin and a generally toxic state. The bacteria can cause ulceration and inflammation in the bowel and lymphatic system and may be characterized by an enlarged spleen (found under the left lower ribs and extending into the upper abdomen). Other common salmonella poisonings are known as paratyphoid, of which there are different types (A B and C), the most frequent of infections being 'food poisoning'. This may be caused by a variety of bugs in the salmonella group, ranging in symptoms from mild diarrhoea and cramps to potentially fatal events.

RECOMMENDATIONS

General Advice

- If a diagnosis of salmonella poisoning is made, see **Poisoning**.
- Typhoid should be treated by antibiotics if a complementary practitioner with experience has not controlled the problem within 24hr.

SHOCK

The term shock is used very loosely by the layperson to denote a strong element of surprise but in medical terms it is the clinical manifestation of a failure of blood to return to the heart. The consequence of this is that the heart has less to beat upon and circulation diminishes.

The most common cause of shock is blood loss, which may be visible or invisible. Internal injuries in the chest or abdomen may allow a bleed of some quantity to occur without any external appearance. The abdomen can hold most of the blood in the circulatory system and the severing of a major artery such as the aorta or one of its main branches can lead to a state of shock within seconds.

The neurological system can induce medical shock by a sudden or severe surprise but it more usually occurs with fear. Fainting is often caused by a sudden drop in blood pressure caused by nervous impulses preventing the right amount of blood from reaching the brain. The nervous

system may affect the arteries, as may toxins such as drugs or chemicals produced by certain bacteria. The effect is to cause marked dilation of the blood vessels, thereby reducing blood pressure and, again, preventing blood flow to the heart. Strictly speaking a heart attack or any condition that affects the beating of the heart can lead to shock.

Recognition of shock is important because rapid intervention may be necessary to save a life. Any bleeding must be stemmed and any suspicion of internal bleeding must rapidly be dealt with by a doctor. First-aid techniques are necessary until such intervention is available. The signs are of pallor, weakness and a rapid heart beat accompanied by sensations of dizziness, confusion, nausea and a need to sit or lie down. If a blood pressure-recording instrument is available, a low blood pressure is usual.

RECOMMENDATIONS

General Advice

- Lower the head below the heart by placing it between the knees in a sitting position or lying flat with the legs raised.
- Remember the ABC (Airways, Breathing, Circulation) of emergency resuscitation and move to stem any bleeding if visible.
- Avoid giving anything by mouth, especially if internal bleeding is suspected because this may interfere with any necessary medical intervention.
- Keep the individual warm, using body contact if necessary.

Herbal/natural extracts

- Despite the recommendation above, it is acceptable to give a few drops of Rescue Remedy or a few drops or pills of Arnica 6 or Aconite 6 under the tongue. Do this every 10min until medical attention is received.

Electric shock

A high-level electricity jolt most commonly will have an effect by interfering with the electrical conductivity of the heart and stopping it temporarily or, sadly, permanently. Electric shock also has an effect on the nervous system through creating peripheral blood vessel dilation so that all of the blood pulls into the surface vessels, thereby reducing the cardiac flow.

Emotional shock
As described above, the word shock is not actually a medical term for an emotional state (*see* **Fright**).

SICK BUILDING SYNDROME
The advent of modern offices geared towards high utilization of space and profits has done away with the more natural and healthy working environment. Sick Building Syndrome was a phrase coined in the late 1970s following a boom in the use of computers and high-tech communications.

Symptoms
Individuals working in these offices may find themselves suffering from the following symptoms:

- Headaches
- Visual and eye problems
- Dry throat and nose (including nose bleeds)
- Congestion
- Asthma
- Skin irritations
- Generalized aches and pains
- Neurological symptoms such as numbness and tingling
- Lethargy and fatigue
- Sleep problems

This syndrome is not well recognized although more companies, especially in the USA, are accepting that more modern working conditions do not necessarily mean healthier working conditions. The problems arise from a variety of different areas within the building and the following only scratches the surface of the problem.

Air
Most offices contain a 'soup' of substances in the atmosphere known as volatile organic compounds (VOC). These arise from the cleaning fluids from the carpets, the dry cleaning substances from our clothes and the chemicals released from the computers and VDUs, such as ozone, negatively charged radicals and gold (yes, gold; it is used to coat certain components within computers) all mixed with our own aftershaves and perfumes. These compounds are absorbed and act as free radicals within the system as well as direct irritants and allergens.

Lighting
Ultraviolet light does not penetrate glass. Light is necessary for the skin to produce vitamin D, which, in turn balances calcium and phosphate levels in the system, both of which are essential for the normal functioning of many biochemical pathways. Muscles in particular are affected by an imbalance, causing a tendency towards aches, pains and strains. The brain chemicals that switch on and turn off our levels of activity (including naturally produced melatonin) are all dependent upon amounts of ultraviolet light. An absence created by being in an environment with no natural light, especially in the darker winter months, leads to fatigue and sleep disturbances.

Noise
Noise from extractor fans, air-conditioning units, traffic, the buzz of computers and the raised voices

of colleagues not only continually activates the brain but sets up vibrations that affect the nervous system and increase the release of VOC from machines.

Sitting position

Chairs are increasingly designed with the user in mind but these are often expensive and most offices are furnished with chairs that encourage bad posture. Stooping over a desk closes up the chest cavity, therefore impeding breathing and applying compression to nerves as they leave the spinal column. This, in conjunction with a lack of exercise and calcium imbalances caused by a lack of natural light, leads fairly swiftly to structural problems. Repetitive strain injury is encouraged by all of this.

Poor nutrition

Many larger offices have canteens where the food may be bought in bulk to save costs and thereby is liable to be non-organic, processed and full of additives. It is likely to be microwaved in its preparation thereby removing some of the vital force (*see* **Microwaves**).

Other factors

See **Geopathic stress**, which may come into play, depending on the position of the office building itself.

RECOMMENDATIONS

General Advice

- *Insist upon fresh air, using suitable filters if necessary.*
- *Insist upon natural light, preferably through open windows or, as a last resort, through natural-light bulbs.*
- *If noise cannot be avoided, spend some time in silence when away from the office. Even relaxing music is stimulatory.*
- *Get outside as much as possible (through breaks or at lunch time), spend time looking at the sky (not directly at the sun) and remember to take off any spectacles.*

- *Ensure that a part of your day is spent at exercise.*
- *A weekly (at least) session with a masseur or Shiatsu practitioner is sensible.*
- *Consider inviting a practitioner with a knowledge of Sick Building Syndrome to visit, along with a Feng Shui practitioner (see* **Feng Shui***).*

Nutritional

- *Ensure an adequate diet (see chapter 7).*

SLEEP PROBLEMS

Sleep is described as a transient, reversible and periodic state of rest in which there is diminution of physiological activity and of consciousness.

The human sleep cycle generally progresses through five stages, stage 1 being light sleep and stage 5 being deep sleep. Following this deep stage, there is an interlude of rapid eye movement (REM) and then the cycle repeats. This REM stage is named after the characteristic bursts of rapid eye movement, which also coincides with the facial muscles becoming floppy and, if one were attached to an electroencephalogram (EEG), a pattern of 'desynchronized' brain waves. It is assumed that most dreams occur in the deeper stages of sleep and in association with REM.

There is a marked decrease in activity throughout the body when asleep. Cell function continues and does not appear to need rest but the diminution in nervous system activity decreases the level and number of commands to stimulate cell metabolism. Why the nervous system needs to sleep is poorly understood. Scientists know the chemicals that are produced in abundance to put us to sleep but why they are produced is not recognized. I have a theory.

Nature is in balance. For every rain shower there is a sunny spell, for every ice cap there is a desert. Activity and rest are simply the night and day of the natural human balance. Sleep is the closest that most people get to a meditative state and it is well established that meditation has a profound effect on well-being if practised properly. Scientists tend to look for a chemical/biological necessity for sleep but in fact it is to do with a spiritual requirement and connection to the source of vital force. Without sleep we die very quickly due to the nervous system's loss of control over vital functions such as digestion and heart rate. There is no neurochemical basis for why rest would 'recharge' nervous cell activity, so the answer will be found when we can better assess the spiritual plane. Sleep is the body's attempt to connect with its God. That moment just prior to falling asleep, if not influenced by our conscious mind, is a very happy moment. I hope this is how we would all feel coming into contact with our 'maker', whatever our beliefs. Awaking from our dream state is often unpleasant.

Narcolepsy

Narcolepsy is a disorder of the body's normal circadian rhythm (body clock) with regard to sleep. Narcolepsy is characterized by uncontrollable attacks of drowsiness or falling asleep in the daytime, a sudden loss of muscular power often associated with emotional experiences, sleep paralysis (*see* **Sleep paralysis** *below*) and frequent vivid hallucinations during sleep.

It is important to differentiate narcolepsy from occurrences such as hypoglycaemia, which may have very mild forms of the same symptoms. Narcolepsy may well be created by damage to the brain through infection, toxins or physical damage. Acute or chronic dehydration may alter the electrolyte balance within the cerebrospinal fluid (the solution that the brain receives its nutrition from). Many cases of narcolepsy have no anatomical or chemical basis and one must return to the spiritual concept and ask why an individual is shutting out their consciousness. We must ask the question why does the sufferer need to escape reality.

RECOMMENDATIONS

General Advice
- *Try to isolate the cause by removing obvious toxins such as cigarettes, alcohol and other drugs.*

If the condition started at a particular point in time, review the events of the previous three months and see if any change in diet (food allergy) or close contact with an environmental pollutant may be relevant (see **Poisoning** *and* **Radiation***).*
- *Ensure that narcolepsy is not being confused for excessive tiredness due to a lack of sleep at the appropriate times.*
- *Ensure good hydration by drinking half pint of water per foot of height as a minimum daily intake.*
- *Consult a physician for a diagnosis if the above measures have not succeeded.*

Supplemental
- *Take a multivitamin/multimineral supplement at three times the daily recommended dose (RDA) for three weeks and see if there is an effect.*

Homeopathic
- *Consult with a qualified homeopath to select a suitable constitutional remedy.*

Orthodox
- *Review any orthodox drugs, as many have a narcoleptic effect. Antihistamines, tranquillizers and hypnotics are all very relevant.*

Sleep apnoea

Sleep apnoea is the cessation or suspension of breathing. Its reversibility separates it from asphyxia, which is effectively suffocation. However, for the few seconds that apnoea occurs, the physiology is moving towards respiratory failure.

The cause is uncertain but for some reason the nasopharyngeal area of the throat (that part behind the nose and mouth) closes up. If the problem is associated with an infection, treatment should be followed as for a common cold, but if it occurs separately and without reason, treatment should be attempted.

Rarely is sleep apnoea a problem for an adult, although partners of those who share a bedroom with the condition often have very disturbed sleep. Symptoms that are characteristic are grunting, snoring and restlessness as the individual attempts to pull air in past the obstruction. Cessation of breathing may occur for several seconds followed by an apparent sleep-state panic, which includes the noises mentioned above plus marked restlessness and an eventual gasp. The individual rarely wakes up and settles to repeat the cycle within a few moments. Periods of sleep apnoea occur throughout the night rather than remaining persistent.

Sleep apnoea in children below the age of two years may lead to asphyxia and is known as sudden infant death syndrome (SIDS) or cot death (*see* **SIDS**).

RECOMMENDATIONS

General Advice

- *Please look up in this book any concurrent problems, such as the common cold, if sleep apnoea is transient.*
- *See* **Snoring**, *because apnoea may be an extension of this condition.*

Homeopathic

- *A constitutionally chosen homeopathic remedy should be selected by a homeopath.*

Herbal/natural extracts

- *The Bach flower remedy Vervain should be taken before bed.*

Sleep paralysis

A most disturbing occurrence is experienced by most people at some time. On awakening, the body is unable to move. This condition rarely lasts for more than a few seconds but can continue for a moment or so. Quite simply the body is unable to move due to some lack of coordination between conscious thought and neuromuscular control. As the condition is sporadic, it is not possible to do studies on this matter but the assumption is made that a chemical disturbance occurs within the cerebellum at the base of the brain, an area that controls coordination.

RECOMMENDATIONS

General Advice

- *The problem is transient and is probably due to an excess of sleep chemicals not being removed from a part of the brain that controls coordination.*
- *If the problem persists, see a neurological specialist.*

Sleep patterns

The biochemistry of the brain is controlled by chemicals that are stimulated by the level of oxygen, glucose and probably other nutrients in the bloodstream. On top of this, the brain responds by producing chemicals such as melatonin in response to sunlight and darkness.

The human being has evolved as a daytime animal and principally we should sleep when the sun goes down and arise at dawn. Our evolutionary ancestors benefited by sleeping longer hours and keeping their metabolic rate low in winter when food was less abundant but could enjoy longer periods of wakefulness through the summer when nature produced its bounty. Having said that, it has recently been established that most teenagers need on average 9¼ hours sleep.

Chinese Energy Clock

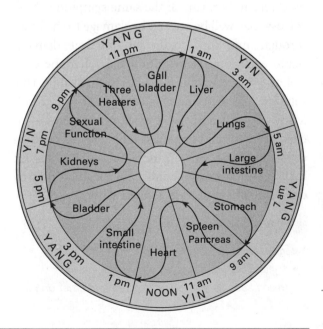

What is more, the production of melatonin, a chemical that helps us sleep, is produced an hour later than might be expected in adolescents, resulting in the fact that teenagers have trouble falling asleep before 11pm and are difficult to rouse early in the morning.

The Eastern philosophies had noticed a time clock and brought it into their medical philosophy well before science discovered chemical 'circadian' rhythms. The diagram opposite is one suggested time clock, which shows when various organs are energized. Sleep is a very active process as far as energy flow is concerned (*see* **Insomnia** *below*).

Insomnia

Insomnia needs to be divided into those who cannot get to sleep (sleep induction) and those who awaken (sleep interruption). The causes may overlap, although psychological stress factors are more likely to stop someone from sleeping than wake them up. Disturbed sleep is the result of a poor production of sleep chemicals (particularly serotonin), an overproduction of stimulating hormones such as adrenaline, cortisol and glucagon (the antagonist of insulin), or of external disturbances.

The causes of insomnia may be divided into the following categories.

Psychological factors

Any cause of stress, fear, anxiety or tension needs to be assessed and dealt with. As with any problem, if it cannot be solved then the individual must learn how to come to terms with it through counselling or relaxation techniques. Other factors include an unfavourable or noisy environment, a change in sleeping venue or a snoring partner. Psychological anxieties may lead to nightmares, sleepwalking, restlessness and sleep talking, which will disturb sleep and potentially awaken the individual.

I have often noticed that sleep may be deprived from an individual if their mind or body is trying to sort out a problem that sleep does not have an answer for. Do not go to bed with an unanswered question, wherever possible, but if this is unavoidable then ensure that 15–20 minutes of a relaxation technique or meditation time is taken to counteract the adrenaline created by the unresolved problem.

Toxins

There are obvious stimulants such as amphetamines and cocaine that keep people awake. Caffeine has some effect on most people and may be hidden in foods such as a bed-time cup of chocolate or tea, as well as coffee and coffee-flavoured ice cream. Less well known are the arousing effects of nicotine, cheese, red meat, alcohol and marijuana. The latter two are often a surprise to the uninitiated, who may confuse passing out with going to sleep. As the alcohol is denatured, a stimulatory effect is created and sleep is disturbed.

Bad habits

Other than those that come under the heading of toxins, such as smoking or drinking coffee, it is worth noting that a lack of exercise will inhibit sleep patterns. Regular exercise for as little as 20 minutes per day will use up excess adrenaline and release endorphins – the body's natural opiates. Having a large meal at night will create a large insulin response to be followed at some point through the night by a reflex hypoglycaemia. When the brain registers a low glucose level it will instruct the body to release adrenaline, glucagon and steroids to raise the blood sugar level but at the same time it will overstimulate itself and thereby disturb sleep.

Ley lines

The earth has energy lines known as ley lines created by the production of positively and negatively charged particles produced by the flow of water. These ley lines can interfere with our own intrinsic electromagnetic pattern and can be very disturbing to sleep. Those with unrelenting insomnia may consider the proximity of water, especially streams, which may be underground. The regional geological Survey Departments or local water companies may be able to furnish you with maps. Treatment is available by moving the bed so that the energy lines move in harmony with the body, rather than contradicting it.

Do not resort to botanical or supplemental medicines unless all the potential causes have been removed because in the long term symptoms will only be suppressed which will show up in another way later on. If the mind does not want to sleep, help it by removing the cause rather than suppressing it. The use of over-the-counter sedatives (usually an antihistamine-type drug) or prescribed sedatives or hypnotics should really be avoided except for very short-term use.

Sleep disturbances

Many conditions, both physiological, and pathological, can disturb sleep: pregnant ladies; weak bladders; gentlemen suffering with prostatism; breathing difficulties from conditions such as asthma or hay fever; vivid or bad dreams.

Simple matters such as ineffective curtains, an uncomfortable mattress or pillow need to be considered and, more unusually, the atmospheric ionic (positive or negatively charged air) effects of nearby or subterranean water flow. If you are near water or there is a suspicion of a subterranean stream, try moving the bed for a few nights to see if there is any benefit (*see* **Ley lines** *above*).

Other factors

The Eastern philosophies believe that specific organs and systems are energized at different times of the day and night. The previous diagram in the section on 'Sleep Patterns' describes different times when different organs are fed with the vital force. The triple heater, which controls the adrenal and thyroid glands, is at its weakest at the end of the day and is replenished between 9pm and 11pm.

The gallbladder and the liver are replenished between 11pm and 1am, and 1am and 3am,

respectively, having spent the day helping digestion and processing toxins.

Between 3am and 5am the lungs receive their energy, so they may be fully active during the day. The energy to the large intestine is replenished between 5am and 7am, which is why we generally evacuate our bowels at that time. Any disturbance to these organs will correspond to a greater or lesser demand for energy, which disturbs the general flow and in turn disturbs sleep.

As we age, we need less sleep. There is no orthodox scientific reason for this although certain chemicals are known to diminish as our cells deteriorate which may have some effect. The Eastern principle considers the diminution in 'vital energy' (life force) to be pertinent. The vital force we have requires less replenishment, and sleep is the time when this most occurs. We require less because we use less by lowering our levels of activity.

There is a condition known as nocturnal myoclonus which is characterized by a muscle group contracting whilst asleep. Like snoring, the perpetrator is unlikely to be aware of the condition and a sleeping partner usually initiates the diagnosis. This condition is similar to the restless legs syndrome (*see* **Restlessness**) and treatment may be needed.

RECOMMENDATIONS

General Advice

- *Eliminate all stimulants from the diet and lifestyle. Once a sleep pattern returns, introduce these stimulants early in the day and monitor whether they disturb sleep. If they do, they have to be cut out permanently.*

- *Assess any stress and deal with this, or learn and practise a good relaxation/meditation technique.*

- *Ensure that the sleeping environment is comfortable, quiet and dark. The reclining Buddha is always seen lying on his right with the right hand under the head. This position* encourages the energy flow needed for sleep and should be practised by everyone.

- Ensure that 20min of exercise is performed each day, and for bad insomnia try doing this again in the evening.
- If the individual is waking at a particular time, please review the possibility of an energetic disturbance in the organ or system that corresponds to that time of night (see the diagram on page 352).
- Move the bed 90° in case ley lines are relevant.

Nutritional

- Look back 6hr from the time of awakening and register what was eaten or drunk. This may be a specific intolerance and should be eliminated.
- Do not eat a heavy meal late at night, and avoid refined sugars at the evening meal.

Supplemental

- The following supplements and extracts can be used in doses as recommended below per foot of height approximately 1hr before going to sleep. Try one of the compounds at a time and add in the next if the effect does not become apparent after five nights: niacin (20mg), vitamin B$_6$ (10mg) and magnesium (60mg).
- The amino acid tryptophan can be taken at 75mg per foot of height, but is difficult to obtain because there is some controversy over the possibility of a toxic effect. Medical practitioners may have access to this amino acid. This should be taken one hour before sleeping with water and no other food or drink.
- Melatonin is being well-hyped as a safe 'supplement'. I put this word in inverted commas because this hormone comes under the licensing of a supplement but is in fact being touted as a medicine. It may well be safe but there is scant evidence to support this. Melatonin is best left alone or used as a last resort under medical supervision.

Homeopathic

- There are many homeopathic remedies that have insomnia or sleep disturbance as part of their symptom picture. Accurate selection is necessary but pay attention to the remedies Aconite, Lycopodium, Coffea and Arsenicum. The remedy opium should also be reviewed but may not be easy to obtain without a homeopath's prescription. All of these remedies should be taken at potency 200 for three consecutive nights and a result may occur immediately or within ten days. Be patient.

Herbal/natural extracts

- Valerian, Passiflora and Chamomile can all be taken but should be administered by a herbalist or knowledgeable complementary practitioner. Over-the-counter supplements may be tried but take care not to exceed the recommended dosage.

SNORING

Snoring is a rough audible sound caused by vibration of the soft palate at the back of the roof of the mouth during sleep. Anything that influences the tension, weight or size of the soft palate will influence snoring. This part of the roof of the mouth is very important in the formation of sound and swallowing and therefore has many muscular connections.

When we sleep, our muscles relax. The deeper the sleep, the more the relaxation and therefore a deep sleeper may well relax the soft palate muscles to such a point that it vibrates through normal breathing. The use of sleep-inducing drugs and, most frequently overlooked, alcohol will relax the tension in this area and cause snoring.

Fat settles around the soft palate and its muscles and an excess will alter the weight of the palate and predispose to snoring. Any condition that may inflame the area, such as the common cold, hay fever or other causes of rhinitis and, very importantly, smoking, can cause snoring.

Noisy breathing through sleep that is not actually soft palate-created snoring may occur with any nasal obstruction. Rhinitis, the common cold, nasal polyps, sinusitis and enlarged adenoids may all produce a snoring sound. The use of the nose to abuse drugs such as cocaine, amphetamines and heroin by 'snorting' will create inflammation and worsen snoring.

RECOMMENDATIONS

General Advice

- *Temporary snoring associated with a common infection may benefit from treatment directed at rhinitis (see Hay fever).*
- *Persistent snoring may be stopped by losing weight, cessation of smoking and stopping alcohol and excessive sweet foods.*
- *The position in which a snorer sleeps may influence the noise. Generally speaking, sleeping on the back makes the problem worse.*
- *There are devices called mandibular advancement devices (MADs), which prevent the lower jaw from falling back, thereby pulling the tongue forward and away from the soft palate.*
- *Continuous positive airways pressure (CPAP) units actually pump air at high pressure into the airways, which may strengthen the musculature.*

Supplemental

- *L-Tryptophan, an amino acid that is difficult to obtain, may well be beneficial if taken in moderate doses because it is turned into serotonin by the nervous system, which enhances muscular tension.*

Homeopathic

- *The homeopathic remedy Opium (often available only on prescription, especially in the USA) can be taken at potency 200 each night for one week.*

Herbal/natural extracts

- *The Bach flower remedy Vervain, four drops before bed, may also influence snoring.*

Orthodox

- *The orthodox world will offer steroid nasal sprays which show some efficacy but need to be used continually.*
- *Surgery may be offered as a last resort. Avoid if at all possible.*

- *A new injectable technique may be available soon. The injection hardens the soft palate and has proven successful in trials with chronic, long-standing snorers.*

SPEECH PROBLEMS – *see* **Stammering** *and* **Dysphasia**.

TINNITUS

Tinnitus is the medical term for a persistent noise heard in the head or in either, or both, ears. Very often tinnitus will disappear if there is background noise but in severe cases it will override even that.

The traditional view is that tinnitus is caused by stimulation of the nerves and structures leading to the auditory centres in the brain and can, therefore, be triggered by inflammation or damage from the eardrum through the ear ossicles (bones) found in the middle ear, through the delicate nerve endings in the inner ear and damage along the nerve pathways into the brain. Continuous and loud noises such as an explosion, infections, head injuries and arthritic conditions of the ear ossicles can all be potential causes. Irritation of the eardrum by ear wax can be an innocent and easily treatable problem. Certain mineral deficiencies may also trigger the problem.

A different view of this is based on the 'Jastreboff model', which was published in a top neurological research magazine in 1990. This suggests that tinnitus is not solely caused by damage, but is the fault of the brain's perception of a background sound that we would all normally hear. The suggestion is that oversensitivity is created by underlying irritation, anger, depression, anxiety or other persistent negative emotions. The parts of the brain that are electrically activated by sound are greatly influenced by the subconscious areas of the brain. If stress chemicals such as adrenaline are creating a belief in our subconscious that we are in danger, our hearing becomes hyper-acute as part of our survival mechanism.

Tinnitus – Ear and Nerves

The vestibular nerve transmits extraneous stimuli to the auditory centres in the brain which we experience as tinnitus.

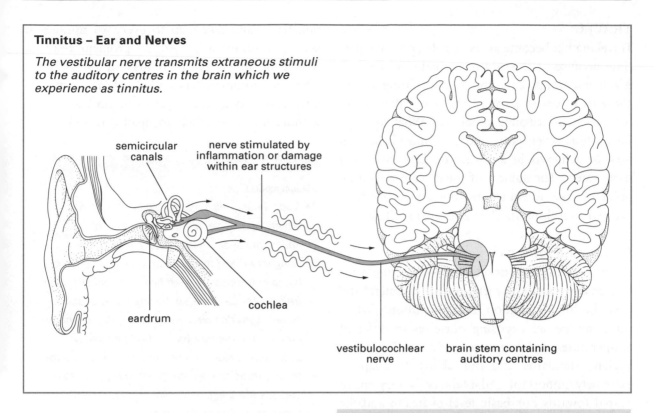

semicircular canals

nerve stimulated by inflammation or damage within ear structures

cochlea

eardrum

vestibulocochlear nerve

brain stem containing auditory centres

Retraining the brain to ignore the persistent sound is the basis of a very specific therapy.

RECOMMENDATIONS

General Advice

- If the following do not help over a few days then a visit to your GP to rule out an obvious and visible cause should be undertaken.
- Chiropractic, craniosacral and cranial osteopathic treatment can all be instantly effective although a few sessions may be necessary.
- It is also wise to remove the amalgam (mercury) from your teeth and ensure that you are not taking in metals from aluminium pans. A metal toxicity test may be beneficial here.
- If tinnitus persists after these measures, then a referral to a neurologist and CT or MRI scanning is advisable to rule out the rare serious causes of this problem.
- Provided that there is no serious problem, try hypnotherapy if it persists.

Nutritional

- Reduce saturated fats and cholesterol in your diet and avoid aspirin.

Supplemental

- Take magnesium and potassium replacements at twice the recommended dose given or eat six bananas per day (two with each meal).
- Vitamin B complex (50mg) or vitamin B_6 (50mg) may help to remove fluid in the middle ear.
- Ginkgo biloba, around 50–60mg a day for an adult, taken in divided doses with breakfast and with supper may be beneficial.

Homeopathic

- The homeopathic remedies Salicylic acidum, Cannabis indicus and Kali iodatum should be reviewed to see if the symptoms are suitable.

Orthodox

- Consider contacting The Tinnitus and Hyperacusis Centre, 32 Devonshire Place, London, W1G 6JL, discussing with an ear, nose and throat specialist, or finding a local specialist by visiting www.tinnitus.org

TRAVEL

Travelling has become an extremely accessible pastime because of the advent of high-speed travel. Airplanes, trains, cars and fast sea-faring vessels allow us to get to parts of the world that would have been inaccessible otherwise. What took Dr Livingstone seven years and cost him his life can now be achieved in a matter of days with a lot more safety. The subject of travel from a medical point of view is enormous, but few books have been written about it. The basics are as follows.

Preparation for travel

When booking the tickets and organizing your foreign currency, it is worth looking at general and basic health preparation and precautions. When travelling we are exposing ourselves to different temperatures, sun exposure, pollution, foods and hygiene standards and our ability to adapt is extremely important. Adaptability is very much geared towards our basic level of health and the more extreme the travel or adventure, the healthier we should be. Those lacking in health should not risk travel to countries that are very different from their own.

RECOMMENDATIONS

General Advice

- *Avoid travelling when your health is below par.*
- *Travel to tropical areas when there is lower risk of infections, such as avoiding the monsoon season in malaria-endemic areas.*
- *A basic check-up with a complementary medical practitioner is a useful starting point and follow their suggestions to achieve and maintain a good level of health.*
- *Take suitable medical supplies as described below.*

Medical supplies for travel

I recommend that the following homeopathic and supplemental remedies are taken and used as described, as well as certain supplements and topical creams. All remedies should be bought at

potency 6 and taken up to every 15 minutes if acute symptoms arise. As the problem resolves, reduce the dose to every 2 hours and stop 24 hours after the condition has settled. Always contact a physician if symptoms worsen or do not resolve within a few doses of a homeopathic remedy.

RECOMMENDATIONS

Supplemental

- *Acidophilus – High-potency yoghurt bacteria tablets should be taken with any sort of abdominal upset. Acidophilus needs to be refrigerated and therefore may survive only a few hours in the heat. Aircraft holds are below freezing temperature so Acidophilus exposed to non-refrigeration on the way to the airport and on arrival, until the mini-bar or a kitchen can be accessed, should be fine. Adults should take two tablets three times a day preferably just before eating something, and children should take one tablet at the same frequency.*
- *A multivitamin/multimineral supplement should be taken at twice the daily recommended dose because travel usually exposes one to processed foods and is unlikely to provide the recommended daily five portions of fresh fruit or vegetable. A change in diet often alters absorptive capacity until the bowel readjusts and a natural food-state multivitamin should compensate. Once the normal diet has been resumed, drop the supplements to just the recommended doses.*

Homeopathic

- *Aconite – for any condition that comes on suddenly and any problem that is associated with fear or agitation.*
- *Apis – for any sting, bite, red or hot area on the skin or in any joint. Bites from unidentified snakes or spiders must be dealt with by a doctor, although Apis may be used prior to consultation.*
- *Arnica – for any shock, psychological or physical. It can be used for any bruise or sprain until a better choice of remedy is available.*

Medical Supplies for Travel

MULTI-VITAMIN

PHILUS OGHURT

CONITE

NICA REAM

CARB VEGA

EPAR L PH

Supplies that should be taken include homeopathic remedies, Acidophilus tablets, Arnica- and Calendula-based creams, and vitamin and mineral supplements. It may also be advisable to obtain prescription painkillers and antibiotics.

* *Carbo vegetabilis – for diarrhoea associated with pain and flatulence. Any upper abdominal symptoms such as heartburn or reflux may benefit from this and Carbo vegetabilis is a good remedy for a stomach upset that is associated with a chest infection. Use this remedy if bowel habit changes because of the type of food eaten rather than for food poisoning.*
* *Hepar sulphuris calcarium – this remedy is useful for any topical infections, such as an abscess or earache, and infections that are associated with glandular swelling, including tonsillitis. It is always wise to use a specific remedy but Hepar sulphuris calcarium is an excellent first-aid choice.*
* *Nux vomica – this is useful in dysentery or diarrhoea following food poisoning. Frequent visits to the toilet or diarrhoea alternating with constipation suggest Nux vomica.*

Herbal/natural extracts

* *An Arnica-based cream should be taken up to four times a day for any penetrating injury or bruises, sprains and ligament or bone injuries.*
* *A Calendula-based cream should be used up to four times a day on any cut, scrape, bite, burn or superficial injury.*

Orthodox drugs for travel

If the travel will be taking the individual out of reach of immediate medical care, then the following prescriptions should be obtained from a GP and packed with the luggage.

RECOMMENDATIONS

Orthodox

* *A paracetamol/codeine mix as a moderate painkiller.*
* *A powerful painkiller (a step below opiates) such as mefenamic acid.*
* *The antibiotic amoxicillin. A broad-spectrum antibiotic which should only be used if an infection has settled in and naturopathic treatments are not working. Use this for any general infection such as a sore throat, tonsillitis or chest infection.*
* *The antiobiotic metronidazole. This is useful in infections by bacteria that do not require oxygen to breed and therefore is potentially useful in severe bowel infections, dental infections, sinus infections or a deep wound.*

Ensure that the doctor or pharmacist labels the maximum allowable dosages of all of these compounds.

Travel vaccinations

I am principally against the use of vaccinations, which I think may be more dangerous than protective in some individuals, unless the traveller is immunocompromised (has a low immune system) or is unlikely to be able to avoid coming into contact with a condition. Most parts of the world only recommend vaccination, although some require it as a prerequisite for obtaining a visa. See **Vaccinations** after finding out your requirements through a local pharmacist or a major airline's medical section.

If you choose, having read the information in this and other publications, not to use vaccinations for travelling you may use the following homeopathic remedies, bearing in mind that their efficacy is not scientifically accepted despite government statistics to the contrary. Alternatively you may take these remedies before regular vaccinations because they may prevent unwanted side effects from the orthodox drugs.

It is acceptable to take all of these together but it would be better to space them out. Start all homeopathic prophylaxis one week before departure.

Malaria prophylaxis is not a vaccination and I generally recommend the use of these drugs if exposure to malaria is probable (*see* **Malaria**).

Travel tips

RECOMMENDATIONS

General Advice

- *If travelling outside of developed countries, drink only bottled water. Even in 'First World' countries, water safety can be suspect. Mediterranean countries and others with hot climates may still carry risks. Sterilization tablets should only be used in circumstances where bottled water is not available because these compounds kill all bugs, including the normal bowel flora.*
- *Avoid foods that have been washed in tap water, such as salads and fruits with edible skins. Peel these and they should be okay.*
- *Try to eat foods that you have seen being cooked. These should be served fresh and not allowed to sit for any length of time. Restaurants in top-class hotels are also permissible dining venues but even these are not likely to be as*

Condition	Remedy	Frequency
Cholera	*Camphora* 200	Weekly
Hepatitis (A, B and others)	*Lycopodium* 200	Weekly
	Chelidonium 200	Weekly
Japanese encephalitis	*Belladonna* 200	Weekly
Malaria	*Natrum muriaticum* 12	Morning and night whilst away and for one week after returning
Meningitis	*Belladonna* 200	Weekly
	Iodoformum 200	Weekly
Polio	*Lathyrus* 200	Weekly
Rabies	*Hydrophobinum* 30	Weekly
Tuberculosis	*Tuberculinum* 200	Every two weeks
Typhoid	*Baptisia* 30	Weekly
Yellow fever	*Arsenicum album* 200	Monthly

The homeopathic remedies that correspond with the infections commonly vaccinated against when travelling. (See **Travel vaccinations**.*)*

safe as the street seller with a boiling vat of lentils.

- Consider going vegetarian, as many dangerous infections are transmitted more easily in meat.
- Consider the cleanliness of the cook or chef. If you have any doubts do not risk him transmitting disease through the oral-faecal route.
- Bottled and carbonated drinks are generally not good but two or three a day in a hot climate will replace sugars and salts that are lost through sweating. These should be taken with water to avoid the dehydrating effect.
- 'Chai' or 'Chaa' is a milky, sweet tea with cardamom and other spices, commonly served on the streets in India and other hot countries. This acts as a marvellous antiseptic for the bowel and the high (unfortunately refined) sugar content replenishes energy that is used up by the sweating process. It tastes nice too.

Air travel

The increasing number of airline passengers has created increased chances of developing health problems in transit. There are two main areas of concern that have been noted by the orthodox scientific world and the passengers themselves, along with the overburdened general practitioner. Mainly they are blood clot formation and increased respiratory tract infections.

Clotting

See **Deep vein thrombosis (DVT)** and **Blood clotting and clots**.

RECOMMENDATIONS

General Advice

- Exercise the legs and calves by doing heel–toe exercises while sitting or walking up and down the aisles – if it is not too inconvenient.
- Avoid dehydration. Drink one litre of water for every six hours of flying. Avoid alcohol.

Supplemental

- Vitamin E 400iu, essential fatty acids 1000mg, and grape seed extract 500mg, all taken daily starting three days before the flight, repeated on the day of the flight, and after six hours on the aircraft if the flight is a long one. Children over 12 can take the adult dosage but those below should take proportionately lower dosages.

Orthodox

- Aspirin 150mg taken the day before and the day of the flight. This should be not be used by asthmatics, by those who have symptoms of indigestion, nor by those who have raised blood pressure.

Respiratory illnesses

While there are no statistics, most general practitioners, as well as airline crews, would admit to noticing an increase in the frequency of coughs and chest infections, sinus and ear problems that seem to be associated with having travelled by air within the previous two to three days. More research needs to be carried out in this area, but I believe that increased efficiency of the aircraft's ventilation systems needs to be considered. In the meantime, following the recommendations below may reduce the chance of infection.

RECOMMENDATIONS

General Advice

- Take fruit and vegetables or multi mineral/antioxidant supplements in high doses the day before and during the flight.

Supplemental

- The following should be started three days prior to travel and continued three days after:
  - Beta-carotene 1000iu per foot of height daily
  - Vitamin C 500mg per foot of height
  - Multi-vitamin B complex, as recommended on the package.

Herbal/natural extracts

- *Consider taking Echinacea or an Echinacea combination at the maximum dose as recommended on the packaging, starting three days prior to travelling and then continuing for three days after.*
- *Take one drop of Tea tree essential oil in a cup of hot water provided by the airline crew inhaled every four hours. A drop or two on a handkerchief or shirt collar will suffice.*

Jet lag

Jet lag is a most disturbing aspect of long-distance travel. It is caused by the alteration of the body's internal clock which throws the chemical, sleep, hydration and elimination patterns out of synchronization. The nervous system adjusts slowly and the trick in avoiding unpleasant patterns is to readjust to these at a quicker pace.

Sleep disturbed through long-haul travel, shift work or partying reduces the amount of a protein called HFF2 that is thought to activate tissue repair in the gut. Missing sleep also lowers the levels of this compound.

RECOMMENDATIONS

General Advice

- *No alcohol for 24hr prior to departure.*
- *If you are crossing more than four time zones (4hr difference) start adjusting a few days before by going to bed earlier or later and getting up at the time the sun rises at your destination.*
- *Try not to travel if you have a cold or ear problems. See a health practitioner if you have.*
- *Avoid the aisle seats. You are invariably going to be disturbed by passengers and staff walking by.*
- *Consider ordering the vegetarian meal – proteins demand more energy to digest.*
- *Ensure that you drink half a litre (1 pint) of water for each 3hr on the plane.*
- *Take healthy snacks with you and eat them at the meal times of your destination.*

- *Broad-spectrum light – BSL – stimulation. BSL stimulates the production of melatonin and, if used at specific times as specified on specialized charts, can maintain the circadian (normal body) rhythm.*
- *Pituitary – light stimulation – visors. There is now a computerized high-tech visor available that delivers a suitable dose of broad-spectrum light. The flight times and appropriate stimulation are delivered via the computer, which sits comfortably in a sport-like sun-visor on the forehead. This stimulates the pineal and pituitary gland to produce natural melatonin and markedly reduces jet lag. These are invaluable to a frequent traveller and may be bought or hired.*

Homeopathic

- *Homeopathic remedies. People who have trouble taking off on a plane should consider the use of Spongia 6, four pills four times a day prior to the flight and every hour starting 3hr before take-off. Those who have trouble landing should consider the remedy Borax 6 at the same frequency. Other remedies that can be reviewed are Arnica, Aconite, Cocculus indicus, Rhus toxicodendron and Nux vomica.*

Herbal/natural extracts

- *Calendula cream is the moisturizer of choice.*

Skin, hair and eye care

RECOMMENDATIONS

General Advice

- *Hair should be washed and conditioned before and after a flight with a non-medicated shampoo.*

Herbal/natural extracts

- *Calendula-based creams can be used as a moisturizer.*
- *Euphrasia (eyebright), one or two drops of a diluted solution, can be dropped into the eye during and after a flight. It may be very helpful for 'red-eye'.*

Relaxation techniques

RECOMMENDATIONS

General Advice

- *Some airlines now have a video or audio channel set aside for passengers who are frightened of flying or who wish to have an audible aid to meditation whilst in their seat. Use this.*
- *A session with a yoga or Tai Chi teacher can give you a personal plan suitable for you to use during and after flights.*
- *Massage. Those lucky enough to fly first class with certain airlines may be offered an in-flight massage. Accept it. For the rest of us, the basic for self-assisted massage using acupressure, stretch techniques and Shiatsu can be taught by a Shiatsu practitioner to help circulation in muscles and lymphatic drainage. Many travellers find that they catch colds and sore throats on long flights. This is partly caused by the air conditioning and the close proximity of infected passengers, but also by the lack of lymphatic flow caused by neck stiffness.*

Treatments and remedies

Several homeopathic remedies and supplements can be utilized, depending upon the individual and their anticipated problems. It is best to discuss matters with a homeopath but the following suggestions can be used safely.

RECOMMENDATIONS

Supplemental

- *A whole amino acid tablet taken with each meal on the day of the flight and the following day supplies the essential amino acids that will help the body to produce its own relaxation and sleep chemicals. This is not a tranquillizer of any sort because one could take the entire bottle and not have any neurological effect. It simply provides the body with the amino acids that it needs to produce its own sleep chemical when it tries to.*

Homeopathic

- *If you are fearful of flying, take Aconite 30 every 4hr starting the day before travel and every half-hour from checking in.*
- *If you suffer from travel sickness, try Cocculus indicus 6 starting half-hour before boarding and taken every half-hour if necessary through the flight.*
- *If you are frightened of landing or nauseous with downward movement try Borax 30. This remedy should be taken every 2hr once on the plane and every 15min as soon as the descent is commenced.*
- *If you are frightened by taking off or frightened of heights, use Spongia 30. Start 6hr before the flight and take a dose every 2hr increasing this to every 15min once on the plane. Once cruising altitude has been reached, take Spongia as infrequently as the fear arises.*

Herbal/natural extracts

- *I currently advise against the use of the new drug melatonin (discussed in chapter 10). It is probably safe and works by mimicking the body's natural melatonin, which puts us to sleep. The trouble is that there has not been enough research to categorically state that it is safe and any drug that takes over from a natural function of the body may, in some way, inhibit normal function. Some people also have side effects such as headaches.*
- *Lavender oil, two drops on a handkerchief or the collar of a shirt, is essential if any congestion is being suffered in order to avoid ear and sinus pain. One drop in hot water (provided by the cabin staff) can be used as an inhalation.*

TUBERCULOSIS

Tuberculosis is caused by a bacterium known as *Mycobacterium tuberculosis*. There are two strains, one human and one bovine (cow), which are spread by inhalation of infected sputum in the case of the former and by drinking infected milk in the case of the latter.

Tuberculosis is generally overcome by an intact

immune system but anyone with a lowered resistance from conditions such as malnutrition, diabetes and drug use (including alcohol or smoking or those taking drugs for immuno-suppression, as in HIV and AIDS) are more likely to succumb if this disease is contracted. Anybody with lung infection or disease is also more prone.

The incidents of tuberculosis remain high in overcrowded and Third World countries, but until recently tuberculosis was on the wane in the Western world. Unfortunately, injudicious use of antibacterial agents has led to resistant strains developing, which are now defeating even the strongest of antibiotics. We appear to be coming full circle (as with syphilis) and returning to a time when individual health and a strong immune system is going to prove of more benefit than drug treatment.

This condition used to be known as consumption because of the symptoms of malaise, weight loss or failure to grow, and a persisting cough with the development of shortness of breath. Many other features are known to physicians and would be looked for at an examination if necessary.

Left alone, the great majority of those who contract the condition will simply defeat the bacteria and leave a characteristic calcified area noted on X-rays. This is formed by the body's attempt to wall in the infection. Tuberculosis may continue to live within this cavity and escape at times when the individual is run down, causing a reactivation of the symptoms.

Investigations include chest X-rays with lesions that usually appear in the upper part of the lungs. Some blood changes may be found, including a positive TB antibody test, but a definitive diagnosis is generally made by culturing sputum or urine samples, depending upon where the infection is, and growing them in special culture mediums.

In a severely ill person, treatment with antibiotics may need to be started before a firm diagnosis is made and before it is known whether the antibiotics being used are in fact going to affect this type of bacteria. Complementary medical treatment may be of benefit in less seriously ill people whilst they await the sensitivity reports so that accurate antibiotic treatment may be given.

RECOMMENDATIONS

General Advice

- *Any persistent illness needs to be checked by a doctor and it is worth reminding physicians in the West, who may not come across tuberculosis, to consider it as part of their differential diagnosis.*
- *If tuberculosis is diagnosed do not rush into drug treatment unless symptoms are causing marked problems. Instead consult a complementary medical practitioner with experience in this field. Self-treatment may not necessarily be the best.*
- *Ensure that a change in lifestyle is made to eliminate all factors that may be reducing immunity, especially bad habits such as smoking and excess alcohol. Any drug of abuse will reduce the body's immune system response.*
- *Prevention is generally the best form of treatment so ensure that health is at an optimum level before visiting areas where tuberculosis is endemic. If optimum health is not present, then see* **Vaccinations** *to decide whether such an inoculation should be used.*

Homeopathic

- *Whilst awaiting specific treatment protocols, use the homeopathic remedy Tuberculinum 200 nightly for three nights.*

Miliary tuberculosis

If tuberculosis spreads through the blood, it can land in any tissue anywhere. Widespread symptoms may occur and the above treatment recommendations should be considered bearing in mind that this condition is far more aggressive and likely to have a poorer prognosis.

TYPHOID – *see* **Salmonella poisoning**

ULCERS

An ulcer can be described as an interruption of an

internal or external surface which is associated with an inflamed middle or base. Ulcers are usually due to some traumatic event or to some toxin directly applied or produced by a disease process.

WATER RETENTION – *see* Fluid retention

WEIGHT LOSS AND OBESITY (OVERWEIGHT)

The word obesity is used by doctors to label those in the population who are 10 per cent above the average. This can be 50 per cent of the population in some parts of the world and, distressingly, is becoming more common in our children. Being overweight is not as simple as having a set ratio of height/weight, because some people with large muscle mass may be overweight but should not be considered clinically obese. Obesity is only a problem if it affects an individual psychologically or is creating a strain on the body. This stress may be a structural one, affecting the joints and circulation or affecting vital organs such as the heart, which has to beat harder to move the blood around the increased size of the system.

Interestingly, most of the charts that doctors use to help an individual determine an ideal weight are based on a population of those who have taken out insurance and remained in good health over a period of years. As most people who take out insurance come from a higher income bracket and are more likely to pay attention to their health, this standard may be incorrect. It may be better to determine obesity by comparing fat with lean weight. This can be done by:

- Skin-fold callipers. This simple piece of equipment measures the thickness of a fold of skin,

most commonly measured below the navel, just below the shoulder blade, above the hip bone and behind the upper arm, by the use of specialized callipers.

Height and Weight Chart

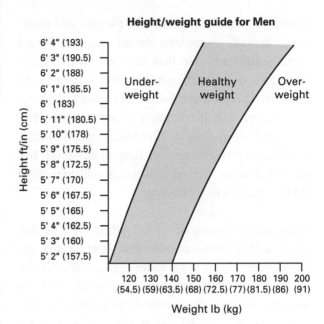

Height/weight guide for Men

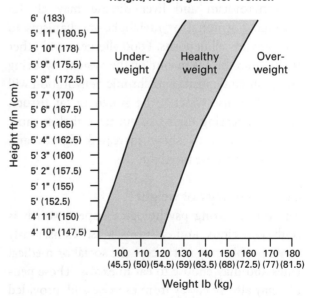

Height/weight guide for Women

While there is no one ideal weight for men and women of certain heights, the above tables show the weight ranges we should aim to maintain.

- Computers are now available in most gymnasiums or diet clinics that calculate the speed of electrical flow, which is different through fat than through lean tissue. By entering height and age into the computer, an extremely accurate lean body/body fat ratio can be calculated.

Obesity is actually governed by the size and number of fat cells. Somehow the cells seem to have a target minimum size that increases with age. If this size is not met then hormones are sent to the brain by the fat cells themselves telling the nervous system that it is hungry. Cravings ensue and increased input results. The biochemistry of this metabolic system is not yet fully understood, but we watch with interest because it will inevitably lead to options in treatment.

There are two types of fat cell: white fat cells that store, and brown fat cells that control storage. Those individuals with more brown fat cells are able to eat large amounts and rarely put on weight, whereas those with little brown fat may behave extremely well dietetically and yet increase in weight. Certain diseases such as diabetes, hypothyroidism and liver disease may all act through hormonal or metabolic mechanisms to increase fat cell deposits. Food allergens and other toxins may be taken out of the system by being stored in fat deposits and chronic dehydration will certainly cause water to be stored in fat tissues, falsely increasing their size but nevertheless causing the scales to show increased figures and clothes to become too tight.

The psychology of weight

There is a strong psychological aspect, which is both conscious and subconscious. Consciously some people may not accept the social or medical rules and may choose to eat in excess. These people may also shy away from exercise and, provided that their obesity is not harming their health and they are happy, there is no reason for them to change their attitudes. The subconscious, however, may not necessarily be making them happy or healthy.

We respond to external stimuli such as the sight, smell and taste of food which can trigger almost addictive tendencies to eating. We are constantly bombarded by advertising and one of the biggest culprits is television. Around meal times advertisers promote their fast-food products, which trigger memories of sweet, fat and other stimulatory tastes. Interestingly, television watching is specifically linked to obesity, not only because of its reduction in physical activity but also because it has a trance-like effect that leaves the brain thinking it needs something and, not knowing exactly what it wants, it decides that food is the easiest answer.

We also have a tendency to reward with food. A visit to Grandma or an outing to the cinema, fun fair or sporting event is usually 'rewarded' with a sweet drink, refined sugar or processed meat snack. This association of food with good times leaves us feeling empty if we are relaxing but not imbibing.

Weight and our habits

At the end of the day, when all is said and done, an increase in fat and weight is due to an excess of calorific input over calorific expenditure. A pound of human fat is equivalent to 3,500 calories and weight reduction can only be obtained if output is greater than input to that degree. In more realistic terms a negative output/input balance of 500 calories is needed per day to lose one pound of weight per week. Running a mile at your top speed will burn up approximately 400 calories but a fast-food hamburger will put on over 450. A large gin and tonic will add over 200 calories, which would take nearly 15 minutes at a fast pace to burn off on an exercise machine. Evolution and nature have remembered days gone by when food was not easily available and the storage mechanisms in the human system were important survival factors but have not yet adapted us to our more affluent lifestyles.

I find it interesting to note that obesity is much more a problem of the developed countries of the world. Primitive cultures that remain untouched by modern advances and refined foods are not overweight. So-called Third World countries that are affected by refined and high-fat foods have much greater levels of obesity and a corresponding shorter life expectancy. Kenya is an interesting example. The Africans who live within the cities tend to be overweight and indeed a culture has developed that regards obesity as an attractive asset. However, the native, indigenous peoples not affected by unnatural foods tend to maintain a healthier, lower weight.

Weight and Qi

The Western world has concerned itself entirely with calories when it comes to obesity. A more holistic viewpoint is that food carries an energy. It is the same vital force that exists in every living cell and is possibly a reflection of the way in which electrons, surrounding their nuclei, move and resonate. The presence or absence of electrons alters the function of any atom and thereby gives it many of its characteristics. This vibration is transmitted to other substances that it may come into contact with. Food created by nature's humours – air, light, water and earth – will carry specific vibrations and building blocks from which we have evolved. Our need to store is less pronounced when nature's balance is allowed to run its course. The vital force within a food substrate may be more relevant than we realize.

Many gurus and their disciples who meditate for many hours of the day require little, if any, sleep and often exist on very small amounts of water and food. Their metabolic rate is reduced but even that cannot account for the reduction in the amount of nutrients and calories upon which they need to survive. The hypothesis put forward by those who have studied meditation is that energy is actually absorbed from the cosmos through the art of meditation. On a more tangible note, I have wondered why individuals expending

the same amount of calorific output and living in similar climates may have such disparate ranges of weight. For example: the population living in Florida are much fatter than people of a similar socioeconomic group who live in, say, Bombay. I have drawn the conclusion that processed foods and nutrients that have been attacked by preservatives, additives and microwave energy lose their vital force. Although the calories and nutrients are available, the vital force is missing and therefore much larger amounts need to be eaten to create a level of satiety. Natural and fresh foods do not lack this energy and create a 'fullness' more swiftly. Ask somebody to eat three bananas and they would be struggling. The equivalent amount of calories would appear in a doughnut or a small bar of chocolate and, more often than not, one is not enough.

Fat storage may, therefore, not simply be a calorific matter but revolve around a quest for energy. Fat stores are not just holding calories but are an attempt to contain a vital force that is not coming into the system regularly or naturally. Stagnation of this Qi is a well-accepted Eastern philosophy and may be to do with a lack of electron movement in 'dead' calories.

Weight and deficiencies

If the body is deficient in a particular nutrient, instructions will be sent via nerves or hormones to the brain advising it to imbibe the missing factor. Instincts and cravings are very accurate in children but alter as we age, mostly by psychological factors. As I have mentioned, the reward and comfort eating of sweet and fatty foods registers in memory banks and the brain correlates these high-calorie foods with types of reward and happiness. We train our children at a very young age by rewarding and congratulating them with sweets, chocolates, French fries and carbonated sweet drinks rather than fruit or other natural sweeteners. This tendency is very much appreciated by the brain which, after its structure is in place, only utilizes glucose to function. Refined foods, sweet foods and fats provide a swiftly absorbed source of glucose that the brain can utilize at a quicker rate than a complex carbohydrate or protein. When a nervous or hormonal instruction is sent to the brain, intending to register a deficiency in a nutrient, the brain cannot differentiate whether this is a need that is easy to fulfil or one suggesting a period of starvation. The brain triggers a response that basically says 'eat' and as the brain itself prefers sugars our tendency is to eat sweet foods. Refined starch comes a close second and fats third because these provide sugars as mentioned above. A deficiency in, say, chromium, may therefore lead to a sugar and starch craving and it is often only by good fortune that the original deficiency is plugged.

Weight loss

Losing weight is achieved by dealing with the following four areas.

Correct diet

This needs to be balanced between protein, carbohydrate and fats and contain the correct amounts of essential trace elements and minerals, vitamins and supplements. A correct dietetic plan may need to be followed and guidelines are set out in chapter 7.

Exercise

When all is said and done, calories and fat cannot be stored if the output of the body is greater than the input. The correct exercise plan is dependent upon an individual's body type and the natural tendency to avoid exercise as we age needs to be borne in mind (*see* Exercise).

Psychological factors

Incorrect attitude and education is the principal cause of obesity from a psychological point of view. Being socially advised, through peer pressure and advertising, to alter body weight leads to weight swings that can alter the body's natural mechanism for achieving satiety when enough calories have been taken in. Reprogramming the consciousness and subconsciousness and removing the reward aspect of calorific foods is extremely important.

Stagnation and deficiency of Qi

This does not only lead to obesity but also to disease processes. Poor dietetic energy input must be evaluated and corrected. This is a concept that is perhaps best taught by meditation teachers and yoga and Qi Gong masters.

RECOMMENDATIONS

General Advice

- *A sudden onset of weight gain or obesity without obvious reason should initially be reviewed by a GP who should check for metabolic disorders such as hypothyroidism and diabetes. The liver is very responsible for much of the body's fat metabolism. Alcohol in particular and other liver-stressing drugs, including orthodox medication, can affect the liver metabolism and thereby encourage obesity. This clearly needs to be reviewed but may require a complementary medical practitioner's assessment as well. Poor digestive capabilities through a lack of hydrochloric acid or pancreatic enzymes may also need reviewing by a non-orthodox practitioner.*
- *Simple analysis of whether obesity is in fact a problem should be undertaken before any attempts are made to lose weight. Trying to keep the body below its preferred size is difficult and will be an uphill and, ultimately, losing battle.*
- *See* **Exercise** *or discuss matters with a gym master. A personal exercise programme should be set up, which should minimally include 20–30min of aerobic exercise at least three times a week and should balance the amount of calorific input.*
- *Depression, anxiety and other strong emotions may lead to comfort eating. Review and analyse attitudes to food with friends and family or discuss the matter with a counsellor. Neurolinguistic programming and hypnotherapy may be of great benefit if craving tendencies are marked.*
- *Do not underestimate the role of Qi or the vital*

force in weight gain. Techniques of yoga, Qi Gong or Tai Chi, and even ballet or martial arts, can offer both an exercise programme and techniques for moving energy through the system.

- Marked weight fluctuation is probably water retention and the most common causes for this are hormonal cyclical changes and dehydration. Do not confuse obesity with water retention and ensure that at least 1 pint of water is drunk per foot of height per day.

- Decrease television watching. More so than other stagnant activities such as reading, viewing of the television has been shown to have a pronounced effect on obesity through factors other than decreased activity. Do not eat in front of the TV.

- Acupuncture may be useful in helping to decrease appetite but should only be used in a programme aimed at dealing with the underlying causes of obesity.

- The Buteyko breathing technique changes the acidity of the blood, creating a weight-reducing biochemical effect. If available, learn the technique.

- Certain weight-reducing diets may advise gentle exercise after a meal. I believe they are wrong. Exercise will interfere with digestion.

- Weight loss may be quite marked in the first week or two because of an initial removal of water stored in the tissues. Do not be down hearted if weight loss seems to tail off. You are now losing fat and not water.

- Gauge weight loss by the comfortable fitting of clothes and a personal impression of the body in a mirror rather than on a scale because exercise may build up muscle mass, which is markedly heavier than fat. A review of the body fat/lean weight ratio is the best guide.

Nutritional

- Establish a suitable diet by reviewing or sitting with a nutritionist.

- Increasing fibre in the diet will suppress appetite without any side effects by swelling the stomach and giving the sensation of fullness. Fibre will also bind to fats and cholesterol in particular, holding them in the bowel for excretion through the faeces. Strictly avoid appetite-suppressant medication. There is inevitably a rebound effect because deficiencies are inevitable and there are serious risks including heart attacks and strokes.

- Avoid crash diets or total fasts as a means of weight reduction. The body registers starvation and will hold onto its fat stores preferring to break down protein (muscle) to provide energy. Some fat stores will, of course, diminish but these will be replaced before the muscle. Weight reduction can only be obtained if carbohydrates and a small amount of healthy fats are absorbed. An ideal weight reduction programme will not encourage weight loss beyond two to three pounds per week.

Supplemental

- A dietary fat, conjugated linoleic acid, an amino acid, L-carnitine, and a salt, potassium hydroxycitrate, have all been shown to help reduce weight. They work separately or in combinations to create an enzyme that breaks down fat stores. Take at the dose recommended on the product label.

THE HEAD AND NECK

BALDNESS

I have not come across any particularly successful treatment for male baldness in the world of alternative medicine. Some people have had some benefit by taking high-dose mineral supplements, oxygen therapies, scalp massage and yogic head-standing techniques, but never to any great degree. If you are genetically predisposed to losing your hair, orthodox non-invasive, surgical and drug treatments are your only option.

RECOMMENDATIONS

General Advice
- See **Hair** for initial advice.

- *Visit a trichologist for supplemental advice and the latest methods of hair replacement and weaving.*
- *If baldness is detrimentally affecting your life, counselling and hypnotherapy may allow you to come to terms with the problem even though it does not solve it.*

Orthodox

- *The drug minoxidil has been hailed as effective. It works for approximately 12 per cent of people but needs to be used continuously; 50 per cent or so have some success and the remainder obtain no benefit. Minoxidil was a hypertensive drug (until withdrawn from the market) that created hirsutism (increase in hair growth) and was experimentally applied topically. It has many side effects, including water retention, weight gain and tachycardia, and should only be considered in full knowledge of these effects.*

Alopecia

Baldness occurring in patches or throughout the scalp, as opposed to male pattern baldness, is called alopecia and is associated with:

- Fungal infections
- Stress
- Drug taking, such as anticancer drugs
- Trauma
- Mineral and protein deficiencies

Hair is dependent upon a good blood supply to the hair follicles. Stress can cut down the blood supply to the scalp, mineral and protein deficiencies can prevent the follicle from forming the hair, drugs poison the follicles. Trauma and fungi inhibit the follicles as well.

RECOMMENDATIONS

General Advice

- *Visit a complementary medical practitioner to establish a cause.*
- *Stop using medicated shampoos unless instructed by a qualified practitioner. Certain*

medications may inhibit folic activity.
- *Gentle massage and yogic headstanding techniques can be beneficial but need to be taught. Too much rubbing may be detrimental.*
- *As in all conditions where stress is relevant, consult with a stress management practitioner.*

Supplemental

- *Replenish the body with high-dose mineral and essential amino acid supplements.*

Homeopathic

- *Homeopathic and herbal treatments are available but are best prescribed by practitioners because they must aim at the underlying cause.*

SKULL FRACTURES

Trauma or, extremely rarely, diseases such as Paget's disease or cancer may cause a fracture to the skull. Treatment is very much dependent upon where the fracture has occurred. Diagnosis is generally made by medical consultation, examination and radiographs (X-rays), and generally hairline or thin fractures are left alone. Care must be taken to observe an individual in case an intercranial bleed (*see* **Bleeding**) has occurred.

Depressed fractures where the skull bone may be pushing down on the brain tissues or fractures which are causing malalignments may need to be corrected surgically.

RECOMMENDATIONS

General Advice

- *Any blow to the head must be examined by a doctor immediately.*
- *Do not refuse X-rays or even CT scans if the doctor is uncertain.*
- *Skull fractures may not be dangerous in themselves but may cause damage to the blood vessels underneath which, should they continue to bleed, may cause pressure on the brain and create symptoms up to two months later (see* **Subdural haemorrhage***).*

THE EARS

LABYRINTHITIS

The labyrinth is a part of the inner ear that contains specialized nerve fibres that send impulses to the brain giving information about the head's position. If the head is tipped, the fluid level within the labyrinth moves and some nerves have more pressure applied while others have less. This combination tells the brain exactly what position the head is in. It assumes that the rest of the body is following suit!

Inflammation of this area causes symptoms of dizziness, nausea and vomiting, which can last anywhere up to one month although the first few days are generally the worst. The infection is generally caused by a viral infection, although dehydration and an acid/alkaline imbalance may also be relevant.

RECOMMENDATIONS

General Advice

- *See **Dizziness**.*
- *It may be necessary to take time off work and stay lying flat because labyrynthitis may cause an individual to fall over and potentially risk injury.*

MENIERE'S DISEASE

This is a disease of the inner ear that is characterized by deafness, vertigo, nausea and often vomiting. Tinnitus (the perception of a buzzing or ringing in the ears) and an involuntary movement of the eyes from side to side may also occur.

The cause is uncertain although infection is possible. There is some evidence for an allergic reaction being the cause but so may dehydration or electrolyte imbalances which cause more fluid

to pass into chambers within the body instead of staying in the tissues or blood vessels.

RECOMMENDATIONS

General Advice

- *See **Dizziness**.*
- *Ensure good hydration by drinking at least half a pint of water per foot of height.*

Nutritional

- *Check for food allergies (see **Food allergy testing**).*
- *Reduce salt intake.*

THE EYES

If you study a horizontal section of an eyeball you will see the complexity of the eye and perhaps, like me, wonder why more things do not go wrong. Light has to travel through the conjunctiva and cornea (the covering layers of the eyeball) through a variety of channels and fluids to affect the retina, which is a collection of nerve endings

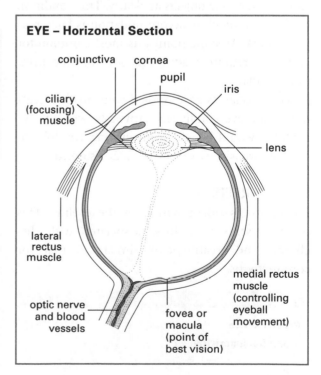

EYE – Horizontal Section

conjunctiva cornea
pupil
iris
ciliary (focusing) muscle
lens
lateral rectus muscle
medial rectus muscle (controlling eyeball movement)
optic nerve and blood vessels
fovea or macula (point of best vision)

and light sensitive cells which are at the end of the fibres which join together and become the optic nerve. These, in turn, transmit the impulses to the optic centres at the back of the brain. Problems anywhere along this pathway will lead to visual disturbance. Neurological diseases such as multiple sclerosis may show up as double vision and specific problems are discussed in this book under their own title.

The function of the eye is to bring the rays of light that enter to a sharp focus on a layer of light-sensitive receptors at the back of the eye known as the retina. Light rays are bent towards the retina mostly as the light passes through the cornea and the anterior and posterior chambers of the eye, which are fluid-filled. However, part of the adjustment occurs through the lens. The lens is itself contractible, controlled by the ciliary muscles. This ability to change the width of the lens is known as accommodation. In our youth the lens is elastic and objects can be sharply focused by accommodation but from the age of eight years onwards and usually by middle age the elasticity of the lens becomes reduced and the unaided eye can no longer see objects as clearly. This condition of diminishing close accommodation is known as presbyopia. At some point it is most common for adults to require reading glasses, for fine print in particular.

Few specialists have studied naturopathic treatments for eye conditions. Anybody with an eye problem would benefit from visiting Dr Roberto Kaplan's website: www.beyond2020vision.com

BLEPHARITIS

Blepharitis is inflammation of the eyelids. This often presents as redness associated with discharge, and treatment is similar to that for conjunctivitis.

RECOMMENDATIONS

General Advice
• See **Conjunctivitis**.

Homeopathic
• Consider the remedies Graphites, Sulphur, Apis and Euphrasia from your preferred homeopathic manual.

Herbal/natural extracts
• The fluid extract of Euphrasia (eyebright) can be used in a dilution of two drops to one eyebath of water.

Orthodox
• Avoid topical antibiotics if possible because these will kill the good bugs as well as the bad and allow the possibility of a difficult bacteria to enter the eye.

BLURRED VISION

A blurring of vision may be created by faulty accommodation but things tend to come back into focus either in the distance or close up, depending on the type of problem. Blurred vision at any distance is liable to be either traumatic or due to a disease process affecting the neurological pathways and should initially be dealt with by a specialist.

RECOMMENDATIONS

General Advice
• Any problem with vision, whether acute in onset or gradual, should be reviewed by a specialist for a firm diagnosis.
• Eye exercises may make a profound difference, especially those known as Bates eye methods. In principle, Bates and other eye training techniques teach the brain to 'see', not 'look', by a series of exercises. The techniques are best taught, although books can be found on the subject but time and patience are required.
• Stress and tiredness cause changes in muscle tension and may therefore affect the shape of the lens, thereby altering an individual's ability to accommodate. 'Eye strain' does not actually exist but persisting anxiety and tiredness may come close to creating something along those lines.
• The use of spectacles and contact lenses should

- *Blurred vision or problems not corrected with spectacles or contact lenses must be reviewed by an ophthalmic specialist.*

Supplemental

- *Take beta-carotene (3mg per foot of height) in divided doses throughout the day and review the diet with a nutritionist to find out why the deficiency has occurred.*

EXOPHTHALMOS

This is a medical term for protruding eyeballs. Genetic or hereditary protrusion is, of course, not a medical problem but the development of exophthalmos usually indicates some pathology. Sadly, the common cause is emaciation of the face, through starvation, but this is not true exophthalmos because it is really only a relative widening of the eyes in comparison to the surrounding tissues.

Unilateral exophthalmos is usually associated with tumour growth in the orbit or eye socket but by far the most common cause of exophthalmos, typically bilaterally, is Graves' disease. This is a condition of hyperthyroidism at its extreme. The raised levels of thyroxine, and in particular another hormone called long-acting thyroid stimulator, encourage the small amount of fat that lies behind the eyeball in the orbit to grow excessively. This increased fatty tissue pushes the eyeballs forward.

RECOMMENDATIONS

General Advice

- *The development of exophthalmos requires a medical opinion.*
- *Once a full diagnosis has been made a complementary medical practitioner may be able to offer treatment for the underlying condition but, unfortunately, exophthalmos is not reversible.*

Orthodox

- *In extreme circumstances operative procedures may be feasible.*

FLOATERS

Floaters are small black dots of irregular shape that are visible by all of us if we look. They are caused by small amounts of debris in the vitreous humour of the eye. Floaters are usually not noticed but trauma or diseases of the retina may cause larger fragments, which become disturbing.

RECOMMENDATIONS

General Advice

- *An increasing number of floaters should be viewed by an eye specialist.*
- *Sadly, I have not come across any alternative or orthodox therapies that can help with floaters. They are often broken down and reabsorbed by the body and may not, therefore, be a persistent problem.*
- *Hypnotherapy may be beneficial in helping to ignore the visual annoyance.*

GLAUCOMA

Glaucoma is an increase in pressure within the eye, usually caused by an obstruction to the outflow of the fluid in the eye. There is, rarely, an increase in production of this fluid, which is not drained quickly enough and this results in an imbalance.

There may be some correlation between long-standing glaucoma and the amount of a type of a protein called collagen found in the tissues of the body, which acts' as a type of scaffolding. An excess of collagen may block the outlet, as may abnormalities in the tissues at the back of the eye. There are two types of glaucoma:

Acute (closed-angle) glaucoma

Acute glaucoma presents with a severe pulsating pain in the eye, blurred vision and, commonly, nausea or vomiting. The pupil will be dilated and fixed and does not respond to light as it should. Acute glaucoma can occur in one eye only.

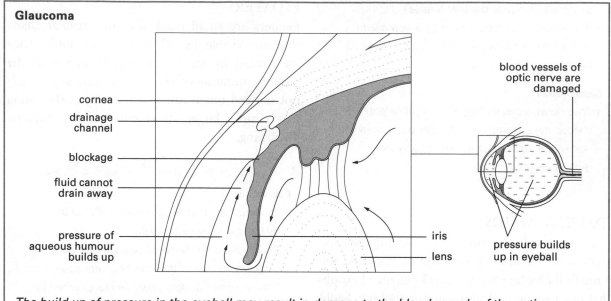

Glaucoma

cornea

drainage channel

blockage

fluid cannot drain away

pressure of aqueous humour builds up

blood vessels of optic nerve are damaged

iris

lens

pressure builds up in eyeball

The build up of pressure in the eyeball may result in damage to the blood vessels of the optic nerve.

Chronic (open-angle) glaucoma

This may have no symptoms until the condition has been present for several years. It is noticed as a gradual loss of peripheral vision and if left untreated will result in tunnel vision, which is exactly as it sounds. If no action is taken then pain, blurring, headaches and nausea will eventually result. I have one patient whose eyeball pressure rose at times of stress. This is not a well-recognized factor, but it may be that stress can cause glaucoma.

RECOMMENDATIONS

General Advice

- *Acute glaucoma is a medical emergency. If untreated, the pain will be excruciating and blindness will ensue. Rush to an emergency department and therapy needs to be started within 48hr.*
- *Any disturbance of vision must be checked initially by an optician who will refer you to your family practitioner who will decide on whether a specialist is required. Do not delay because many conditions can progress rapidly to blindness.*
- *Learn a relaxation/meditation technique.*

Nutritional

- *Many studies support the belief that allergy may play a major part in chronic glaucoma. Food allergy testing is a highly recommended procedure.*

Supplemental

- *Vitamin C is known to reduce inner eye pressure and in chronic glaucoma should be used at a dose of 1g (1,000mg) per 10kg of body weight in divided doses with meals through the day. One gram of vitamin C can be taken every 15min in acute glaucoma and every hour once treatment has been initiated. Take natural food state vitamin C, otherwise at these levels you are guaranteed to upset your digestion.*
- *Blueberry extract – anthocyanoside, 15mg per foot of height taken three times a day initially may be used in chronic glaucoma. Continued use of this compound should be monitored by a complementary practitioner with experience in this area.*

Homeopathic

- *Homeopathic remedies may be chosen on the symptoms but the remedies Spigelia and*

MYOPIA (SHORT-SIGHTEDNESS) AND HYPERMETROPIA (LONG-SIGHTEDNESS)

A normal eye produces a sharp image on the retina of an object at a distance by not bending, or accommodating, the lens at all. However, not all eyes are the same. Some are too long from front to back and the focus forms in front of the retina causing a blurred vision (myopia). This can be corrected by providing the individual with a concave (known in optical circles as a negative) spectacle or contact lens.

Other eyes are too short, in which case they form the positive image behind the retina once again causing blurring (hypermetropia). This problem is corrected by a convex or positive spectacle or contact lens.

Not all blurred vision is created by defects of light refraction, and disease or damage to the retina or optic nerves may be the reason. Vitamin C and nutritional deficiencies can also cause problems, as can tiredness and stress.

Any visual problem can reduce confidence and, in the case of short-sightedness, close the world around an individual. Simple pleasures like going to the theatre, a football match or taking part in field games become more difficult and a vanity concerning wearing glasses or contact lenses can often lead to mild but repairable psychological difficulties. Children in particular may not wish to disclose their 'failing' and an eye test is advisable for any child who is failing at school or is

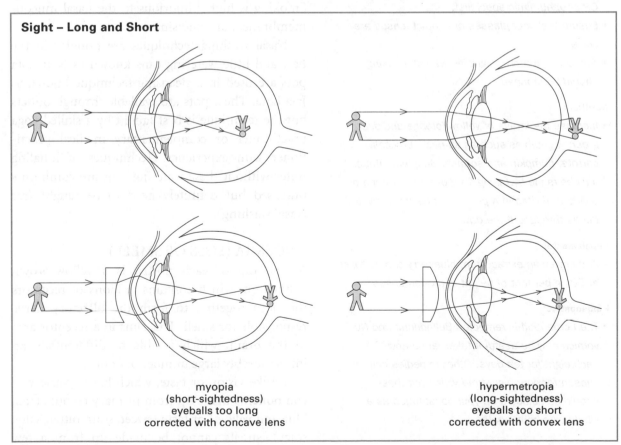

Sight – Long and Short

myopia
(short-sightedness)
eyeballs too long
corrected with concave lens

hypermetropia
(long-sightedness)
eyeballs too short
corrected with convex lens

becoming less sociable. A change in hand–eye co-ordination may well be a visual problem.

One must always ask the question when confronted with a visual problem: 'what do I not want to see?'

NIGHT VISION

Difficulty in seeing at night or in a darkened environment may be a matter of becoming short-sighted (myopic). However, deficiency of a chemical called rhodopsin, which is found in association with vitamin A, may stop the specialized pigment cells in the retina (back of the eye) from working properly. Other causes include glaucoma and decreased circulation to the retina. The symptoms may be most noticeable when driving at night.

RECOMMENDATIONS

General Advice

- *Any problem with vision should be checked by a GP or ophthalmic specialist.*
- *Ensure that your glasses or contact lenses are correct.*
- *Tobacco can affect night vision and smoking should be stopped.*

Nutritional

- *Increase the intake of yellow/orange and deep-green vegetables such as spinach, broccoli, carrots, pumpkin and squash. Supplementation may be made by taking 1mg of beta-carotene or 2,000iu of vitamin A per foot of height in divided doses throughout the day.*

Supplemental

- *Anthocyanidin extract from blueberry can be taken at 20mg per foot of height in divided doses.*

Homeopathic

- *The homeopathic remedies Belladonna and Nux vomica may be useful if taken at potency 30 each night for ten days. Other remedies can be chosen for poor night-time vision but these should be selected on your constitution as a whole by a homeopath.*

THE NOSE

The nose is the preferred entrance for air to enter the lungs. It is a longer route than breathing through the mouth and thereby the air is warmed and cleansed more effectively by the nasal hairs. The nasal membranes are sensitive to pollutants and produce mucus to trap foreign material and protect the delicate lung tissues. The sinuses – air spaces within the skull bones – are mucous membrane-lined cavities that drain fluid into the nasal passages.

CARE OF THE NOSE

The nose is very much self-repairing and provided that it is not damaged will look after itself. Damage can occur from trauma and, becoming more common, from the inhalation of drugs of abuse such as cocaine, heroin and amphetamines. Smoking is highly injurious to the nasal mucous membrane, hairs and sinuses.

Nasal washing techniques are popular in the East and little watering cans known as Neti Lota pots are used in a cleansing technique known as Jala Lota. These pots are available through outlets but the technique is best taught by a skilled yoga practitioner or complementary medical practitioner with experience. Techniques of inhaling water without these watering cans are commonly practised but definitely need to be taught (*see* **Nasal washing**).

ANOSMIA (LOSS OF SMELL)

At the top of each nostril is a yellow-brown epithelium, which contains millions of receptors that join together to form the olfactory nerve responsible for smell. This runs to a receptor area in the brain, which is able to differentiate an immeasurably large number of odours.

Unlike vision or taste, which have a variety of components made up from primary colours (red, blue and yellow) or taste (sweet, sour, bitter, salty, spicy), smells cannot be made up from a few components. Each olfactory receptor may have its own specific odour molecule to recognize and it may mean that thousands have to be activated before the brain recognizes a smell.

As an aside, smells may be unrecognized but nevertheless noticed. Insects in particular are known to give off pheromones (airborne chemicals) that attract members of the opposite sex. It is probable that human beings recognize or pick up airborne chemicals from others without registering them consciously as a smell. The phenomenon whereby women placed in a dormitory or in close proximity will all eventually have their periods at the same time suggests a pheromone activity. (Either that or there is a non-measurable energetic transmission from some part of the brain, probably the pituitary gland, or an area that is considered by Eastern philosophies to be the centre of the highest chakra.)

A loss of smell occurs due to any interference with the transmission of impulses from the receptor to, and including the olfactory centre in, the brain.

Transient or temporary loss is often noted with colds or inflammation of the nasal membranes. Conditions such as hay fever or nasal polyps, whereby the mucous membranes swell and may engulf the olfactory receptors may appear permanent until the season changes or the polyps are cured. A more permanent anosmia will occur if the olfactory receptors are damaged, as they are by pollution, smoking and the inhalation or 'snorting' of narcotics such as heroin, cocaine and amphetamines. Glue-sniffing is a sad and rapid cause of olfactory receptor damage. Trauma or infection such as meningitis or encephalitis can damage both the olfactory nerve and the brain centre, as can tumours.

RECOMMENDATIONS

General Advice
- *A transient loss due to an obvious cause should be treated as per the recommendations in the appropriate section in this book.*

Nutritional
- *In chronic cases food allergy must be considered and blood testing to isolate culprits is recommended. Ingestion of allergens may create a permanent inflammation in the membranes, which envelop and block the olfactory receptors.*

Homeopathic
- *Homeopathic remedies may be of use and should be chosen based on the constitution of an individual by a homeopath.*

Herbal/natural extracts
- *The Eastern philosophies, especially Tibetan medicine, believe that the loss of one of our senses is an indication of a very deep disorder. It does not mean that it is particularly life-threatening but simply that treatment may be difficult and require much discipline and therapy. Referral to a Tibetan physician is recommended but if none are available then Chinese or Ayurvedic physicians may help.*

Orthodox
- *A gradual or persistent loss of smell should be examined by a doctor with referral to a nose specialist or neurologist. Testing will be carried out by asking an individual to smell coffee, almond, tar and lemon, all of which are generally pungent and easily recognized. Foul-smelling compounds such as asafoetida, which possesses a smell so unpleasant that the nose will wrinkle uncontrollably, are used to determine whether anosmia is complete or not.*

BROKEN NOSE

A broken nose is a common injury, especially in people who play a lot of sport. It is a painful occurrence and very often the softer cartilage at the front of the nose is itself fractured or fractures away from the bone. The nasal bones may be broken and very often the swelling will hide any marked deformity. Radiographic examination is often required but, because little is done to treat a broken nose until the swelling has subsided, this may not take place for a couple of days. The nose is a highly vascular area and bleeding is often very profuse.

RECOMMENDATIONS

General Advice
- *If a broken nose is suspected it should be reviewed by a GP or accident and emergency doctor.*

Homeopathic
- *Administer the homeopathic remedy Arnica 6 every 10min for five doses and then every 2–3hr for 2–3 days. If the damage is severe, alternate the Arnica with Symphytum 6 every 3hr for one week.*

Herbal/natural extracts
- *Apply an Arnica-based cream around the damaged area.*

Orthodox
- *An operative procedure may be necessary (see **Operations and surgery**).*

EPISTAXIS (NOSE BLEEDS)

The cause of nose bleeds is often trauma such as a direct blow or persisting inflammation in the nasal passages caused by infection or irritants which may be as innocuous as pollen in hay fever sufferers.

Rarely is a nose bleed serious although it can be associated with diabetes and hypertension. Sinusitis and nasal polyps are less serious conditions but also need to be considered. Problems with the clotting system may often show up as more bleeds.

In children, ensure that there is no foreign body in the nose and do your best to stop any picking!

RECOMMENDATIONS

General Advice
- *Sudden, unexpected, persistent (more than 25 minutes) or bright red bleeding should be examined by a physician since cauterization (sealing of a blood vessel by heat) may be necessary.*
- *Remove any foreign object if necessary.*
- *Keep the head tipped forward and apply pressure*

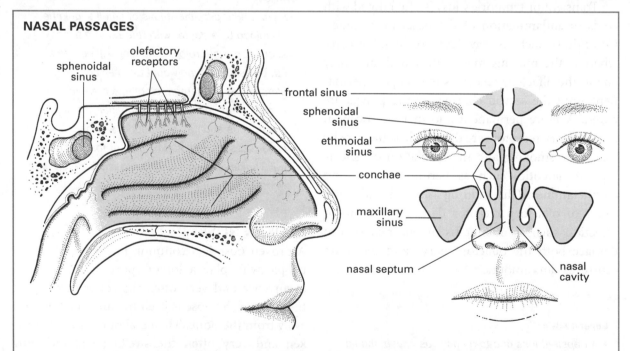

NASAL PASSAGES

sphenoidal sinus

olefactory receptors

frontal sinus

sphenoidal sinus

ethmoidal sinus

conchae

maxillary sinus

nasal septum

nasal cavity

Incoming air is filtered of dust and foreign bodies by hairs inside the nostrils. The air then passes over the mucous membranes in the sinuses between the bones of the nasal conchae. The mucus carries away microorganisms, and warms and humidifies the air before it passes into the lungs.

to the soft lower part of the nostril or nostrils.

- Apply a cold compress on the bridge of the nose and the back of the neck. This may help to stem the flow by decreasing blood flow.
- Avoid swallowing blood by spitting out.
- If no obvious cause is apparent consult a complementary medical practitioner and check for vitamin and mineral deficiencies.

Supplemental

- Recurrent nose bleeds, with no established serious cause, should be treated with treble the recommended dose of a multimineral and vitamin supplement. Beta-carotene 2 mg per foot of height should be taken in divided doses through the day. Recurrent nose bleeds should also be examined by an ear, nose and throat specialist to isolate any defective or weak blood vessels or other underlying health problem.

Homeopathic

- The following homeopathic remedies can be employed and taken every ten minutes at potency 6. Bright red blood – Phosphorus, bright blood with steady flow – Ferrum phos, Following injury – Arnica.

NASAL BLOCKAGE

The nose can be blocked by a foreign object, inflammation, growths or polyps. Inflammation is most commonly caused by pollutants, including smoking or drugs of abuse, or infections such as the common cold.

RECOMMENDATIONS

General Advice

- See the appropriate section when underlying cause of an obstruction.
- A foreign body may be easily removed but if not see a doctor.

NASAL POLYPS

Nasal polyps are actually fluid-laden, mucous membrane 'sponges' usually created by persistent irritation from an external pollutant such as pollen, mechanical fumes or drugs of abuse. Smoking in particular is a major cause. There is a correlation with hay fever, asthma and other allergic responses and it may be triggered by food allergies. Hypoglycaemia encourages membrane swelling and mucus production and is often an overlooked reason for polyp production. There is some hereditary predisposition. The nasal passages swell in response to tears and emotional suppression is another overlooked cause of polyp growth.

Nasal polyps are most often protruding from the sinuses, especially the ethmoid and frontal sinuses. Their presence causes nasal obstruction, mucus excess and diminution in smell and taste.

RECOMMENDATIONS

General Advice

- Any persistent discharge or congestion should be examined by a GP.
- Avoidance of any nasal pollutants, including smoking, should be encouraged.
- A nasal washing technique should be learnt (see **Nasal washing**).
- Any repression of sadness or tears needs to be brought to light and neurolinguistic programming or hypnotherapy prior to counselling may be a curative.

Nutritional

- Diets high in sugars and refined foods should be adjusted. Spicy foods and alcohol should also be avoided.
- Specific food allergy testing should be undertaken to identify any negative response.

Supplemental

- The following supplements should be taken in divided doses throughout the day at the following levels per foot of height: beta-carotene (1mg), vitamin C (1g), chromium (twice the daily recommended dose of a good-quality product) and zinc (5mg taken before going to sleep).

These levels should be tried for one month in conjunction with homeopathic remedies.

Homeopathic

- *Homeopathic remedies should be considered, in particular Calcarea carbonica and Teucrium. These should be taken at potency 30 twice a day for two weeks.*

Herbal/natural extracts

- *Herbal treatments may be of benefit but should be prescribed by a specialist. These include nasal sprays of herbal and homeopathic remedies. Try them, they may work.*

Orthodox

- *Steroid drops prescribed by a GP and taken without fail four times a day for one month may be curative if the underlying cause is removed. At the very least steroids will be effective at relieving the congestive symptoms. Do not exceed the recommended two drops per nostril because some absorption will take place through the membranes and a considerable amount may be swallowed unless the head is in the correct position. This requires an individual to kneel and place the vertex of the skull on the floor and stay in that position for a couple of minutes. Do not sniff and swallow afterwards, instead preferably blow the nose gently.*
- *Refined endoscopic techniques are now available for surgical polyp removal and should be insisted upon if other treatments do not work and surgery is required. Bear in mind that 40 per cent of polyps will recur and that the procedure is an uncomfortable one and should really be left until other avenues have failed.*

Nasal washing

Nasal washing is best done by the use of a Neti pot (a small watering can available at many health-food stores and clinics) and the technique from yoga known as Jala Lota.

For Jala Lota prepare a saltwater solution using a teaspoonful of salt in a cup of warm water. Fill the Neti pot and, standing by a sink or a bath, place the top of the head pointing directly down. Breathe through an open mouth slowly and pour the water through the Neti nozzle up one nostril and out of the other. Ensure a continuation of breathing as this creates a negative pressure and may help to pull the fluid into the sinuses. Repeat this technique four times a day.

POSTNASAL DRIP

A postnasal drip may be recognized as a sensation of fluid at the back of the nose, but is often un-recognized. Whilst upright and awake a postnasal drip tends to be swallowed or coughed out, but at night when asleep or in a horizontal position, the trickle may descend into the lungs, causing a night-time cough. If the postnasal discharge is infected, then sore throats, loss of voice and bronchitis may be created. Most postnasal discharge comes from the sinuses.

RECOMMENDATIONS

General Advice

- *See **Sinusitis**, but bear in mind that sinus discharge is not necessarily associated with infection and therefore may not be painful.*
- *Adenoids (lymphatic glands at the back of the nose) may also become inflamed and create mucus as may the nasopharynx mucous membrane. If sinuses are not a problem (see **Coughs** and **Colds**).*

Nutritional

- *Pay special attention to food intolerances, cow's milk products, alcohol and sweet foods, as all these encourage mucus production.*

SINUSITIS

The skull bone is extremely heavy and if it were not for the air-filled cavities known as sinuses it would be too heavy for the neck to support. These hollows are lined by mucous membranes that pro-duces secretions to protect the bones from infection and trap airborne invaders. If these

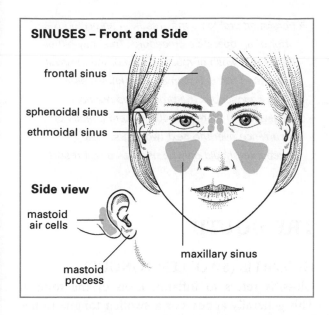

SINUSES – Front and Side

frontal sinus

sphenoidal sinus

ethmoidal sinus

Side view

mastoid air cells

mastoid process

maxillary sinus

swimming pools, may all trigger a non-infected inflammation. Fatigue, fever and discharge are associated and a yellow or green mucus is usually indicative of a bacterial infection.

Frontal sinus headaches have a peculiarity of developing midmorning. I am uncertain why this occurs but it seems that there must be some body clock mechanism. Nostrils tend to fluctuate in their patency due to vasoconstriction altering throughout the day and Ayurvedic philosophy suggests that more energy is absorbed through the left nostril than the right. (This is why all effigies of Buddha in a reclining position have him on his right side.)

Rhinitis created by allergies is a frequent initiator of acute sinusitis and the chronic state may be encouraged by food or airborne allergies. Low blood sugar levels trigger mucous membrane inflammation and mucus production so any factor affecting or causing hypoglycaemia must be taken into account. Toxic bowels can often induce sinus irritation.

The diagnosis of sinusitis is frequently clinical but investigations such as CT scans or fibre optic endoscopy can be utilized. Sinus X-rays are frequently useless and provide a dose of radiation that is not likely to be of benefit.

membranes become inflamed, the condition of sinusitis occurs.

Sinuses can be very extensive and travel back into the skull bones. They interconnect and all the sinuses drain into the nasal cavity except for the mastoid sinus, which drains into the middle ear. Inflammation of the drainage channels can lead to back-pressure, which is extremely painful. Diving or rising or descending in a poorly controlled pressurized aircraft leads to a differentiation of pressure, which can cause pain. The Valsalva movement (pinching the nose and blowing) is most commonly used to free any blockages in the Eustachian tube, but can be used to open up the passages to the sinuses.

Sinus infection may be either acute or chronic. Pain is usual in chronic sinusitis but is not always present and the site is dependent upon which sinus is affected. Most commonly infection will trigger inflammation, viral and bacterial being more common than yeast or fungal, but the latter two are often overlooked. The maxillary sinuses may, one time in four, be inflamed because of inflammation in the upper teeth, gums or jaw.

Inhalation of noxious substances, which include smoking, inhaled drugs of abuse such as cocaine and amphetamine, strong industrial fumes, pollution and even the chlorine from

RECOMMENDATIONS

General Advice

- Attempt to keep the mucus thin and less viscid by ensuring good hydration by drinking plenty of water (one pint per foot of height a day) and avoiding dry atmospheres such as air conditioning.
- Hot showers or hot compresses over the inflamed area will be beneficial.
- In acute infections, see **Colds** for treatment.
- If problems continue, nasal washing techniques may be of use. Sniffing salt water by blocking one nostril and inhaling water until it reaches the back of the throat and blowing it out can clear the nasal passages but does not encourage the solution to enter the sinuses. It is better to use a small watering

can device that is often available at healthfood stores known as a Neti pot. This technique is known as Jala Lota (see Nasal washing).

- *See Allergies and Postnasal drip.*
- *Consider counselling and hypnotherapy to remove underlying or suppressed sorrow or grief.*

Nutritional
- *Establish any food allergies by exclusion diets or food allergy testing and avoid any allergens.*

Supplemental
- *Chronic infections may benefit from using the following supplements in the following dosages per foot of height in divided doses throughout the day: beta-carotene (2mg), vitamin C (1g), chromium (20µg) and zinc (5mg before bed).*
- *The following may be used to thin mucus and act as anti-inflammatory agents: N-acetylcysteine and bromelaine, each at 400mg per foot of height in divided doses throughout the day.*

Homeopathic
- *Homeopathic remedies can be used in both acute and chronic conditions. Selection of a remedy should be based on the site and type of pain, type of discharge and other associated symptoms.*

Herbal/natural extracts
- *Attempt to soothe sinus inflammation with inhalations of lavender, chamomile or Olbas by putting two drops of the essential oil into a bowl of steaming water.*
- *Infectious causes may be benefited by taking Echinacea and Golden Seal at twice the recommended dose on a proprietary brand.*

Orthodox
- *The orthodox use of painkillers is sometimes necessary because sinus pain can be most debilitating. Steroid drops and sprays with or without antibiotics may be offered and are usually used if the sinusitis is related to polyps (see Nasal polyps).*

- *Persisting problems may result in an orthodox offer of an operative procedure. This may either be a sinus wash or mucous membrane removal performed through a small tube known as a sinus endoscope. The procedures are not pleasant and there is a 40 per cent chance of recurrence over the next two years. This procedure should only be used as a last resort.*

THE MOUTH

GLOSSITIS (SWOLLEN TONGUE)

Glossitis refers to inflammation of the tongue. This generally appears as a swollen tongue rather than a painful or red tongue, although these may be in association.

It is important to remember that the mouth is the top end of a 30-foot tube that ends at the anus. Like a hose pipe, holes may occur anywhere along its length but the two ends receive most of the attention and can reflect the integrity of the whole pipe.

The Eastern philosophies of medicine pay special attention to the tongue and a swollen tongue may be very helpful in diagnosing any underlying conditions.

The tongue will swell in response to trauma, such as accidental biting or bee stings. Allergic reactions can cause the tongue to swell to such an extent that it may obstruct breathing and very rapidly this may become a serious medical emergency. The tongue may also swell in rare medical conditions. A swollen tongue is viewed by holistic practitioners as being an indication of swelling elsewhere or throughout the bowel. This may occur in any inflammatory problem such as ulcerative colitis, Crohn's disease or peptic ulcers. The bowel may also swell when absorption is poor as a reflection of more blood being pushed into the bowel in an attempt to absorb more nutrients. Swelling of the tongue may show as indentations along the edge caused by long-term pressure on the teeth.

General Advice

- *A rapidly swelling or persistently swollen tongue needs to be reviewed by a doctor as a potential emergency. It may only take a few minutes or even seconds for the tongue to swell to a level that obstructs breathing.*
- *Review any intake, such as food or drugs recently imbibed before swelling was noticed. Particularly salty or acidic food may be a cause.*
- *Rinse the mouth with a strong salt solution but do not swallow. Gargling, provided that it does not cause retching, is beneficial because the tongue starts halfway down the throat.*
- *A more persistent swollen tongue should be reviewed by a complementary medical practitioner with knowledge in either herbal or homeopathic medicine.*

Homeopathic

- *The homeopathic remedy Aconite 6, should be taken every 10min with an acutely swollen tongue or Apis 6 every 10min for a tongue swelling secondary to an insect bite or sting.*

SALIVA AND SALIVATION

Saliva is a secretion from specialized glands around the jaw that should be clear, tasteless and slightly acidic. The functions of saliva include moistening and lubricating the food before swallowing, initiating digestion (it contains an enzyme called ptyalin which breaks down starch to simple sugars) and acting as an antiseptic. Saliva enhances the taste of food by its initial breakdown action on sugars making the molecules more available for the taste buds.

Saliva is produced in the parotid, submandibular (below the jaw) and sublingual (below the tongue) glands. Two little holes (punctae) in the cheeks are the end points of the parotid duct and may be isolated by gently sucking and feeling the slightly cool saliva entering the oral cavity. Two little fronds are felt at the front of the mouth under the tongue which are the end points

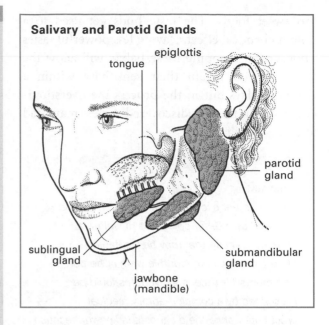

Salivary and Parotid Glands

tongue — epiglottis — parotid gland — sublingual gland — submandibular gland — jawbone (mandible)

of the other glands. The glands are under the control of the nervous system, which may be stimulated by the sight and smell of food and even by the sound of cooking. This is a conditioned reflex much studied by Pavlov (the scientist who noted that a dog salivated more when he rang the dinnertime bell regardless of whether the dogs were fed or not). Once food is in the mouth, other nerve reflexes continue saliva production.

Hypersalivation (excess salivation)

Excess salivation is most commonly associated with a hypersensitivity of smell and taste. This commonly occurs with fevers and in pregnancy due to heat or to hormones sensitizing the nervous system. Injury or pain in the mouth, such as in teething in infants or disease at a later age, will also initiate hypersalivation. Any disease of the nervous system that causes impulses to be poorly controlled may also stimulate salivation. Such conditions are most commonly seen in Alzheimer's and motorneurone disease. Dyspepsia (burning pain in the upper abdomen) and other digestive problems may increase secretions throughout the gut, including the mouth.

Taste and smell may be diminished by habits such as smoking or persistently eating too spicy or too sweet foods. The taste buds get used to a potent chemical effect, leaving less powerful tastes unobserved. Stopping these habits will allow the taste buds to regain their sensitivity within a matter of days but in the process the overstimulation from these rediscovered tastes may lead to excessive salivation.

RECOMMENDATIONS

General Advice

- *Any persistent excessive salivation should be reviewed by a GP or specialist to isolate an underlying cause that may be treatable.*
- *More intensive homeopathic work or herbal treatments for excess salivation should be prescribed by a complementary medical practitioner once the diagnosis is known, because suppression of the symptom by a 'drying' action may suppress an early symptom of a condition better treated in its early stages (ie gum disease).*
- *Certain drugs, especially chemotherapeutic drugs, can create hypersalivation through their effects either on the nervous system or on the blood supply, causing an overstimulation of the salivary glands.*
- *Pseudosalivation may occur not because of an excess production but because the saliva cannot be swallowed. This is usually associated with neuromuscular conditions which may be very difficult to treat.*
- *Acupuncture may relieve symptoms but should be used in conjunction with herbal treatments as prescribed by a complementary specialist.*

Homeopathic

- *Occasional bouts may be relieved by the homeopathic remedy Mercurius 6, four pills four times a day for three days.*

Hyposalivation (lack of saliva)

Hyposalivation occurs because of damage to the salivary glands or a diminished nerve or blood supply to them. This may occur through age or disease as the nerves become less sensitive, especially those of taste. Disease processes such as sarcoidosis may directly affect the salivary gland tissue as may viral infection. Diuretics, antihistamines, certain heart drugs and most drugs that affect the neurological system (including drugs of abuse) can have an effect, although usually temporary.

Adrenaline and other catecholamines – the stress chemicals – all suppress bowel activity, including the production of saliva. This is very marked in moments of extreme fear, when the mouth can become parched, but it will have a general effect to some degree in people who are nervous or anxious.

Dehydration will, of course, lead to a dry mouth and this is part of the first recognition mechanisms (*see* **Dehydration**). Please note that smoking may have a drying effect as may the intake of any 'heat'-increasing compounds, such as spicy food. High sugar levels will encourage a dehydrating effect and saliva may thicken, causing a dry effect without any actual diminution in production. We all notice a dry mouth after sucking on a sweet or eating an ice cream.

RECOMMENDATIONS

General Advice

- *Isolate the cause by discussions with a complementary medical practitioner or a GP. Treat the underlying cause, bearing in mind that the cessation of doctor-prescribed drugs may be dangerous.*
- *Ensure adequate hydration. Drink half a pint of water per foot of height per day.*
- *Learn and practise a relaxation or meditation technique or consider counselling if anxiety is a notable aspect of the personality.*

Homeopathic

- *There are many homeopathic remedies for a dry mouth and the correct one should be selected on general symptoms. Whilst assessing the underlying cause try Nux moschata 30 four times a day.*

SWOLLEN TONGUE – *see* **Glossitis**

THE THROAT

DYSPHAGIA

This is the medical term for a difficulty in swallowing. If it should occur for no particular reason or it is persistent, then see a physician or go to the hospital emergency room immediately.

Dysphagia can occur for either a physical or mental reason. The throat is a central chakra point in Eastern medicine and, whatever the immediate cause of the dysphagia might be, one must ask whether there is a build up or deficiency of energy in that area causing a blockage or an inability for the oesophagus (food pipe) to swallow.

Physical causes may include inflammation of the oesophagus, causing the food pipe to close up, external pressure from, say, an enlarged thyroid or lymphatic glands, but more sinister obstructive causes such as tumours need to be excluded in a persistent difficulty in swallowing.

Many people with dysphagia may have an associated eating disorder or a strong subconscious ability to stop a food allergen entering the system. Anxiety in general may create difficulty in swallowing, as may excitement or fear.

RECOMMENDATIONS

General Advice
- *Persisting dysphagia for no apparent reason must be examined by a GP and possibly a specialist.*
- *Emotional causes of dysphagia should be dealt with by a counsellor.*

Homeopathic
- *The homeopathic remedies Aconite and Stramonium, at potency 6, can be taken every 15min in an acute episode or whilst on the way to the doctor.*

DYSPHASIA

Dysphasia is the medical term for difficulty in the ability to use language; aphasia is the complete loss.

In reality, laryngitis may be classed as a dysphasia, as indeed may any condition ranging from inflammation, infection or even tumour that affects the vocal cords and throat. It is wiser, however, to rule out any serious illness of the area or of the nervous system when dealing with an inability to speak.

Dysphasia may be created by damage to the nervous system, in particular to the speech centres, by events such as stroke, encephalitis, meningitis and diseases of the nervous system such as motorneurone disease. These need to be established.

RECOMMENDATIONS

General Advice
- *Any dysphasia that persists or does not have an obvious cause should be reviewed by a GP.*
- *Follow through with specialist investigations, including CAT and MRI scans, to rule out or establish the cause. A complementary medical practitioner can then be confronted once a firm diagnosis has been made.*

HOARSENESS

A coarse voice caused by inflammation of the vocal cords is responsible. *See* **Sore throats** and **Loss of voice**.

LARYNGITIS AND PHARYNGITIS

The larynx lies protected behind the Adam's apple. The area above this, leading up to the tonsils, is known as the pharynx. Inflammation in these areas cause a sore throat and can lead to hoarseness and loss of voice.

RECOMMENDATION

General Advice
- *See* **Sore throats**.

LOSS OF VOICE

The loss of the voice is most commonly associated with laryngitis (*see* **Sore throats**). The larynx

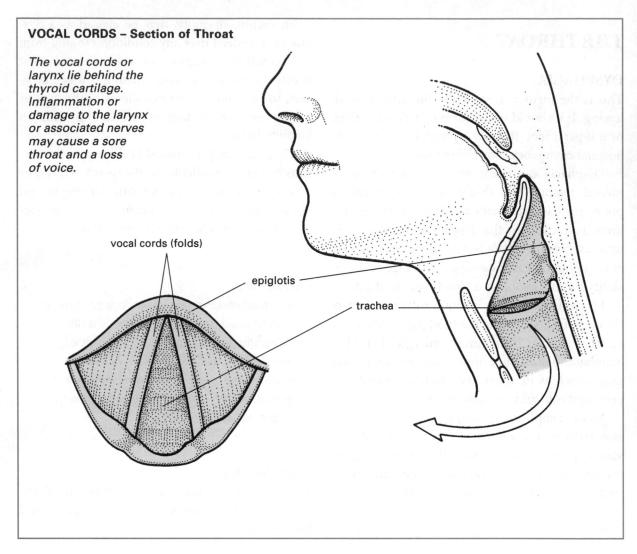

VOCAL CORDS – Section of Throat

The vocal cords or larynx lie behind the thyroid cartilage. Inflammation or damage to the larynx or associated nerves may cause a sore throat and a loss of voice.

vocal cords (folds)

epiglotis

trachea

is colloquially known as the voice box and is protected by cartilage, which can be felt superficially as the Adam's apple. The larynx is composed of two leaves of mucous membrane containing muscle that is very finely innovative and controlled by different laryngeal nerves that are branches of the vagus nerve. A loss of voice may therefore not only be caused by infection and inflammation but by any damage to these nerves. Trauma, tumours and nerve disease may all result in the loss of voice. Any condition that may apply pressure to the larynx must also be considered, especially an enlarged or inflamed thyroid gland. A loss of voice may be a sign of hypo- or hyperthyroidism. Toxins such as pollution and smoking may also create inflammation leading to a loss of voice.

RECOMMENDATIONS

General Advice

• *Isolate the cause. Recurrent or persistent sore throats that do not appear to be associated with inflammation or infection may be an early sign of an underlying disorder and a doctor's investigations are required.*

• *A loss of voice caused by infection should be treated by referring to the section on sore throats (see **Sore throats**).*

SORE THROATS

A sore throat can, of course, occur at any age from a variety of causes. There may be acute (sudden) and chronic (longstanding) and, broadly speaking, sore throats may be internal or external. Most sore throats are caused by bacterial or viral infections affecting the membranes (an *internal* sore throat) or affecting the tonsils and neck glands (an *external* sore throat).

Trauma, tumours, tonsillitis and diseases of the thyroid gland can all be the cause of a sore throat. Laryngitis (inflammation of the voice box) and pharyngitis (the area between the tonsils and the larynx) are simply medical terms to isolate the exact whereabouts of inflammation in this area.

In the case of chronic sore throats a cause is usually apparent, such as smoking or the overuse of the vocal cords in singers, but is sometimes overlooked, as is the case of people who have many hot drinks throughout the day. Alcohol and fizzy drinks may also be culprits. Persisting sinusitis may lead to a postnasal drip causing sore throats. This is quite common in smokers. Persisting sore throats that do not have an obvious answer need to be examined by a doctor to rule out less common and more dangerous causes. Remember that the throat contains a lot of organs, not just the food and wind pipes, and there are also residual pouches such as the brachial and pharyngeal pouches that exist as little pockets where infection can sit very tenaciously. These pouches have no apparent use but are present because of our evolutionary development, a bit like the appendix.

RECOMMENDATIONS

General Advice
- Remove any obvious cause of a sore throat, such as smoking, shouting and excessive hot drinks.
- Use saltwater gargles if the throat is sore at the back of the mouth. Do not swallow this.
- Both internal but especially external sore throats may be soothed by wrapping around a silk scarf.

- See **coughs** and **colds** if the sore throat is so associated.
- A persistent sore throat or one without obvious cause needs to be reviewed by a physician to rule out more serious underlying reasons.

Supplemental
- For any inflamed membrane use beta-carotene (2mg per foot of height) in divided doses throughout the day.

Homeopathic
- The following homeopathic remedies may be beneficial: Aconite 6 every 2hr for sudden onset of a sore throat regardless of the symptoms; Spongia 6 for a dry barking cough associated with loss of voice; Aconite, Hepar sulphuris calcarium or Nitric acid, potency 6, every 2hr for splinter-like pains on swallowing; Lachesis for sore throat resulting from overuse of the voice. Splinter-like pains on swallowing.
- There are many different homeopathic remedies that may be chosen depending on the specific symptoms, such as if it feels better for hot and cold drinks, feels worse in a draught, or has an associated cough. Please refer to your preferred homeopathic manual.

Herbal/natural extracts
- Chop up some fresh root ginger into a hot mug of water and sip at a comfortable temperature. Honey and lemon may be added if the ginger is an unpleasant taste. You may gargle with this solution before swallowing it.
- The ginger solution mentioned above, lavender, or a mix of cloves and cinnamon can be placed in steaming water and inhaled in the case of a sore throat secondary to sinusitis. This tip is useful in cases of laryngitis or voice loss.
- Take comfortably warm or iced drinks of chamomile tea as preferred.
- A teaspoonful of turmeric powder in half a pint of skimmed milk with a half teaspoonful of butter and a teaspoonful of honey brought to a simmer, then drunk when at a comfortable temperature may be instantly soothing and curative of sore throats.

THE CHEST

BREASTS

General care

There has been some recent controversy on the efficacy and necessity of breast self-examination. Whatever the statistical evidence eventually shows, I am of the firm opinion that care and attention paid to the breasts makes a substantial difference to their well-being. I am not a great supporter of the mammogram (*see* **Mammograms**) and I have therefore encouraged self-examination throughout my career and many lumps have been found and dealt with, including cancers, which, when caught early, can mean the difference between health and illness.

The breasts are very much under the influence of the female hormones and there are nervous and hormonal reflexes associated with touching the breasts that may contribute to keeping them healthy. Love and attention from both the individual and partners may have a profound effect.

BREAST – Four Quads and Axilla

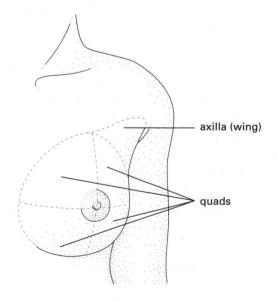

axilla (wing)

quads

Self-examination

Self-examination should be performed on a regular daily basis.

In the bath or shower imagine a line drawn from the middle of the collar bone down through the nipple to the lower rib and another line bisecting this perpendicularly across the chest at the level of the nipple. We have now imaginarily divided the breast into four quadrants. There is a fifth section that requires attention called the 'wing'. This is the section from the upper outer quadrant stretching back to the armpit or axilla.

Using the palm of the hand in a rotating motion examine the left breast with the right hand, and vice versa. Place the palm in the middle of each quadrant initially but move the palm so that it covers the entire area. Repeat this in all four quadrants. Lumps are very noticeable in the palm of the hand and cannot slip between the gaps in between fingers. The same should be done with the wing of the breast, although fingers must come into play nearer the armpit. Special attention should be paid after this initial examination to the nipple and areola. Gentle palpation with the fingertips all around and directly below the nipple is recommended.

All breasts have lumps. Examining the breast daily will allow the individual to get an idea where these lumps are and whether they change at different times of the cycle.

Breast tissue is very often granular, either generally or at particular times of the cycle when the breast is most under oestrogen effect (two weeks prior to the period). Establishing a knowledge of what your breasts feel like will remove the likelihood of your missing an unusual textured lump or of worrying unnecessarily. I encourage partners to examine the breasts regularly to offer a second opinion. The use of doctors and gynaecologists is essential but should not be considered a completely safe option. Whilst doctors may have more experience, a yearly all-clear does not take into account the lump that develops two months after the examination. A clear examination is not complete security for the year.

Remember that most lumps are harmless and that bringing a lump to the attention of the doctor does not usually return a verdict of cancer. Developing the 'ostrich syndrome' by burying your head in the sand and ignoring a possible cancer can lead to a poor outcome. Breast cancer, if caught early enough, is treatable and curable.

RECOMMENDATIONS

General Advice

- *Self-examination should be done daily.*
- *Note lumps and bumps mentally or keep a note if necessary and compare at different times of the month.*
- *Bring any hard or persistent (present for more than one month) lump to the attention of your GP.*
- *Bring any nipple changes or breast shape changes (unless in both breasts and associated with the cycle) to a doctor's attention.*
- *Cancer lumps generally do not alter on a cyclical basis, although the tissue around them may. A lump that comes and goes is not likely to be dangerous. Do not worry, but get it checked.*

BREAST CANCER

The UK has the highest incidence of breast cancer in the world. More than 25,000 women receive a diagnosis of breast cancer each year and 15,000 die from it. It is the leading cause of death among women aged 35–54 years. The devastation to family life is enormous. The figures in Europe and the US are lower but still dramatic, whereas Japan has a strikingly low incidence of breast cancer. These statistics and other evidence indicates that nutrition and environmental pollutants are very likely to be relevant. Women who smoke have a higher incidence of breast cancer and those with low fat and higher antioxidant intake have lower incidence.

There is also an increased rate in those who suffer from constipation. This may be due to an unexplained raised oestrogen level or a simple increase in body toxins. One professor has published a book relating cow's milk and its products to an increased risk of developing breast cancer. The compound in question is IGF-1 (insulin growth factor) and this is present at high levels in cow's milk and causes cells to divide and reproduce at a fast rate. There are probably other chemicals, including prolactin, that may 'confuse' regular cell growth.

Also, an epidemiological study has suggested that women who have used tricyclic antidepressants for two years or more are twice as likely to develop breast cancer than women who have not used antidepressants.

The breast is made up of several types of tissue. Cancers can occur in any of these and treatments and considerations are dependent upon which site the tumour has developed in. The two more common terms are adenocarcinoma (the bulk of the breast tissue) and intraductal carcinoma (within the milk ducts).

Cancer is suspected because of three major tell-tale signs:

- An unexpected lump, which is most often harder than other lumps found in the breast and is occasionally immobile.
- Retraction or inversion of the nipple.
- Discharge or blood seepage from the nipple.

Any of these signs must be brought to the attention of a doctor who has preferably also qualified as a complementary practitioner. I say this because of the current attitude of most specialists to use the mammogram as the principal diagnostic tool.

Investigations

If a breast lump is found that does not disappear at certain times of the cycle, is hard, seems to be fixed to the underlying rib cage or is distorting the skin or nipple area, investigations are warranted.

Medical examination

Most gynaecologists will have vast experience in examining breasts and will be able to give a 'best guess'. If the specialist is not suspicious then neither should you be. Most will err on the side of caution and may suggest further investigations.

Blood tests

There is a compound that can appear in some breast cancers known as CA_{153}. The presence of this 'marker' in the bloodstream is indicative of a breast cancer but unfortunately the reverse is not necessarily true because many cancers do not produce this chemical. A negative test, therefore, does not mean that the breast is clear.

The Humoral Pathological Laboratory Test – high magnification of blood cells – should be considered if available. This test can show changes in the red and white blood cell patterns in the bloodstream and, although not well substantiated through scientific experimentation yet, is a useful addition to the equation.

Ultrasound

As ultrasonography is becoming more accurate, this test is a non-invasive and harmless investigation. A small probe is run over and around the breast tissue and sound waves are bounced off the regular breast tissue and any lumps. A computer will rearrange the sound waves into a picture and, in the hands of an experienced technician, the density and consistency of the breast lump should be easily noted. Any suspicion should lead an individual into further

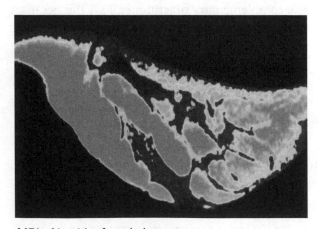

MRI of healthy female breast.

investigations, such as magnetic resonance imaging or lumpectomy.

Magnetic resonance imaging (MRI)

Details of this test can be found in chapter 8. Magnetic resonance imaging is a highly sophisticated, non-X-ray technique that at this time has less evidence of being dangerous than an X-ray. It is my preference, at this time, to recommend MRI before mammograms (*see* below). This technique can image a lump and give a clear indication of the possibility of a cancer and can also be used to test the axillary (armpit) nodes for the possibility of spread.

Mammography

I am fearful that mammograms may be more harmful than beneficial and I suspect that doctors and the public are not being given all the information concerning their efficacy and safety. Despite sophisticated technology, mammograms are not faultless. The machinery may emit far higher levels of radiation than necessary and give a dose above that which is safe.

The images may suggest a cancer that, after operative procedures, proves to have been wrong. There is considerable evidence of inaccuracy. This may be partially because of misreading but also because dense breast tissue is hard for the X-rays to penetrate. The use of HRT increases breast tissue density and makes the identification of lesions more difficult.

There is no doubt that radiation is toxic and can cause cancer. The amount of radiation in a mammogram is unlikely to trigger this but radiation has a cumulative effect. Twice the amount of radiation emitted in a mammogram is obtained in a transatlantic flight; however, regular flying and mammograms may build up radiation within the system. Up to three per cent of the population carry a particular gene, the ataxia-telangiectasia (AT) gene which is seemingly extremely sensitive to radiation and can alter into a cancerous state. The AT gene can be tested for, although at about

£600 the cost is prohibitive and the test is not easy to obtain. Perseverance through a private laboratory may provide an answer for those who can afford it.

Statistically, the orthodox world will point out that mammograms do spot cancerous lumps sooner than women who only self-examine. I could find no study that compared mammograms with ultrasound, however. If a mammogram does find a cancer, if the woman is below the age of 50 years it is unlikely to make a difference to the outcome. Put another way, a cancerous lump found by mammogram will receive treatment sooner but have little effect on the rate of survival of a woman who discovers the cancer through a self-examination if she is under the age of 50 years. Once over 50 years there is some statistical significance but, again, the studies have flaws because they do not take into account the overall health of the individual, nor do they compare a group of women whose breast cancers were found by ultrasound.

Further doubt has been cast following a major study from Canada which suggests that mammograms are no better at detecting cancer in women aged 50–59 than regular examinations by nurses and the women themselves. This is a particularly interesting study since a 1998–9 study conducted in the UK suggested that self-examination was pointless. It is astonishing how figures can be arranged to come up with the result required. It also beggars belief that it should be considered sound medical advice that women should not bother examining themselves.

Mammography is an aggressive and uncomfortable technique. The breast is squashed quite tightly between two X-ray plates and then held in that position for a few moments. It is well established that crushing and manipulating a tumour lump may encourage its spread and whilst the orthodox world is very swift to condemn the use of massage in cancer patients (quite unjustly, as qualified masseurs would not massage a cancerous lump nor lymph nodes that may be involved),

they have no criticism of applying pressure to a potentially cancerous lump.

Biopsy

A biopsy of a lump is an outmoded diagnostic technique but is still used by some practitioners. A needle is passed into the suspicious area and a sample of tissue taken. The needle may miss the lump altogether or hit a part of the lump that does not have any cancerous cells. This will provide a false negative result. Alternatively, if the needle does pass into a cancerous area, as it is withdrawn cells may be seeded into a higher level of the breast or even into the skin, where the spread may be much more profound. I do not support biopsies and think that further investigations should be done through lumpectomy.

Lumpectomy

A lumpectomy is the procedure of removing a lump. It can occur anywhere in the body but is commonly used for the removal of breast lumps. This usually requires a general anaesthetic, although smaller lumps may be done under a local anaesthetic. The lump is isolated and tissue about 1cm around the lump is taken out with it. Very often this is sent down to the laboratory immediately, while the patient is still under anaesthetic and if a cancer is found a wider excision or mastectomy takes place. This is always discussed with the patient before the operation.

Lymph node sampling

At the time of the lumpectomy, or separately, any enlarged or suspicious lymph nodes may be dissected and sent away for examination to see if any cancer has spread through the lymphatic system. This procedure often leaves the lymph drainage of the arm compromised and can cause swelling (lymphoedema) and damage to the nerves in the area, leading to partial paralysis and persistent pain. These side effects are rare but must be taken into account when giving permission for an operative procedure.

Studies are currently underway to support the excision of one principal lymph node in the axilla area that is thought to collect all the lymph draining from the breast before it distributes this solution to other nodes. A cancer will spread to this node first and, therefore, may prevent more aggressive or more numerous lymph gland removal. This procedure is not in common use and will not be until further trials have taken place, which may take 2–3 more years.

RECOMMENDATIONS

General Advice

- *Perform self-examination.*
- *Obtain a medical opinion.*
- *You will note that at no point do I suggest that mammography should be undertaken.*

Orthodox

- *Routine screening through blood tests as described above is sensible.*
- *Ultrasound examination on a yearly basis is safe and sensible.*
- *Any suspicious area found on ultrasound should be examined by MRI.*
- *Any continued suspicion after MRI should lead to a lumpectomy. Do not biopsy.*

Treatments

The wide variety of cancer treatments and preventative measures are discussed in the section on cancer (*see* **Cancer**). Breast cancer is preventable and is treatable but, as in most serious conditions, requires the best line of treatment to be decided in consultation with a complementary practitioner.

RECOMMENDATIONS

General Advice

- *See* **Cancer** *and follow the advice described there.*
- *Establish the percentage success rate of any*

treatment you are offered. Correlate this with the lifestyle changes and toxicity of the course you are recommended and in consultation with a medically qualified complementary practitioner discuss your options. One year of normal life with a possibility of a complementary treatment may be better than two years in and out of treatment centres with all the associated side effects.

- *Please refer to the various sections in this book discussing complementary therapy alongside the treatments (see* **Operations and surgery***, and* **Radiotherapy***).*
- *Always obtain a second or even third opinion.*
- *Visit the library and bookshop and read a couple of books on the subject from a complementary angle.*

Nutritional

- *Broccoli contains a sulphur compound which has been shown to protect against breast cancer in animal studies. Regular intake may help.*
- *Some breast cancers are oestrogen-dependent. This means that they grow quicker in the presence of oestrogen. There is some debate at the moment about whether plant oestrogens act by stimulating cancer growth or by blocking the oestrogen receptors on the cancer cells, thereby preventing oestrogen from influencing the growth rate. Until this debate has been resolved, all women with oestrogen-dependent tumours should avoid plant oestrogens and the foods in which they are contained, such as hops, soya products, celery, fennel and rhubarb. Those with breast tumours that are not oestrogen-dependent should use phyto-oestrogen supplements as they may hinder breast tumour growth.*

Herbal/natural extracts

- *The use of natural progesterone cream should be encouraged but prescribed by a complementary medical practitioner with experience in this area.*

Orthodox

- *Orthodox treatment – apart from the use of*

mammography, the orthodox approach to breast cancer has been proven to be very effective over the last two decades. The treatment protocols include:

(a) Surgery includes removal of the lump (lumpectomy), removal of part of the breast (partial mastectomy) and total mastectomy. Lymph glands in the armpit (axilla) are often removed, which can lead to the side effect of poor lymph drainage causing limb swelling, but radical mastectomy (total removal of the breast and all lymph glands) is now rare. Some studies have suggested that an operation on a breast cancer is less likely to recur if it is performed in the two weeks before the next period. The higher progesterone levels at this time may have a protective influence.

(b) Radiotherapy. Certain types of tumour are susceptible to radiation but first one should insist upon genetic testing for the ataxia-telangiectasia (AT) gene, which makes people more sensitive to cancer formation from radiation.

(c) Chemotherapy. The advent of oestrogen receptor-blocking drugs has so far proved to be effective in tumours that are oestrogen-sensitive. These drugs, such as Tamoxifen and Megace, have side effects and block all oestrogen effects, thereby leading to menopausal-type symptoms and improved survival rates, although they are not, so far, proven to be curative by themselves. Other chemotherapy protocols are available in abundance. One major criticism is that despite the liaison and ability of breast cancer specialists there are currently over 50 different protocols, none of which seem to be more or less favourable than the others. Clearly some unity is needed.

• Mention to your specialist about testing for HER2 protein/receptors. A new treatment, herceptin, maybe be beneficial if HER2 positive.

BREAST DISCHARGES

Discharge from the nipple at any time other than when breast-feeding, and even then only breast milk should be leaking, is a sign of pathology and must initially be assessed by a GP or gynaecologist.

Breast discharge may be related to:

• Hormonal fluctuations
• Inflammation and infection
• Mastitis and abscesses
• Intraductal carcinoma

RECOMMENDATIONS

General Advice

• Book an appointment with the doctor who deals with your gynaecological matters.
• Once a cause has been established, see relevant section in this book.

Homeopathic

• Whilst awaiting diagnosis, a discharge of pus can be treated with Silica 6 (four pills every 3hr), that of blood with Phosphorus 6 and a milky discharge with Calcarea carbonica at the same potency and frequency.

BREAST ENLARGEMENT OR REDUCTION

I do not support cosmetic surgery for the sake of vanity but if an individual's life is being negatively affected and counselling cannot change this, then augmentation or removal of breast tissue is to be considered as an option.

SILICONE IMPLANTS

At the time of writing, silicone breast implants have been banned in the United States after 20 years of use. There is strong evidence to suggest that these implants may promote autoimmune disease although this has yet to be proven conclusively. There has been some correlation between silicone implants and cancer. New implants containing other compounds are available and discussion with at least two cosmetic surgeons should be considered before a decision is made.

RECOMMENDATIONS

General Advice

- *Ensure that the plastic surgeon is a specialist in this area.*
- *Following a recent scare of the potential cancerous effects or immune-suppressing effects of implants made from silicone, consider other implant options until this debate is concluded and silicone is found to be harmless.*

Orthodox

- *See* **Operations and surgery**.
- *See* **Plastic surgery**.

calcarium, Apis and Bryonia. Phytolacca is a master remedy if the mastitis is associated with a lump or lumps.

Herbal/natural extracts

- *Gently massage in an Arnica-containing cream. Do not massage too hard or frequently because this may increase inflammation.*
- *Phytolacca (pokeweed root) – one teaspoonful in a mugful of water, simmered for 15min and taken three times a day or $\frac{1}{2}$ ml of the tincture with water three times a day – is worth trying before an antibiotic is taken.*

MASTITIS AND BREAST ABSCESS

'Mast' is the abbreviation for one of the medical terms for breast, and 'itis' means the inflammation of. Mastitis presents as an area of redness, heat, pain and tension. There may be associated streaks as the inflammation travels along the lymphatic vessels to the lymph glands in the armpit (axilla). If left untreated, this may lead to an abscess.

Mastitis more commonly occurs during lactation and a breast duct becomes clogged, but it may occur away from breast-feeding when the cause is either trauma or, more commonly, an infection that has tracked up from the openings in the nipple. Mastitis is rarely a presentation of cancer.

RECOMMENDATIONS

General Advice

- *Apply hot and cold compresses to the area.*
- *Place cabbage leaves from the fridge or freezer, over the inflamed area.*
- *Persistence or any associated nipple discharge other than breast milk should be brought to the attention of your GP. If you are breast-feeding, express the milk from the affected breast but do not feed it to the child.*

Homeopathic

- *Consult your homeopathic manual and consider remedies such as Belladonna, Hepar sulphuris*

BREAST LUMPS AND SWELLINGS

Breast lumps are most commonly caused by swelling of the breast tissue in response to the hormone oestrogen and are known as breast mice, fibroadenomas or fibrocystic disease. They are generally harmless and have no greater tendency to become cancerous than regular breast tissue but cancer needs to be ruled out (*see* **Breast cancer**).

Generally speaking these lumps are symptomless but they can be tender and even painful, especially close to a period. Provided that they come and go and your doctor, gynaecologist (with confirmation by an ultrasound) consider the lump or lumps to be innocent, the following basic recommendations can be beneficial.

RECOMMENDATIONS

General Advice

- *See the section on 'General Care and Self-examination'.*

Nutritional

- *Avoid coffee and caffeine in general – they cause breast lumps.*
- *Reduce dietary fat if the fibroadenomas are sensitive or preferably before they are due to become so if there is a cyclical pattern.*

PAINFUL BREASTS (MASTODYNIA)

Painful breasts are not uncommon leading up to a period. All the advice given in the section on mastitis can be utilized.

NIPPLE PROBLEMS

Nipples can become painful, sore and cracked for reasons of friction, infection, trauma and skin disorders such as eczema and psoriasis. Breast-feeding is notorious and special attention should be paid to the nipples during this period.

BREATHLESSNESS – *see* Shortness of breath

BRONCHITIS

Bronchitis is inflammation of the bronchial tree (the tubes to the lungs). It can be acute (short term) or chronic (long term).

Acute bronchitis

Often created by viral or bacterial infections, acute bronchitis can be associated with colds and flu. The symptoms are irritation, with cough and often pain. The bronchitis may be dry or productive and, as a rule of thumb, if the sputum is clear the problem is viral and if it is coloured it is bacterial or fungal. Please note that this is not always the case.

LUNGS – Bronchitis

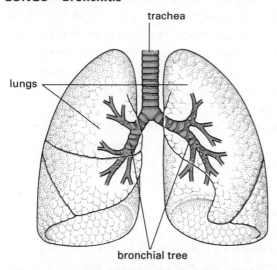

trachea

lungs

bronchial tree

RECOMMENDATIONS

General Advice
- With persistence of symptoms over a week, symptoms that disrupt sleep or your lifestyle and any sign of blood in the product, please go to see your complementary practitioner.
- Acupuncture can be instantly relieving.

Supplemental
- Beta-carotene, 2mg per foot of height in divided doses with three meals per day.
- Vitamin C, 2g with each meal.
- Zinc, 15mg at night.

Homeopathic
- Consult a homeopathic manual for the best remedies concurring with your symptoms.

Herbal/natural extracts
- Herbal drinks or steam inhalations with the essential oils of the following can be very beneficial: hyssop, mullein, thyme, squill and especially lobelia. Seven drops of any of these in water may be drunk and can be most relieving. Make sure first that the product is suitable for internal use.

Orthodox
- Avoid the use of antibiotics unless a sputum culture is carried out. This is because many bronchitis attacks are viral and antibiotics may make the situation worse.

Chronic bronchitis

Chronic bronchitis is usually associated with persisting lung infections, often found in smokers or people subjected to airborne industrial pollutants such as asbestos. Here the inflammation has become deep-seated and usually bacterial infection abounds. The true definition of chronic bronchitis is a productive cough lasting for more than three months.

RECOMMENDATIONS

General Advice
- All the aspects of treatment in acute bronchitis can be utilized.
- In addition, learn a breathing technique and consider regular treatment from a physiotherapist for air passage clearing, and a Shiatsu practitioner for chest-opening bodywork.
- The practice of yoga and Qi Gong is very rewarding.
- See **Breathing**.

Homeopathic
- Homeopathic and herbal treatments must be based on your constitution and best selected by specialists in that area.

CARDIOMYOPATHY

This is the medical term for a pathological problem with the cardiac muscle. It is a specialist diagnosis.

RECOMMENDATION

General Advice
- There is no self-help for this condition and consultation with a complementary medical therapist will help you find the better treatment courses using homeopathy, herbal medicine, diet and exercise.

CHOKING

Choking occurs if an inhaled object or food travels down the trachea (windpipe).

General Advice

- *Try to remove the obstruction with your fingers. If you cannot reach it, move to the next step.*
- *If by yourself, punch yourself one inch below your sternum (chest bone). This will be painful but will throw the diaphragm into spasm which in turn causes a strong exhalation of air, which may force the obstruction out. If somebody is with you, indicate the need for a slap between the shoulder blades hard, three or four times.*
- *If the above procedures do not work, try the Heimlich manoeuvre.*

Heimlich manoeuvre

Move behind the person and interlock your fingers. Place your encircled arms over the head and shoulders until the knuckles are facing towards the person about one inch below the sternum (chest bone). Pull inwards and upwards sharply, three or four times. This will cause the diaphragm to spasm and force the obstruction out of the airway.

Do not practise this technique on those not choking. If the patient has lost consciousness at any point,

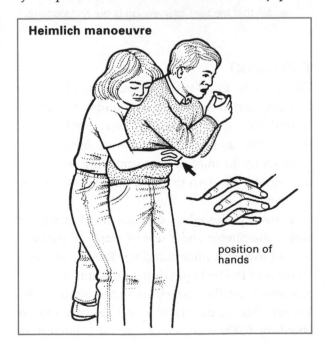

Heimlich manoeuvre

position of hands

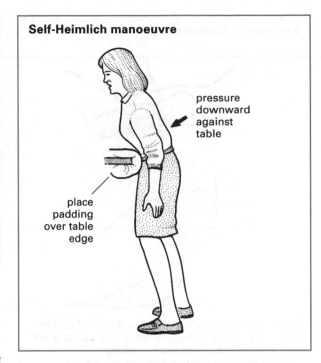

Self-Heimlich manoeuvre

pressure downward against table

place padding over table edge

then once the obstruction is removed initiate artificial respiration.

Self-Heimlich manoeuvre

Move to the corner of a table. Swiftly place something soft and thick (such as your jumper or shirt) over the corner. Lower yourself to a suitable height, placing the corner one inch below the diaphragm and lean forward heavily. Repeat this three or four times with enough force to expel the air in the lungs swiftly.

Do not employ this technique if somebody else is around to perform the above procedure.

EMERGENCY TRACHEOTOMY

A tracheotomy is the formation of an opening into the trachea generally performed under medical supervision when obstruction to breathing has occurred because of trauma to the trachea or mouth above the level of the Adam's apple. In an emergency situation where medical help is not available and an individual is not breathing because of obstruction, it may be necessary to undergo the following emergency procedures.

Emergency Tracheotomy

In an emergency tracheotomy, as described in the recommendations above, a tube is inserted into the trachea to allow breathing.
This procedure should only be carried out when absolutely essential.

This technique should only be employed in exceptional circumstances. Other options, such as the Heimlich manoeuvre, must have failed and medical personnel not present before this procedure is considered. The individual must be completely unable to breath as shown by no movement of the chest, blueness around the lips or cardiac arrest.

Ensure that someone has called the ambulance or emergency service.

- Obtain a tube, such as the outer casing of a pen, and a sharp instrument.
- Lie the patient flat on the floor and extend the neck by tipping the chin backwards.
- Locate the Adam's apple and below the prominent notch there will be a noticeable dip, approximately half-inch wide in an adult.
- Whilst applying adequate pressure, insert the sharp object through this cricothyroid membrane horizontally and, once through the thickened membrane and into the trachea, turn the object vertically.

- There may be a surprising amount of blood.
- As swiftly as possible insert the tube in the gap either side of the sharp object and, when in place, remove the sharp object.
- Bubbling should be heard as air enters the lungs through the tube and also through the inevitable blood in the trachea.
- If this is not heard ensure that respiration is taking place and commence artificial respiration using the tube instead of the mouth.
- Attempt to stem any bleeding with gentle pressure.
- Clean the area as well as possible and tape the tube into place.
- Breathe into the tube if artificial respiration is needed.
- Transport the individual to a medical centre as soon as possible.

RECOMMENDATIONS

General Advice

- *Do not perform a tracheotomy unless it is absolutely essential, and this should be based on the fact that there is no respiration despite attempts at mouth-to-mouth resuscitation.*
- *Do not perform a tracheotomy unless you are certain that medical intervention is not forthcoming.*

THE HEART

The heart is, from an orthodox point of view, a four-chambered muscle that pumps the blood around the system. Despite every author and poet being aware that a broken heart is an inevitability for most of us at some time in our life no credibility is given to the emotional aspects that surround it.

Eastern philosophies describe heart energy as both a distributor and a seat of emotion, particularly of love and understanding. Blood nourishes all parts of the body providing nutrients and oxygen which are the material manifestations of the 'energy' that the Eastern philosophies have spoken about for 5,000 years. Once again it is interesting

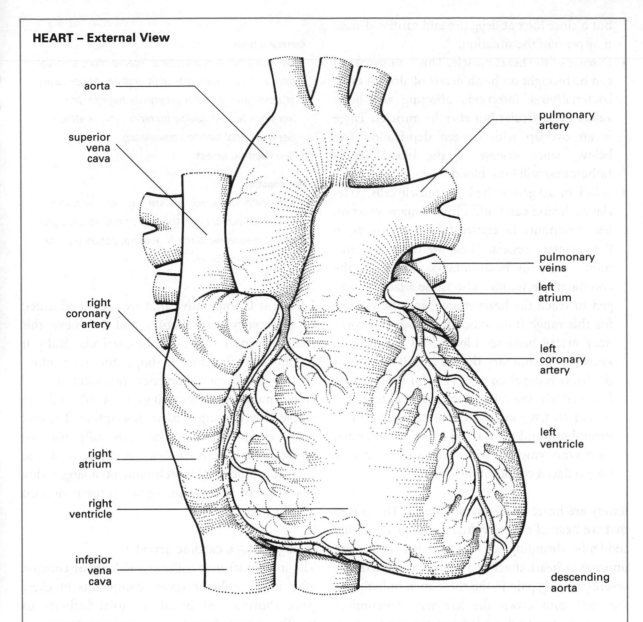

HEART – External View

aorta

superior
vena
cava

right
coronary
artery

right
atrium

right
ventricle

inferior
vena
cava

pulmonary
artery

pulmonary
veins

left
atrium

left
coronary
artery

left
ventricle

descending
aorta

The heart, showing its four chambers (the atriums and ventricles) together with the major blood vessels. The aorta and vena cava carry the blood to and from the body respectively, while the pulmonary arteries and veins go to and from the lungs. The coronary vessels service the heart.

to see how modern science is slowly but surely reaching the same conclusions that have been around for millennia.

Heart attack
A heart attack is the lay-person's term for a pathological cessation of the normal function. If the heart stops beating, the blood (life force?) can no longer circulate and death will ensue within 2min due to a deprivation of oxygen to the brain. The heart will stop for only a few reasons.

- A fault in the electrical conduction system, the causes of which are emotional shock, electrical shock, certain drugs and diseases. There is little that can be done to prevent the sudden shocks but a close look at drug use and cardiac disease may prevent the situation.

- Disease of the heart muscle. This is unusual but can be brought on by an excess of alcohol or by bacterial/viral infections affecting the heart valves in particular but also the muscles. There is an overlap with oxygen deprivation (*see* below) since disease of the blood vessels (atheroma) will limit blood flow.
- A lack of oxygen to the heart muscle cells. Arterial occlusion can build up over many years or, less commonly, be caused by a clot forming in the coronary vessels. These are the most common causes of heart attacks. Spasm of the coronary arteries may also cause a lack of oxygen to reach the heart muscle and the reasons for this range from shock to toxins. If a coronary artery becomes blocked by a clot, it is known as a coronary thrombosis. If an area of the heart is deprived of oxygen for more than a few seconds, the cells will die off and that area is said to have infarcted. The terms coronary thrombosis and myocardial infarction are often used synonymously with heart attack but may only reflect a couple of the causes.

Rarely are heart attacks symptomless. The stories that we hear of an individual in the prime of life suddenly dropping on the squash court are unusual. A heart attack is usually pre-empted by a severe gripping pain in the chest often radiating to the neck and down the left arm. Discomfort through to the back and down the right arm is less common. Dizziness and nausea are frequent and all of these symptoms are associated with a shortness of breath. Many other reasons for chest and upper abdominal pain may mimic mild heart attacks and an interesting differentiating point is the marked fear that is most frequently mentioned by those who have had heart attacks. The orthodox world offers no explanation but if one assumes that the centre of emotion sits in the heart then perhaps the Eastern philosophies do explain the presence of fear with a heart attack.

RECOMMENDATIONS

General Advice
- *Without emergency medical intervention, survival from a major heart attack is unlikely. Minor heart attacks have a better prognosis but are dire warnings for a probably imminent major attack. Seek medical advice immediately.*
- *See* **Cardiac arrest**.

Homeopathic
- *Once orthodox medical care has been obtained or the individual is on the way to the hospital give the homeopathic remedy Aconite, potency 30 or lower, every 15min.*

I think it is imperative that we are all educated in emergency resuscitation and I believe this should be part of all school curricula. Sadly it is not and therefore I hope the description in this book on emergency resuscitation and cardio-pulmonary resuscitation (CPR) will be ample in providing a basic description. I would recommend that everyone, especially parents, spend some time on a first-aid course or at the very least practise this technique on a large teddy bear! Do not practise emergency resuscitation on a well person.

Recognizing a cardiac arrest
The individual may collapse suddenly or collapse after initial mild or severe complaints of chest pain, shortness of breath or total inability to breathe or pains into the neck or down the arm.

Resuscitation concerns ABC (Airways, Breathing, Circulation):

A – Check that there is no visible obstruction in the mouth or the throat.
B – Watch the chest for no more than 10 seconds to see if there is any movement. You may also listen to the mouth and nose for any air passage sounds.
C – Place three fingers in the space between the Adam's apple and the strap muscle of the neck (the sternocleidomastoid). Move the fingers

around a little bit whilst applying moderate, but not strong, pressure to see if you can feel any pulsation in the carotid artery.

You may then proceed to the following steps.

General Advice

- *Send somebody for medical assistance but do not go yourself if you are alone. Hopefully someone will turn up. The delay you may create by going for help may cost the individual's life.*
- *Follow clearly the instructions to establish whether emergency resuscitation is required.*
- *Follow the instructions for CPR in chapter 4.*

Homeopathic

- *Once the patient has been resuscitated you may give Aconite 6, four pills under the tongue, but nothing else. (A physician may well administer an injection of an anticlotting compound called streptokinase or give oral aspirin.)*

Heart failure

There are two functional sides to the heart: the right side collects blood that has been around the body prior to pumping it into the lungs, and the left side receives the oxygenated blood prior to pumping it through the aorta to the rest of the body.

The term 'heart failure' means just that. If severe it may be life-threatening but, if mild, symptoms occur depending on which side of the heart is failing. Right-sided failure will lead to a back-up of blood in the venous system, leading to water retention and most commonly oedema in the legs. Left-sided failure will not allow oxygen to reach the part of the body and this, in combination with the lungs not being able to empty, will cause shortness of breath (dyspnoea), lethargy and tiredness. Persistent left-sided failure will eventually lead to right-sided congestion and a

failing on that side as well.

Heart failure is a consequence of heart muscle disease, heart attacks, infections, pollution, deficiencies and certain drugs. High blood pressure, heart valve disease and congenital defects such as hole-in-the-heart can all cause heart failure.

General Advice

- *Symptoms suggestive of heart failure need to be reviewed by a GP and a cardiac specialist.*
- *Treatment for heart failure should be under the care of an experienced complementary medical practitioner.*
- *Avoid straining the heart but ensure that correct exercise programmes are undertaken. Yoga, which pays special attention to the concept of a heart chakra, is essential.*
- *Spend time with a meditation teacher or religious advisor to establish the underlying causes of emotional blocks. Suppressed emotion and rage are two underlying factors for the heart to fail.*

Nutritional

- *Correct diet must be low salt, low alcohol and include no caffeine.*

Herbal/natural extracts

- *Discuss with your health carer the use of herbal treatments such as Crataegus, and other herbal mixtures. Homeopathic remedies such as Digitalis, Cactus and Aurum metallicum are amongst those that have a strong cardiac influence. Selection must be accurate to be effective and a homeopath should be consulted.*

Orthodox

- *Undergo blood tests to isolate deficiencies, particularly in iron and its carrier-protein ferritin, calcium, magnesium and potassium. Also check for environmental pollutants through blood and bioresonance techniques.*

Heart beat – irregular or blocked (arrhythmia)

Arrhythmia is the medical term for an irregular heart beat. The heart beat is generally not felt but at times of stress, whether physical from exercise or mental from anxiety, the tension in the diaphragm and chest muscles and the increased frequency and strength of the heart itself can lead to the beat becoming noticeable. 'Irregularity' can be noted on inspiration when the heart rate slows, and on expiration, when it may speed up. This is a physiological (normal) variation and not considered an arrhythmia.

Arrhythmias can take the form of increased beats, decreased rate or missed beats. Please learn how to take a pulse. Place your middle and index finger on your wrist below the creases of the wrist on the side of the thumb. Apply gentle pressure and you will feel the radial pulse. This should be beating at a rate of 60–75 beats per minute although a rate of 50 is acceptable in very fit athletes and up to 85 if anxious or having mildly exercised. Outside this range it should be considered too slow (bradycardic) or too fast (tachycardic).

The heart has a comparatively simple electrical system that initiates and controls the beating. A small section of tissue known as the sinoatrial node builds up and releases a charge at around 70 impulses per minute. This spreads through electrical conducting tissues known as Purkinje fibres, which travel to the atrioventricular node before distributing to all of the heart muscles. This atrioventricular node also has an intrinsic beat of around 40 impulses per minute and acts as a fail-safe should the sinoatrial node fail. The autonomic (uncontrolled) nervous system sends impulses through the vagus nerve from the brain, controlling the heart rate acccording to our oxygen demand, in other words whether we are at rest or exercising.

Any interference with this electrical system will cause an irregularity in the beat. Anxiety and fear will stimulate a faster rate by blocking the suppressive action of the vagus nerve. Hormones or

HEART – Conduction System

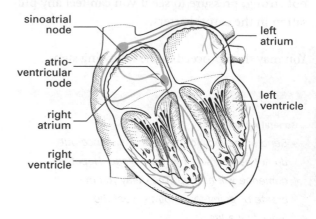

sinoatrial node
atrio-ventricular node
right atrium
right ventricle
left atrium
left ventricle

The electrical conduction system of the heart.

other chemicals such as drugs can have a direct affect on the sinoatrial node. Trauma such as an electrical shock and disease processes including myocardial infarction can lead to interruption or disturbance of the electrical system.

If overstimulation occurs then palpitations and a fast heart beat can be registered or, alternatively, if the action of the interference is suppressive then a slower beat or a heart block may occur. There are many types of heart block depending on whether the individual is simply missing one beat every five, for example, or depending on which fibres are blocked. One may have right- or left-heart fibre bundle branch block, which are simply medical terms to indicate the area of obstruction.

Symptoms of heart block are varied. Some may not be noticed unless a routine (electrocardiogram) is performed, whereas others are severe enough to cause heart failure or even a heart attack.

RECOMMENDATIONS

General Advice

- *Orthodox medical investigation is essential and avoidance of any obvious causes a must.*
- *Complementary treatment must only be initiated by an experienced complementary practitioner because many herbal treatments prescribed in the wrong way may be dangerous.*

- *Yoga is essential because it works on the heart muscles from an aerobic point of view and also because of its effect on any heart chakra weakness or excess. It is best to have an exercise programme set by a cardiologist if more aggressive exercise is desired.*
- *Any heart problem is frightening. Talk about your fears with your GP.*
- *One study has shown that stress can directly produce lethal arrhythmia. Learning a meditation or relaxation technique is essential.*

Nutritional

- *Diet is important and the restriction of alcohol, caffeine and other neuro-affecting substances are all very important.*

Tachycardia

Tachycardia is excessive beating of the heart at a rate above that expected for the level of activity. Exercise may raise the heart rate to above 200 beats per minute but should lower swiftly. If it does not then a tachycardic state is said to exist (*see* the above section on irregular **Heart beat**).

Palpitations

Palpitations are the experience of feeling the heart beating in the chest. There are a variety of sensations, some of which are physiological and not to be worried about. Heavy exercise can induce a fast heart rate (tachycardia), which is felt because of tension in the diaphragm and chest wall muscles. Palpitations must be considered pathological if the sensation is one of an irregular nature. The heart should beat rhythmically at varying speeds, depending on the level of oxygen requirement but an irregular heart beat is inevitably pathological. This does not mean that it is dangerous because several conditions, such as atrial fibrillation (*see* **Fibrillation**), can create an irregular heart beat that may be recognized as a palpitation without it being life-threatening.

The rate of the heart is controlled by nerve tissues within the heart which are in turn controlled by two nerve centres known as the sinoatrial and the atrioventricular nodes.

Further control is exerted by the autonomic (involuntary) nervous system through the sympathetic (speeds up) and parasympathetic (slows down) nervous system. The sinoatrial node sends out impulses that cause the heart muscles to contract at a rate of approximately 70 beats per minute. Should this node fail for any reason, the atrioventricular node will cause the heart to continue to beat but at a slower rate. Any disease or traumatic condition that affects the nodes or conducting system, the central nervous system or the hormones that have an effect on nervous tissue, such as adrenaline and thyroxine, can create an irregular beat. Thyroxine in particular can trigger atrial fibrillation producing an irregular palpitation.

Diseases of the heart muscles, often created by a lack of oxygen following a heart attack or by the build up of atheroma, can cause areas of heart muscle to release their own impulses, triggering contraction of the whole heart.

The autonomic nervous system can be affected by anxiety, phobias and depression, all of which can create a palpitation either by directly interfering with the heart rate or by creating tension within the thorax (chest). The heart and nervous system are sensitive to toxins, and a variety of drugs such as caffeine, nicotine from cigarettes, amphetamines, cocaine and other drugs of abuse may trigger palpitations. Thyroxine replacement and other doctor-prescribed medication may also have an effect. Hypertension (high blood pressure) may lead to palpitations because of an increased heart muscle size or the need for the heart to beat with more strength to get the blood past obstructive blood vessels.

The actual sensation of a palpitation is created by tension within the chest, therefore any levels of anxiety or nervousness may make an individual aware of the heart beat.

As with any heart problem, according to Eastern philosophies the difficulty is not with the heart itself but with the energy to the heart. Heart energy reflects fear and emotions usually associated with relationships and these aspects must be addressed for any other treatments to be effective and permanent.

RECOMMENDATIONS

General Advice

- *Any sensation of an irregular heart beat that is not associated with exercise or a sudden shock, and palpitations that are persistent, must be seen by a GP.*
- *If a palpitation occurs that is irregular in nature or is associated with shortness of breath or chest pain, this must be treated as an emergency. On the way to hospital apply gentle pressure with two fingers just to the side of the Adam's apple where the pulse in the carotid artery can be felt. There are two nerve centres either side of the Adam's apple, which, if stimulated, can slow down the heart. This technique should not be employed if the palpitation is noted to be slow.*
- *Try to isolate any causative factor such as a food, drink or drug that may create palpitations. Food allergy testing may be required.*
- *If no reason for palpations is found, consult a complementary medical practitioner with experience in pulse, tongue or other diagnostic techniques.*
- *Palpitations may be created by conscious or subconscious anxiety and a meditation or relaxation technique would be preferable. Counselling may be required.*
- *For palpitations that are irregular, see* **Heartbeat – irregular**.

Homeopathic

- *Aconite 6 should be taken every 5min until medical attention is received.*
- *The homeopathic remedies Crategus, Digoxin and the snake poisons Naja or Lachesis may be reviewed. Any heart problem should be dealt with by professionals and a homeopathic opinion is best sought.*

Herbal/natural extracts

- *Self-prescribed herbal treatments are best avoided, but in the hands of an expert herbal treatments may be used with comparative safety.*
- *Chinese or Tibetan herbal medicine may be associated with acupuncture. Masters in the art may actually insert an acupuncture needle that will touch the heart. Be very wary!*

Orthodox

- *An ECG will trace the electrical system's effects on the heart and, occasionally, if the palpations are sporadic throughout the day a Holter monitor may be employed which measures the electrical system throughout a 24hr period.*
- *Cardiac drugs or other medication, depending upon the cause, are generally effective and potentially life-saving. These should not be ignored or avoided if prescribed.*
- *Rarely, cardioversion using electrical shock may be required or a pacemaker may need to be fitted. The latter is a small electrical device that instructs the heart and nervous system to beat at a set rate. Surgery is infrequently required for palpations.*

Heart transplant

This life-saving interventional surgery is one of the major successful advances in modern medicine. There is, obviously, no alternative treatment but *see* **Atheroma** and **Cholesterol** to avoid congesting the new heart's blood vessels. There are causes other than coronary thrombosis that lead to the requirement of a heart transplant and again prevention is the best cure.

RECOMMENDATIONS

General Advice

- *See* **Atheroma** *and* **Cholesterol**.
- *See* **Operations and surgery**.

LUNG DISEASE

Pulmonary oedema

Pulmonary oedema is a medical term describing build-up of fluid in the lung tissues caused by a back-pressure from a failing left side of the heart. Fluid is pushed out of the blood vessels, causing the lungs to become like a sponge, thus inhibiting breathing. The symptoms are breathlessness and a cough, which initially may be dry and will produce a frothy pink sputum. Valvular disease and heart attacks are the most common causes.

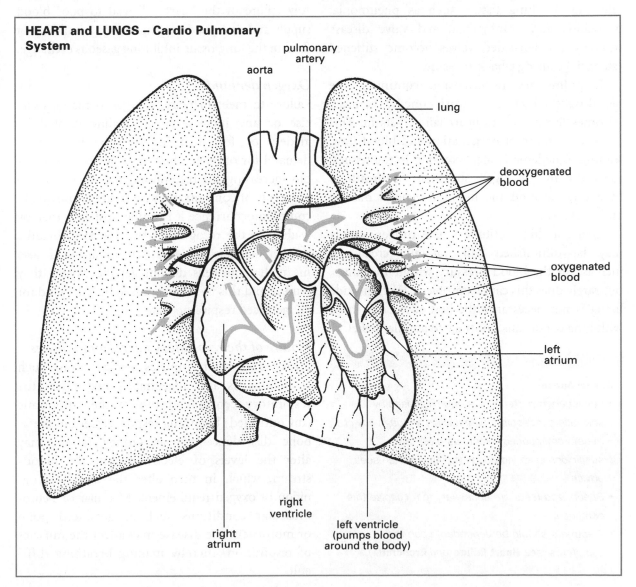

HEART and LUNGS – Cardio Pulmonary System

- aorta
- pulmonary artery
- lung
- deoxygenated blood
- oxygenated blood
- left atrium
- right atrium
- right ventricle
- left ventricle (pumps blood around the body)

Pulmonary hypertension

Pulmonary hypertension is the term used to describe an increase in pressure in the blood vessels of the lung. The right side of the heart pumps blood into the lungs which, once oxygenated, will flow into the left side of the heart to be pumped out through the body.

Any condition that diminishes oxygenation of the blood will encourage the body to send out impulses to the right side of the heart to make it beat faster and harder. This increased flow of blood to the lungs raises the pressure. Conditions that do this are diseases causing anaemia, diseases affecting the lung tissue, such as pneumonia, bronchitis and emphysema, and valve disease whereby the left-sided valves become stiffened (stenosis) causing a back-pressure.

If pulmonary hypertension continues, the blood vessels thicken, the work done by the heart becomes too great and heart failure sets in. This leads to a failure of oxygenation and blood flow, leading to oedema (water retention in the tissues, especially in the legs), shortness of breath, a blue tinge around the lips and general malaise and weakness.

Living at high altitude where oxygen supply may be diminished will naturally create an increase in the blood pressure within the lungs, but rarely does this cause a problem. High-altitude living is not necessarily the best advice for those with lung conditions, contrary to popular belief.

RECOMMENDATIONS

General Advice

- *Pulmonary hypertension is only diagnosed by specialists in respiratory medicine, although any of the aforementioned symptoms must raise suspicions in an individual who should then seek advice.*
- *Specialized tests are necessary to recognize this condition.*
- *Treatment should be dependent upon the symptoms (see **Heart failure** and **Bronchitis**).*

SHORTNESS OF BREATH

Shortness of breath can occur for four reasons.

The lungs

Any disease process that damages the lungs or the blood supply (to and from) will lead to shortness of breath. Obstruction of the upper airway through trauma, asthma, bronchitis, pneumonia, emphysema or lung collapse (pneumothorax) are the most common causes of lung-induced shortness of breath.

The heart

Any failure of the heart will lead to poor blood supply and decreased oxygenation or a build-up of fluid in the lung tissue inhibiting gaseous exchange.

Oxygen demand

Failure to meet increased oxygen demand, exercise or any increase in adrenaline created by anxiety or fear will increase the body cells' demand for oxygen, which may not be met without increasing the respiratory rate. Very often in moments of concentration we forget to breathe (a common occurrence if running upstairs), thereby leading to the recognition for a need to breathe quicker. Deficiencies that create anaemia also mean that the cells do not get the oxygen they require and this too is recognized by a demand for an increased respiratory rate.

Failure of the respiratory nerves and muscles

Stroke and brain injuries or infections such as meningitis and encephalitis may affect the respiratory centre and inhibit the autonomic (uncontrolled) breathing response. Certain metabolic disorders such as kidney failure may alter the levels of electrolytes in the bloodstream, which in turn alter the brain's recognition of oxygen requirement. Muscular or neuromuscular conditions such as advanced polio or motorneurone disease may affect the muscles of respiration, thereby making breathing difficult.

General Advice

- *Isolate the underlying cause of the shortness of breath and treat appropriately.*
- *See* **Breathing**.

THE DIGESTIVE SYSTEM

ACID REFLUX

Acid reflux is caused by a weakness in the musculature at the lower end of the food pipe (oesophagus) and in the stomach being weak. There is actually no valve *per se* as there is for example in the bladder or at the other end of the stomach before the duodenum. The muscles of the oesophagus act as a partial valve. If the acid in the stomach travels up the oesophagus, it is due to either a hiatus hernia (*see* **Hiatus hernia**), an over-filling of the stomach or intra-abdominal fat putting pressure on the stomach contents.

The symptoms are usually a burning sensation

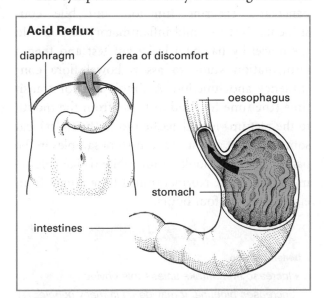

Acid Reflux

diaphragm · area of discomfort

oesophagus

stomach

intestines

Acid reflux occurs when acid from the stomach travels up the oesophagus. The resulting burning sensation is known as heartburn.

or, less commonly, a tightness felt at the top of the abdomen or behind the sternum. The burning can extend into the throat.

General Advice

- *See* **Hiatus hernia**.
- *Consult your GP if the symptoms persist.*

Homeopathic

- *The homeopathic remedies Nux vomica, Carbo vegetalis, Lycopodium and Arsenicum should be reviewed in your homeopathic manual.*

Orthodox

- *The occasional use of antacids is not unwarranted.*
- *Milk may give immediate relief but it stimulates acid production and can worsen the condition if taken persistently.*

BELCHING

Belching or burping is the release of gas from the stomach through the mouth. There is generally an air bubble floating at the top of the stomach contents, kept in by the weak valve at the base of the oesophagus (food pipe) and the tightness created by the diaphragm where the oesophagus passes through it. It is perfectly normal to belch and only needs to be taken as a pathological problem if it is excessive or foul smelling. Eighty-five per cent of air in the gut is swallowed and the other 15 per cent is created by bacteria or the release of gas from food fermentation.

General Advice

- *Try not to talk whilst you are eating or, more accurately, prior to swallowing.*
- *If the belching is foul smelling (see* **Bad breath**).
- *Diaphragmatic tension can squeeze the air bubble at the top of the stomach, so excessive stress can cause belching.*
- *Very rarely, an irritation in the stomach lining can create a sensation of needing to belch.*

- *Belching can also be a habit, which may require hypnotherapy or analysis to resolve.*

Nutritional
- *Cut back on foods that contain air, such as leavened bread, fizzy drinks and pulses.*

BLOATING

Bloating is one of the most common presentations to a general practice and it generally refers to a swollen abdomen. The most common cause is a build-up of flatus (abdominal gas or 'wind'), but the most serious causes must be eliminated before treatment is considered. Unless belching or passing wind from below relieves the situation then the problem should be assessed by a physician, especially if it is of sudden onset and associated with pain or if it is persistent and recurrent. The doctor needs to rule out more serious conditions, such as inflammatory bowel disease (IBD), diverticular disease or even cancer. Uterine fibroids and growths in other abdominal organs can also be mistaken for gaseous bloating.

Up to 85 per cent of gas in the bowel has been swallowed. This is either taken in routinely and unconsciously when swallowing to moisten the food pipe or swallowed as a constituent of food (bread, for example, is very airy). Poorly chewed food often takes with it a lot of air. Swallowing air is also an involuntary action of anxiety and nervousness. Oxygen tends to be absorbed into the bloodstream, so the main component of bowel gas is nitrogen. Nitrogen has no smell and the unpleasant odour comes from only about 1 per cent of the gas. This is caused by sulphur-based gases that tend to come from the bacteria in the bowel as well as from foods containing high levels of sulphates, such as vegetables, and, especially, beans, bread and beer. Sulphur is also contained in many proteins, so foods such as meat and lentils also increase the odour.

Bloating tends to occur when the gases cannot be passed and, having ruled out an obstructive disease, this tends to occur if the bowel is moving slowly due to mild dysfunction. The common causes are: poor digestion requiring the food to stay in the bowel longer to be broken down and therefore to become absorbable; poor hydrochloric acid or pancreatic enzyme production from the stomach and pancreas respectively; a reduction in bile production through mild liver dysfunction. A mild inflammatory response in the bowel may stop a portion of the bowel from contracting as it should which then interferes with peristalsis (the contractile movement of the bowel), thereby slowing down the movement of gas.

The normal bowel flora, made up of bacteria and, to a lesser extent, yeasts, fungi and viruses, are essential for the breakdown of foods. An imbalance or a lack of bowel bacteria can lead to poor digestion and poor peristalsis thereby causing bloating. An overgrowth of yeast in the bowel, most commonly *Candida*, can also be responsible for slow peristalsis and excess gas production.

Investigations may be required if the recommendations below do not solve the problem. Consider discussing suitable tests with a complementary medical practitioner for assessing hydrochloric acid production in the stomach, pancreatic exocrine function and bile constituents. Test for mild inflammatory response in the bowel by having a leaky gut test and then a fermentation study to assess bowel flora constituency and function. A simple test for transit time (the time for food to travel from the mouth to the rectum) is to defecate (go to the toilet), eat some beetroot and study your stool samples in the pan of the toilet looking for a blood-like colouring of the water. Normal transit time ranges from eight to twenty four hours.

RECOMMENDATIONS

General Advice
- *Increase fibre intake unless this obviously increases bloating. It may do so in many people.*
- *Increase daily exercise.*

- Ensure good hydration by drinking ½ pint (¼ litre) of water per foot of height per day.
- See **Flatulence, Candidiasis** and **Constipation** if relevant.

Nutritional

- Many of us are lactose (milk sugar) intolerant and bacteria act upon this non-dissolvable sugar and they in turn release gas. Cut milk out.
- Remove foods that you recognize as causing bloating.
- Consider removing high protein foods such as red meat and large portions of lentils from your diet. Avoid excess legumes and beans and the cruciferous vegetables, such as broccoli and cabbage.
- Avoid fizzy drinks, especially beer.
- Avoid foods containing yeast, such as bread, beer and mushrooms.

Supplemental

- Take a good quality acidophilus with each meal or last thing at night.
- Preferably after testing, consider using hydrochloric acid supplements with main meals and pancreatic enzyme supplements with all meals.

Homeopathic

- Consider any of the following taken at potency 6 every one to two hours, reducing frequency as improvement occurs:
- ○ Carbo vegetabilis – heaviness, fullness and burping.
- ○ Chamomilla – distending with griping in the middle of the abdomen.
- ○ Lycopodium – bloated and full immediately after a meal, a right to left shooting pain.
- ○ Nux vomica – distended with spasmodic pains, a shortness of breath and a desire for stool.

Herbal/natural extracts

- Aloe vera extracts, liquorice and slippery elm are all easily available. A combination of two

teaspoonfuls chamomile, one teaspoonful sage and one teaspoonful rosemary brought to the boil in one pint of water and left to simmer for ten minutes can be drunk, one cupful every half hour for immediate relief.
- Charcoal absorbs gases, especially sulphurous ones, therefore reducing odour. It is found as charcoal biscuits in most health food stores. Follow the instructions on the packet.

Orthodox

- It is important to eliminate any underlying pathology. Laxatives and antacids should be avoided but simethicone, which theoretically allows the conglomeration of trapped gas particles that then pass more easily, could be considered.

BOWEL POLYPS

A polyp is a smooth, round or oval mass that projects from the bowel membrane. These may be broad-based, but are generally on a stalk. There is a genetic trait in some cases and then this condition is known as familial polyposis coli when numerous polyps are found throughout the bowel. There is an inevitable change in polyposis coli from a benign to a malignant polyp in this condition and treatment is currently considered to be a total colectomy (removal of the colon). Most polyps in the bowel are not dangerous except in this condition. Found in the colon on investigations such as colonoscopy or barium enemas, polyps are often removed because of a risk of malignant change.

Investigation is usually initiated because of blood or mucus found in the stool or a change in bowel habit. Polyps may be found quite coincidentally or may be the cause of these symptoms. It is rare but they may enlarge to a point that obstructs the bowel, creating symptoms of bloating, constipation and painful distension.

Bowel polyps are considered by the holistic world to be created through poor diet and a tendency to a retentive body type, which holds toxins in the system and encourages irritation of cells, which then proliferate.

General Advice

- *Any change in bowel habit or the presence of blood or mucus should be investigated by a GP and a specialist if necessary.*
- *A polyp is a warning of lifestyle and diet faults. Increase fibre and water intake and reduce smoking and refined foods.*
- *Polyps are generally an indication of a retentive tendency, and psychological and spiritual changes to encourage a more outgoing personality and expansive spiritual belief must be encouraged.*
- *Pre- and postoperative care should be followed (see **Operations and surgery**).*

Homeopathic

- *Homeopathic and herbal treatments may be considered and attempts to remove the polyps without surgery are possible but they require expert treatment from a homeopathic practitioner for constitutional prescribing and from an experienced herbalist.*

Orthodox

- *A polyp is best removed because of its potential for change into a bowel cancer.*

CANDIDIASIS

There are shelves of libraries full of books containing evidence of the ill-effects of *Candida* and a myriad of treatments against this yeast. The most common form is *Candida albicans*, which lives within most of us. Fifty per cent of women will house *Candida* in the vagina. *Candida* is not a particularly virulent organism, thriving only when our own immunity is low. When this occurs, however, *Candida* can be most devastating in its effects.

Orthodox medicine does not consider it to be a particularly relevant aspect of ill-health. The alternative bandwagon has enjoyed portraying *Candida* as the potential cause of many and variable ailments. As always, the answer lies in a balance between the two extremes. It is important not to get drawn into the 'germ theory' that the orthodox approach portrays so fully. *Candida* itself is not particularly troublesome, it is the lack of immune system response and generalized ill-health within the system that makes it more aggressive.

Very often a diagnosis of exclusion (ruling other causes out) is the only way to diagnose this condition. *Candida* in the system may not pass out through the urine or stool and may not be found floating freely in the bloodstream via blood tests. Diagnosis is often made by:

- Experienced diagnosticians
- Bioresonance techniques
- Exclusion of other causes

The symptoms of candidiasis are so varied that to list them would inevitably lead to missing some out. Any organ or system can be affected, either directly by the presence of *Candida* or by the toxins that *Candida* produces. Mental symptoms such as tiredness and lethargy may be produced by the poisonous effects of a small colony of *Candida* existing in the colon. More commonly symptoms such as vaginal thrush, rashes in infants, diarrhoea and itching may result from direct infection. A persistent presence of *Candida* in the bowel may activate the immune system in such a way that it overreacts to other things and can therefore be an indirect cause of allergies.

General Advice

- *Ensure an accurate diagnosis by some form of investigation. Many alternative practitioners have jumped on the bandwagon, suggesting that Candida is the cause of all problems and sadly often overlooking simpler and more easily treatable conditions.*
- *Swabs from the vagina and stool and urine tests may isolate Candida. Blood tests may show antibodies to Candida. If these orthodox*

investigations prove negative, then consider the Humoral Pathological Laboratory Test or bioresonance – see chapter 8.

- *In principle, Candida is not a problem to the body unless the immune system is low and bacteria that compete with Candida for food are run down. The use of antibiotics and laxatives, which affect the normal bowel flora will allow Candida to flourish because of greater availability of food.*

Nutritional

- *Candida, more than other organisms, flourishes on high levels of sugar and carbohydrates and these foods should be reduced, if not cut out, once a diagnosis has been made.*
- *Avoid foods containing yeasts such as bread and live cheeses. Many yeasts excrete compounds that help yeast growth.*

Supplemental

- *If over the age of 14 years, take 30mg of zinc each night. Below that age, discuss the matter with a complementary medical practitioner.*
- *Caprylic acid (approximately 700mg) can be taken 15min before each meal and Lactobacillus acidophilus (2 billion organisms) can be taken with the meal.*

Herbal/natural extracts

- *The fluid extract of broom – one teaspoonful 20min before each meal in a glass of water – or a low iron supplement (5mg) can be taken daily.*

Anti-*Candida* diets and treatments

There are many anti-*Candida* diets on the market. My experience is that they are difficult to follow and the above recommendations often work without ripping into an individual's lifestyle and preferred dietetics.

I do *not* recommend the use of anti-*Candida* drugs such as nystatin. Like most drugs, they kill the majority of the *Candida* colony but encourage the breeding of resistant strains, which will then multiply because nothing has been done to encourage the bowel bacteria or immune system.

This gives a false sense of security, making the individual feel better for a short time but inevitably leading to a recurrence. The recurrence will be with a much tougher strain of *Candida*, which can lead to worse symptoms or new problems.

The same can be said for colonic irrigation. Whilst this does not confer the likelihood of resistant strains, it is often a temporary measure and should only be used in conjunction with anti-*Candida* therapy as recommended above.

CHOLECYSTITIS

Cholecystitis is the medical term for inflammation of the gallbladder and its main ducts. This inflammation is caused by blockage of the tube leading from the gallbladder to the duodenum causing an increase in pressure, or directly by infection that tends to occur in association with a drainage blockage. Blocking of the bile ducts usually occurs due to small gallstones but can occur because of more sinister conditions including cancer of the pancreas.

The symptoms of chronic cholecystitis are a dull but persistent ache on the right side of the abdomen underneath the rib cage. This ache has acute exacerbations, which can be incredibly severe and unrelenting. Very often these pains are brought on by eating, most commonly, fatty foods.

Acute cholecystitis (sudden and severe) may require an emergency operation to relieve the pain, so any suggestion of aches and pains in that area needs to be investigated thoroughly.

RECOMMENDATIONS

General Advice

- *See your GP who will examine you and organize blood tests and an ultrasound at least.*
- *Having ruled out more sinister problems (see* **Cholelithiasis***).*
- *The discomfort can be markedly relieved by squeezing two teaspoonfuls of lemon juice into warm water and drinking.*

Nutritional
- *Until the problem is diagnosed and treatment initiated, do not eat any fatty foods.*

Supplemental
- *Stop taking any fat-soluble vitamins such as vitamins A and E, cod liver oil and Evening Primrose Oil.*

Homeopathic
- *The homeopathic remedies Berberis vulgaris 6, Chelidonium 6 and Lycopodium 6 can be taken every 10min and may relieve the discomfort.*

CHOLELITHIASIS (GALLSTONES)

Gallstones are found in approximately 1 in 5 women in the West and 1 in 10 men. They are generally made out of cholesterol, liver breakdown products known as bile pigments, calcium and other minerals or, most often, a mixture of the above. They are generally asymptomatic, sitting in the gallbladder quite innocuously.

Gallstones develop when the bile (the compound made by the liver that is responsible for the breakdown of fats) becomes too concentrated. This may also occur because too much cholesterol and pigment is being made. The former indicates excess activity by the liver on dealing with toxins in the system, and the latter indicates dehydration (*see* **Cholesterol** *and* **Dehydration**).

Symptoms, if they occur, are caused by the stones moving from the gallbladder into the bile ducts, causing obstruction and pain as they travel down the tubes. The absence of bile in the bowel because of the obstruction will lead to poor digestion causing abdominal distension, burping and flatulence, nausea and potentially vomiting. The discomfort is usually in the right side of the abdomen although it can radiate to the back, which is sometimes a tell-tale sign of gallbladder disease or gallstone obstruction. An experienced physician will be fairly accurate about the diagnosis but firm assurance can be obtained by using ultrasound.

Prevention of gallstones is much easier than treatment. Principally this is because a gallstone in the gallbladder is not a problem and the larger it is the less likely it will escape into the narrow bile duct tube. Treatments that reduce gallstones are therefore potentially hazardous and best left in the hands of complementary medical practitioners who can support and monitor the situation. As a rule of thumb, therefore, I recommend that anyone who has a diagnosis of gallstones through a screening test (ultrasound) or who has had one attack should endeavour not to reduce their gallstones but to prevent further gallstone growth or formation.

Those who have recurrent or frequent attacks and who are being threatened with surgical procedures should come under the care of an experienced complementary practitioner, who will use specific treatments to reduce gallstones and at the same time encourage the patient to maintain a low-fat (not fat-free) diet, thereby inhibiting any aggressive contraction by the gallbladder (in response to fatty foods) which may dislodge a gallstone. It is because of the need to be monitored that I have chosen not to mention the details of specific treatments, which if effective

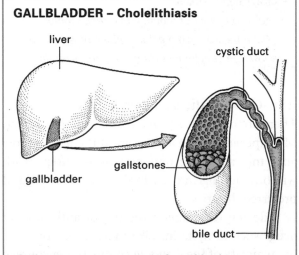

GALLBLADDER – Cholelithiasis

liver

cystic duct

gallstones

gallbladder

bile duct

Gallstones are commonly found in the gallbladder and cause few problems. However, they may be the source of much discomfort if they become lodged in the bile duct.

may reduce the size of the gallstone and lead to the potentially serious medical condition of a blocked bile duct and cholecystitis.

There is a popular gallstone treatment called the olive oil liver flush. There are variations of this but they all revolve around an olive oil mix with lemon juice. Patients have proudly presented saying that they found green stones in their stool. This is not the case. What has been produced is a complex of minerals, fats and acid which form within the gut. The treatment is *not* a good idea. The extra oil can cause the gallbladder to contract and the oleic acid in olive oil may be a cause of gallstone formation.

RECOMMENDATIONS

General Advice

- *See* **Cholecystitis**.
- *For recurrent chronic gallstone-related problems, consult an experienced complementary medical practitioner for specific therapies.*
- *Perhaps most importantly, ensure good hydration so that the bile is not encouraged to become concentrated (see **Dehydration**).*

Nutritional

- *Reduce the input of foods containing saturated fats, refined sugars, cholesterol and fried foods. Animal protein should be kept to a lean minimum. Increase the intake of fibre through fruits and vegetables.*
- *Check for food allergies (see **Food allergy testing**). Eggs, pork, onion, dairy produce and caffeine are all documented as being relevant to gallstone formation.*

Supplemental

- *Vitamin C and vitamin E deficiencies have been noted as increasing gallstone formation: vitamin C (500mg per foot of height in divided doses) and vitamin E (50iu per foot of height in divided doses) should be taken.*
- *If an individual has had one attack or falls into the risk categories mentioned above, then the following compounds should be taken prophylactically on a daily basis per foot of height: phosphatidylcholine (100mg), choline (200mg) and L-methionine (200mg).*

Herbal/natural extracts

- *When discussing the situation with your complementary practitioner, ensure that the following herbs are considered in the treatment: Taraxacum, Cynara, Scolymus and Silymarin.*

Orthodox

- *There are pharmaceutical medications that can dissolve some types of gallstones but this has to be discussed with your GP and only as a last resort because it does not deal with the underlying cause or tendency.*
- *Surgical intervention may be required and, at the time of writing, laparoscopic gallbladder removal is the favoured method. This avoids major abdominal incisions and reduces the length of time an individual needs to stay in hospital. Ensure that the procedure is performed by a surgeon with experience in this area.*
- *One may be offered lithotripsy, a sound-wave procedure that shatters the gallstones. This is losing favour in some parts of the world because the small particles tend to reform into a larger number of gallstones. This would certainly be the case if the underlying causes of the predisposition, such as dehydration or overactive liver function, were not dealt with. Keep this technique at arm's length.*

CIRRHOSIS

This is the medical term given to the replacement of damaged liver tissue by scar tissue. This tissue is non-functional and blocks the liver cell ducts and the blood supply. The most popular concept for the cause of cirrhosis in the West is alcoholism, but worldwide the most common cause is malnutrition and hepatitis. Drugs and heart failure (causing a back-pressure of blood on the liver) are also causes.

The liver is a phenomenal organ and the body

may notice very little change in its well-being until 80 per cent of the liver is non-functional. It is this principle that is paramount in complementary medical treatment because medicine has no method of preventing cirrhosis from spreading through the liver once it has started. Helping the healthy and non-affected cells of the liver to work at their hardest encourages both well-being and longevity.

Diagnosis of cirrhosis is made by liver biopsy, which is usually performed after your GP has established that there are incorrect liver function tests. These are performed after an individual presents with excessive tiredness, jaundice, digestive problems, nausea, vomiting or a combination of any of these. Cirrhosis is not a painful condition unless associated with inflammation of the liver, such as in hepatitis.

RECOMMENDATIONS

General Advice

- *Any jaundice or suspected liver problem should be assessed by a GP initially.*
- *Cessation of any liver-insulting habits, such as the use of alcohol and drugs, smoking, bad diet and stressful living, is essential.*
- *Remember that the liver, according to Eastern philosophies, represents indecision and irritability and so these emotions may well be prominent after cirrhosis sets in but are more likely to have been present to allow cirrhosis to have occurred and must, therefore, be confronted through counselling.*
- *The use of detoxifying regimes (see chapter 7) are most beneficial and should be used on a monthly basis.*

Nutritional

- *Do not add salt to food, absolutely no alcohol, no fat from red meat and no dairy products, although fish oils and vegetable oils are essential.*

Supplemental

- *The use of magnesium, zinc and multi-trace-mineral supplement and a vitamin B complex is beneficial but correct dosage is best assessed*

by a naturopath. The liver is the main chemical factory of the body and too high a dose of any of the necessary compounds can be a strain on the healthy liver cells.
- *Beta-carotene rather than vitamin A should only be used after recommendation by a naturopath.*

Homeopathic

- *Homeopathic remedies based on the individual's constitution can be taken but special attention should be paid to Berberis vulgaris, Natrum sulphuricum and Lycopodium.*

CONSTIPATION

Constipation is a condition in which the bowels are evacuated at long intervals or with difficulty. The body will do this for several reasons:

- because the bowel does not contract well enough;
- because the bowel is moving more slowly to allow longer for food and water absorption;
- because the stool lacks bulk;
- because the stool is too large or hard to pass through the anus without pain.

There is no ideal number of times to evacuate the bowels. Everyone has a rhythm and it is important to keep that stable. A change in bowel habit that persists needs to be reviewed by a GP. Everybody will go through constipation and other bowel changes on occasions, and treatment should only be considered if the problem persists or is uncomfortable.

A lack of fibre in the foods we eat causes stool to become soft so that when peristaltic waves in the colon try to flush the faeces towards the anus, some of the stool will pass in the opposite direction. If the body is deficient it may slow down the movement of food through the small intestine to allow more time for absorption to take place. This can appear to be constipation simply because there is nothing to pass out. The colon (large bowel), which makes up the last four feet of the bowel is where most of the water is absorbed from our food and drink. If we are dehydrated, and I think most of us spend our lives in a state of partial dehydration, the colon will move more slowly to allow more time for water absorption.

Because constipation may be due to body deficiencies or dehydration and involve soft stool or hard stool there is no single treatment that will benefit all patients. It is important to know the cause of the constipation so that correct treatment can be chosen. Problems not relieved by the following recommendations should be taken to a nutritionist or herbal medicine practitioner. Ayurvedic and Tibetan practitioners have a very good grasp of this matter.

RECOMMENDATIONS

General Advice

- A change in bowel habit that persists must be referred to a GP for assessment.
- Ensure that you are drinking 2–3 pints of water per day away from food.
- Avoid dehydrating conditions, such as exercising without fluid intake, alcohol, caffeine and an excess of spicy or sweet foods. The latter pulls water into the bowel and prevents the tissues from receiving it.
- 'Natural' laxatives are available at healthfood stores and may be used if constipation is infrequent but having to use a natural laxative more than three times in any month requires investigation with your complementary medical practitioner.
- Stool softeners and stool bulk-formers should be used only as a last resort.
- Do your best to avoid regular laxatives, which can have a long-term debilitating effect on the colon and its musculature. Long-term laxative abuse is treatable under the care of a nutritionist, herbalist or homeopath.
- Colonic irrigations are fine on occasions but they should not be considered as a treatment for constipation.
- Three finger-widths below the navel is the Sea of Energy acupuncture point, which if you gradually apply more pressure on it for 2min whilst you are in a lying down position may be beneficial if practised twice a day.
- Constipation following cessation of smoking is treatable by herbalists, who will replace the nicotine effect on the bowel contraction with a healthier herb, which they will reduce over a period of time. You may try taking one teaspoonful of Cascara sagrada 1hr before going to bed.

Nutritional

- Ensure that you have adequate fibre in your diet (see chapter 7).
- Please establish, by reading chapter 7 or by having a consultation with a nutritionist/dietician, that your diet is satisfactory.

Supplemental

- Gut bacteria are essential to the digestive process. Poor diet and the use of antibiotics, directly from pills or indirectly through eating foods containing such drugs, can alter the bowel flora and lead to constipation. Correct this with a good quality Acidophilus (2 billion organisms with each meal) for at least one month.
- Two grams of vitamin C with each meal can act as a natural laxative and can be used for short periods if a problem persists. Children below the age of 14 years need to take half that amount.

Herbal/natural extracts

- Try six drops of rosemary oil in half a cup of olive oil, rubbed in a clockwise motion around the abdomen twice a day.
- Two apples freshly squeezed in combination with a teaspoonful of fresh ginger juice diluted with a little water, taken three times a day before meals, can be effective.

DUODENAL ULCERS AND DUODENITIS
– *see* Peptic ulcers

DYSPEPSIA

Dyspepsia is a medical term for disturbed digestion but is generally used to describe a burning or acid sensation in the upper abdomen or lower chest that often radiates up the throat. Generally, dyspepsia, also known as heartburn and indigestion, is caused by inflammation in the lower part of the oesophagus (reflux oesophagitis), the stomach or duodenum. All these conditions can be precursors to peptic ulcers (*see* **Peptic ulcers**).

As a rule of thumb, pain occurring after a meal is gastritis, discomfort associated with bending down or lying down is acid reflux (often associated with a hiatus hernia) or, if occurring 2–3 hours after a meal or around 2.00am in the morning is duodenitis.

It is commonly assumed that the problem is caused by an excessive amount of stomach acid, although the exact opposite may also be true. A paucity of acid (hypochlorhydria) prevents food from leaving the stomach because it has not been broken down and this persistence causes an irritation in the stomach lining. Yeast and, more recently discovered, *Helicobacter pylori* and other bacterial infection may colonize the stomach and cause problems.

Anxiety and tiredness will lead to a tightening of the diaphragm, which may pinch the top part of the stomach and force acid up into the oesophagus (*see* **Acid reflux**).

RECOMMENDATIONS

General Advice
- *A persistent or severe dyspepsia should be examined by a doctor to rule out any serious condition.*
- *See* **Gastro-oesophageal reflux disorder (GORD).**

Nutritional
- *Recognize and remove any foods that commonly cause problems, specifically alcohol, caffeine and refined sugars.*
- *Persisting problems may require food allergy testing via bioresonance techniques or blood tests. Consult your preferred complementary medical practitioner.*

Supplemental
- *Calcium carbonate tablets are freely available and should be used, ensuring that they do not contain any aluminium. Only use half or even a quarter of a tablet at a time because this can often be sufficient.*
- *Discuss with your holistic health practitioner the use of hydrochloric acid tablets with or without pepsin (a protein enzyme) because low stomach acid may be the cause. I recommend taking a minimal dose before one meal (if any worsening of symptoms occurs then do not consider this as a treatment). Slowly increase the frequency to before each meal and then increase the amount over a period of two weeks. Suddenly using a large quantity of hydrochloric acid can create discomfort or worse.*
- *Take high dose antioxidants as these protect against acid damage and increase membrane repair.*

Homeopathic
- *Homeopathic remedies need to be chosen on the symptoms and reference should be made to your preferred homeopathic manual, paying attention to the remedies Aragonite, Carbo vegetalis, Calcarea carbonica and Nux vomica initially.*

Herbal/natural extracts
- *Liquorice root, aloe vera and slippery elm are all soothing and can be used at the maximum dose recommended on any proprietary product.*
- *Avoid mint or peppermint, despite its effectiveness, because this will render homeopathic treatment useless.*

FLATULENCE

Flatulence is the passage of gas (flatus) from the intestine through the anus. Individuals of all ages should pass wind between 5 and 15 times a day. There is no right or wrong concerning the amount that is passed from a health prospective. In the West, passing wind is, arguably, not socially acceptable. Healthwise it is not a serious matter to withhold the passage of gas but this often leads to abdominal aches and pains. Eighty-five per cent of gas in the intestinal tract is swallowed and 15 per cent is produced by bacteria. The swallowing of air is most commonly associated with eating rapidly and talking whilst masticating (chewing). Most food has air as part of its cellular components or structure and chewing crushes this out. Poor chewing, therefore, allows air to pass into the stomach and thereafter the rest of the intestine.

Bad bacteria (those that are not commensal – meant to be with us) often produce more gas and are the cause of an excess in a few per cent of cases. Our natural bowel flora produce gas and the rate at which they do so will be dependent on the contents of the colon. Higher sugar levels will increase the bacteria's metabolic rate, thereby increasing their gaseous biproduct. Bacterial gas accounts for the characteristically unpleasant smell which will vary depending on the food eaten and its enhancement of bacterial activity. Flatulence is not a medical problem unless it is associated with bowel pain, is sociably unacceptable, too frequent or bad smelling.

RECOMMENDATIONS

General Advice

- Eat food more slowly, chewing well and avoiding talking whilst masticating and swallowing.
- Avoid overeating or eating late at night.

Nutritional

- Review the diet in association with the amount or odour of the flatus and see if specific foods can be isolated as a cause of any problem. Cut down on refined sugars and excessively sweet foods.
- Review the amount of fibrous foods and ensure that the diet is not too heavily weighted in foods that are hard to digest, such as raw vegetables.

Supplemental

- Yoghurt bacteria tablets such as Lactobaccillus acidophilus or Probifidus can alter the bowel flora in the colon and have a mild effect on unpleasant flatus.

- Consider the use of hydrochloric acid tablets with a pancreatic enzyme supplement since poor digestion may allow undigested foods to reach the bacteria in the colon which then feast. If things improve with this treatment consider visiting a complementary medical practitioner for a discussion on why the digestive process is lacking.

FOOD POISONING

Food poisoning is a broad definition little used by the medical profession. It is most commonly created by the ingestion of a bacteria from the *Salmonella* group but may also be created by other bacteria, viruses, yeast and fungi. Symptoms may vary from mild nausea through to severe vomiting, diarrhoea and abdominal pain. The severity is often associated with the amount and type of toxins that the bacteria produce whilst in the bowel. Local inflammation may be caused by the bacteria affecting the walls themselves, but any form of systemic condition, such as fever or rashes, is due to these enterotoxins. Fungi, in particular, including yeasts like *Candida*, may produce chemicals known as aflatoxins that have mild or severe toxic effects ranging from fevers to nervous collapse and paralysis. Chronic fatigue syndrome may often be associated with these infections.

RECOMMENDATIONS

General Advice

- Avoidance is the best treatment. Do not eat food that may have been unrefrigerated or prepared in unhygienic conditions. If you have any doubts, throw the food away.
- Food poisoning creates many symptoms and reference to the various symptoms in this book, such as fever, vomiting and diarrhoea should be reviewed.
- It is important to drink at least one pint of water per foot of height to help flush the bowel, keep toxins diluted and avoid dehydration.
- See **Gastroenteritis** below.

Supplemental

- Remember to replenish normal bowel bacteria by using high doses of Acidophilus or other yoghurt bacteria supplements during and after any food poisoning.

Homeopathic

- If the causative agent is known, then the homeopathic preparation at potency 30 (such as Salmonella 30, Escherichia coli 30) should be taken every 3hr.

GASTRIC ULCERS AND EROSIONS
– *see* **Peptic ulcers** *and* **Dyspepsia**

GASTRITIS – *see* **Dyspepsia**

GASTROENTERITIS

Gastroenteritis is inflammation of the inner lining of the stomach and the intestines, which can occur at any age for a variety of reasons. Symptoms may be mild or severe and range from abdominal aches and nausea to vomiting and diarrhoea, all may be with or without fever. These 'tummy upsets' can be very serious in children, the elderly or the infirm because associated fluid loss from vomiting and diarrhoea can lead to dehydration and biochemical changes. Gastroenteritis can be caused by:

- Viruses and bacteria that are ingested;
- Drugs (especially antibiotics which destroy the bowel's normal flora);
- Alcohol;
- Excessively spicy foods;
- Even a change of diet for those particularly sensitive;
- Stress, which causes an excess of acid production in the stomach can lead to inflammation through the entire intestinal tract.

RECOMMENDATIONS

General Advice

- Any persisting abdominal complaints or symptoms that are sudden or severe must be reviewed by a physician to rule out any other cause.
- Ensure adequate replenishment of water and fluids with natural sugars and salts. Proprietary electrolyte replacement fluids are fine but natural alternatives include thin broths and soups, dilute fruit juices and herbal teas.
- Ensure that the individual washes the hands after going to the bathroom because transmission of the causative organism in gastroenteritis is quite common.

Nutritional

- Avoid foods that are hard to digest, such as proteins, fats and fried foods. Milk, alcohol and caffeine should all be avoided.

Supplemental

- Yoghurt bacteria tablets (preferable to live yoghurt, which may not survive the acid and alkaline environment in the intestine) may be beneficial. Take 250,000 units of any Acidophilus or derivative per foot of height three times a day.

Homeopathic

- Homeopathic remedies are beneficial but need to be selected based on the symptoms. Please review the sections in this book on whichever other symptoms are prominent or refer to your preferred homeopathic manual.

Herbal/natural extracts

- A hot drink made of two teaspoonfuls of chamomile and one teaspoonful each of rosemary, sage and honey in one pint (500ml) of boiled hot water, a cup of which should be drunk every 15min to half an hour, is of benefit.
- Half a tablespoonful of fennel seeds with dried peppermint leaves and a pinch of sodium bicarbonate may be relieving but cannot be used if a homeopathic remedy is employed.
- Berberis fluid extract (1 teaspoonful in a cup of water) can be drunk four times per day.

Gastro-oesophageal reflux disorder (GORD)

GORD has been established as one of the most common medical conditions in Western society. Affecting around one in three people the condition is characterized by a burning or acid sensation in the upper abdomen or lower chest.

It is caused by inflammation occurring at the lower end of the oesophagus (food pipe) due to acid from the stomach refluxing up the tube. Orthodox treatment generally comprises antacid treatment to reduce the amount of acid that refluxes. However, a diet high in antioxidants or supplementation with vitamin extracts can be curative.

RECOMMENDATIONS

General Advice

• See **Dyspepsia** for further information and recommendations.

Supplemental

• A combined high dose antioxidant containing Vitamins A, C, E and CoQ10, and the minerals selenium and zinc should be considered.

Herbal/natural extracts

• Artemisia asiatica, the recommended dose on the product packaging, may be useful due to it containing a powerful antioxidant (DA-9601).

HAEMORRHOIDS OR PILES

A haemorrhoid, also known colloquially as a pile, is a vein or veins that become dilated, engorged, inflamed, painful and occasionally thrombosed or clotted. Symptoms range from mild itching to severe pain or bleeding. There is a thin line where the skin of the buttocks meets the membrane of the anus, known as the anorectal line. Haemorrhoids that originate below this line are called external haemorrhoids and those above the line are called internal haemorrhoids. Internal haemorrhoids may well extend down past the anorectal line.

HAEMORRHOIDS – Internal and External

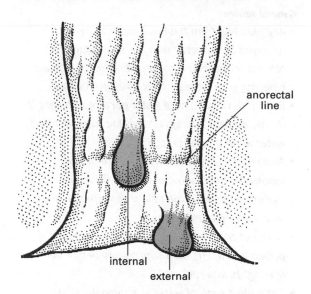

A breach or weakness in the anal muscular wall is the cause of a haemorrhoid. Weakness may occur through a lack of dietary fibre, deficiencies (particularly of vitamin C, bioflavonoids and proteins) that reduce the strength and amount of the connective tissues in the muscular walls, and through trauma from a penetration of the anus. Medical conditions that can cause haemorrhoids are a build up of pressure from straining, constipation and an obstructed bladder outlet. Pregnancy, obesity and an increase in pressure in the veins from obstruction in the abdomen or an enlarged liver blocking the main vein of the body, the vena cava, are also causes. Sitting on a cold surface can cause constriction of the muscle and straining after this may push a vein through the wall, or prolonged sitting or sitting on a warm surface may draw blood into the veins, which may then pass through weakened muscle walls. Treatment and avoiding recurrence requires consideration of all these factors.

A pile may bleed gently and appear only as a smear on the toilet paper, or may bleed more aggressively and may show as bright blood in the toilet. Provided that the bleeding stops, neither is a serious condition although a persistently heavy-bleeding pile may require surgical treatment.

RECOMMENDATIONS

General Advice

- Any bleeding from the back passage must be reviewed by a doctor, with the possibility of a referral for proctoscopy or colonoscopy because bleeding may represent colitis or even cancer.
- Ensure that one pint of water per foot of height is drunk, spaced throughout the day. Avoid drinking water around meal times.
- Avoid caffeine and alcohol until the problem has resolved. These substances dehydrate and therefore increase the risk of constipation and also weaken muscular walls.
- Core out an index finger-size portion of raw potato and insert as a suppository before bed five nights in a row.
- Sitting in a bath of water at around 40°C (or 103°F) may offer relief.
- Haemorrhoids are a varicose vein, see **Varicose veins** for further medicinal treatments.

Nutritional

- Ensure an increase in dietary fibre by eating more fresh fruit and vegetables, lightly cooked. At the time of the pile, one or two teaspoonfuls of psyllium husks twice a day, shaken vigorously with 8oz of water and drunk immediately, will help prevent constipation.

Homeopathic

- Homeopathic remedies may be of benefit. Aesculus 6 four times a day for itching, Hamamelis 6 for bleeding with a bruise sensation and Capsicum 6 if the sensation is of burning. Other remedies may be chosen depending on the variety and severity of symptoms.

Herbal/natural extracts

- Peppermint oil (1 drop in 10 drops of olive oil; dilute further if stinging occurs) can be applied with a clean finger.
- Witch-hazel or Hamamelis fluid extract (diluted one teaspoonful to three tablespoonfuls of boiled water) should be soaked into a flannel and the flannel wrapped around an ice cube and applied to the anus.
- A cream containing Arnica or Calendula (or both) should be applied before and after each stool and before bed (before inserting the potato strip).

Orthodox

- Surgical treatment may be required but before this takes place, see if you can find a practitioner who uses monopolar direct current therapy, which can be applied with local anaesthetic. Operative procedures may include banding, where an elastic band is place around the base of the engorged vein, or injecting with a sclerosing fluid (a chemical irritant that produces an inflammatory reaction with subsequent scarring) that causes the vein to collapse and stick together, thereby not allowing blood into the protruding area. If either technique is not convenient or suitable then a haemorrhoidectomy (removal of the vessel) and surgical sealing of the vein may need to be carried out (see **Operations and surgery**).

HEARTBURN – *see* Dyspepsia *and* Peptic ulcers

HELICOBACTER PYLORI

Helicobacter pylori is a bacterium that is found in the stomach and is capable of surviving the high acidity therein. It is thought to be acquired in childhood, probably from a parent, and is associated with gastritis, ulcers of the stomach and the duodenum and it may be of concern in both gastro-oesophageal reflux disease and dyspepsia. Curiously, over 50 per cent of people born before 1950 are thought to have this organism in their stomachs as opposed to 20 per cent born after that date. Developing countries have an infection rate of over 80 per cent.

It is worth noting that developing countries have a far lower level of gastric ulcerations than those in the West. I think this is a most important point since it would suggest that factors other than *H. pylori* are the underlying cause of problems. It is probable that *H. pylori* is a mere bystander and may, in fact, be doing a protective job by battling other bacteria. We may be worsening the situation by eradicating it. It is hard to get good statistical analysis because the pharmaceutical industry, which carry out most of the tests and studies, make so much money from the sale of drugs designed to eradicate this germ.

About 15 per cent of people infected with *H. pylori* will develop a peptic ulcer and 1 per cent will go on to develop cancer of the stomach. There is some indication of a correlation between *H. pylori* infection and cardiovascular disease, but this has yet to be corroborated.

Naturopathic treatments have yet to be put through scientific studies, but attempts to eradicate the organism naturally may be considered with your physician's consent. Since it is rarely an urgent matter, bearing in mind that the bacteria have probably been in the stomach for many years, waiting a few more weeks to see if a naturopathic approach might do the trick is unlikely to do any harm. That may not be the case if the infection has been discovered with a serious concern such as an active ulcer. However, since orthodox treatment is primarily by the use of antibiotics and antacids, avoiding this would be preferable when looking at general overall health.

RECOMMENDATIONS

General Advice

- *If you have a past history or family history of indigestion or worse, consider having a* H. pylori *breath test which is the main diagnostic investigation.*
- *Avoid foods that irritate the stomach lining, such as caffeine, alcohol and spicy foods. Strictly avoid smoking.*
- *Antacids are recommended in orthodox treatment and may enhance pain relief if indigestion is present. Whether it is necessary to eradicate* H. pylori *is uncertain.*

Nutritional

- *Theoretically reducing the body's acidity may help eradicate* H. pylori. *Consider a predominantly vegetarian/vegan diet or follow the Hay diet (food combining) as this may reduce stomach acidity.*

Supplemental

- *A good acidophilus compound may be beneficial. There is some evidence that acidophilus is active in the stomach and may compete with* H. pylori.
- *High-dose antioxidants are beneficial in membrane growth and may reduce the damaging effects of* H. pylori.

Homeopathic

- *The homeopathic preparation of H. pylori potency 30 can be taken four times a day in conjunction with other complementary therapies. Take it for 2 weeks as part of an eradication treatment.*

Herbal/natural extracts

- *Allicin, found in garlic, has been shown to inhibit* H. pylori.
- *Berberine from berberis may inhibit* H. pylori *if taken as a fluid extract, diluted x3, daily.*
- *Slippery elm or liquorice in powdered or liquid form can be taken prior to meals as a 'cover' for inflamed areas, thereby reducing the damaging effect of* H. pylori.

Orthodox

- *There is some debate between what is known as triple or double therapy and whether one or two week regimes are necessary. Triple therapy is a combination of two antibiotics with an antacid, usually, bismuth or a proton pump inhibitor. Double therapy is less effective but does cut down the amount of antibiotic used.*

HEPATITIS

Hepatitis is inflammation (itis) of the liver (hepar). There are a multitude of causes of hepatitis, the most common of which is viral. Hepatitis can be, however, caused by drugs, alcohol, bacteria, tumours, heart problems and food allergy or intolerance. Hepatitis may cause jaundice (yellowing of the skin) but does not necessarily need to do so.

Symptoms of hepatitis may be nothing more than a general ache in the upper right abdomen but may also include fevers, gastrointestinal symptoms such as vomiting and an inability to eat, fatigue and jaundice. With jaundice, dark urine and pale stools may be symptoms, along with a yellowing of the whites of the eyes.

Hepatitis A

This virus is caught by ingesting food that has been contaminated. This contamination usually comes from food containing faecal matter, often from the unhygienic unwashed hands of people preparing food. Transmission through water is possible if people have defecated in the source of the water in question. It takes two to six weeks to cause the physical symptoms – this is termed the incubation period.

Hepatitis A in a healthy being is an uncomfortable and unpleasant illness but rarely serious or fatal. It never becomes chronic, although it can leave the individual unable to tolerate alcohol or fats for up to one year.

Hepatitis B

Hepatitis B is transmitted through infected blood, saliva and sexual secretions such as vaginal or seminal (sperm) fluids. This is the type that is transmitted through sexual intercourse, particularly anal intercourse, intravenous drug abuse and transfusions. The incubation period is six weeks to six months; the infection is serious, causing death in around one per cent. In ten per cent of cases the infected person may not destroy the virus completely, which then settles into the cells of the liver and persists in causing no problems or only mild problems. This medical situation is called a chronic carrier state and leaves the individual potentially capable of infecting others and also with a 10 per cent risk of developing cirrhosis over the following 30–40 years.

Hepatitis C

This is similar in its transmission to hepatitis B, although up to 40 per cent of those infected can develop the chronic carrier state. This type of hepatitis is found more commonly in patients who have had blood transfusions. The incubation period is thought to be between two weeks and five months and some studies have suggested that acute hepatitis C may actually have a fatality rate of 10 per cent.

Hepatitis D, E and others

There are many more rare forms of viral hepatitis, probably mutated from the other three. Little is known about them and more is being discovered regularly. From the point of view of classification, Epstein-Barré virus, more commonly associated with glandular fever, is a cause of a hepatitis similar to hepatitis A. Cytomegalovirus is another uncommon but established cause.

Vaccinations for hepatitis

Hepatitis A is treated with a gamma globulin (an artificial chemical compound based on the body's natural immunoglobulin production that attacks hepatitis A) that is available against hepatitis A and is often called a vaccination even though it is not.

Hepatitis B has a vaccination that is encouraged by governments and health officials to be used by those at risk, such as hospital and careworkers. Vaccinations and treatments for other types of hepatitis causing viruses are not yet established.

Investigations

Anyone suspecting that they have hepatitis should be investigated by their GP and will be tested for raised liver-function tests (chemicals found in the bloodstream), a variety of tests for different parts of the hepatitis-causing viruses, such as the Australian antigen in hepatitis B, and urinalysis to establish what liver functions are not being performed. Those interested may choose to have a bioresonance or humoral blood test to help establish liver cell damage.

General Advice

- Any liver area pains that persist, or any suggestion of yellowing of the skin or sclera (the whites of the eyes), must be taken to a GP or other doctor for full evaluation. Remember that you may be transmitting and passing on a dangerous virus unwittingly.
- Once hepatitis has been established, consult your complementary medical practitioner because self-help is not generally enough.
- See **Vaccinations**.
- A period of fluid fast or following the basic Detox diet in chapter 7 should be considered if the appetite is poor or vomiting is preventing ingestion (see **Detox diet**).
- Avoid strenuous exercise, lack of sleep and undue stress. The liver breaks down adrenaline and the more you produce, the harder the liver has to work.
- Those with hepatitis A should not cook for others and should be particularly careful with their hygiene. Those with other forms of hepatitis should avoid unprotected intercourse until the incubation period is over and they are assured that they do not have a carrier status, which can only be assessed through blood tests.
- A relaxation or meditation technique must be practised daily.

Nutritional

- Avoid alcohol, caffeine, saturated fats (butter, lard and animal fats), additives, preservatives and overeating. Remember that the liver is the chemical factory of the body and everything you eat passes through it before reaching any other part of the body.

Supplemental

- The liver is required for the manufacture of several essential compounds and therefore the following should be taken in doses recommended by your specialists: vitamin B complex, vitamin C, coenzyme Q10 and all amino acids particularly methionine, choline and lipoic acid (100–200mg three times a day for most adults in this case). Specific treatments should include the use of milk thistle, Cheledonium (Celandine), the Ayurvedic herb Phyllanthus amarus and the widely available Ayurvedic formula called Liv 52.
- Intravenous vitamin supplementation can be of great benefit but needs to be administered by a doctor. The liver may not be processing correctly and direct introduction into the bloodstream of necessary nutrients can be very rewarding.

Homeopathic

- Constitutional homeopathic remedies with specific remedies against hepatitis are beneficial and an eminent naturopath recommends a particular homeopathic remedy that is specially made up: two drops of the patient's first morning sputum, two drops of the first morning urine and two drops of blood all added to 34 drops of water and succussed down to potency 6. Four drops are then given nightly.

HIATUS HERNIA

The definition of a hernia is an abnormal protrusion of a part of an organ through the containing wall. The hiatus (a space or opening) in this case

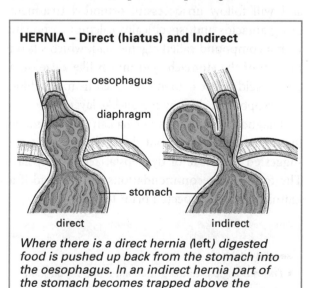

HERNIA – Direct (hiatus) and Indirect

oesophagus

diaphragm

stomach

direct   indirect

Where there is a direct hernia (left) digested food is pushed up back from the stomach into the oesophagus. In an indirect hernia part of the stomach becomes trapped above the diaphragm.

is in the diaphragm muscle where the oesophagus passes from the chest to the abdominal cavity. There are two types. In the first the diaphragm is simply weak and when the stomach contracts to push the digested food through into the duodenum, it refluxes back up into the oesophagus (*see* **Acid reflux**). The second situation is one where the upper part of the stomach becomes trapped above the oesophagus, either permanently or temporarily, the diaphragm tightens and the acid flows into the lower part of the oesophagus directly.

Treatment must vary depending on the individual situation. Toning of the diaphragm is vitally important and very often overlooked by the orthodox world. A diaphragm that is too tight because of hyperventilation and stress requires relaxation techniques, whereas a diaphragm with a weakened opening needs some tightening. Fortunately, yoga breathing techniques with specific relaxation teaching will cover both angles by toning the diaphragm. Excess acidity may also be a cause, as may obesity. The amount of fat visible on the outside of a body is often reflected within, and fat in the abdominal cavity will push upwards on the stomach, encouraging acid to flow the wrong way and the stomach to be forced through the diaphragm.

Persisting discomfort may require an endoscopy and will follow unsuccessful orthodox treatment using antacids and, specifically, calcium carbonate with a compound called algenic acid, which sits on the top of the stomach acid, much like algae on a pond. Acid reflux is then prevented from touching the oesophageal sides by the oil-like layer.

Diagnosis of a hiatus hernia can only be made through an endoscopy but the symptoms that are suggested are those of dyspepsia (*see* **Dyspepsia**). The following recommendations can be used if a hiatus hernia is suspected prior to endoscopy.

RECOMMENDATIONS

General Advice
• *Learn a yogic breathing technique and meditation exercise.*

• *Any suggestion of being overweight – try to lose it.*
• *Do not stoop, preferably learn to pick things up by bending at the knee. Raise the head of the bed by placing two bricks at the head end – this will allow gravity to pull the stomach and contents downwards.*
• *Avoid antacids as much as possible and certainly do not use anything containing aluminium. Algenic acid is a godsend in acute or night-time situations and can be used until other techniques bear fruit.*
• *Do not eat late at night or lie down within 2hr of eating. Siestas should be had in an upright position if this is your custom.*

Nutritional
• *Alcohol, smoking, caffeine and refined sugars all increase stomach acid production and will worsen a hiatus hernia. Specific food intolerance may be noted and food allergy testing through bioresonance or blood tests is recommended. Food allergies can weaken musculature and may be the underlying cause of the failure of the diaphragm to work as an effective valve.*

Herbal/natural extracts
• *Use slippery elm compounds or pure slippery elm (one teaspoonful mixed into a thin paste with water) before bed, after meals and if uncomfortable up to a maximum of six times per day.*

Orthodox
• *Operative procedures may be necessary in severe cases when the above recommendations and both naturopathic and orthodox drug treatments have failed. If so (see **Operations and surgery**).*

INDIGESTION – *see* Dyspepsia *and* Peptic ulcers

NAUSEA AND VOMITING
Nausea is the brain's way of telling us that we

have taken in something potentially toxic, as in food poisoning, or a warning that we are doing something that may be injurious. In the case of taking an exam, where our adrenaline levels may be too high, this is a fair but unnecessary warning. Motion or travel sickness is an unnecessary warning (*see* **Motion sickness**). Nausea is the most common early-warning symptom issued by the brain to advise us of an incorrect situation. Diseases of any part of many major organs, such as the kidney, liver, gut or even the heart, may be heralded by nausea. Persisting nausea may represent cancer. Obstruction by stricture, inflammation or tumour anywhere in the gastro-intestinal tract can lead to, and be a cause of, vomiting.

In principle any toxin in the system, whether it is created by, say, a failing kidney or liver, the ingestion of bacteria, such as in food poisoning, or excess alcohol, will cause nausea or potential vomiting.

The act of vomiting generally suggests that the body has reached a toxic state and is trying to rid itself of a poison. Vomiting is often associated with sweating, another eliminatory process, and may be accompanied by a need to urinate or defecate. If the toxin is in the stomach or the upper part of the intestine then the vomiting may be curative, but very often the poison lies in the bloodstream, has influenced the vomit centres in the brain and is therefore of no direct use. Vomiting without an obvious cause, or a persistence of vomiting, must be assessed by a GP.

Another of the most common causes of nausea is low blood sugar. Often associated with hunger, low blood sugar levels can trigger nausea. This is an odd paradox because nausea usually reduces appetite. I suspect that nausea is a more aggressive way for the brain to attract attention to the need for food when hunger pangs have failed. The feeling of an impending vomit is not necessarily a digestive problem. However, the emptying of the stomach contents is.

RECOMMENDATIONS

General Advice
- *Nausea or vomiting without any obvious cause that is sudden, copious or persistent must be reviewed by a GP to rule out a more serious underlying cause.*
- *Once the cause has been established, certain techniques listed below can be utilized but the principal treatment should be against the underlying cause.*
- *There is an acupressure point that may be very beneficial in nausea or vomiting. Place three fingers up the forearm starting at the wrist crease. The third finger will lie over a sensitive point, which should have pressure applied to it for approximately 1min.*
- *If the nausea is associated with not having eaten for several hours or following a particularly sweet meal (there is inevitably a reflex low blood sugar or hypoglycaemic state), eat a piece of fruit and see what happens.*
- *See* **Motion sickness** *if relevant.*
- *Persisting nausea despite the above recommendations should result in a consultation with a complementary medical practitioner.*

Nutritional
- *Correlate with the possibility of a food intolerance or allergy if the nausea is sporadic.*

Homeopathic
- *The homeopathic remedies Ipecacuanha, Nux vomica and Carbo vegetabilis may help. Try one of these remedies at potency 6 every 10min and if there is no response after three doses, try the next.*

Herbal/natural extracts
- *Half an inch of fresh root ginger chopped into a mug of boiling water may be drunk when the temperature is acceptable.*
- *A combination of chamomile tea (two teaspoonfuls) with a teaspoonful each of sage and rosemary per pint of boiling water can be very soothing if drunk every 15min.*

OBSTRUCTION OF THE BOWEL

An obstruction anywhere from the throat to the anus is not a matter of self-help unless it is caused by an easily reachable foreign object. Specific conditions should be referred to in this book and include cancer, toxic colon, volvulus (a twist in the gut) and hernia. Intussusception and foreign objects are the most common causes in infants and children.

The symptoms are pain and bloating, usually associated shortly after with vomiting and, of course, an absence of bowel motions. An inability to pass wind in association with these symptoms must immediately arouse suspicion.

RECOMMENDATIONS

General Advice

- *Any suggestion of a bowel obstruction must be examined by a GP.*
- *Please refer to the relevant section in this book to deal with the cause of obstruction.*
- *Do not eat or drink anything until a diagnosis has been established.*

Homeopathic

- *The homeopathic remedies Carbo vegetabilis or Cinchona can be considered at potency 6 every 10min until a doctor is seen, and thereafter a suitable remedy should be chosen by a trained homeopath.*

Orthodox

- *Do not try any form of laxative because this will make things worse.*

OESOPHAGEAL PROBLEMS

Oesophageal achalasia

This is a condition whereby the nerves controlling the rhythmic peristalsis that allows food to travel down the oesophagus are absent or diminished. This causes food to stick in the oesophagus which leads to pain.

The orthodox world has no specific cause for this isolated symptom, although it can be associated with serious neurological problems such as multiple sclerosis or motorneurone disease. Vitamin E deficiency may be related.

The Eastern philosophies consider this to be a severe loss of energy in the throat chakra, usually caused by a block in the lower energy centres. Severe emotional stress is often associated, although it may be deeply buried and require hypnotherapy to illuminate.

In itself the condition is unpleasant, leading to pain and halitosis (bad breath), but if not treated the individual will lose their appetite and malnutrition will ensue. Orthodox treatment includes investigation with barium swallows and endoscopy, often associated with special dilating techniques, cutting of the oesophageal muscles at the lower end of the oesophagus or even removing part of the tube. Before this, antispasmodic drugs will be recommended and should only be used after the alternative recommendations have failed.

RECOMMENDATIONS

General Advice

- *A sudden or persistent inability to swallow or oesophageal pain should be reviewed by a throat or gastric specialist.*
- *Consider underlying stresses, especially anger, and if none are apparent consider hypnotherapy to illustrate the cause and to help relax the spasm in the muscles.*

Nutritional

- *Persistent ingestion of food allergens (foods that the body does not like) may cause a mind–body reaction leading to the oesophagus refusing entry into the system. Food allergy testing by bioresonance or blood testing might well be appropriate.*

Oesophageal pain

Pain in the oesophagus can occur simply from swallowing a solid bolus of food such as a boiled sweet, the oesophageal muscle then cramps but this pain passes swiftly. If a tear or cut occurs, the pain may be persistent. Unlike tears in other parts of the body, the pain is often described as a cramp rather than a sting. This can be very severe and may even mimic more serious problems, such as a heart attack.

A persisting pain with no obvious reason needs to be investigated because conditions such as cancer may give rise to this discomfort. Oesophageal spasm can occur through anxiety or persisting oesophageal reflux (*see below*).

Oesophageal reflux

The refluxing of stomach acid into the lower part of the oesophagus may occur from overeating but most frequently is associated with a hiatus hernia. For treatment of this condition (*see* **Hiatus hernia** *and* **Acid reflux**).

Oesophageal stricture

Stricture of the oesophagus presents as pain or an inability to swallow. A build up of mucus or vomiting immediately after swallowing food or drink may be an early sign. Strictures may be acute, caused by a spasm of the oesophagus that is, in turn, often caused by swallowing something too hard, which causes a small nick in the oesophageal membrane. More serious conditions of stricture occur as a result of cancer or long-term reflex oesophagitis, secondary to a hiatus hernia.

THE PANCREAS

The pancreas is found as an axe-shaped organ behind the upper part of the abdomen behind the small intestine and the stomach.

It has two principal functions, both glandular.

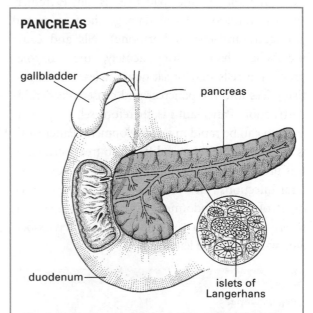

PANCREAS

gallbladder

pancreas

duodenum

islets of Langerhans

The islets of Langerhans produce insulin which controls sugar levels in the blood. The pancreas also makes enzymes to aid the digestive process.

As an endocrine gland (passing a hormone into the bloodstream), the pancreas produces insulin from special cells known as the islets of Langerhans. Insulin controls the sugar levels in the bloodstream. The exocrine (production of chemicals *not* into the bloodstream) function is to produce digestive enzymes that pass into the small intestine. These juices pass down the pancreatic ducts and join the common bile duct before entering into the duodenum.

The pancreas sits in that part of the body often referred to as the solar plexus. It lies under main acupuncture points along the vessel of conception and is tied into a theoretical axis running from the pituitary through the thyroid itself and down to the uterus and prostate. This axis is sensitive and a problem with any one organ may lead to a problem with another. Pregnancy is a prime example of triggering both thyroid and pancreatic deficiencies for no orthodox reason. These problems must therefore be viewed from a deep energetic angle as well as the practical, scientific one.

Pancreatitis

Inflammation of the pancreas is an extremely serious condition. It can damage the insulin and glucagon (anti-insulin hormone) cells and cause metabolic chaos. More acutely, the enzyme-producing cells may break down, release the digestive juices into the pancreas and cause considerable destruction. Pancreatitis is, therefore, self-perpetuating and can be rapid in its development. Pancreatitis is extremely painful and difficult to treat because of this process. Usually triggered by alcoholic excess or viral infections, the symptoms may be the gradual onset of upper abdominal discomfort or a sudden severe pain. Nausea and vomiting are often associated with profound lethargy.

RECOMMENDATIONS

General Advice
- *Pancreatitis must be diagnosed and treated by doctors. A specific blood test for a compound*

known as amalyse is diagnostic, along with the symptoms of pancreatitis.
- *Follow the advice given by the hospital and specialists accurately.*
- *The pancreas is associated with the vessel of conception and therefore any energetic form of treatment is liable to be beneficial. Consider acupuncture initially.*
- *Yoga and polarity therapy will affect the central energy store or chakras and benefit the condition.*

Homeopathic
- *Consult with a complementary medical practitioner with experience in this area for homeopathic treatment. Only the most experienced of naturopaths should be allowed to treat pancreatitis with medication.*

Pancreatic cancer

This is a most serious cancer because it produces the complications of malignant disease but also pancreatitis at some stage. Cancer of the head of the pancreas can obstruct the flow of bile from the liver and gallbladder, and therefore one of the initial symptoms may be jaundice.

RECOMMENDATIONS

General Advice
- *See **Cancer**.*
- *See **Pancreatitis** above.*

PROLAPSED ANUS

This is the extrusion of the lower part of the intestinal tract through the sphincter of the anus. This condition is generally created by a weakness of the anus through trauma or marked intra-abdominal pressure. Severe infections such as cholera, which may create marked weakness within muscles and frequent diarrhoea, may cause a prolapse. Pressure from a tumour or strain from chronic constipation may cause an anal or even rectal prolapse.

PEPTIC ULCERS

The word 'peptic' is derived from the Greek term meaning 'pertaining to or promoting digestion'. It is the medical term for ulceration that occurs in the mucous membranes of both the gastrum (stomach) and duodenum.

Treatment of peptic ulcers therefore also covers gastric ulcers, duodenal ulcers and the precursors to this condition: gastritis and duodenitis. Some inflammations and ulcers in this area are 'silent' – have no symptoms – but these are rare and because they are not spotted early are usually serious. Most ulcerative and pre-ulcerative conditions in this area present as a burning sensation in the upper abdomen radiating, occasionally, through to the back. The pain may also radiate into the chest and give rise to symptoms similar to heart pains. (The reverse is true and symptoms suggestive of bowel disease are often found to be emanating from the heart.) Silent ulcers are generally due to the inflammation or erosion not affecting the nerve endings. These ulcers may eat into blood vessels causing bleeding, which if profuse may cause vomiting of blood (haemetemesis) or if not so profuse a black tarry stool called melena, created by the digestion of red blood cells.

The stomach is lined by cells that produce a thick mucus, which protects the stomach lining from the very aggressive hydrochloric acid produced to break down our food. A failure to produce this mucus or an overproduction of acid will lead to inflammation and potential ulcer formation. The duodenum is bathed in a strong alkaline solution, which neutralizes the small amounts of acid that are released through the pyloric sphincter, but the small intestine also has a protective mucus layer against the strong alkaline that it comes into contact with from the pancreatic juices. Excess acidity passing into the duodenum will override these defensive measures and, again, cause inflammation and the predisposition to ulcer.

Excessive hydrochloric acid is often produced in response to food allergy/intolerance, alcohol, caffeine, tobacco and excess adrenaline created by stress. Damage to the protective mucosa and thereby a reduction in the protective mucus can occur through any of the above, plus excessive eating or the embibement of hot and spicy food. Aspirin, non-steroidal anti-inflammatory drugs, steroids and other less commonly utilized drugs can all predispose to pre-ulcer conditions.

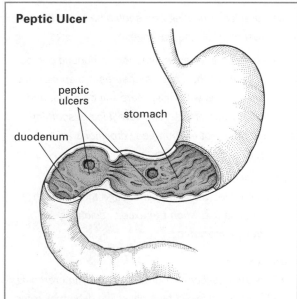

Peptic Ulcer

peptic ulcers

stomach

duodenum

Peptic ulcers may occur either in the stomach or the duodenum.

Helicobacter pylori

Recently, a specific bacterium called *Helicobacter pylori* has been associated with a higher chance of ulcerative and pre-ulcerative conditions. Indeed, most individuals with ulcers will have *H. pylori* in attendance, but by no means all. Conversely, many people carry *H. pylori* and have no problems with ulcerative conditions. A holistic practitioner should therefore continue to ignore the persistence of the orthodox world which supports the 'germ' theory and instead understand that *H. pylori* may exacerbate a situation but is probably not the cause. Treating *H. pylori* is effective but recurrence usually occurs if the underlying weakness or dietetic problem is not dealt with. This is, of course, a good thing for the pharmaceutical industry, who encourage the frequent and costly use of two antibiotics with a powerful antacid.

RECOMMENDATIONS

General Advice
- *Persistent burning or discomfort in the upper abdomen, chest or surrounding area should be considered a pre-ulcerative condition and treated accordingly.*
- *Keep the same diary as the nutritional one below for times of stress.*

Nutritional
- *Keep a diary of foods in association with the discomfort and isolate and eliminate any causative substances.*
- *Specifically avoid hot, spicy, fried and refined foods. Avoid alcohol, caffeine and refined sugars until the condition settles and then keep a close eye on which of these brings the symptoms back.*
- *Foods that are hard to digest, such as raw vegetables, abrasive foods such as nuts and non-soaked wholegrains, wholemeal bread and oats should be avoided until the condition settles, despite their nutritional value.*
- *Aim at more easily digestible foods such as*

soups, diluted fruit juices, soaked grains, fish and chicken. Cook your vegetables for slightly longer than one would normally encourage.*
- *Avoid milk. It may give a temporary relief due to its alkaline properties but this causes a rebound acid production and the casein in the milk is hard to digest, encouraging more acid production.*
- *If the above measures are not effective, then consider some basic treatments as follows:*

(a) *Make fresh cabbage juice and drink one glass before meals for two weeks. It contains vitamin P which is shown to help the healing of ulcers. Do not use this technique if you suffer from a hyperthyroid condition.*

(b) *Take the following supplements, which are known to help membranes heal, in the following amounts per foot of height in divided doses with meals: beta-carotene (2mg) or vitamin A (5000iu), vitamin E (100iu) and buffered vitamin C (1000mg); also take zinc (5mg per foot of height) before bed.*

(c) *Slippery elm or compounds containing this should be taken as prescribed on the package (it very much depends on the percentage of the compound).*

(d) *Liquorice is healing and should be taken as prescribed on the package.*

(e) *A half-tablet of an indigestion compound can be used whilst the above measures are employed, although, as with milk, there will be a rebound hyper-acidic effect. Aloe vera juice is soothing and does not encourage hydrochloric acid production in the same way.*

(f) *Meditation and the associated breathing techniques that gently massage the stomach are essential when the excess acidity is stress-associated.*

Orthodox
- *Persisting discomfort or any difficulty in breathing should be reviewed by a physician, who may refer the individual to a surgeon for a gastroscope or*

barium studies. These should be considered only in acute situations or in persistent cases where the above measures have not helped, because the treatment will inevitably be drug-induced antacid treatment with medications such as ranitidine, cimetidine or omeprazole. If H. pylori is found then triple therapy – two antibiotics and bismuth – will be employed which may be curative but very often is not for the reasons described above.

PILES – *see* **Haemorrhoids**

THE UROGENITAL SYSTEM

BARTHOLIN'S CYSTS

Bartholin's glands are found on both sides of the lateral vaginal walls. They generally secrete part of the vagina's protective lubricant. Occasionally the gland can become inflamed and/or the duct that carries the secretions out can become blocked.

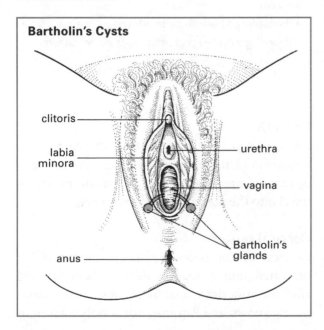

Bartholin's Cysts

clitoris

labia minora

urethra

vagina

Bartholin's glands

anus

Bartholin's cysts present as painful (though not always) swellings or pea-like lesions on either side of the vaginal opening. These are often noticed on intercourse.

RECOMMENDATIONS

General Advice
- *Any swelling in the genital area that does not respond to basic treatment after 48hr should be viewed by a GP or gynaecologist.*
- *Apply hot and cold compresses to the area.*
- *Intercourse should be avoided.*
- *Avoid pressure on the area. Squeezing will not release the blockage.*
- *If the problem persists the orthodox world would encourage the use of antibiotics, but before you use these, consult a complementary medical practitioner for herbal or homeopathic alternatives.*

Homeopathic
- *The homeopathic remedy Hepar sulphuris calcarium 30, four pills every 2hr can be utilized.*

Orthodox
- *An operative procedure is rarely required but if it is then pre- and post-operative precautions should be taken (see* **Operations and surgery***).*

BLADDER PROLAPSE

Bladder prolapse appears as a bulge of the front aspect of the vagina, usually with marked protrusion of the urethra. It is associated with increased frequency of urination, incontinence, and, frequently, cystitis symptoms. It is generally caused by a weakening of the ligaments that hold the bladder in place and these are generally compromised by pregnancy or pelvic tumours.

RECOMMENDATIONS

General Advice
- *Pelvic floor exercises from yoga, Qi Gong or basic physiotherapy may help a mild prolapse.*

- *Avoid allowing the bladder to overfill with urine by urinating frequently.*

Orthodox

- *Vaginal pessaries are rarely beneficial and operative procedures are frequently required (see* **Operations and surgery***).*

CANDIDA AND THRUSH – *see* Candidiasis

Thrush is an irritating, itching condition of the vagina. There may be an accompanying cheesy, white or pale-yellow creamy discharge that clings tenaciously to the vaginal walls. There may also be an associated slight fishy smell but generally this is not caused by the thrush but by other organisms. The irritation may be bad enough to cause scratching, which leads to bleeding, and also the *Candida* itself can cause superficial cuts that bleed.

Some women will notice some or all of the symptoms mildly leading up to their periods. The vaginal flora is sensitive to the changes in oestrogen and progesterone levels.

As discussed more fully in the section on candidiasis, thrush is encouraged by a decrease in the normal vaginal flora. Antibiotics, poor diet, excess white sugar and poor hygiene all encourage this condition.

RECOMMENDATIONS

General Advice

- *Visit your GP, family planning nurse, midwife or gynaecologist to establish a firm diagnosis.*
- *Wear loose clothing around the groin.*
- *Avoid deodorants or medicated soaps in that area or generally if bathing.*
- *Unless all else fails, avoid strict dietetic advice because this is troublesome and not generally effective.*
- *Adding one cupful of sea salt to bath-water may prove soothing.*
- *See* **Vaginal douching** *and* **Candidiasis**.

Nutritional

- *Avoid refined sugars throughout the time of irritation.*

Homeopathic

- *Obtain a homeopathic remedy after consultation with a homeopath and/or a herbal treatment from a herbalist. Self-prescribing is somewhat hit and miss, although you can review the homeopathic remedies Sepia, Arsenicum album, Lilium tigrinum, Calcarea carbonica and Silica.*

Herbal/natural extracts

- *Tea tree pessaries with or without lavender can be used nightly for seven nights.*
- *If available, Calendula and/or Hydrastis pessaries can be used for three nights in succession and then, one week later, for three nights again.*
- *Obtain a douche bag or 50ml syringe. Mix one tablespoonful of cider vinegar in a mug of water and douche each evening before retiring. One tablespoonful of live yoghurt culture mixed thoroughly in one mug of water should be used as a douche each morning. If no improvement is forthcoming after one week, please see your healthcare practitioner.*

Orthodox

- *If antibiotics have to be used, ensure vaginal douching with live yoghurt culture as described above.*

CERVIX

The cervix is the name given to the part of the uterus found at the top of the vagina and in which there is an opening (the os) up which the sperm travel into the uterus in search of an egg.

Cervical cancer

Cervical cancer is an aggressive tumour if left untreated and a regular Papanicolaou (named after an American anatomist) test, more commonly known as a Pap smear or simply a smear, is

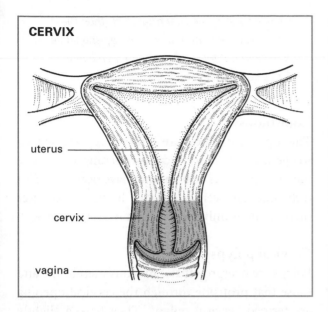

CERVIX

uterus

cervix

vagina

through intercourse, making this cancer a potentially transmittable one. Like any internal cancer it is often 'silent', giving no symptoms. But unlike other cancers, a regular check-up can find precancerous cells or early cancer well in advance of there being any major risk. A specific gene may have recently been found which predisposes a woman to cervical cancer. Over the next few years this gene may be tested for as a routine, highlighting those women at risk. Cervical cancer is more common in the sexually active for this reason.

essential. In the UK the National Health Service encourages a Pap smear every three to five years. This is a bureaucratic decision that has no medical standing. A cancer can develop overnight, and waiting three years for a diagnosis is liable to be a fatal decision. I recommend that a woman has a smear every year after she has lost her virginity and every six months if she changes her sexual partner during that time.

The medical world divides changes in the cells of the cervix into precancerous and cancerous cells. Precancerous cells are further divided up into dyskaryotic cells – cells that look, under the microscope, unusual but not cancerous – and cervical interstitial neoplasia (CIN) I, II and III cells with premalignant changes. The numbers I, II and III represent the depth to which the precancerous changes are occurring in the walls of the os from where the smear is taken.

If any unusual cells are found then a further investigation, called a colposcopy, is performed. This is a specialized scope that can travel into the opening of the cervix (the os) and takes biopsies to establish the severity of the changes.

There is an association between two types of human papilloma virus (HPV) and cervical cancer. These viruses are commonly transmitted

Cervical incompetence

The cervix is the lower part of the uterus found at the top of the vagina. In the centre of the cervix lies an opening called the os, which allows access for the sperm to the eggs travelling down the Fallopian tube into the womb. The os is generally closed, except at childbirth and under hormonal and nervous controls during intercourse.

Cervical incompetence can occur for traumatic reasons and represents the condition of a persistently open and loose cervical os. This is in no way a problem until childbearing is required, when a patent (open) os may allow the product of conception to fall out of the uterus.

General Advice

- *If you are advised that your cervix is incompetent then a gynaecological opinion must be sought. There is no complementary or orthodox treatment other than surgical treatment, where a Shirodkar stitch is placed around the opening and tightened.*

Orthodox

- *As with any operation (see **Operations and surgery**).*

Cervical interstitial neoplasia (CIN)

Cervical interstitial neoplasia is a term that describes a precancerous change in the cervix. Cervical smears should isolate these changes, which are more likely to become cancerous than dysplasia and should be treated accordingly.

Cervical interstitial neoplasia is divided into groups I, II and III. They do not represent the severity of the changes but merely the depth to which the pre-cancerous cells are buried in the walls of the os (the opening to the uterus).

General Advice

- *A pre-cancerous change should be dealt with by a complementary medical practitioner with experience in this area.*
- *To avoid this situation in the first place and certainly if a condition of CIN has been described, condoms or a cap should be used when having intercourse.*
- *See **Vaginal douching** and replace the cider vinegar with a teaspoonful of Arnica and Calendula fluid extracts.*

Nutritional

- *High-dose antioxidants and a health diet must be discussed with your practitioner.*

Orthodox

- *Unless there is a reduction in the CIN number, ie from CIN III to CIN II, within two months of*

complementary medical treatment, then the orthodox treatment of laser therapy should be considered. If there is a change then continue with treatment and test again.

Cone biopsy

This operative procedure removes a cone-shaped wedge around the cervical os opening to remove the pre-cancerous changes that have occurred. This technique has been superseded by the use of laser therapy and is only used in certain circumstances.

Cervical polyps

Polyps are overgrowths of mucous membrane and those that protrude through the cervical opening are termed cervical polyps. They have a slightly increased chance of becoming cancerous, more so than any other part of the mucous membrane and they may bleed which can cause concern.

Cervical polyps are generally discovered on a routine examination because they are usually symptomless. Gynaecologists and GPs will have a tendency to suggest their surgical removal and this should only be considered if complementary medical techniques fail to resolve the problem. Any polyp is considered to be an excess of damp in the body and correct dietetics and homeopathic and herbal treatments are often effective.

General Advice

- *Obtain a gynaecological opinion but avoid surgery except as a last resort.*
- *Consult with a complementary medical practitioner with experience in this area.*

Nutritional

- *Discuss with your preferred practitioner a low refined sugar diet and ensure that you are not dehydrated. Consider the homeopathic remedy Thuja 30, one dose three times a day for two weeks, or preferably seek advice from a homeopathic prescriber.*
- *Consider following the Hay diet (see chapter 7).*

Herbal/natural extracts

- *Ayurvedic, Tibetan and Chinese medicine may be successful in removing the excess damp that creates polyps.*

Orthodox

- *If the above recommendations do not solve the problem then surgical intervention should be considered because a polyp may represent a higher risk of uterine cancer.*

Cervical smears (Papanicolaou, Pap smear)

A cervical smear is a simple although invasive procedure. The cervix is one of the more common areas for cancerous changes to take place and examination of this part of the uterus is a recommended process.

Bureaucracy has governed that a cervical smear should be performed every 3–5 years, depending on which part of the country the woman lives and the habits of the general practice. I believe this to be too long a gap. A cancer may develop overnight and waiting three years will certainly allow a spread of this disease. Sexually active women should have a cervical smear every year and virgins or non-sexually active women should have this investigation performed every 18 months. After menopause, a two-yearly gap is acceptable. I recommend a cervical smear within three or four months of changing a sexual partner. Women with more than one sexual partner should have a cervical smear every six months.

Dysplasia

Dysplasia is the medical term for abnormal cells. It is not a precancerous condition, although it may require more frequent examinations to ensure that precancerous changes do not occur (*see* **Cervical cancer**).

GENITAL HERPES – *see* Herpes

INTERCOURSE (PAINFUL) – *see* Dyspareunia

INTRAUTERINE DEVICE (IUD)

This contraption is more commonly known as the coil. These multishaped devices are inserted by a doctor or gynaecologist into the cavity of the uterus. They set up a mild inflammatory response simply by irritating the inner lining of the uterus, which creates an environment in which a fertilized egg is not likely to implant. The fertilized egg will therefore pass out through the cervix or be expelled at the next period, although nature may override this inflammation and pregnancy can take place.

It is important to note that if fertilization of an

IUDs

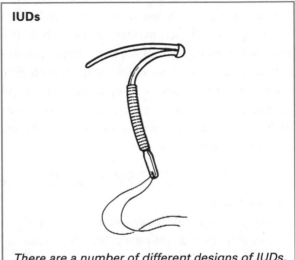

There are a number of different designs of IUDs, in this case a copper '7'. They seem to inhibit the implantation of a fertilized egg in the uterus.

IUD in position

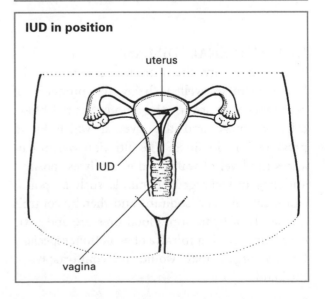

egg does take place and if religious doctrine or personal beliefs do not allow the intentional cessation of life, then this form of contraception should not be considered.

There are other reasons why a coil or IUD should be used as a last resort. Infection may enter with the insertion of a coil or settle around this foreign object. Should the infection travel down the Fallopian tubes, it may block them and create sterility. Very often insertion is not recommended until the woman has had as many children as she wishes.

A common concern of alternative practitioners, although dismissed out of hand by the orthodox medical world, is the use of copper in coils. This encourages the inflammatory response but may allow some absorption of copper. Copper poisoning can lead to muscular and neurological conditions even as severe as epilepsy. There is no scientific evidence to suggest that a coil may create such toxic levels but minor effects may be created that we are unaware of.

RECOMMENDATIONS

General Advice

- *The coil should only be considered as a form of contraception once the woman has had as many children as she wishes.*
- *Insist on a non-copper coil.*
- *Ensure that the coil is changed every two years.*

KIDNEY (RENAL) DISEASE

The kidneys are the filtration system for the bloodstream as well as being the producer of hormones that govern the amount of red blood cells we make and the level at which blood pressure is maintained. The filtration system balances the level of water and electrolytes (positive and negative charged chemicals such as potassium, calcium and sodium) and thereby controls our levels of hydration, blood pressure and toxic excretion. This is a miracle of evolution, especially for an organ that would fit comfortably in the hand.

KIDNEYS – Position in relation to other organs

The kidneys act as a filtration system, removing toxins from the bloodstream together with excess water. They also maintain the balance of acidity and alkalinity of the blood and control levels of salts and minerals.

For some reason, the translation from Eastern to Western understanding has labelled the body's energy store as the 'kidney' energy or meridian. The organic function of the kidneys and the Eastern philosophy of kidney energy are not compatible but nevertheless the term kidney energy is often used by those who follow the principles of energy flow. When a practitioner of complementary medicine says that your kidney energy is weak or in excess, this does not represent, necessarily, there is a disease process within the organs themselves. Interestingly, however, disease of any organ is likely to leave the individual tired but an incapacity of the kidneys seems to result in a much greater weakness within the system as a whole than most other organ problems.

Glomerulonephritis

Glomerulonephritis is an inflammatory disease of the kidney affecting the glomeruli – part of the filtering system. Symptoms may vary from severe pain, blood in the urine, water retention and headaches in an acute inflammation, to no symptoms at all as the process slowly but surely damages the kidneys.

RECOMMENDATIONS

General Advice

- A tell-tale sign is froth in the toilet bowl that persists for more than 60sec (caused by protein in the urine) or blood. Straight to the doctor please.
- Persisting water retention or oedema or the discovery of high blood pressure will lead to your doctor checking your urine because protein and blood may be present but not obviously visible.
- This condition may lead to permanent kidney damage and should not be treated without expert advice. After initial treatment or advice from an orthodox kidney specialist, discuss the matter with a complementary medical practitioner with experience in the area.
- Consider consulting a homeopath, nutritionist or herbalist before taking orthodox treatment which will include antibiotic or even steroid use. Complementary naturopathic treatment should run alongside these drugs and, in the hands of a medically qualified complementary specialist, may even help avoid the use of orthodox drugs.
- See an acupuncturist.

Supplemental

- There is overwhelming evidence that vitamin E is effective at levels of around 100–200iu per foot of height in this condition.
- The Omega 3 fatty acids EPA and DHA at levels of 30mg per foot of height and 25mg per foot of height (respectively) have been shown to be of benefit in a wide range of immune disorders and specifically IgA nephropathy.

Herbal/natural extracts

- See a Chinese herbalist, preferably a doctor.

Orthodox

- Your nephrologist will consider specific blood pressure medications such as ACE inhibitors and beta-blockers as a therapy, regardless of blood pressure levels. This should be accepted, especially if there is any suggestion of high blood pressure. (See **Hypertension**).

Infection of the kidneys – *see* Pyelonephritis

Inflammation of the kidneys
– *see* Glomerulonephritis

Kidney stones (renal calculi) and renal colic

Sudden and severe, often described as excruciating, pain that strikes anywhere from the small of the back around the sides and down into the groin or vagina/penis/testes may be renal colic and is most likely to be caused by the passage of a stone. These are usually composed of calcium, oxalic or uric acids and phosphates. These compounds normally remain in solution but a change in the acid/alkaline status of the urine or the presence of a foreign body may cause these to precipitate out and start a stone or 'calculus' formation. If the stone is small it will travel out of the kidney, down the uretha, through the bladder and out, but if it lodges in one of the fine tubules in the kidney it will slowly grow in size.

A calculus forming within the kidney may grow to a very large size before it will cause any problems and even these may not be noticed because the pressure, whilst destroying that kidney will have no effect on the other one which will deal with the filtration of the body quite happily without its partner. If, however, a stone moves, then nature has, for some reason, made the urethra a most sensitive passage. Liken the pain to dragging a small rock across an eyeball.

This severe pain will be associated with nausea, if not vomiting, generalized weakness and the characteristic fevers and rigors of kidney problems. It is estimated that six per cent of the Western population will develop kidney stones. This is much higher than in other parts of the world. The inevitable conclusion is an association with some part of the

Western lifestyle, although orthodox renal specialists will not hear of there being any association with diet. This is because a couple of trials have removed the major foods containing calcium and uric acid and found no appreciable difference. Of course they will not if other factors such as dehydration, deficiencies and heavy metal poisoning are not also taken into account. Studies have shown that vegetarians have a decreased risk of developing stones, as also have those with reduced sugar intake (insulin is very relevant to calcium levels through indirect metabolic pathways) and the presence of low levels of citric acid (from oranges, grapefruits, lemons and limes). An excess intake of milk and alkali foods including antacids, can cause stones. This condition is known as the milk–alkali syndrome. An excess of vitamin D (not uncommon in countries such as the USA, which fortify their milk with vitamin D) are also at risk because this increases the absorption of calcium thereby causing an increase in urinary calcium.

Several serious medical conditions can cause an excess secretion of calcium, oxalate and uric acid and all these need to be reviewed if a stone is passed.

RECOMMENDATIONS

FOR AN ACUTE ATTACK

General Advice

- *If a sudden excruciating pain should occur and a stone is suspected, ensure that all urination is done through a sieve to catch the calculus.*
- *A castor oil pack on the front, side and back of the side that is hurting may be beneficial. It is worth remembering that a pain anywhere from the kidney to the tip of the urethra may be reflected from the stone being anywhere along that passage. The brain is not good at isolating the exact point of urogenital pain.*

Supplemental

- *Beta-carotene and vitamin C should be taken as follows to help the healing of the damaged kidney*

and urethra: beta-carotene (2mg) and vitamin C (500mg), both per foot of height in divided doses with food throughout the day.

Homeopathic

- *The homeopathic remedies Aconite and Hypericum, both at potency 6, should be alternated every 10min until the stone has passed or adequate pain relief has been given, usually through an injection of pethidine.*

Herbal/natural extracts

- *Lobelia tincture (three drops in warm water) every hour may make a considerable difference. A tea made from the leaf of Uva ursi (available from herbal shops) can be drunk to relieve the pain and it also acts as a mild diuretic. Ensure that plenty of water is taken.*
- *A stone may lodge in the urethra due to spasm. A herb known as Kella was used 4,000 years ago by the Egyptians in the treatment of kidney stones. Dosage depends on the purity and it is best prescribed by a herbalist. More easily available are Aloe vera products, which may actually reduce the size of a stone if taken at a level high enough not to cause diarrhoea.*

Orthodox

- *Visit your GP, preferably with the passed stone. If the stone has not yet left the body, admission into hospital will be preferable for adequate pain relief. Full metabolic investigations must be undertaken and renal X-rays should be undergone, including those using special X-ray opaque dyes to ensure that the passing stone was not part of a larger calculus.*
- *If the presence of Kella, Aloe vera and high water intake do not remove a lodged stone, the orthodox world will suggest the use of a ureter basket to remove it. This is a specialized instrument that is passed into the bladder via the urethra and up the ureter. At the level of the*

stone a small nylon net is ejected from the end, passes around the stone and, when tightened and withdrawn, will bring the calculus with it. This method has now been surpassed by the use of ultrasound, which shatters the stone, but this is not available in all hospitals.

RECOMMENDATIONS

FOR PREVENTION OF STONE FORMATION

General Advice

- *There is an increased chance of a stone or calculus reforming unless the following lifestyle changes are considered.*
- *Ensure that someone analyses the type of stone you have produced because dietary restrictions will be recommended around the type of compound that created the calculus.*
- *Do not cook with aluminium pans.*

Nutritional

- *Remove high protein, fat and refined sugar from the diet. Eliminate caffeine, alcohol and manufactured soft drinks, which generally contain phosphoric acid.*
- *Avoid beetroot, spinach, nuts, cabbage and rhubarb. Special mention should be made of cranberry and sesame seeds, both of which are considered to be 'healthy' for kidney problems but are contraindicated in renal calculi.*
- *If the stone has calcium involved with it, increase the intake of wheat bran, corn, potatoes, bananas, avocado, brown rice, soya products, oats and rye, all of which have a high magnesium/calcium ratio.*
- *Ensure that you are not taking any regular vitamin D compounds and watch out for those fortified foods.*

Supplemental

- *Vitamin B_6 (10mg) and magnesium (50mg), both per foot of height in divided doses throughout the day, can reduce oxalic acid.*

- *Take the daily dose as recommended on your chosen product.*
- *Discuss with a complementary medical practitioner the correct doses for the use of vitamin B_6, vitamin K, glutamic acid, magnesium and potassium.*

Nephrotic syndrome

Nephrotic syndrome is characterized by the finding of protein in the urine with consequential low protein levels in the bloodstream that lead to a tendency for oedema or water retention within the tissues. Other findings include high fat levels in the blood. There are often no symptoms, and other tests including blood pressure are normal. This condition results from damage to a part of the kidney that allows proteins to leak through when they should not.

Nephrotic syndrome may occur for no apparent reason in pregnancy but is probably associated in non-pregnant patients with an asymptomatic infection or toxic intake, such as chemicals, additives, pollutants, smoking, alcohol and other drugs.

RECOMMENDATIONS

General Advice

- *This condition is usually diagnosed by a simple urine test and the physician who performed this is liable to do extensive tests on the kidneys because protein in the urine may represent more sinister conditions such as infection or tumours. It is important to rule out any other condition.*
- *See recommendations for the prevention of kidney stone formation.*

Nutritional

- *Follow strictly the advice of a kidney specialist. There is some debate whether a high or low protein diet should be followed, but whichever belief your kidney expert expounds, the protein intake should be organic and pesticide-free.*

Pyelonephritis

Pyelonephritis describes infection of the kidney and is derived from nephron (a minute filtering structure in the kidney) and pyelo (meaning pus within). An infection may be acute following bacterial infection up from the bladder, or invading the kidney via the bloodstream. Direct trauma may also cause an acute infection. Chronic pyelonephritis is the same situation but usually with less aggressive bacteria and simply means a prolongation of the initial infection. A chronic condition may flare up repeatedly and can be created due to a weakness at the valves in the bladder end of the urethra, which allows bacteria to travel up.

The symptoms are of tiredness and pain in the small of the back, usually one-sided but often bilateral. There is often a waxing and waning of fever and an almost characteristic condition known as 'rigors' which are simply uncontrolled shivers. Kidney infection is usually associated with cystitis and therefore painful urination and blood in the urine are often seen (*see* **Cystitis**).

RECOMMENDATIONS

General Advice

- *The kidneys can be damaged very swiftly and if untreated renal failure is a possibility. If the alternative medical suggestions below do not seem to have an impact within the first few hours of treatment then a medical opinion, including the use of antibiotics, should be considered with appropriate complementary medical care aiming at preventing antibiotic effects or a condition becoming chronic.*
- *Take a sample to your GP for culture, microscopy and sensitivity (CMS).*
- *Whilst awaiting the results of the CMS ensure good hydration. Start antibiotics if kidney pain is present whilst awaiting urine sample report. Drink one pint of water per foot of height in divided doses throughout the day.*
- *Follow the recommendations in this book for cystitis (see* **Cystitis***).*

- *See recommendations for the prevention of kidney stone formation.*

Homeopathic

- *Whilst awaiting the outcome of the urine investigations, use Aconite 6 every 2hr. A more specific remedy may be chosen by consulting your preferred homeopathic manual.*

Renal failure

The failing of the kidneys is an extremely serious condition that requires emergency medical attention. Complementary medicine can only be of benefit in supporting the technical expertise of the nearest hospital with facilities to deal with such an emergency. If the kidneys shut down, the body's metabolism will become out of balance within a couple of hours and death will ensue within two to three days.

The symptoms of renal failure are nausea, vomiting, drowsiness, confusion, water retention, headaches, diarrhoea, itching skin and eventually coma. These are created by metabolic changes and the failure to excrete the natural waste products of our normal metabolism. Urine is named after its main component, urea, which is a nitrogen-containing compound derived mostly from a breakdown and utilization of proteins. An increase in the amount of urea in the blood leads to a condition known as uraemia, which is toxic to the functioning of the nervous system and brain.

Acute renal failure

A sudden drop in blood pressure, usually resulting from trauma or peripheral blood vessel dilation following a toxic ingestion, will lead to a sudden, acute renal failure. A less common cause is the formation of a blockage to the urethra, by a stone, tumour or trauma, which causes a back-flow of urine up the urethra into the kidneys with resulting severe dilation and pressure necrosis. A severe infection may also cause a sudden shutdown of the kidneys.

Chronic renal failure

Chronic renal failure may exhibit all the signs and symptoms as mentioned above but tends to develop more slowly. A partial obstruction may lead to a partial hydronephrosis but recurrent infection or slow-growing tumours may also cause this problem. Untreated or unrecognized high blood pressure or diabetes will damage the blood flow to the kidneys and slowly but surely cause renal failure.

The insidious onset of chronic renal failure will create an imbalance of electrolytes and thereby create new diseases or worsen current ones. An inability of the body to control its sodium levels will lead to higher blood pressure, calcium and iron deposits will settle around the system because the kidney cannot remove these. As I mentioned above, the kidney also has functions in directly controlling blood pressure through a hormone called angiotensin. Another hormone called erythropoietin is a controlling mechanism for the amount of red blood cells we make. Raised blood pressure and anaemia are two of the more common conditions associated with renal failure.

RECOMMENDATIONS

General Advice

- *The recognition of renal failure, either acute or chronic, is made by a GP. Emergency orthodox medical treatment must be followed.*
- *Utilize alternative or complementary medical techniques, depending on the underlying cause, symptoms and treatments.*
- *See recommendations for the prevention of kidney stone formation.*
- *Do not underestimate the speed with which a kidney problem can deteriorate and do not try to treat renal failure without expert complementary medical guidance. Medically qualified nutritionists, homeopaths and herbalists are the only people who should be involved initially.*
- *Acupuncture and healing can be utilized once under proper orthodox medical care.*

- *End-stage renal failure is the gruesome term used to describe exactly that. Sadly, 75 per cent of those with chronic renal failure will succumb unless a renal transplant is possible. Dialysis may only be usable for a few years because certain toxins cannot be removed and kidney functions just cannot be replaced. The use of the homeopathic remedy Arsenicum album 30, four times per day, will ease the passage from this life to the next.*

Nutritional

- *Specific diets will be recommended by the nutritionists or dieticians associated with the renal unit. Follow these guidelines strictly, even if they go against your preferred or previously recommended dietetics.*

Homeopathic

- *If acute renal failure is recognized, use the remedy Aconite 30 every 20min for the first 2hr and then drop it to every 4hr until a suitable homeopathic remedy has been chosen by a practitioner.*

Orthodox

- *Do not hesitate to use renal dialysis. This may require your visiting a hospital for attachment to a specific machine, but nowadays special small machines are being used at home with training for an individual to attach themselves to the life-saving device every 6–8hr. This is known as ambulatory dialysis.*

THE TESTICLE

As far as the genes and natural selection are concerned, the body is a life support system for the testicles or testes! Their function is to produce sperm, which when transmitted through sexual intercourse will continue procreation. Failure of the testes to develop may lead to a lack of puberty and maturation (*see* **Undescended testes**) and it is possible, following the work of a professor in Zurich, to assess the chances of hypogonadism by comparing the size of the testes to a string of increasing-sized beads known as an orchidometer.

Sperm counts are, apparently, falling, possibly due to pollution and toxins within the food chain, and it may be that the size of the testes will diminish accordingly. Our professor in Zurich will keep an eye on this.

TESTICULAR SWELLING

In the same way that women should be encouraged to examine their breasts on a regular basis, so should males examine their testes through the scrotal sack. Testicular tumours (using the word tumour in its broadest sense – swelling) are most often benign but an unrecognized and untreated cancer is dangerous.

Coele is the medical term for lump and is prefixed by whatever has caused it. Hydro- (fluid), spermato- (sperm), varico- (a swelling of a vein) or haemato- (blood filled) are all examples. Most often these fluid filled sacks are caused by trauma but many arise spontaneously or with associated diseases such as infections or cancers.

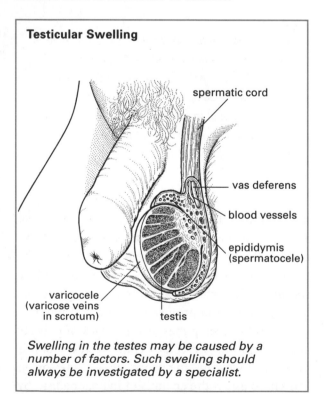

Testicular Swelling

spermatic cord

vas deferens

blood vessels

epididymis (spermatocele)

varicocele (varicose veins in scrotum)

testis

Swelling in the testes may be caused by a number of factors. Such swelling should always be investigated by a specialist.

A testicular swelling may prove to be a cancer. There are different types, some of which are more aggressive than others, but orthodox medicine has a good success rate if a testicular tumour is caught early.

URINE AND URINATION

Urination is the product of the passage of blood through the kidneys, which acts as a filtration system taking out most toxins. Urine is predominantly water with a variety of minerals and compounds known as electrolytes, which include sodium, potassium, hydrogen and chloride. These, more so than the minerals such as calcium, magnesium and sulphates are sacrificed in an attempt by the kidneys to keep the blood at a balanced level of acidity:alkalinity. Urine obtains its name from the presence of urea, a nitrogenous waste product of the body's metabolism.

Because the body generally produces acid in its metabolic pathways, the urine removes this and is

Urinary System

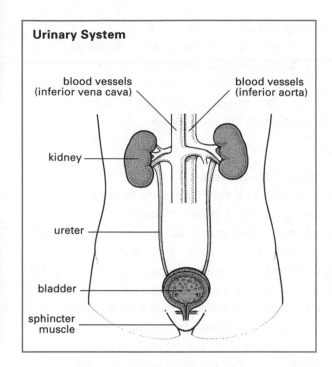

blood vessels
(inferior vena cava)

blood vessels
(inferior aorta)

kidney

ureter

bladder

sphincter
muscle

such as multiple sclerosis and tumours, either benign, such as fibroids in the uterus, or cancerous.

The urethra has sensitive nerves that, if irritated, can send impulses to the brain recommending urination. The intention is to have a flow of urine pass over the irritated area to try to wash out any causative agent.

therefore usually mildly acidic. This is an important factor because many bacteria prefer an acidic environment and changing the pH to make it more alkaline may be an effective treatment for bladder and urinary problems.

Urination is the outflow of this waste product and can amount to between one to two and a half litres in a normal, healthy adult. The more we drink and the more diuretics we take in the form of caffeine, alcohol and refined sugars, the more we pass urine.

The need to urinate is governed by stretch receptors within the bladder wall. A full bladder will take the stretch of these neurones beyond a threshold and an impulse will be sent to the brain saying 'empty'. Our consciousness registers a discomfort and we generally make our way to the bathroom. Stretch receptors may be influenced by pressure from outside of the bladder as well as from inside. Any 'growth' in the lower pelvis may trigger the desire to urinate. Pregnancy, enlargement of the prostate and obesity are common factors. A full rectum or lower 'sigmoid' colon can apply pressure, as can an enlarged prostate. More sinister causes include nerve damage from diseases

Incontinence

The inability to hold urine is known as incontinence. An overfilled bladder in association with increased abdominal pressure from sneezing or laughing may cause a natural incontinence. Attention should be paid if a mild rise of abdominal pressure by coughing, laughing or sneezing creates a leakage. This is known as stress incontinence. Pregnancy and pelvic tumours may cause pressure that overwhelms the valves, causing incontinence. Inflammation of the urethra or bladder, as in cystitis, will encourage urinary flow to flush out any irritant.

Neurological problems may affect both the voluntary and involuntary valves, and in men inflammation or enlargement of the prostate may alter the valve control. Incontinence is part of the picture of prostatitis (*see* **Prostatitis**). Women may have weakness of the muscles and ligaments that hold the uterus in place, especially due to overstretching in pregnancy or to the diminution in oestrogen levels following menopause. If the uterus should drop down it would put pressure on the bladder, thereby encouraging incontinence. The bladder itself may lose its supports for the same reasons and a bladder prolapse may also be a cause.

Anxiety and nervousness may trigger bladder emptying by a mechanism described in the section on stress (*see* **Stress**). Very often this may create such an impulse to urinate that a dash to find a toilet is inevitable. This is known as urgency incontinence. (*See also* **Incontinence** in chapter 6.)

RECOMMENDATIONS

General Advice
- *Obtain the opinion of a urological specialist if urination or incontinence is a problem.*
- *If a specific cause is isolated, try to remedy it by following the instructions in the appropriate section in this book.*

Homeopathic
- *The homeopathic remedies Ferrum phosphoricum or Causticum, potency 30 taken four times a day, may be beneficial until a more specific homeopathic remedy is selected.*

Painful urination

Urination should never be painful. Elimination from the body is usually an enjoyable experience and a mildly pleasant sensation is usually associated, although not noticed until it is pointed out! The body likes to have its toxins removed and the nervous system generally says thank you.

Painful urination must thereby be considered an important warning. Generally, inflammation in the bladder or the urethra is the cause but tumours and neurological diseases need to be excluded if the problems do not resolve under basic medical care.

RECOMMENDATIONS

General Advice
- *Painful urination that does not respond to the advice given in the section on cystitis must be reviewed by a GP initially (see* **Cystitis***).*

Homeopathic
- *Homeopathic remedies Berberis, Juniper and Cantharis may be used at potency 6 until a definite diagnosis has been made and more specific homeopathic remedies are chosen on the symptoms as a whole.*

Retention of urine

Retention of urine is the inability to pass the bladder contents. A desire to urinate usually occurs when the bladder is holding approximately a pint of urine (half a litre). Pain will increase if the bladder is not emptied when approximately one and a half pints is retained. The bladder can stretch and accommodate up to five pints of urine but the pain becomes excruciating.

The reason is due to outlet obstruction and needs to be treated as an emergency because the back-pressure from the full bladder up the ureters (the tubes from the kidneys) will lead to the kidneys developing hydronephrosis (kidneys filled with urine) that in turn will damage the kidney function.

Obstruction may slowly develop due to an enlarged prostate in males or an increased worsening of bladder or uterine prolapse in women. Strictures from a chronic infection or acute inflammation of the urethra and prostate may all obstruct the flow. Rarely, but more frequently in children, foreign objects may impede urine flow. Trauma to the urethra from external injury or internally from operative procedures or catheterization may anatomically block the flow or encourage inflammation. Tumours at the neck of the bladder or, very rarely, in the urethra may be a problem.

RECOMMENDATIONS

General Advice
- *An inability to pass urine must always be seen by a doctor immediately. A catheter may need to be passed.*
- *If retention is noted, stop drinking until attention is sought and found.*

Urine quality

The urine should have a clear yellow colour. The presence of any opacity (cloudiness) or a darkening or redness of the urine is abnormal. The colour and viscosity (dilution) is dependent upon the food eaten and those who take vitamin B complexes will note that their urine may appear a much darker yellow or even a light orange. A reason for colour change must be obvious otherwise it should be assumed that blood is present and this is pathological. Colourless urine is associated with overdilution and is triggered most frequently by drinking diuretics such as alcohol and caffeine. Provided that an obvious reason for this colour deficiency is apparent, then no further action needs to be taken.

RECOMMENDATIONS

General Advice

- *Any change in colour of the urine that is not clearly related to a dietetic change must be reviewed by a physician.*
- *Any sign of orange, brown or pink blood in the urine, bleeding within the urogenital tract must be assumed and investigated.*
- *Always take a first-morning urine sample and refrigerate if the appointment with your physician is not within 3hr. In any case, collect the next urine sample after any abnormality is noted.*

Homeopathic

- *Until a firm diagnosis is made, any suggestion of blood in the urine should be treated by the remedy Phosphorus 6, one dose every hour.*

Urinary urgency

Urinary urgency is an uncontrollable desire to empty the bladder. It is a sensation unlike any other and is controlled by information from the nerves in the area. The brain can sense urgency because of an over-stretched bladder, inflammation of the bladder or urethra or by injury or stimulation of the nervous system between the bladder and the brain.

Inflammation caused by infection will encourage the bladder to empty in an attempt to flush out the invading organism but often irritation from trauma or overly acidic or alkaline urine may have the same effect. In males, an enlarged prostate will push up on the bladder exit and send false information about the bladder fullness to the brain. A tilted pelvis or misaligned lower spine may pinch the sensory nerves of the bladder, telling the brain that the bladder is full when it is not. Spinal injury or problems within the brain itself may also do this.

When nervous or under stress the body produces adrenaline, which moves blood to areas such as the muscles, heart and lungs in preparation for fight or flight. This blood has to come from somewhere and will be taken from the skin (we go pale), the bowel (we feel butterflies in our abdomen) and the bladder (we need to pass urine). Stress and anxiety will encourage the desire for urination and may be the cause of urgency. The brain is sensitive to habit and once a problem with the bladder has been triggered the consciousness is concentrated on this area and an individual becomes even more sensitive.

RECOMMENDATIONS

General Advice

- *Ensure good hydration because a concentrated acidic or alkaline urine will trigger urgency.*
- *Isolate the possibility of any psychological stress or nervousness and use relaxation, meditation or counselling techniques to remove this.*
- *If problems persist, take a first-morning urine*

sample to a GP and ask for an assessment and examination.

- *Please refer to the relevant section in this book if any underlying cause is discovered.*
- *Any undiagnosed situation or one that is associated with back pain should be seen by an osteopath or chiropractor to assess the structural position of the lower back and pelvis.*
- *Hypnotherapy may be of benefit if no physical or obvious psychological cause can be isolated.*

Nutritional

- *If the problem is sporadic, consider a food allergy or intolerance (see **Food allergy testing**).*

Homeopathic

- *Please refer to the following homeopathic remedies in your preferred homeopathic manual: Cantharis, Kreosote, Petroselinum and Sulphur. If the desire is nocturnal, consider Causticum, Graphites, and Pulsatilla as well as those above.*

Weak urinary flow or stream

A weak flow is an indication of nerve damage to or from the bladder muscle or a partial obstruction, which may be due to a developing stricture, inflammation or tumour but is most frequently associated in men with an enlarging prostate. The enlargement narrows the urethral lumen.

RECOMMENDATIONS

General Advice

- *Attention should be paid to any cause of a weak flow; if uncertain, please see a doctor or urological specialist.*
- *Please treat the underlying cause by following instructions from the relevant section in this book.*

UTERINE PROBLEMS

Hydatidiform mole

A hydatidiform mole is a benign (it does not spread) tumour that forms in the part of a fertilized ovum that attaches to the uterine wall that will become, or already is, the placenta. Hydatidiform moles can mimic pregnancy (by being initially discovered because of a missed period and a positive pregnancy test) and may be dangerous because of the potential for a serious haemorrhage. If caught early (by ultrasound scan), treatment is by dilatation and curettage (D and C), but those that are not noticed may require a hysterectomy. Clearly, this is a devastating condition to have and I believe one that should be dealt with by modern medicine.

RECOMMENDATIONS

General Advice

- *A hydatidiform mole is likely to be spotted only by an experienced physician or an ultrasound. Follow orthodox advice.*
- *Consult a complementary medical practitioner for constitutional support.*

Orthodox

- *See **Operations and surgery**.*

Uterine prolapse

A prolapse is the falling or sinking of a part or the whole of an organ.

Uterine prolapse is the displacement of the uterus downwards through the vagina. A mild prolapse may not be noticed and is quite common after several pregnancies but may descend to fill the vaginal vault and even become exposed. The latter produces several problems as the cervix and the lower part of the uterus will be exposed and lose its moist, protective environment. As the uterus descends it puts pressure on the bladder, causing a frequent desire for urination and incontinence. Pain may be formed by the pressure.

Prolapse is usually the outcome of a weakening of the ligaments that hold the uterus in the pelvis. This may be due to an overstretching following pregnancy or through a diminution in the tensile strength because of a loss of oestrogen. Prolapse is therefore more common following multiple pregnancies or menopause.

Normal and retroverted uterus

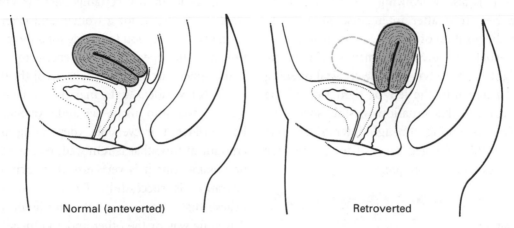

Normal (anteverted)　　　　　Retroverted

The illustration on the left shows the uterus tilted in the normal position. On the right is the almost vertical position of a retroverted uterus.

RECOMMENDATIONS

General Advice

- *Any discomfort or symptoms in the vagina or pelvis that do not resolve need to be examined by a gynaecologist.*
- *Pelvic floor exercises taught through yoga, Qi Gong or basic physiotherapy may support and correct a mild prolapse.*
- *Before any operative procedure is considered, please see a complementary medical specialist with an interest in herbal medicine and acupuncture because the two in combination may tighten up the ligaments more so than exercises alone.*

Orthodox

- *More severe prolapses may be corrected by the insertion of a ring pessary that is fitted and placed at the top of the vaginal vault by a gynaecologist.*
- *Surgical repair may be necessary and this is performed by tightening up the uterine ligaments or, radically, by a hysterectomy.*

Uterine retroversion/anteversion

When standing erect a woman should find her uterus in a position with the cervix pointing downwards but the top of the uterus pointing forwards.

This anteverted position of the uterus to some extent prevents gravity from pulling down the fertilized egg and has been enhanced through natural selection during human evolution. Many women, however, have a uterus that is more erect in its position and this condition is called a retroverted uterus. It is an anatomical anomaly and not a disease condition and only rarely causes problems, such as pressure on the sacral nerves leading to discomfort in the lower back, pelvis and legs or infertility. It is caused by a tightness or shortness of the supporting ligaments.

I recommend that all women have a gynaecological examination specifically to ascertain the position of the cervix in relation to the uterus. Ultrasound may be very beneficial as well. Unexplained back pains may be associated with this and prolonged and invasive techniques for investigating infertility may be avoided. As you can see from the diagram, if the cervix is pointing too far forward then there is a strong suggestion of a retroverted uterus. Conception may prove difficult because the sperm will pool at the back of the vagina and not have easy access to the cervical opening, the os. In such cases, sexual intercourse with the female on all fours or face down will allow the weight of the uterus to fall forward, therefore bringing the cervix more into a mid-line and available area. It is also worthwhile for the woman to sleep on her front after intercourse in order to maintain the position of the os (*see* **Conception**).

In unusual cases the uterus may be lying to the left or right in the pelvis and the cervical opening will be pushed into the left or right side of the vagina. Again, if this situation is established then corrective positioning through intercourse may well deal with prolonged cases of infertility. (*See* **Sexual position and technique.**)

RECOMMENDATIONS

General Advice
- *Obtain a gynaecological assessment to recognize the uterine position.*
- *Strengthen pelvic floor muscles through yoga or Qi Gong techniques because this may pull the uterus into a less retroverted position.*
- *In infertility, consider using a variety of positions both for intercourse and sleeping after sex.*
- *For backache, etc consult an osteopath/chiropractor and use in combination with yoga or Qi Gong.*

Orthodox
- *In extreme cases and where necessary, consider operative procedures (see* **Operations and surgery***).*

VASECTOMY

A vasectomy is the voluntary surgical interruption of the vas deferens from both testicles. It is a simple procedure whereby a surgeon will create a small opening in the scrotum, locate the spermatic cord, isolate the vas deferens (the tube up which the sperm travels) and remove a section. Both ends are sealed and from then on any sperm produced cannot gain access to the seminal fluid and prostate and will be reabsorbed by the body.

Sperm and testicular function are unaltered, although there have been some recent studies suggesting that vasectomies may cause cancer. These have been further researched and refuted.

Vasectomy is generally performed on a man who

has established his family arrangements, having had enough children. It is certainly safer for a man to be sterilized than it is for a woman and is an effective form of contraception (allowing for a short period of time after the operation when sperm may still exist in the upper part of the vas deferens or the urethra).

The downside is that a man may be able to father a family well into his dotage and a vasectomy must be considered irreversible (depending upon the amount of tube that is removed, reconnection may be possible but it is very rare that such a reversal operation is successful). There is no reason to believe that a vasectomy will alter libido or sexual drive one way or the other and a lot depends upon the psychology of the individual and the reasons why a vasectomy was performed. I have come across no spiritual reasons to interrupt a man's fertility.

RECOMMENDATIONS

General Advice
- *The operation is under local anaesthetic and therefore the insult to the system is reduced.*

Herbal/natural extracts
- *Prepare the scrotum by applying an Arnica-based cream twice a day for five days before the operation.*

Orthodox
- *Please follow the pre- and post-operative suggestions (see* **Operations and surgery***) to help healing because this is a tender operation although discomfort is generally held at bay by the use of Arnica 6 and a painkiller.*

STRUCTURAL MATTERS

ANKYLOSING SPONDYLITIS (AS)

This is an autoimmune disease affecting the joints between vertebrae. It generally starts in the lower spine and presents as backache and stiffness with referred discomfort such as chest pain, leg pains and sometimes breathing difficulties.

General Advice

- *Osteopathy and acupuncture are essential for both pain relief and potential curative treatment.*
- *Daily exercise is essential to keep the muscles from going into spasm. Yoga and the Alexander Technique should be considered.*
- *Regular visits to a Shiatsu or Rolfing practitioner are most relieving, as is basic massage and physiotherapy.*
- *As with any back problems, ensure that you sleep on a hard mattress. Practise the neutral position (head raised on one or two telephone directories and the knees raised until the small of the back is flat on the ground) several times a day.*

Homeopathic

- *Homeopathy needs to be considered and specific remedies should be based on the type of discomfort. The remedy Calcarea fluorica 30 taken every 2hr can be very beneficial in acute attacks.*

Herbal/natural extracts

- *Specific herbal treatments, especially Chinese and Tibetan, can be most beneficial.*

BACKACHES

Backaches will affect most people at some time of their lives. It is most commonly associated with years of incorrect posture whilst sitting or walking and also with poor abdominal musculature. If you consider the trunk of the body as a tube and imagine cutting out the lower half of one side, you have a good description of a human body with weak abdominal muscles. The strain is all placed on the back muscles, which invariably maintain a level of tension that is much easier to strain or pull.

Structural abnormalities such as retroverted uterus or kidney inflammation are a cause and more chronic conditions such as arthritis of the spine, ankylosing spondylitis and ruptured discs must be ruled out, but for basic backaches that are not recurrent or persistent, certain rules can be used.

General Advice

- *Apply heat in the form of a hot water-bottle wrapped in a towel, or hot baths.*
- *Regular body work is recommended. Massage can work wonders. Polarity therapy, the Alexander Technique, yoga and Qi Gong are all useful to correct posture if backaches are recurrent.*
- *Debilitating backaches should be assessed by an osteopath or chiropractor.*
- *Persisting problems not amenable to osteopathy or chiropractic should be referred to Rolfing or Shiatsu practitioners and have some relief.*
- *Common sense. If you have a weak back, do not pick up heavy objects and do not spend time in a stooped position.*
- *Sleep on a hard mattress, preferably face up, without a pillow.*
- *Avoid orthodox painkillers because removing the pain will allow a continuation of the bad posture or injury which may therefore worsen.*
- *Assessment from an orthopaedic specialist is a last resort.*
- *Recurrent or persisting backache should be assessed by a specialist in gait (posture and physical structure) as some experts believe that up to 90 per cent of back problems emanate from incorrect posture. These are often chiropractors or osteopaths.*
- *See an Alexander Technique teacher.*

Homeopathic

- *Homeopathic remedies to be considered are Arnica, Magnesia phosphorica, Rhus toxicodendron and Ruta. These are a few common remedies amongst the vast array. Refer to your preferred homeopathic book.*

Herbal/natural extracts

- *Herbal treatments such as strong chamomile tea, aniseed (which cannot be used in conjunction with*

homeopathy), caraway seeds (chew three teaspoonfuls or infuse in a mug of hot water) and Passiflora (30 drops in water every hour) are a few of the antispasmodic herbs.
- Devil's claw has been shown to act as an anti-inflammatory with far fewer side effects than conventional medicine.

BUNIONS

A bunion is the swelling of a small sac that is lined with synovial membrane. Synovial is the medical term for the inner lining of all the sacs that surround the joints in the body. The term bunion is usually associated with a swelling at the base of the great (big) toe and is associated with a thickening of the overlying skin and a forcing of the great toe across the other toes.

It is usually created by prolonged use of tight footwear, including socks, and if not noted early and treated correctly, surgery is the only option.

RECOMMENDATIONS

General Advice
- Avoid wearing tight, pointed shoes.
- Spend as much time in bare feet as possible, especially if a bunion is appearing.
- Apply cotton wool between the big toe and the fourth toe to try to correct the angle for as much of the day as possible.
- Have your blood checked for levels of uric acid by your GP in case you have gout.

Supplemental
- Try eicosapentaenoic acid and Bromelain at twice the recommended daily dose of a good natural product.

Homeopathic
- If inflammation sets in use the homeopathic remedy Apis 6, four pills four times a day; if things do not settle within five days or if the problem worsens, consult a complementary medical practitioner.

Herbal/natural extracts
- Apply Arnica creams frequently.

Orthodox
- If an operative procedure is necessary (see **Operations and surgery**).

BURSITIS

Bursae are the small sacs that surround the joints in the body. They contain a nutrient and lubricating fluid called synovial fluid and the inner lining of these bursae is known as the synovial membrane.

Bursitis is inflammation of this membrane and is usually caused by injury or persistent use of the tendons that lie above the bursae. Housemaid's knee is the most famous condition, although sportsmen and women can develop inflammation here as well.

RECOMMENDATIONS

General Advice
- Submerge the inflamed area in hot and cold water, 2min in each for 20min. Repeat this process three or four times a day.
- Rest the area. You may need to immobilize the area with a bandage or sling for anywhere from 10 days to 6 weeks. In the case of a bursitis in the knee, avoid kneeling.
- A persisting bursitis should be seen by an acupuncturist/osteopath for very effective and swift treatment.

Homeopathic
- A red, swollen, hot joint will benefit by the homeopathic remedy Belladonna 6, four pills every hour, but a persistent discomfort requires a specific remedy and you should refer to your homeopathic manual, paying attention to the remedies Apis, Bryonia, Pulsatilla, Rhus toxicodendron and Ruta.

Herbal/natural extracts
- Apply Arnica creams to the area.

CARPAL TUNNEL SYNDROME

The carpal tunnel syndrome (CTS) is the most common of the repetitive strain injuries. It is usually brought about by overuse of the wrists in an incorrect position and therefore found commonly in typists, computer users and keyboard players. It is less frequently found in workers who use their wrists and hands in a repetitive manner.

Carpal tunnel syndrome may be associated with conditions such as rheumatoid arthritis and other autoimmune diseases, hypothyroidism, calcium deficiencies, certain drugs (especially the oral contraceptive pill and HRT) and, not uncommonly, pregnancy. These conditions lead to a deficiency of vitamin B_6 which is relevant to the condition.

The condition is characterized by pain, pins and needles, and loss of sensation in the thumb, index finger and third finger as well as the palm and, to some extent, the back of the hand and the wrist. A diagnostic technique is to flex the wrist (pull the hand back) for about 1min, which should bring on or intensify the symptoms, and then extend the wrist to relieve the symptoms.

Carpal tunnel syndrome is caused by swelling of the tendons that control the flexion of the wrist and fingers. Overuse causes extra blood to be pulled into the area to supply the muscles with oxygen and this swelling puts pressure on the median nerve that nestles in-between these tendons. All of these, along with other nerves, veins, arteries and the lymphatic system, are sheathed in a tight covering that does not allow the swelling to move outwards and therefore causes pressure directly applied to the nerve.

RECOMMENDATIONS

General Advice

- *A persistence of this problem needs to be checked by a GP to rule out any underlying condition such as those mentioned above.*
- *Ensure that the position of your chair, when at a computer, typing or at a keyboard, is such that your wrists are at a slightly higher level than the keyboard.*
- *It may be necessary to avoid the repetitive action that triggered the problem for up to six weeks which may be inconvenient for many professions. A persistence of the problem will require this as a medical necessity and if not heeded can lead to permanent damage which will require surgical intervention.*
- *Acupuncture and osteopathy in combination is most often curative.*
- *Hot and cold applications around the wrists and up the arm and also gentle massage of Arnica cream can be swiftly relieving and even permanently curative.*

Supplemental

- *Supplement your daily diet with vitamin B_6 (50mg) and calcium (400mg) at each meal.*

Homeopathic

- *Homeopathic remedies Magnesia phosphorica, Hypericum and Nitric acid can all be used at potency 6, one dose every 2hr for three days during an acute attack and then one dose twice a day for ten days.*

Herbal/natural extracts

- *Use a teaspoonful of turmeric (the Indian spice Haldi) mixed with half a pint of skimmed milk four times per day.*
- *Chinese, Tibetan and Ayurvedic herbal medicines can be of benefit and should be used before considering surgery.*

Orthodox

- *If you are taking any drugs, check that they do not cause vitamin B_6 or calcium deficiency.*
- *Avoid oral contraception or HRT, any colourings in foods and an excess of protein in the diet, all of which can reduce vitamin B_6 levels.*

GANGRENE

Gangrene is an emotive word that, quite rightly, strikes a note of fear.

Gangrene arises in tissues that have been deprived of oxygen due to a loss of circulation from such things as frostbite, trauma, diseases that compromise the circulation, such as Buerger's disease in smokers and diabetes, and age-related conditions such as arteriosclerosis. Blockages in arteries known as emboli are also a common cause. Prior to gangrene setting in, the tissues become painful and if not treated immediately will turn black and, mercifully, numb. This situation is known as *dry gangrene,* so called because it is not infected. *Wet gangrene,* which has a 'wet' appearance, is created when anaerobic (not requiring oxygen) bacteria invade the dead tissue. If these produce a foul-smelling gas then the condition is known as *gas gangrene.* Wet and gas gangrene produce toxic chemicals that will lead to septicaemia (blood poisoning) and shock.

RECOMMENDATIONS

General Advice
- *Seek medical attention immediately.*
- *Refer to the sections in this book to treat any underlying condition.*

Homeopathic
- *The homeopathic remedy Bothrops or Lachesis, potency 30 taken every 15min, can be used for dry gangrene whilst awaiting further medical intervention.*
- *Echinacea and Tarantula cubensis can be used at potency 30 every 15min for wet or gas gangrene (again, whilst obtaining medical treatment).*

Orthodox
- *Surgical debridement and possible amputation may be necessary, along with antibiotics and medical wound treatment.*

GOLFER'S ELBOW – *see* Tendonitis

GOUT

Gout is an inflammatory joint condition caused by a build-up of uric acid crystals in and around the joints. Symptoms can vary from mild to severe and they present as intermittent or persistent joint pains, swelling, redness and deformity. A characteristic of gout is the heightened sensitivity that does not allow even the weight of a bed sheet to rest on the joint without pain. The most frequent site for gout is the big toe joint, but gouty arthritis can affect anywhere and the possibility should be considered in any painful joint.

Initial testing for gout is carried out by a blood test looking for raised uric acid levels. If this is equivocal then joint fluid can be removed as an aspirate by a fine needle and uric acid crystals looked for under a microscope. X-rays are often taken but it is not always possible to differentiate one cause of arthritis from another.

Uric acid is a naturally occurring substance created by the breakdown of proteins known as purines. The uric acid should be excreted in the urine but failure to do this or an excessive production of uric acid may lead to gout. Direct causes include dehydration, excessive alcohol or diets high in foods containing purine, poor kidney function and drugs such as diuretics. Aspirin is also associated with gout.

Gout is 20 times more common in men than in women. It has an association with being overweight and 10 per cent of cases have a hereditary or genetic pattern.

Conventional treatment is aimed initially at taking away the pain with the use of anti-inflammatory drugs, followed by the use of dietetic advice and long-term preventative drug use.

RECOMMENDATIONS

General Advice
- *Avoid excessive alcohol consumption, especially of red wine or port.*
- *Ensure good hydration as concentration of the blood encourages crystal deposition. Drink at least ½ a pint (¼ litre) of pure water for each foot of height per day.*

Nutritional

• Avoid red meat (especially offal), broths, gravy, anchovies, sardines, scallops and coffee. Unfortunately, peas and beans are also potentially high in purines, as is poultry. These latter foods should be avoided during acute episodes and only eaten in moderation if the problem is recurrent or genetic.

Supplemental

• See **Arthritis,** but specifically consider anthocyandins (particular antioxidants found particularly in certain berries), taken at the maximum dose recommended on the product label.

Homeopathic

• All of the remedies below can be taken at potency 6 every hour initially, and then reduced as the discomfort abates:

○ Colchicum used at the onset of the inflammation and especially if the pain moves from joint to joint and is associated with an irritable patient.

○ Urtica urens, particularly if burning or itchy as well as swollen.

○ Belladonna when the joint is extremely tender and feels hot and swollen.

Herbal/natural extracts

• There are many herbs that benefit arthritic conditions. An established treatment is mixing birch leaves, sallow bark, alder, buckthorn bark and nettle leaves in equal parts in a mug of boiling water taken two to three times a day. I only recommend the use of such herbal treatments under the instruction of a qualified herbalist or with a doctor's consent after orthodox medication is not working or cannot be used.

Orthodox

• Non-steroidal anti-inflammatory drugs or Colchicine deal with acute attacks. Side effects are generally associated with the dosage so the lower the

amount used the better. Allopurinol lowers uric acid levels by inhibiting its formation and is used in chronic or recurrent gout. Probenecid and sulphinpyrazone increase the excretion of uric acid and tend to be used in prevention. All of these drugs have side effects ranging from fatigue and numbness through to liver damage. The latter two drugs can cause kidney stones.

HAMSTRING INJURY

The hamstrings are the large muscles found below the buttocks, behind the thigh bone that causes the knee to flex. These immensely powerful muscles are frequently injured by athletes, who will be seen suddenly pulling up, usually after a sudden movement. Ironically, the more finely tuned the athlete and the stronger the muscle, the more likely the fibres are to tear. Hamstring injury is generally very painful and if the muscle is ruptured a lump will be felt. Relief is obtained by relaxing the leg and the pain is made worse by trying to flex the knee.

RECOMMENDATIONS

General Advice

• Avoid hamstring injury by stretching out thoroughly before and after exercise. Place the outstretched leg on a support at hip height or sit on the ground with the leg splayed. Keep the knee slightly bent and aim at placing the forehead on the knee. Do not bounce but apply gentle pressure, count to eight and return to an upright position. Repeat this process eight times.

• Apply heat or ice, depending on whichever is soothing, for relief of the immediate pain. If the injury is due to cramp then heat will be of benefit; if the muscle has torn and inflammation has set in, then ice will be the choice.

• Apply ultrasound via a physiotherapist or body worker with suitable equipment.

• Acupuncture, Shiatsu and massage techniques will all speed healing.

- *Osteopathy and chiropractic may be of benefit but must be considered if the injury is longstanding. Extra weight will be placed on the other leg and pelvic malalignment is inevitable but easily adjusted.*

Supplemental
- *The fluid extract Ruta should be taken (one teaspoonful in water) three times a day until the injury has healed.*

Homeopathic
- *The homeopathic remedy Arnica 6 should be taken immediately every 15min. Consider Ruta and more Arnica on a four-hourly basis, depending on the symptoms of the injury.*

Herbal/natural extracts
- *If an injury has already been sustained, apply an Arnica-based cream regularly to the entire muscle, paying special attention to the area around the injury.*

HERNIAS – *see* Hiatus hernia

A hernia is the protrusion of an organ from its own cavity or space into another. This usually occurs through muscle but can also occur through any membrane.

There are over 170 areas where a hernia may occur. The most common are inguinal hernias (groin), a hernia following pregnancy down the midline of the abdomen and incisional (postoperative) hernia. All these occur because of a weakening of the abdominal muscles with a protrusion of the bowel or the omentum – the fatty tissue that carries all the blood vessels, nerves and lymphatic system to and from the bowel itself. These are all, effectively, external hernias. Internal hernias may be just as common, as in a hiatus hernia, which is a protrusion of the stomach through the diaphragm.

Most hernias are repairable, usually by surgery and more rarely by exercise techniques and naturopathic medicines that strengthen musculature.

Hernias only become serious if the organ that is herniating is a vital one, such as the brain, which can herniate down through a membrane that effectively divides the brain into an upper and lower part. Hernias that obstruct or pinch an organ, thereby compromising its normal function or blocking its blood flow, can lead to gangrene, which can be fatal if not treated.

Inguinal hernia

The inguinal hernia deserves a special mention because it is the most common and the most commonly referred to. There are two types: *indirect* and *direct* inguinal hernias.

The indirect inguinal hernia occurs because of a weakening at the top end of a small canal down which the testicle descends from the abdomen into the scrotal sac in the latter stages of foetal development or the early part of life. A membrane forms but this can be torn with excessive internal pressure, often created through pregnancy, excessive coughing or strain.

The direct hernia occurs usually because of a muscular strain, often by incorrectly picking up an object that is too heavy. Here, the abdominal wall tears and the gut protrudes through. In both cases the hernia may be reducible or not, depending on whether the lump can be reduced. The danger signs are a non-reducible lump that becomes painful, apart from the initial tear that may occur with the strain. This suggests a compromised blood flow and must be treated as an emergency.

RECOMMENDATIONS

General Advice
- *All lumps and bumps that are unexplained, persistent or painful should be reviewed by a GP. Surgical intervention may be necessary (see* **Operations and surgery***).*
- *A small muscular tear may repair but at least six weeks of very careful non-exertion of the muscle group must be maintained.*
- *Discuss options for strengthening the muscle*

group with an osteopath or a sports injury physiotherapist.
- *Acupuncture may speed up the healing.*

Homeopathic
- *If the initial strain is painful, use Arnica 6 every 15min for up to 2hr.*

Herbal/natural extracts
- *Applications of Arnica creams four times a day to the area may be beneficial.*

HIP PROBLEMS

Arthritis of the hip
Arthritis of the hip deserves special mention, simply because of its prevalence in our elderly population. Treatment at any stage of the disease may be effective but very often a replacement is in order.

The operative procedure for an arthritic hip is very successful and recent changes in surgical technique encourage the patient to be up and out of bed within 48 hours. Complications are rare but poor fixing of the ball and/or socket components does occur and this operation is notorious, especially if the individual does not get out of bed swiftly, for producing blood clots that can lead to pulmonary emboli. These risks are, however, small and the techniques are improving. Twenty years ago it would be necessary to consider replacing a replacement within 5–7 years but now, with techniques and components at a much higher standard, a hip may last up to 20 years.

RECOMMENDATIONS

General Advice
- *See **Arthritis** for information on how to avoid the necessity of an operation.*
- *See **Operations and surgery** if an operation is required.*
- *Ensure that good physiotherapy, osteopathy and yoga are all employed before and after any operation. Strengthening the muscles around the*

hip joint and ensuring re-alignment of the inevitably dislodged pelvis speeds healing and will maintain the joint at a better level of health.

Hip fracture
Gravity has a profound effect on everything and the calcium in our bones is no exception. As we age, the protein matrix in which the calcium sits in bones diminishes, in part due to lack of exercise, decreased oestrogen and, especially, progesterone levels and, for many reasons, the Western diet. The outcome in the longest bone in the body – the femur or thigh bone – is that the top end (the hip) becomes less dense. For a variety of reasons, including a loss of control in the balance centres in the brain and weakening muscles, elderly people have a greater tendency to fall and this, in combination with the weakened neck of the femur, makes hip fractures one of the two most common breakages in the elderly (the other being a Colles' fracture of the wrist).

A hip fracture may sever the artery leading to the head of the femur which, having cut off the blood supply, will cause a necrosis (death) of the

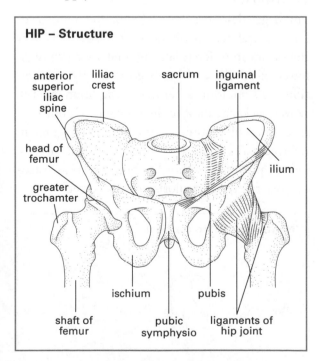

455

top part of the bone. This can become extremely painful eventually and can also lead to gangrene, which could be fatal.

RECOMMENDATIONS

General Advice

- *Any trauma that leads to an immobile or painful hip must be reviewed by an accident and emergency department and X-ray investigation should be undertaken.*
- *See **Operations and surgery** if surgery is required.*
- *See **Arthritis of the hip** for recommendations and pre- and postoperative care.*
- *Prevention is the best form of medicine. Unfortunately, bone density is often determined in our teens and by the time a hip threatens to fracture interventional treatment is necessary (see **Osteoporosis**).*

Homeopathic

- *The homeopathic remedies Arnica and Symphytum at potency 30 should be taken every 2hr, decreasing to every 4hr after medical intervention has ceased.*

LUMBAGO

Lumbago describes backache in the lumbar or lumbosacral region of the lower back. It is very important to differentiate any underlying cause of lower backache, and lumbago is simply a definition of a symptom rather than a condition in itself. Lower backache may be the outcome of poor posture, muscular strain, structural malalignment, referred pain from abdominal or pelvic organs, disease processes within the bones such as osteoporosis, rarely tuberculosis or even cancer.

'Neutral' position for back

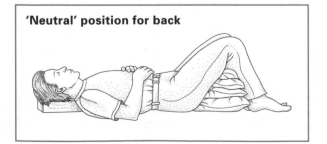

In Ayurvedic medicine sexual energy lies in the pelvis at the base of the spine and is known as *kundalini*. Spiritual or psychological problems involving sexuality may lead to persisting lumbago. Chinese practitioners consider the lower back as representing many acupuncture points on the bladder meridian. Bladder Qi is strongly affected by fear, suspicion and jealousy, as well as being an organ that removes 'dirty' fluid waste. Any of these emotions may be related to lumbago and need to be assessed in a holistic treatment.

Excessive abdominal weight or pregnancy in association with weak abdominal musculature will put extra pressure on the back muscles and allow either muscular strain or malalignment in the lumbosacral area. The fused joints between the hip bones and the sacrum, known as the iliosacral joints, are often slightly malaligned. In pregnancy and during menopausal changes, raised or lowered oestrogen levels will alter the flexibility of the pelvic ligaments (the more oestrogen, the more supple), which can alter the pelvic bone positions. Inflammation can occur in the lower back joints through osteoarthritis, rheumatoid arthritis, ankylosing spondylitis and certain infections, all of which have to be assessed before a correct treatment can be established.

RECOMMENDATIONS

General Advice

- *Use simple measures such as the application of heat or ice (whichever feels relieving) and spend time in the 'neutral' position: with the head raised by a telephone directory (two if you live in a small country!) and four pillows under the knees.*
- *Gentle stretching exercises (best taught by a body worker or gym master) may be relieving.*
- *A visit to an osteopath or chiropractor for a diagnostic consultation should be considered if problems persist.*
- *Polarity therapy, the Alexander Technique, yoga and Qi Gong should all be considered as part of a long-term preventative package.*

- *Shiatsu and massage will be relieving, if not curative, as may acupuncture in association with other body work.*
- *Please review the relevant sections in this book if a specific condition is causing the lumbago.*

Homeopathic
- *Back pain through pregnancy or menopause may be hormonally related and should be treated by a complementary medical practitioner with an understanding of naturopathic treatments affecting hormones. Homeopathic remedies will be of benefit and should be chosen depending on the symptoms. Arnica, Bryonia, Rhus toxicodendron and Ruta should all be considered.*

NAILS

Care of the nails

The nails are scaled down versions of claws which were once very necessary for survival. They are created by uniting the epithelial or surface cells, integrated with a protein called keratin. The nail grows from the nail bed, which is a very vascular part of modified skin. The half-moon is paler in colour because it is less vascular but is nevertheless an important growing part of the nail. It takes approximately 3–4 months for a nail to grow from

its base to the loose distal border in the finger, and about 6–8 months in a toe nail.

The nail is derived from a modified type of skin surface or epithelium and therefore any compounds that can benefit the skin can benefit the nails and their strength. Keratin is derived from amino acids, so any deficiency in protein intake is also liable to cause skin problems. Although the function of the nails has diminished as we have developed over the ages, their use as an ornament in women is well-respected by the cosmetic industry and indeed a well-manicured finger has its attractions and can reflect a subconscious attitude of the owner for neatness or tidiness. Bitten or chewed nails may show a nervous disposition and dirty nails may be a comment on personal hygiene (with apologies to those farmers and mechanics whose profession may not allow an alternative to dirty nails!). Health is certainly reflected by deformities, ridges, the nails being brittle and the colour of the nail bed.

Nails grow forwards on a flat plane unless the nail bed has been damaged or infected. Keeping the nails trimmed to the level of the end of the fingers offers protection to a very sensitive part of the body and protects against injury. Compression of toes can cause the soft pulp around the nails to overgrow or cut into the nail, which will be painful and lead to infection. When cutting nails it is best to create a small V-shape in the middle section (*see* **Ingrowing toe nail**) to encourage growth forwards rather than sideways.

There is no health risk or disadvantage in using nail varnish or strengthener provided that the nail bed and its surround are not infected.

Abnormal nails

An abnormality in shape, colour or texture of the nail can all be indicative of underlying disease or deficiency.

Biting the nails

Biting the nails is not a problem, although it usually includes nibbling at the surrounding skin and cuticle. This needs to be stopped if it is painful or

---

NAILS – Structure

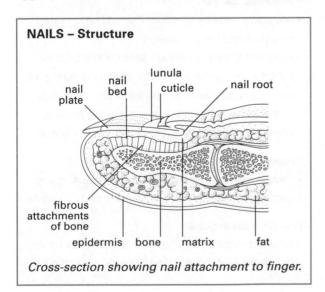

Cross-section showing nail attachment to finger.

predisposing to infections. Nail biting does suggest an underlying anxiety or nervous disposition, which will benefit from a relaxation or meditation technique. Hypnotherapy and counselling may also be required.

Deformed nails

Deformed nails usually occur because of damage to the nail bed through injury.

Discolouration of the nails

Discolouration of the nail itself usually occurs because of fungal infection, which tends to make the nail yellow. Rarely, toxins in the system will be eliminated in the nails and create a change in colour. Little black specks are indicative of a condition known as bacterial endocarditis and represent small clots. This is a serious condition and needs to be dealt with by a physician immediately. White patches are indicative of deficiencies in calcium, zinc or vitamin A. These are not uncommon in growth spurts in children but in adults usually represent dietary deficiency or drug-induced calcium loss.

Changes in the colour of the epithelium underneath the nail can show anaemia if pale, jaundice if yellow and the rare condition of excess iron ingestion if brown. A bruised nail will appear purplish or black.

Fungal infection

Fungus has a propensity to settle in nail beds, causing deformity by either killing off the growth area or causing a faster rate of growth leading to thickened nails (*see* **Fungal infections**).

Ingrowing toe nail

This painful condition is caused by the edges of the toe nail growing downwards and thereby cutting into the soft pulp of the toe. It is most commonly found in the big toe and is predominantly created by injury or persistent compression through tight-fitting footwear.

An ingrowing toe nail that is uncared for will minimally inflame but may also create an area of

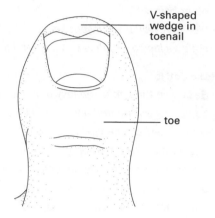

INGROWING TOE NAILS – Treatment

V-shaped wedge in toenail

toe

Do not cut back the problem nail area too far. Cutting a V-shaped wedge will encourage growth away from the affected area.

infection that, if left untreated, could jeopardize the toe nail or possibly allow gangrene to set in.

RECOMMENDATIONS

FOR INGROWING TOE NAILS

General Advice

- *Ensure from an early age that loose-fitting shoes are worn and that as much time as possible is spent barefoot. Remember that tight-fitting socks can be just as compressing.*
- *See* **Feet, care of**.
- *Any injury involving a toe nail should be reviewed by a podiatrist or chiropodist.*
- *Ensure that the toe nails are kept cut short. Do not cut back too far the area of the nail that is cutting into the toe because this may, paradoxically, encourage further growth at a faster rate. It is better to cut a small V-shaped wedge in the middle of the toe nail.*

Homeopathic

- *Review your preferred homeopathic manual, paying specific interest to Arnica, Hypericum and Calendula.*

Herbal/natural extracts

- *Soak some cotton wool and compress in an Arnica or Calendula lotion and wedge gently under the nail.*

- *Apply an Arnica or Calendula cream around the inflamed area.*

Orthodox

- *Any persisting problem, or one that is inflamed or infected despite the above treatments, should be seen by a podiatrist or GP, who may remove part or all of the nail under a local anaesthetic.*

Infection around the nail (whitlows, paronychia)

Medically termed paronychia or whitlows, this is colloquially known as Mother's Blessing and is a painful red or pus-filled infection occurring at the side of the nails and extending underneath on occasions. These infections are painful, usually because of the pressure build up, and treatment is recommended at an early stage as described in the recommendations below.

Ridging of the nails

This can represent deficiencies in the vitamins A, B complex and D, calcium, zinc and essential fatty acids.

RECOMMENDATIONS

General Advice

- *When cutting the nails, create a small V-shape in the middle to encourage forward growth.*
- *Avoid tight footwear, which will encourage the nail surround to be cut by the edges of the nail.*
- *Discolouration of the nail without an obvious cause should be presented to a GP for diagnosis.*
- *Brittle, ridged or cracking nails are usually indicative of deficiency or heavy metal toxicity and a suitable blood and hair analysis should isolate the specific compound, which should then be replenished. You can try supplementation of the nutrients mentioned above but, because any of them may be the problem and an improvement may not be seen for 3–4 months (the time it takes for a nail to grow), this is an expensive*

method of correcting the fault.

- *A bruised finger may be painful because of the pressure built up under the inflexible nail. Place the digit in iced water in an attempt to take down the swelling. Application of an Arnica-based cream may be beneficial. It may be necessary for a doctor to pierce the nail to release the blood underneath. If a doctor is not available, place a sewing needle in boiling water for a few minutes, remove it and hold the needle over an open flame (ensuring not to burn your own fingers because both ends of the needle will heat up). Whilst the needle is still hot, apply gentle pressure through the nail, making sure that the needle does not penetrate into the very sensitive epithelium below. Ensure that the nail is thoroughly cleaned, preferably with alcohol, before inserting the needle. The homeopathic remedy Arnica 6 should be taken every hour for three doses and then every 3hr until better.*
- *Nail biting may benefit by applying an unpleasant tasting substance around the nails or may be stopped by hypnosis.*
- *Ridging may represent deficiencies that should be assessed by a complementary practitioner.*

Homeopathic

- *Paronychia or whitlows should be immersed in hot and then iced water alternately for about 5min. An Arnica- or Calendula-based cream can be applied and the homeopathic remedy Hepar sulphuris calcarium 6 should be taken every hour. A persistence should be seen by a complementary medical practitioner.*
- *Any injury to the nail or fingers will benefit from the homeopathic remedy Hypericum 6, either taken every hour or alternating with the remedies mentioned above.*

NECK PROBLEMS

The neck is notorious as a site for aches and pains, which can occur at any age. There are numerous neck muscles that control the movement of the head, and the skull being a heavy object demands

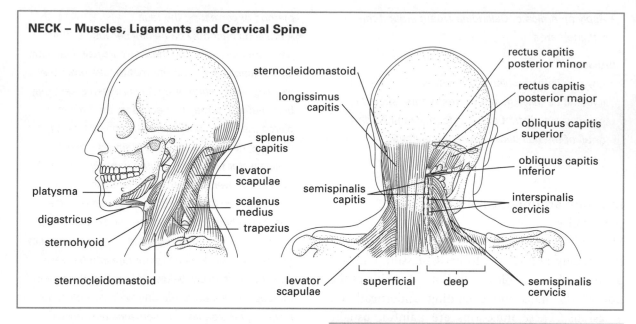

NECK – Muscles, Ligaments and Cervical Spine

much effort on these muscles. The cervical spine is flexible and, more than any other part of the spinal column, undergoes a lot of movement.

The neck muscles are constantly under tension to pull the skull up, and anxiety and nervousness tighten them more. This makes the muscles more prone to being strained than others and aches and pains are therefore frequent. The constant movement within the cervical vertebrae leads to a tendency for arthritis to set in, more readily in older age.

The Eastern philosophies consider that several meridians travel through the neck muscles. The large and small intestine, bladder, gallbladder and triple heater all have acupuncture points along the surface of the neck muscles. Weakness in any of these organs or systems can lead to dysfunctional muscles and thereby problems. I find it fascinating that the triple heater, which may represent the adrenal gland and therefore represent stress, should pass through the neck and over the shoulders. I believe that this accounts for why we feel tension in these muscles and benefit so readily from a shoulder rub rather than other muscles such as the thigh, buttocks or lower back, which carry far more weight and should theoretically tire out much more easily.

RECOMMENDATIONS

General Advice

- *For specific spinal problems, see the appropriate section.*
- *Neck pains associated with any trauma, such as a road traffic accident or sport injury, must be seen by a doctor initially in case the spinal column is damaged.*
- *Apply heat or ice, depending on which is most soothing and does not leave the neck in a worse state of spasm.*
- *Spend as much time as possible in the neutral position; the head supported by two telephone directories and the knees raised so that the small of the back is flat on the floor (see **Lumbago**).*
- *Consider a neck brace if moving the neck is painful, although there is some debate whether neck braces should be used. Discuss this with your health professional.*
- *Osteopaths, chiropractors, craniosacral therapists, Shiatsu practitioners and other masseurs who have experience in this field will all have techniques to resolve neck injuries.*
- *Acupuncture may be instantly relieving.*
- *Neck problems with no obvious cause may be related to acupuncture meridians and a*

consultation with a complementary medical practitioner with expertise in this area may lead to a diagnosis of weakness within the large or small intestine, gallbladder, bladder, adrenal or thyroid glands.

Homeopathic

- Use the remedy Arnica 6 every 15min after the injury for three doses and then every 2hr for the next 24hr. Thereafter take Arnica 30 every 6hr until the discomfort is relieved. Massage in an Arnica-based cream three or four times a day and any gentle massage offered should have a downward motion.

Orthodox

- Injury, especially whiplash, may be investigated by radiography (X-ray). Avoid this unless injury to the spinal column is suspected or the problem is persisting.

Broken neck

The term 'broken neck' is a broad term that may indicate a crack within a vertebra or the severance of the spinal cord.

General Advice

- Any neck injury that has any neurological symptoms associated with it, such as numbness, tingling, loss of sensation, odd sensations or paralysis, must be reviewed by a doctor.
- Immediately immobilize the neck (see **Spinal injury**).
- Please refer to the relevant section depending upon the injury such as fracture, pain or paralysis.

Whiplash

Whiplash is a syndrome that includes headache, pain and tenderness of the neck and the supporting muscles of the head and neck. Whiplash is a hyperflexion of the neck, usually caused by travelling in a vehicle that suddenly stops or is hit from behind or in front. The forward motion of the motor vehicle encourages the head to travel in that direction at that speed and any interference will cause the neck to flex. Most commonly, when hit from behind, the car seat pushes the body forward leaving the head behind, thereby creating a whip-like movement and injury. The damage is usually caused by a strain on the muscles holding the vertebrae together and the

HEAD AND NECK – Acupuncture Points and Meridians

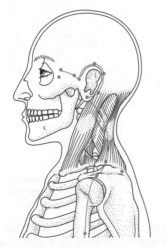

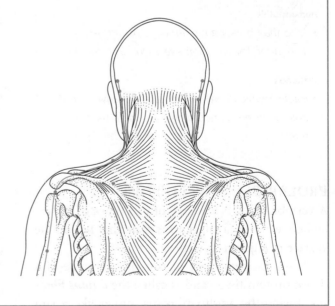

The large and small intestine, bladder, gallbladder and triple heater meridians have acupuncture points on the head and neck.

other neck muscles that tense in an attempt to protect movement. Trying to move the head against these cramped muscles causes pain as well as the strained vertebral muscles.

Other than the pain, neurological symptoms may be present if the spinal column was bruised in the incident. This may range from tingling and numbness through to partial or even total paralysis, which is usually transient.

PROLAPSED ('SLIPPED') DISC

A vertebral disc is a wedge of two types of material between the cartilagenous plate that lies on the surface of adjacent vertebrae.

The peripheral part of this disc is made of a dense protein tissue and is called the *anulus fibrosus*. Inside the anulus fibrosus, much like a jam

doughnut, lies a gelatinous material called the *nucleus pulposus*. The anulus fibrosus is tightly attached to the vertebrae through the cartilage plate and is the main reason why the vertebrae can only move small degrees. The elasticity of the disc absorbs a large part of any strain put through the vertebral column. If a stress is greater than the strength of this disc, the anulus fibrosus may rupture and the nucleus pulposus may herniate. This is described as a prolapsed or slipped disc.

There is usually excruciating pain and any movement makes the situation worse. The characteristic 'locking' in a bent position is because a disc usually slips when a heavy weight is lifted and the strain is taken at the vertebrae rather than at the knees as in a straight back lift.

The spinal column, in Eastern philosophies, represents an anatomical signpost for the major flow of energy through the system. This is especially true in Tibetan medicine. A weakness in a disc, therefore, is associated not only with a bad injury but is also a fundamental weakness in the energy as a whole. It may take an incorrect lifting

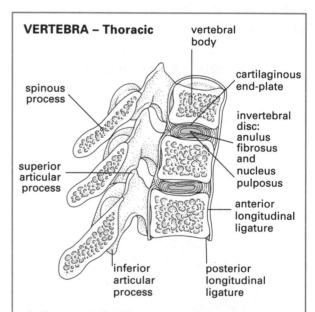

VERTEBRA – Thoracic

vertebral body
spinous process
cartilaginous end-plate
invertebral disc: anulus fibrosus and nucleus pulposus
superior articular process
anterior longitudinal ligature
inferior articular process
posterior longitudinal ligature

A disc may 'slip' if excess strain is put on the spine. The dense outer layer of a disc, the anulus fibrosus, *may rupture allowing the gelatinous inside layer, the* nucleus pulposus, *to herniate.*

position to trigger the event, but the underlying weakness is the reason why the injury occurs. This is particularly relevant if the injury is recurrent or chronic.

A slipped disc may be difficult to diagnose because pulled muscles and nerve entrapment may mimic the symptoms. An experienced osteopath or chiropractor is likely to be able to differentiate, but sometimes an X-ray is required.

RECOMMENDATIONS

General Advice

- *Application of heat through a wrapped up hot water-bottle or heat pad may be instantly soothing. Settle into the most comfortable position and get the opinion of an osteopath, chiropractor or experienced Shiatsu practitioner.*
- *Osteopathic, chiropractic or Shiatsu treatment may supersede physiotherapy in alleviating discomfort and the associated muscle spasm that follows a ruptured disc.*
- *Acupuncture may be instantly relieving.*
- *Any nerve entrapment or associated injury should be dealt with by referring to the section on nerve injury (see* **Nerves***).*
- *Always pick up heavy objects with the back straight, taking the weight on the knees.*
- *Regular exercise and stretching will keep muscles toned and limbered.*
- *Yoga and Qi Gong are essential to prevent recurrence.*
- *Avoid painkillers, because more damage will be done if movement is continued.*

Homeopathic

- *The immediate use of Arnica 6 every 10min is a homeopathic essential.*

Orthodox

- *A doctor can administer an injection by local anaesthetic.*
- *Surgical intervention is a last resort. Techniques are now performed under fibre optic conditions (a small tube is passed in through the back and the operation is done as 'keyhole' surgery), although major operations may be required. In extreme cases the disc is removed and the vertebrae fused so that the joint becomes immovable.*

REPETITIVE STRAIN INJURY
– *see* **Tendonitis**

SACROILIAC PAIN
Of all backaches, this requires a brief but special mention. The pelvis is surrounded by several bones (*see* diagram of pelvis, below). Where the iliac bone connects with the sacrum is known as the sacroiliac joint.

This joint is fused but has enough flexibility to dislodge itself and become malaligned which it does frequently. Even slight movements can strain the ligaments and the result is either a short period of discomfort or longer lasting and more severe pain. The inner aspect of the joint is associated with a muscle that bends up the thigh at the hip, known as the psoas. Through and around the psoas travel most of the nerves from the lower lumbar and sacrospinal cord. Any inflammation of the sacroiliac joint may cause inflammation in

PELVIS – Structure

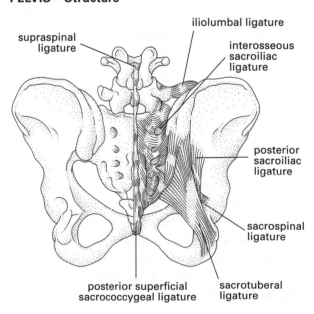

supraspinal ligature

iliolumbar ligature

interosseous sacroiliac ligature

posterior sacroiliac ligature

sacrospinal ligature

posterior superficial sacrococcygeal ligature

sacrotuberal ligature

this muscle or these nerves, leading to a variety of symptoms including sciatica. Abdominal discomfort and hip pain, as well as pains and neurological symptoms throughout the legs, buttocks and lower back, are all associated therefore with the sacroiliac joint.

The ligaments of the pelvis are very much under the influence of oestrogen, which will loosen them, especially in preparation for pregnancy. Women are therefore prone to sacroiliac displacement when oestrogen levels are high during the monthly cycle and are more prone to straining the joint as the ligaments tighten during menopause. Certain activities, especially if muscular stretching has not been undertaken beforehand or if heavy weights are lifted without the back being straight, will all entice sacroiliac strain.

RECOMMENDATION

General Advice
- *See **Backache**.*

SCIATICA

Sciatica is the medical term for a pain that travels from the lower back down the back of the leg, through the calf and to the outer aspect of the foot. It is caused by inflammation of the sciatic nerve, which is the largest nerve in the body, the main nerve of the lower limb, and has branches coming from the spinal column from the spaces between lumbar vertebrae four and five (L4–5) all the way down to sacral outlet three (S3).

Depending upon which part of the nerve is inflamed, a pain may be felt anywhere along the sciatic nerve line, such that a discomfort in the foot or calf may be a sciatic inflammation. The diagnostic test is to lie down and pull the toes backwards which stretches the sciatic nerve. A worsening is probably sciatic discomfort. The same will occur if the leg is raised with the knees straight.

The cause is usually a malaligned vertebra or inflamed muscles through which the sciatic nerve

passes. A prolapsed disc or arthritic condition may be responsible and, rarely, viral and supplemental deficiencies can trigger inflammation.

RECOMMENDATIONS

General Advice
- *Apply heat through a wrapped hot water-bottle or heat pad to the area.*
- *Osteopathy, chiropractic, Shiatsu and acupuncture may all be instantly relieving and perhaps preferable to physiotherapy initially.*
- *Any one of yoga, Qi Gong, Alexander Technique and Polarity therapy may be considered to train and strengthen the back muscles to protect the sensitive nerves.*
- *Two handfuls of white bread mixed with a heaped tablespoonful of cayenne pepper and enough water to make a dough-like consistency can be placed over the lower back and held on by a wraparound. Remove this after 20min because it may burn the skin, but if it is effective then repeat every 6hr.*
- *Avoid orthodox painkillers if possible because a removal of the pain may encourage movement, which will further damage an inflamed nerve.*

Supplemental
- *Use Vitamin B$_1$ (15mg per foot of height) with the next meal after the problem starts. Then take 10mg per foot of height with each meal for three days maximum. Any nausea or dizziness associated with taking this compound is an indication to stop.*
- *Bromelaine (150mg per foot of height in divided doses) with meals is a very good naturopathic anti-inflammatory.*

Homeopathic
- *The homeopathic remedies Colocynthis or Lycopodium may be used if the discomfort is in the right leg and Carboneum sulphuricum if the pain is on the left. Take potency 6 every hour. A more accurate selection of remedy should be made, depending upon the symptoms, from your preferred homeopathic manual.*

SEVERED TENDON – *see* Achilles tendon

The partial or complete severance or rupture of a tendon is a painful and serious condition. It most commonly occurs with the Achilles tendon behind the heel. When this tears, a severe and marked pain is suffered and if the tendon ruptures there is often a loud crack and an individual feels as if somebody or something has hit the back of his leg. The foot becomes flexed if the entire tendon is ruptured or only a limited amount of extension is possible if some of the fibres are still intact. Tendon rupture elsewhere may not be all this dramatic but is equally painful.

SLIPPED DISC – *see* Prolapsed disc

SPINAL CURVATURE

As the diagram overleaf shows, the spine has a natural curvature that is principally controlled by the muscles running alongside and in-between each vertebra.

This natural curvature can be disturbed by disease processes such as tuberculosis, ankylosing spondylitis and osteoporosis, but most usually is affected by bad posture.

Little or no training is given in the West to good posture, whereas the Eastern philosophies, either through the martial arts or simply by a differing view of etiquette, encourage us at a younger age to keep the back erect. Hard mattresses (or the floor) have been replaced by soft ones and only in the last decade or so has the concept of an orthopaedic mattress been recognized in helping bad backs. Poor spinal curvature and lack of good muscular support is the cause of most backaches, whether initiated by trauma or not.

Lordosis

This is a forward curvature of the lumbar (lower) spine. This increase in the concave natural bend is usually created by carrying excess weight in the abdomen in association with poor abdominal musculature.

Kyphosis

Kyphosis is a forward bending of the spine in the thoracic (mid-back) area, involving a few or many vertebrae. Our literary friend Quasimodo, the Hunchback of Notre-Dame, is an extreme example of kyphosis, which is more often seen in elderly women with osteoporosis. Again poor posture through our youth is a more common cause of mild kyphosis, which can be a persistent cause of aches and pains in the upper back and shoulders. It is interesting to note that kyphosis is more common in left-handed people.

Scoliosis

This is a lateral curvature of the spine, which is

THE SPINE

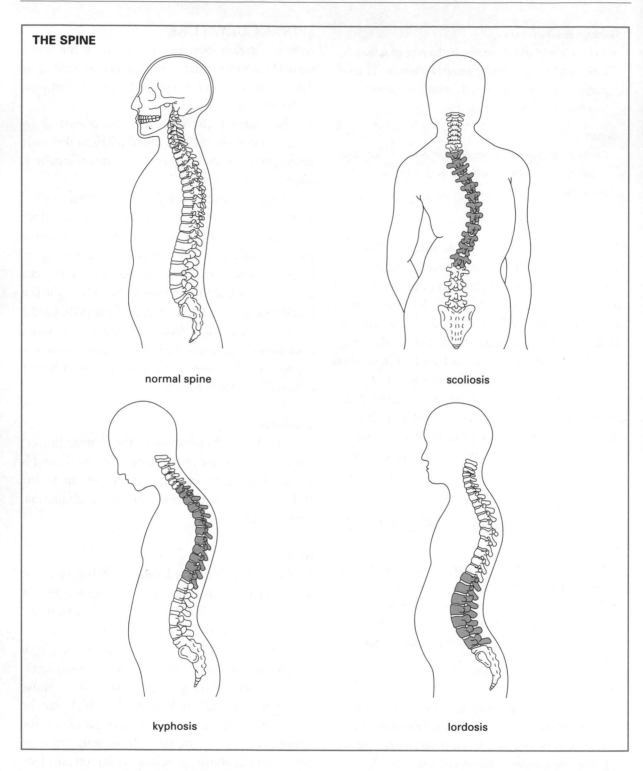

normal spine

scoliosis

kyphosis

lordosis

named according to the location and direction of the convexity (the direction in which the bending is occurring). Unlike other curvatures in the spine, scoliosis may be genetically inherited or caused by trauma that allows a malalignment that is not corrected. Disease processes such as osteoporosis may also cause this problem.

All Eastern philosophies consider the spinal

column to be associated with the main flow of energy through the system. A correctly positioned spine is therefore essential for the free flow of energy.

SPRAINS

A sprain is the wrenching of a joint, producing a stretching or laceration of the ligament. A ligament holds one bone in association with another and is made of flexible, tough, dense, white, fibrous connective tissue.

The most common sprains occur in the ankle, fingers and toes. A mild sprain may require rest for a few days but a serious tear may require an operative procedure. Ligaments are strongly connected to the bones that they attach and a tear may actually cause a splinter or a chunk of bone to be fractured as well.

It is difficult to differentiate clinically between a sprain and a muscular strain. Both are painful although ligament damage is often more so. Swelling and limitation of movement will occur in both injuries but the latter is generally more painful than a ligament injury. The term 'more painful' is rather subjective and only experience might help us differentiate here.

A sprain (or strain) is liable to become recurrent if not healed properly. The recurrence may be associated with a weakness in the underlying energy or meridian line and this needs to be looked at. The mind–body connection should also be considered.

TEMPOROMANDIBULAR JOINT (TMJ) SYNDROME

This condition is hard enough to say and attempting to would make any sufferer worse. The TMJ is where your lower jaw (mandible) joins the skull and is operated by one of the most powerful muscles in the body, the masseter muscle. Any malalignment of the joint or spasm of the muscle will create a pain that affects the jaw, the temples, the teeth and the cheeks. The discomfort can extend down the neck and around the skull, being a cause of headaches and migraines.

Clicking of the jaw joint may be an indication of the development of TMJ dysfunction or may be associated with discomfort. The cause is generally an improper alignment of the teeth or injury to the area. Problems with the parotid gland may cause inflammation creating a tension within the masseter that will pull the jaw out of place; age-related arthritis (osteoarthritis) is another rare cause.

RECOMMENDATIONS

General Advice
- *See a cranial osteopath as a primary referral.*
- *Relaxation and meditation techniques to take the tension out of the masseter is recommended and for a few days try to eat soft foods only. Please note that a lack of chewable foods in the diet may give rise to the problem in the first place.*
- *If there is a painful spot just forward of the angle of the jaw, gentle pressure may relieve the discomfort.*
- *The application of heat to the area may relieve the symptoms.*
- *Acupuncture may be added to any of the above if the problem persists.*
- *Persistence may be due to an orthodontic difficulty and dentists who specialize in this condition should be consulted. It might be necessary to alter the bite or remove molar teeth that may have erupted incorrectly.*

Homeopathic
- *Homeopathic remedy Arnica 6 can be taken*

every hour in an acute situation and four times a day to carry on treatment once relief is obtained.

TENDONITIS

Tendonitis is the medical term for inflammation of that part of a muscle that attaches to bone which is known as a tendon. (Ligaments attach bone to bone.) The most common forms of tendonitis are tennis elbow, golfer's elbow and Achilles tendon. Repetitive strain injury (RSI) is also included within tendonitis – this being inflammation of the tendons of the forearm muscles that control the fingers.

The symptoms are usually that of a sharp pain associated with a persistent ache. The pain is worse on movement – the more work being done, the more pain being expressed.

A persistent tendonitis that is resistant to treatment may be associated with the overlying meridian or energy channel. An assessment by a complementary medical practitioner with a knowledge in this area is of use.

Tenosynovitis

Around most joints lies a nutrient and lubricating fluid called the synovial fluid. This is encased by a membrane known as the synovial membrane. Very often when a tendon or a joint area becomes inflamed the synovial membrane follows suit. This condition is known as synovitis and when in conjunction with an inflamed tendon is termed tenosynovitis.

Trigger finger

Trigger finger is a condition in which the flexion or extension of a finger is at first obstructed but suddenly accompanied by a jerk or a sweep that is usually painful. It is due to a chronic tendonitis.

RECOMMENDATIONS

General Advice
- *Either ice or heat will relieve discomfort. Try both to see which is best.*

- *Rest the area as much as possible. Do not work the muscle beyond endurance.*
- *Both acupuncture and acupressure can be curative, especially in association with osteopathy. Tendonitis can lead to a poor use of that muscle group, leaving the other side of the body more dependent and therefore leading to structural malalignment.*
- *Before resorting to anti-inflammatory drugs, you might consider bee venom injections. This requires a specialist to administer and be careful if you have any form of sensitivity.*

Supplemental

- *Select a vitamin B complex and take the daily recommended dose with each meal for three days. For those aged 14 years or more, manganese (20mg) and vitamin C (1g) should be taken with each meal. An Arnica cream can be applied three times a day to the injury and if this is not available take one teaspoonful of cayenne pepper to two tablespoonfuls of a vitamin E cream (or simply olive oil), mix thoroughly and apply to the area once a day, leaving it on for 20min. Wash this off and be careful not to allow the compound to enter cuts because it will sting.*

Homeopathic

- *Consult your preferred homeopathic manual and pay attention to Arnica, Bryonia, Rhus toxicodendron and Ruta.*

TENNIS ELBOW – *see* Tendonitis

VARICOSE VEINS

A varicose vein is most commonly found in the calf and thighs and appears as blue-tinged lumps or streaks. These are vessels that have become abnormally dilated and tortuous due to a weakness in their walls or, more commonly, the valves within their lumen. The outcome is that blood that is being gently returned to the heart under low pressure falls downwards due to gravity, pools and stagnates. The expansion of the vein makes it visible and, because of the loss of surrounding tissue, it is more prone to being injured and thereby becoming inflamed. If the blood flow is stopped then a clot may occur leading to a venous thrombosis. Strictly speaking, haemorrhoids (piles) are varicose veins also.

Statis and clotting are generally not problems in superficial veins but can be fatal if they occur in a deeper vein. This condition has its own section (*see* **Deep vein thrombosis**).

The cause of varicose veins is generally multiple. A hereditary weakness is usually exacerbated by long periods of standing or increased abdominal pressure through pregnancy or heavy lifting. Poor protein intake may weaken the wall structure and toxins that affect the structure of surrounding tissues may be relevant.

Although varicose veins are principally an anatomical defect, alternative or complementary medical treatments may be of benefit.

RECOMMENDATIONS

General Advice

- *Avoid the possible causes of increased abdominal pressure, such as straining, standing and compression on leg veins through sitting with the legs over a hard edge.*
- *Increase any exercise that involves the leg muscles, particularly the calf muscles, which encourages squeezing of the veins and the upper movement of blood flow.*
- *See* **Leg ulcers.**

Nutritional

- *Increase the fibre in the diet along with vegetable proteins to ensure good muscular wall and surrounding tissue strength.*

Supplemental

- *Bioflavonoids from blueberries, cherries and other blue/red-coloured berries may be beneficial. Supplements at a dose of 150mg per day per foot of height in divided doses with meals will increase the strength of the vein walls.*

- *Bromelaine (100mg per foot of height) three times a day but not with food reduces fibrin breakdown. Fibrin is one of the proteins that holds veins within their tissues.*

Herbal/natural extracts

- *The herbal intake of Aesculus (horse chestnut) may be beneficial because it has anti-oedema and anti-inflammatory properties. Take the extract of the root three times a day at a dose of 200mg per foot of height.*

WATER ON THE KNEE

The term 'water on the knee', also known as housemaid's knee, is actually an inflammation of the fluid pads that protect the knee joints. It is triggered by trauma, usually by prolonged rubbing as was found in servants who scrubbed floors (*see* **Bursitis**).

WOUNDS

A wound is a broad term for any injury but usually refers to a cut or penetrating injury.

RECOMMENDATIONS

General Advice

- *See* **Cuts**.
- *Other wounds, especially deep penetrating ones, need to be treated by a medical practitioner but the basic complementary therapies are the same as for a cut.*

THE SKIN

The skin is a multifunctional organ the primary function of which is to encase and protect tissues and organs of the body. The skin also provides sensory information and in its waterproof and insulating capacity acts to keep the external environment out and warmth in.

The skin contains two types of glands: the

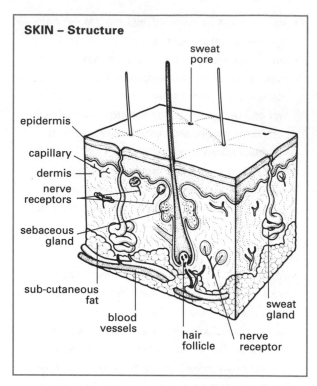

SKIN – Structure

sweat pore
epidermis
capillary
dermis
nerve receptors
sebaceous gland
sub-cutaneous fat
blood vessels
hair follicle
nerve receptor
sweat gland

sweat glands (*see* **Sweating**) and sebaceous glands (*see* **Sebaceous cysts**).

The basal layer of cells grow and move towards the surface, becoming thicker as a protein known as keratin is laid into and between the cells. This keratinized layer is thicker on the feet due to persistent pressure from the weight of the body. It is this layer that offers the greatest protection from the elements. Within the deeper layers lie the sweat glands, involved with cooling the body and eliminating toxins, and the sebaceous glands, which produce the oily secretion that helps keep the skin moist and contains immunoglobulins to fight infection.

There are certain cells in the skin known as melanocytes that contain a chemical called melanin, which darkens in the presence of sun. This darkening is triggered by absorbing what would otherwise be harmful rays of the sun, in particular ultraviolet light. The more melanocytes, the darker the skin and the better the protection.

Disease or dysfunction of the skin may be a topical condition or reflect systemic or internal problems. The skin is dependent on good nutrition and hygiene, more so than the many other parts of the body that it protects. Specific problems are discussed throughout this book and should be looked up according to the disease process.

Through the layers just below the skin travel the major energy lines or meridians that the Eastern philosophies of medicine consider to be integral to health. A weakness in these energy lines by disease processes of particular organs or systems may reflect through the skin. Conversely, damaged skin may lead to a block in the energy flow and thereby cause disease.

CARE OF THE SKIN

RECOMMENDATIONS

General Advice

- *Keep the skin as clean as possible. Most of the world will achieve this with water but if soaps are available non-medicated types are the best. The skin pores will react to medication by assuming that it is a foreign body and, even if there are no symptoms, energy is expelled defending itself. Except in circumstances where skin may be sullied following sport or by dirt from the workplace, the skin should only be washed once a day. More frequent washing will lead to a loss of the natural skin oils (in the sebum) and diminish quality and the skin's immune response.*
- *Avoid applications of deodorants and make-up beyond that which are socially necessary.*
- *Remember that the surface of the skin is only one of many layers and that skin integrity is dependent on nutrition, hydration and oxygenation from within.*
- *The integrity and tension of the skin is dependent upon nutrients to form elastin and collagen – the tissues underneath the skin that prevent wrinkling. As we age or damage the skin through sunlight and chronic dehydration, these fibres diminish causing the characteristic changes of wrinkled skin and cellulite.*

- *Massage, saunas and exercise all have a closing effect on the skin by either increasing blood flow or encouraging natural excretion. All these should be practised frequently.*

Nutritional

- *A well-balanced diet is essential for skin well-being and nutritional lack may well show up in a variety of skin conditions initially.*
- *High levels of refined sugars and fats will find their way to the skin, providing surface bacteria with excess nutrients, and cause an increased rate of growth. Sugar will also attract moisture and therefore prevent correct distribution of fluid to the skin tissues.*

SKIN CONDITIONS

Dry skin

The skin maintains its moisture by protecting itself through the outer epidermal layer and by producing sebum from sebaceous glands. Sebum is composed of fat, proteins, keratin and hyalin, and cellular debris. The production of this compound is dependent upon the quality of oxygenation and nutrition supplied by an adequate blood flow to the sebaceous glands in the deeper layers of the skin. Poor nutrition or oxygenation will prevent sebum production and lead to dry skin.

The sebum travels up the hair follicle from the sebaceous gland and any blockage by dirt or infection prevents the natural moisturizer from reaching the surface layers. Without it, essential defence immunoglobulins are absent and infection is more likely to set in.

Excess heat externally will dehydrate the sebum and a lack of water intake will do the same. The Eastern philosophies would express the view that anything that heats the body, such as stress, excessive exercise, hot drinks and spicy foods, will also dehydrate the sebum and may result in dry skin.

General Advice

- *Consider rehydrating from within rather than applying topical moisturizers. A skin that is dry but falsely moistened will not send out reflex nervous responses to try to pull more fluid into the area. (This is most commonly noted by those who use chapsticks for dry lips. The more you use, the more you need.)*
- *A cigarette burns at over 250°C. This heat is absorbed into the bloodstream rapidly through the lungs and heats the body. It is a potent dehydrator and a commonly overlooked cause of dry skin.*
- *Avoid any contact with oils or chemicals that may block the skin pores. This includes most roll-on and spray deodorants.*
- *Do not use antiperspirants.*

Nutritional

- *Ensure an adequate supply of fats and oils in the diet. Low fat diets are notorious for causing dry skin.*
- *Remove heating foods such as hot drinks, alcohol, pepper, chillies and other spicy foods.*

Homeopathic

- *Homeopathic remedies may be very beneficial and those that should be reviewed in your preferred homeopathic manual are Calcaria carbonica, Graphites, Petroleum, Silica and Sulphur. Use low potencies for an acute condition, six or twelve four times a day, or higher potencies 30 and 200 less frequently if the condition is longstanding.*

Wrinkles

The fullness and turgor of skin is maintained by the level and quality of the interstitial tissues (the connective tissues), made up of protein and fats. Special tissue components known as collagen, fibrin and elastin give the tissues of the body its support and elasticity. These tissues are dependent upon good oxygenation, nutrition and hydration. Absence of the first two will lead to a breakdown of the protein structure and lack of water will damage the cells; the outcome will be similar to a grape becoming a raisin, or a plum becoming a prune.

Wrinkles are, therefore, not strictly a skin problem although the effect is reflected on the outer layer. Anything that dehydrates or depresses nutrition and oxygenation to the tissues will result in wrinkling.

Wrinkles are a natural part of ageing and are in no way a disease condition. They are generally only noticed by those who feel that their looks are suffering. Naturopathic attempts at repair or skin rejuvenation may have an effect but it is unlikely that the skin will ever return to its former glory. With wisdom comes wrinkles, and hopefully the reverse is also true.

General Advice

- *Repair of wrinkled skin is much more difficult than prevention.*
- *Encourage persistent good blood supply by avoiding those conditions that block arteries. Avoid smoking, high fat foods and a lack of exercise.*
- *Encourage oxygenation by frequent exercise. Yoga and Qi Gong are appropriate but should be supplemented at least three times a week by aerobic exercise.*
- *Ensure that a breathing technique is practised; this will be enhanced by using a meditative or relaxation technique.*
- *Massage will encourage blood flow and specific Ayurvedic facial massage using acupressure points is particularly useful because it is wrinkles on the face that create the most despair.*
- *Perhaps most importantly, ensure that at least half a pint of water per foot of height is drunk as a general rule and increase that by 50 per cent when actively dealing with skin problems.*
- *Sunlight is damaging only if taken in excess and exposure should not be discouraged but monitored carefully.*
- *Avoid cosmetic creams because they tend to*

increase fluid levels below the area to which the cosmetic is applied. They have an artificial 'de-wrinkling' effect which diminishes once the product is stopped. Whilst using such products, the body may stop nutrition and fluid moving into that area because it apparently does not need it. This creates a dependency upon the application.

Nutritional

- *Ensure a daily intake of vegetable protein through beans, lentils, nuts or soya.*
- *Do not avoid fatty foods but ensure that they are vegetable-based and poly-unsaturated fats.*

Supplemental

- *Please use the supplemental recommendations for atherosclerosis (see **Atheroma**) at reduced rates, depending upon the amount of fresh fruit and vegetable eaten. Five portions of fruit or vegetable should not require any supplementation and add in one-fifth of the recommendation for every portion not eaten each day.*

Herbal/natural extracts

- *The use of Arnica- or Calendula-based creams may be of benefit because this will attract blood and nutrients into the area.*

Orthodox

- *Surgical repair (plastic surgery) is an option that may be very effective.*

BASAL CELL CARCINOMA (RODENT ULCER) – *see* Cancer of the skin

CANCER OF THE SKIN

There are three forms of skin cancer.

- Basal cell carcinoma (rodent ulcer)
- Squamous cell carcinoma (SCC)
- Melanoma

Recognizing skin cancer

Skin cancer may be present if any of the following simple observations are noticed:

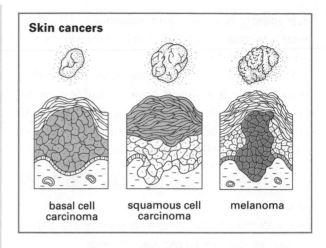

Skin cancers

basal cell carcinoma   squamous cell carcinoma   melanoma

- Any lesion that grows;
- Any lesion that changes colour or has different colours within it;
- A persistently itchy or painful lesion;
- A lesion that bleeds;
- Any lesion that recurs.

Basal cell carcinoma

Basal cell carcinoma or rodent ulcer develops from the lowermost level of the skin and tends to be slow growing and does not spread. A rodent ulcer can be recognized as a rough or scaly bump or as a small ulcer. They generally form where skin meets membrane at the corner of the eye or mouth. This flesh-coloured, painless lesion rarely grows beyond 1cm in diameter without being noticed and dealt with.

Squamous cell carcinoma

Squamous cell carcinoma (SCC) usually arises due to skin damage from heat, ultraviolet light, chronic infection or compromised blood flow, such as in association with arteriosclerosis or venous ulceration. This tumour is invasive to local tissues, ulcerates easily and appears as a friable lesion that bleeds easily. Squamous cell carcinoma does metastasize (spread) and can settle in the lymph glands and other parts of the body.

Melanoma

Melanoma is discussed in its own section (*see*

Melanoma). Basal cell and squamous cell carcinoma are named after the cell from which the cancer initially developed.

However, SCC is less dangerous than melanoma because it is slower growing and less apt to spread and usually tends to produce some local symptoms. It is also amenable to chemotherapy and radiotherapy if the need should arise.

RECOMMENDATIONS

General Advice

- *Pay attention to the above-mentioned criteria and have any such lesion removed. However experienced a practitioner might be, only the microscope can discern a cancerous cell.*
- *Any skin lesion that does not resolve easily must be considered to be a type of skin cancer and excised.*
- *Squamous cell carcinoma and melanoma must be treated with respect and the advice given for general cancer should be adhered to (see **Cancer**).*
- *Basal cell carcinomas need only have local treatment but a tendency to recurrence suggests an underlying tendency to cancer that may exhibit itself elsewhere in a more serious form.*

CELLULITE

Cellulite is not strictly a medical term but has entered the domain of medicine through plastic and cosmetic surgeons who are faced with an increasing number of individuals, 95 per cent of whom are women, who struggle with this deforming condition.

Cellulite is a rippling formation in the deeper layers of the skin, found predominantly in areas where fat is deposited. Cellulite can be symptomless and simply disfiguring, or may cause discomfort, a feeling of tension or tightness and, rarely, pain.

Below the superficial (epidermis) and dermal layers of the skin lies a layer of fat. This is more prominent in women of any age and therefore the condition is more common in this sex. The fat cells are kept apart by a type of tissue called connective tissue, which literally connects the different types of tissues throughout the body. Certain foods and conditions cause this connective tissue to degenerate, pushing the fat cells together in an irregular shape and closer to the surface of the skin.

Cellulite is divided into three groups:

- Stage one – the skin is smooth until it is pinched, when the pitted effect becomes visible.
- Stage two – the pitting becomes visible on tensing the underlying muscle or on standing.
- Stage three – the pitting is visible at all times.

RECOMMENDATIONS

General Advice

- *Reducing the fat content in the body will reduce the fat layer under the skin and thereby reduce the cellulite effect.*
- *Strengthening the muscles underneath the area where cellulite is prominent will increase blood flow and maintain or even repair the loss of connective tissue in that area thus reducing the fat stores as mentioned above.*
- *Massage of the area, both professionally and by the individual, will help to break down some of the fat conglomeration and also increase blood flow and support the connective tissue structure.*
- *Many cosmetic preparations are based on hydrating the area, which simply pushes water into the pitted skin causing it to swell and lose some of its unsightly appearance. Once you stop using the application, the problem will return within a few days.*

Nutritional

- *An interesting paradox. There is a compound called Cola vera that contains 14 per cent caffeine. Applied in a solution up to 1.5 per cent locally it can be beneficial. However, caffeine has been cited as being a cause of cellulite if taken orally and it is important for anyone fighting a cellulite battle to avoid coffee, tea, caffeine-containing canned drinks and chocolate.*

CORNS

A corn, medically known as a clavus, is usually a cone-shaped area of hardened skin with an associated growth of a horny substance, found most commonly around the toes. It is caused by frictional pressure.

FISSURE AND FISTULA

Fissures are cracks in the skin or ulcers that form on mucous membranes. Fistulas are small fissures. In medical parlance these are most commonly referred to when painful, and occasionally bleeding lesions occur around the area of the anus.

Fissures and fistulas are most often caused by trauma. This may be from the outside, as in anal intercourse, or caused by passing hard stools, often associated with straining as in constipation.

This latter tendency often associates fissures with haemorrhoids.

There are certain conditions such as Crohn's disease that can have an association with anal fissures and therefore a persisting irritation or discomfort should be investigated. Fissures and fistulas can occur at any age although adulthood is the most common time. Any such injury in a child, however, must sadly bring to mind the possibility of abuse, which must be addressed immediately.

HIVES

Hives are an allergic reaction characterized by a red, raised, itchy or irritating circumscribed lesion that appears anywhere on the body, usually in groups but occasionally isolated.

Hives are a response caused by the release of histamine and similar chemicals, which cause small blood vessels (capillaries) to leak causing swelling of the tissues. These substances also encourage the opening of the small arteries, causing more blood to flow in because the body has sensed a 'foreign' invader and is trying to flush it away.

Hives may be triggered by allergies, which in turn may be caused by any number of things, ranging from toxins, the foods we eat, the drugs we take and infections such as yeast or fungi. It is well documented that stress can cause a hive reaction and needs to be considered if more material causes cannot be illustrated.

RECOMMENDATIONS

General Advice
- *Pay attention to possible triggers especially drugs such as antibiotics that may appear in processed meats.*
- *See **Allergies** for treatment.*
- *Try applying ice, onion juice or an Urtica (nettle) solution.*
- *Ensure to sustain a high intake of water to flush the system.*

Supplemental
- *An Acidophilus supplement may be curative if the problem is a reaction to one's own bowel yeast population.*
- *Quercetin (500mg per foot of height) in divided doses with food throughout the day may be effective.*

Homeopathic
- *Homeopathic remedy Urtica urens 6 taken every 15min may remove the irritation.*

INFECTIONS OF THE SKIN

The skin has a very strong protective ability. It is water resistant and therefore bacteria and other ineffective agents find it difficult to penetrate. The top layers of the skin are dead cells and therefore viruses cannot live within them. The skin surface is a precarious habitat because our own bacterial flora competes for food with harmful bugs and attacks them directly. The sebum contains immunoglobulin A, a defence chemical that attacks foreign bodies. The deeper layers of skin are packed full of white blood cells and the basement membrane upon which the skin basement cells grow is another fairly impenetrable barrier of fat and protein.

For infection to set in, damage must first be made to the integrity of these barriers or the protective secretions. Once an infective agent penetrates, it can set up home and feed off the nutrients in the blood. Infections will benefit by the sugar content in the bloodstream which is promoted by ingestion of refined sugars and fats.

If the body's defence mechanism is low or an infection is left untreated, abscesses and boils may form. Infections within the bloodstream may be expelled through the skin, as in chickenpox, measles or more serious infections caused by bacteria in the bloodstream (septicaemia). Staphylococcal and streptococcal infections may cause a condition called impetigo.

RECOMMENDATIONS

General Advice
- *See **Care of the skin** to avoid infections and assess why an infection has set in.*
- *Please refer to the specific section in this book for conditions such as abscesses, boils and impetigo.*
- *Persisting skin infections need to be assessed by a GP to find underlying causes, although treatment is best offered by complementary medical practitioners.*
- *Ensure good hydration by drinking one pint of water per foot of height throughout the day to ensure dilution of sebum, which may thicken, especially if there is fever.*
- *Avoid topical antibiotics, which will kill off the good skin bacteria as well as the bad and may encourage resistant strains.*
- *Avoid steroid applications, which may take down the level of inflammation but in the process remove the body's defence mechanism.*

Nutritional
- Review and pay attention to general nutritional status because the skin may reflect any deficiencies before other organs.

Herbal/natural extracts
- Use Calendula-based creams on the site of infection.
- Manuka honey is a wild honey produced in New Zealand that is proven to have antibacterial antiseptic and anti-inflammatory effects. It has been shown to be effective in tests against methicillin resistant Staphylococcus aureus (MRSA) infections. Look out for Comvita manuka honey as this is a better tested and more effective product.

ITCHING SKIN

An itch is, medically speaking, a low level of pain. It is created by some irritation in the nerve endings that is not enough to send a pain impulse but enough to act as a warning. The nerve endings are affected by any obvious external irritant including chemicals, inflammation through trauma or infection, irritants that have been eaten and are coming out through the sweat, histamine release from a food allergy or insect sting, a metabolic disorder such as jaundice and eczema or dermatitis.

RECOMMENDATIONS

General Advice
- Isolate the cause or consult with a complementary medical practitioner initially to diagnose an underlying condition. Remove the cause where possible.
- Persistent itching should be reviewed for diagnosis by a GP.
- Hot or cold applications may be very beneficial.
- In isolated or small areas the application of either a potato or an onion may be relieving.
- Bathing in water containing a tablespoonful of almond oil may help. Do not rub off the oil but preferably dab or air dry.

- Many cases of itching skin are allergic related (see **Allergies**).
- See **Pruritis**.

Homeopathic
- Please refer to your preferred homeopathic manual and isolate one of the many remedies associated with itching.

Herbal/natural extracts
- Herbal treatments may be utilized but because they act as a type of anti-histamine they are best taken under the instruction of a herbalist.

KELOIDS

A keloid is an overgrowth of scar tissue. Most commonly found following trauma or surgery, the formation of excess scar tissue has uncertain origins. Generally the body has a mechanism by which it prevents an excess of scar tissue being created and this mechanism is faulty in those who develop keloids. It is most often found in black-skinned people. I have yet to find any complementary therapy that can alter this defect, which is probably genetic.

A silicone derivative applied to an adhesive gel sheet has been developed that is claimed to work by flattening, softening and fading red and raised scars. This has been shown to work in scars up to 20 years old, and, as usual, is declared to have no risks. Its action is by hydrating the scar area which helps to reduce the size and redness of a scar and can improve elasticity of the tissue. The compound is traded as CICA-CARE.

RECOMMENDATIONS

Homeopathic
- If a trauma occurs or an operative procedure is inevitable in a keloid-forming individual, then consider using the homeopathic remedy Silica 30 twice a day starting one week before the operation and continuing for three weeks after the procedure or any trauma.

Herbal/natural extracts

- *A Calendula cream may be of benefit and can be applied frequently to a keloid-susceptible site.*
- *Aloe vera, sulphur containing compounds such as MSM, and vitamins A and E can all be used and are occasionally found in combination. Apply this three or four times a day to any scar that is not healing properly.*

Orthodox

- *Surgical treatment of a keloid may offer temporary relief but a keloid will form around the scar created by the operation.*
- *The use of injected steroids may be of benefit and the experience of individual plastic surgeons or dermatologists is the guiding light.*
- *Please consider the use of CICA-CARE.*
- *A patented adhesive known as the 'Elastoplast Scar Reduction patch' is available in the UK and it is claimed to be able to flatten, soften and fade both recent and old scars by activating the skin's own healing process.*

rapidly. Melanomas are occasionally spotted on routine eye examinations as they can form in the retina but, like most internal cancers, unless spotted through a routine examination may not show symptoms until the spread has taken place.

RECOMMENDATIONS

General Advice

- *See **Cancer**, **Cancer of the skin** and **Operations and surgery**.*
- *Research is currently underway to produce a vaccine prepared from melanoma cells that triggers a body response to attack melanoma generally. It is in its early stages yet, and we watch with interest.*

Herbal/natural extracts

- *Specific attention may be paid to the herbs Astragalus, containing the alkaloid swainsonine, and Chaparral, both of which have been shown through scientific studies to have an effect on this type of cancer.*

MELANOMA (MALIGNANT MELANOMA)

Malignant melanoma, more commonly known simply as melanoma, is a cancer that is initiated in the melanin-containing cells in the lower layer of the skin. It is characterized by a brown or black mole-like lesion. Like any skin cancer, ominous signs to help recognize this condition are an increase in size (usually expansive rather than raised), a darkening or variation in the colour of the lesion, itching, bleeding or an associated lump in the closest lymph gland group (usually found at the nearest joint).

Unfortunately melanomas do not always fall into this category and can be pale and quite unnoticeable. These are, however, rare. Individuals who have many moles have no greater risk of any mole becoming a melanoma but have more moles and therefore have more lesions to be wary of.

A malignant melanoma may remain localized for a few months but if left unattended will generally spread and grow in other parts of the body

PAPILLOMAS

A papilloma is a growth of surface cells that is differentiated from a wart simply by having a more vascularized core of tissue (*see* **Warts**).

PRICKLY HEAT

This is a condition characterized by itchiness in association with small non-infected pimples that can occur anywhere on the body. Most commonly found in fair-skinned individuals in hot conditions, prickly heat is exacerbated by humidity. The cause is overheating, which triggers a histamine-like chemical release in conjunction with a blockage of the sweat glands.

RECOMMENDATIONS

General Advice

- *See **Sweating**, **Hives** and **Heat stroke**.*
- *A complementary medical practitioner with*

expertise in this area may lead to a diagnosis of weakness within the large and small intestine, gallbladder, bladder, thyroid or adrenal glands.

Homeopathic

- *The homeopathic remedy Sol (a remedy made from sun energy), potency 6 taken every 10min, can be markedly effective.*

Herbal/natural extracts

- *Apply Aloe vera gels or lotions if the area of prickly heat is small, otherwise take the maximum amount of Aloe vera as recommended on the product.*

RASHES

A rash is a lay-term used for nearly any skin eruption, but more commonly for a patch of skin that is red. A rash may also be inflamed and hot, flat or raised, dry or wet, and associated with other symptoms or not.

Many infections, either topical (local) or systemic (through the system), can be associated with a rash. Measles, chickenpox and rubella (German measles) are common examples of infections that are not too serious. However, a rash caused by a bacterium such as streptococcus, as in association with a 'strep' throat, or meningitis, as found on the thighs of infants in particular, is a much more serious condition.

Contact dermatitis (inflammation of the skin due to an irritant) is frequent such as in the rash from a stinging nettle or from a chemical at work, or a rash may be associated with an allergy, be it from contact, ingestion or inhalation. Insect bites can commonly create a rash, especially ticks or fleas. A heat rash may be associated with excessive exposure to sun.

More serious conditions such as blood clotting disorders or leukaemia may present as a rash. A rash is a form of superficial inflammation. Irritation or damage to cells creates a release of chemicals such as histamine that encourage blood flow, which in turn brings in white blood cells for defence and nutrients for repair. A rash is generally a warning or healing process and rarely the end stage of a serious

condition. 'Heed the warning and encourage the repair' should be your motto for any rash.

The Eastern philosophies consider a rash to be associated with excess heat in the system and underlying causes should be illustrated rather than paying special attention to the rash. Homeopathy considers skin to be a very important organ of excretion. Disease conditions move from the inside out and they are often at the end point of resolution when a skin rash appears. Incorrect treatment may suppress the underlying condition, inhibiting repair.

RECOMMENDATIONS

General Advice

- *Please refer to the relevant section if a cause is known for the rash.*
- *A rash may be soothed by cold applications.*
- *An oat poultice, made by soaking oats in water for a few minutes and compressing, can draw heat from an area.*
- *Drink plenty of water to flush the system. This should be neither too hot nor too cold because the former puts extra heat into the body and the latter causes the body to respond by producing more heat.*
- *A persistent rash with no obvious cause should be reviewed by a GP to rule out underlying disease. Special attention should be paid to rashes that are not red or not improving after 48hr. Refuse treatment with steroids or other drugs until alternative treatments have failed.*

Homeopathic

- *A homeopathic remedy may be selected according to the site and type of rash by reference to your preferred homeopathic manual or a homeopathic practitioner.*

Herbal/natural extracts

- *Calendula or Urtica cream should be applied to an area that is irritated.*
- *An application of a strong chamomile tea or oats soaked in chamomile as above can be soothing.*

Orthodox

- *Investigations such as blood tests may be necessary and, at an extreme, a biopsy of the rash may be of benefit to the dermatologist.*

RAYNAUD'S DISEASE

Raynaud's disease, named after a French physician, is repeated episodes of pallor and blueness or redness of the fingers, toes or both, usually induced by cold or emotion. The condition may be secondary to many diseases but most often to chronic arterial occlusive disease such as diabetes, arteriosclerosis or the smoking-related Buerger's disease.

The condition, which is not uncommon, is often noted simply by an individual digit going a different colour, most commonly white. It is caused by the arterial supply being obstructed, which is usually due to nervous control of the artery either from within its own nerve plexus or from the central nervous system. Other than the condition being painful or indicating an underlying disease, the problem is not serious, although in severe cases gangrene or ulceration may occur due to a lack of blood supply for a prolonged period.

The fingers and toes represent different organs, humours (elements) and systems, depending upon which of the Eastern philosophies you study. Most correlate to some degree and the Ayurvedic principle, shown in diagrammatic form opposite, gives an example.

RECOMMENDATIONS

General Advice

- *Infrequent Raynaud's phenomena require no medical investigation but persistent or painful episodes should initiate a consultation to rule out any underlying disease.*
- *Common sense attitudes such as wearing gloves or warm socks and not gripping objects for too long must be remembered.*
- *Avoid smoking – this causes peripheral vascular constriction. Alternatively, an alcoholic drink daily or just prior to an event liable to trigger Raynaud's disease will help to encourage peripheral dilation.*
- *During an attack you may increase circulation by swinging or rotating the arms and legs.*
- *Biofeedback and meditation training can have a swift effect and should be practised daily, regardless of the condition, for those whose problem is severe.*
- *Pallor or pain that is unresolved after a few hours should be examined by an emergency doctor. Paralysis or intolerable pain should be dealt with swiftly. Drugs for peripheral dilation may be administered in acute or severe chronic cases.*

Nutritional

- *Spicy food, especially cayenne pepper, taken regularly may reduce occurrences. Cayenne capsules may be used if spicy food is not enjoyed. The dosage should be as recommended on the product bought, but if no effect is forthcoming then double the dose, being wary of any sensation of burning in the stomach: if this is present the treatment cannot be used.*

Supplemental

- *Vitamin E (100iu per foot of height) taken in divided doses throughout the day may encourage vascular potency.*

Homeopathic

- *Many homeopathic remedies are of benefit and suitable. Choices should be made according to the symptoms by referring to your preferred homeopathic manual. For frequent sufferers who may have burning or aching digits, keep the remedy Cactus 6 in your pocket and take a dose every 15min until the problem resolves.*

Herbal/natural extracts

- *Ginkgo biloba extracts containing 25 per cent by weight of the key active ingredients can be taken twice a day and may increase blood flow to the extremities.*

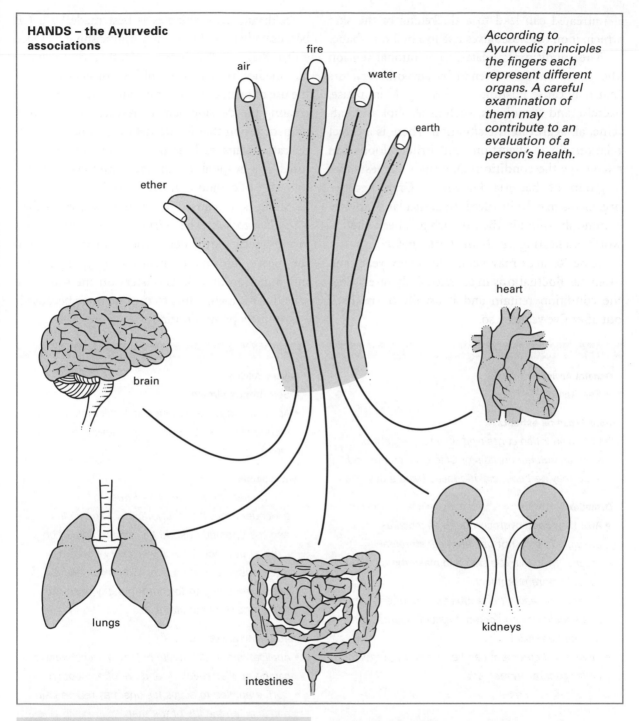

HANDS – the Ayurvedic associations

air

fire

water

earth

ether

According to Ayurvedic principles the fingers each represent different organs. A careful examination of them may contribute to an evaluation of a person's health.

brain

heart

lungs

intestines

kidneys

ROSACEA (ACNE ROSACEA)

Rosacea is minimally a persistent flush usually of the face and mostly over the cheeks, bridge of the nose and forehead. It is often associated with raised spots (papules) and whiteheads (pustules). The condition frequently occurs in middle age and if untreated can lead to a thickening of the skin which, if on the nose, gives rise to a bulbous shape.

The condition is related to emotional tension and stress but is worsened by any other factors that may cause flushing or blushing. Menopause, exercise and stimulants, such as alcohol and caffeine, all aggravate the situation. There is a direct relationship to digestion, and irritant foods can encourage the condition. One study suggests that a group of bacteria known as Gram-negative organisms may be involved. In particular, *H. pylori*, commonly found in the stomach has, been cited as worth eradicating (see ***Helicobacter pylori***).

Acne Rosacea may persist for many years and often has fluctuations in severity. Only rarely does the condition remain and it usually burns itself out after five years or so.

RECOMMENDATIONS

General Advice
- *See* **Acne.**

Herbal/natural extracts
- *Calamine lotion containing about 1 per cent of sulphur, sulphur creams or Calendula cream and soap may be beneficial if applied twice a day.*

Orthodox
- *Avoid low-dose hydrocortisone as much as possible and do not use stronger steroidal cream. It will thin the skin and make the dilated vessels more prominent.*
- *Tetracycline and other antibiotics are often given and should be considered if natural approaches are not beneficial.*
- *Severe disfigurement can be treated by surgery under general anaesthetic.*

SHINGLES

Shingles is an aggressive, painful, blister-like rash that can occur in any part of the body but tends to travel along a band of skin associated with a particular branch of the nerve and only occurs on one side of the body.

A diagnosis of shingles is best made by a GP because other conditions may mimic shingles. Once a firm diagnosis has been made, then complementary medical treatment should be considered before the use of orthodox antiviral drugs. These drugs are creating the development of resistant strains. Any herpetic lesion that is internal or is associated with delicate organs such as the eyes should be monitored by a hospital doctor; these are the exceptions to the use of orthodox antiviral drugs.

Shingles is caused by a herpes virus called *Varicella zoster*. The virus, typical of herpes viruses, settles in a nerve root and travels along the nerve and its branches causing pain and inflammation as well as blisters on the skin. The sensitivity is a guideline to the diagnosis because it is extremely painful initially.

RECOMMENDATIONS

General Advice
- *See* **Herpes simplex**.
- *Applications of ice wrapped in a silk material and then applied can be extremely relieving for a few moments.*

Homeopathic
- *The homeopathic remedies Rhus toxicodendron, Kali muriaticum, Ranunculus and the specific nosode Variolinum can all be used at potency 30 or lower every hour for three doses and then every 2hr in an acute phase, reducing to four times a day once the initial attack is subsiding.*

Herbal/natural extracts
- *Applications of Calendula or Urtica urens creams can be applied regularly and are often soothing.*
- *Coffee applied to active lesions may relieve pain and shorten the life of the rash.*

Orthodox
- *Analgesic relief with regular drugs is acceptable in the acute phases due to the potentially intense pain.*

SKIN DISCOLOURATION

Discolouration of skin is usually a temporary change caused by an alteration in blood flow: too little makes the skin go pale, too much makes it go red. Physiological causes such as embarrassment and excess heat need to be balanced against pathological causes such as rashes. People may go a slight greenish hue in association with motion sickness. (I have absolutely no idea why this is and would be grateful if somebody who has some information on this would let me know.) Brown discolouration may occur through changes in oestrogen levels and may be noted during pregnancy or the menopause. The latter are often known as liver spots but have nothing to do with the functioning of the liver.

Certain metabolic disease processes may alter the skin colour in a more permanent manner. An excess of iron may stain the skin brown and jaundice may cause yellowing.

Tinea nigra

This condition, also known as pityriasis nigra, which is common in the East and the Americas and is characterized by a black or dark brown colouration predominantly on the trunk, neck or palms. It is created by a fungal infection and specific antifungal creams are needed to destroy it.

Tinea versicolor

This is a chronic superficial fungal infection of the skin, which is caused either by a fungus known as *Trichophyton* or *Malassezia*. These fungae cause smooth-edged, usually round or oval lesions of pale skin. The fungus affects or destroys melanocytes, which colour the skin, and creates pale lesions. It is usually transmitted from towels or by skin contact and is common in the Mediterranean and West-coast beaches of America.

RECOMMENDATIONS

General Advice
- Apply a selenium-containing shampoo to the lesions three nights in a row. Wash off in the morning. At any suggestion of an irritation, wash the shampoo off and discuss other treatments with a complementary medical practitioner or physician.

Supplemental
- Take selenium – 20mg per foot of height in one dose with the evening meal.

SKIN GRAFTING

The skin, because of trauma or burns, may need to be replaced by a skin graft. A patch of skin approximately the size of the area that has been damaged is removed from a healthy area, ensuring that the basal (the growing layer) level of cells is removed. This must be accompanied by some subcutaneous tissue to encourage new blood vessel growth into the area to feed the basal cells.

RECOMMENDATIONS

General Advice
- See **Operations and surgery**.
- See **Eczema** and follow the guidelines for supplemental and herbal support.

Herbal/natural extracts
- Once the graft has taken, application of Arnica- and Calendula-based creams would be beneficial.

URTICARIA

Urticaria is the medical term for hives and nettle rash. It is a condition characterized by the appearance of intensely itching welts or weals, usually with a raised centre and surrounding red skin. They appear in the area where an irritant may have come into contact with the skin or in crops, widely distributed over the body surface if the reaction is created by the ingestion or injection of a toxin. Urticaria generally disappears within a day or two.

RECOMMENDATIONS

General Advice
- *See* **Hives**, **Rashes** *and* **Itching skin**.
- *Immediately apply a solution made up of iced water with a tablespoonful of sodium bicarbonate per pint of water.*

Homeopathic
- *Use the homeopathic remedy Urtica urens 6 every 10min until a more suitable remedy, if necessary, is found through your preferred homeopathic manual.*

VITILIGO

This is a skin disease characterized by the loss of pigment, leading to the presentation of white patches. These are highlighted by hyperpigmented areas around the edges in many cases.

Vitiligo occurs in many cases in association with certain diseases including hypothyroidism and pernicious anaemia. Occasionally the body forms antibodies against its own melanin-forming cells (melanocytes) but the most common cause is skin fungi. Nutritional deficiencies may cause vitiligo, especially in children.

If no underlying condition is found, then preventing this disease process is unlikely. The Eastern philosophies consider the loss of normal colour in skin or hair to be an indication of a profound lack of vital force. I am not sure if this is a fair assumption because most prematurely grey individuals do not seem to fare worse in longevity or health stakes than others. Without underlying disease vitiligo is not likely to cause long-term health problems in other areas.

RECOMMENDATIONS

General Advice
- *Any underlying condition must be treated.*

Nutritional
- *Any deficiencies should lead the individual to a nutritionist to discuss whether their diet is poor or their absorptive capacity weak. Digestive enzymes may be required but this really should be determined by a professional.*

Supplemental
- *Take a multi-B complex supplement at four times the recommended dose for one week and then twice the recommended amount for a further month.*
- *Beta-carotene supplements (2mg per foot of height) should be taken twice a day for one week and then daily for three months. At this level yellowing of the skin is not likely but if there is any suggestion, or if pregnant, reduce the dosage by half.*
- *Hair, sweat and blood analysis should be undertaken to assess mineral deficiencies, which should be corrected by taking twice the daily recommended dose for one month.*

Orthodox
- *Topical antifungal creams should be tried. Naturopathic ointments may be recommended but in my experience do not show good results.*

WENS

A wen is actually a sebaceous cyst that most commonly appears on the scalp (*see* **Sebaceous cysts**).

XANTHELASMA

These are yellowish raised plaques that occur around the eyelids and result from lipid-filled cells in the skin. They were considered to be an indication of raised cholesterol and higher risk of atheroma; this is not strictly true in most cases, but may be a sign of raised fats in the blood.

The orthodox world cannot explain why these form in this particular area of the body, although the most reasonable hypothesis suggests that it is a thin area of skin and therefore has smaller vessels, which may become blocked with fatty deposits. A more holistic consideration is the fact that small intestine and stomach meridians connect in this area and are responsible for the absorption of fat.

General Advice

- *Xanthelasma may be a reflection of lipid (fat) levels, so triglyceride and cholesterol blood levels are worth measuring.*
- *Ensure that good hydration is encouraged by drinking at least half a pint of water per foot of height and double that if xanthelasma has formed.*
- *Consult a complementary medical practitioner for an overview of your constitution, which may be showing a tendency to retention.*

Nutritional

- *Review the diet and reduce fat intake.*

Homeopathic

- *The homeopathic remedy Calcarea carbonica taken at potency 6 twice a day for two weeks and repeated in one month if no effect is forthcoming is recommended by one source.*

Herbal/natural extracts

- *Application of Arnica-based creams may help break down the stores and in severe cases laser therapy may be available.*

THE NERVOUS SYSTEM

BELL'S PALSY

Named after the doctor who first described it, Bell's palsy is a paralysis of the muscles, usually unilaterally on one side of the face, due to trauma or inflammation of the facial nerve which exits at the base of the skull and travels across the face. It is often associated with trauma, strong draughts such as those experienced by hanging the head out of a moving vehicle, viral infections and very rarely more sinister causes such as tumours.

Bell's palsy may resolve within a few days, whilst other palsies may never repair completely.

General Advice

- *Consult a cranial osteopath for treatment.*
- *If resolution is not forthcoming within a few days, discuss the matter with a medical practitioner for investigations via a neurologist.*
- *Having established that the cause is not serious and if homeopathy and osteopathy have failed, consider acupuncture with or without the concurrent use of Chinese herbs.*
- *Until discussed with an acupuncturist or Shiatsu practitioner avoid rubbing the area, as this may worsen the matter.*

Supplemental

- *Use vitamin B_1 (100mg with each meal) for three days only in combination with lecithin (1000mg with each meal), a multi-B complex, folic acid (400µg) and extra vitamin B_{12}, all for one week.*

Homeopathic

- *Consult a homeopath for a suitable remedy.*

NERVE DAMAGE

A damaged nerve may cause pain, paralysis, paresthesia (altered sensation) or an alteration in perception in any of the five senses. The effects will depend on which nerves are damaged and treatment is adjusted depending on the site.

Nerves are divided into those in the brain and spinal column, known as the central nervous system, and those on the outside of these areas, known as peripheral nerves. Every part of the body is innervated except for thickened skin, hair and nails, but very often their surrounding parts compensate by being extremely sensitive.

Nerves are further divided into motor and sensory, which control movement and sensation, respectively. A further subdivision is made in the motor nerves: those that are under our control and those that are not. The *autonomic* (non-controlled) nervous system governs the beating of our heart, our non-conscious respiration, our involuntary bladder valves, etc. One may come across the terms *sympathetic* and *parasympathetic* nerves, which are part of this system and act in opposition to each other. For example, the parasympathetic nervous system slows down the heart, whereas the sympathetic nervous system speeds it up. Adrenaline and noradrenaline are the most common catecholamines or neurotransmitters that affect the sympathetic and parasympathetic system in different ways. The ins and outs of biochemical control are complex and not particularly relevant when treating damaged nerves on a self-help basis.

Treatment must depend on the actual problem and, as always, the underlying cause of the nerve damage must be alleviated where possible. The principal causes are:

- Direct injury – injury to a nerve may be partial damage or a partially or completely severed nerve.
- Deficiency – the nerves are made up of proteins and specialized fats as well as vitamins and other nutrients; very common deficiencies are vitamin B_{12}, folic acid and essential fatty acids.
- Disease processes – multiple sclerosis, other sclerosing diseases, infections and metabolic disorders such as diabetes or hypothyroidism. Specific infections such as tetanus, polio and shingles are notorious for causing either pain or paralysis by damaging the nerves.
- Toxicity – alcohol, drugs, smoking and agrochemicals are all culprits. Lead, mercury, aluminium and, rarely nowadays, arsenic are all known to cause nerve damage and, interestingly, an excess of vitamin E may cause problems.

We are told by the orthodox world that nerves do not regrow. This is not strictly true and some nerve transmission may be reconstructed even in a completely severed nerve if the opposing ends are joined either naturally or by a surgical technique. More importantly, the body has the ability to grow new nerves or retrain other nerves to innervate the area that the damaged nerve has ceased to affect.

NEURALGIA

This is the medical term for nerve pain and is most commonly associated with trigeminal neuralgia or sciatica (*see* **Trigeminal neuralgia** *and* **Sciatica**).

RECOMMENDATIONS

General Advice

- *Pain relief with orthodox drugs may be a necessary first-line treatment because of the severity of nerve pain associated with injury.*
- *Any loss of movement or change in sensation, such as numbness or tingling, should be reviewed by a medical practitioner for a firm diagnosis. Remember that many neurological symptoms are not due to nerve damage but are associated with muscular or vascular conditions.*
- *Acupuncture and mild electro-acupuncture treatment can be instantly relieving and help healing.*
- *Marma massage and other Ayurvedic-derived techniques, such as neurotherapy, can be of benefit.*
- *Alexander Technique, yoga and Qi Gong may all help in the redevelopment of innervative areas.*

Supplemental

- *These supplements may be utilized in the following doses per foot height, divided with meals throughout the day: manganese 0.5mg, magnesium 100mg, lecithin 200mg. If there is no improvement within a couple of days, please contact a complementary medical practitioner initially and consider specific deficiency tests through blood or hair analysis.*
- *Take twice the recommended daily allowance of a multivitamin B complex. Chromium (40µg per foot of height in divided doses) can be taken with food three times a day.*
- *Extract from the common oat (Avena sativa) can be taken as a fluid extract – 1 teaspoonful with water every 3hr.*

Homeopathic

- *The homeopathic remedies Hypericum, Arsenicum, Ranunculus, Aconite and Iris should all be reviewed in your favourite homeopathic manual.*

NUMBNESS

Numbness is known in medical parlance as paresthesia. It describes a sensation of partial or local anaesthesia or a deficiency of sensation. The term can be used for a psychological experience but this is not strictly medical.

Numbness occurs because of interference with nerve function and is generally caused by injury, inflammation, infection or disease, affecting the nerve directly or interfering with the blood supply.

RECOMMENDATIONS

General Advice

- *Persistent numbness should be examined by a GP with possible referral for investigations through a neurologist. Conditions such as multiple sclerosis and diabetes may initially present as numbness and, especially in the case of the latter disease, early diagnosis and treatment can make a profound difference in the long term.*
- *See **Neuralgia** and also **Atheroma** if a compromised blood flow is associated.*
- *Osteopathy and chiropractic may relieve pressure if the numbness is coming from a structural origin such as a malaligned spine or cramped muscle.*
- *Numbness may be associated, as may any neurological disorder, with a stagnation of Qi (energy). Acupuncture and Shiatsu may relieve this, as may specific Chinese or, preferably, Tibetan herbal treatments.*

Supplemental

- *Numbness may be an indication of a deficiency in minerals or vitamins, especially vitamin B_{12}.*

Blood and hair analysis are recommended before supplementation.

Homeopathic

- *Several homeopathic remedies are indicated and referral to a homeopathic Materia medica or a homeopath is recommended. The remedies Argentum nitricum, Gelsemium, Lycopodium and Rhus toxicodendron are all commonly found in a home remedy kit and can be used at potency 6 every 3hr until a suitable remedy is selected. Please refer to your preferred homeopathic manual for an initial choice.*

PAIN

Pain is a localized or diffuse sensation ranging from discomfort to agony. It is caused by stimulating special nerve endings known as pain fibres. Trauma or disease irritates these nerves either directly or through the release of chemicals, which include arachidonic acid (AA) or substance P. There are four stages in pain recognition. Mild stimulation or the presence of only small amounts of these chemicals may create an itch or irritation, but as the stimulation increases pain occurs. This process is known as *Initiation*.

Next comes *Transmission*. The ends of these fibres send off chemical impulses along the peripheral nerve into the central nervous system in the spinal column. On the way the chemical messages pass through junctions known as synapses between nerves. Some of these connections are equivalent to checkpoints. A certain amount of chemical messenger has to be accrued before the next nerve will transmit. These junctions are known as pain gates. Once these pain gates are overcome, transmission terminates at the pain centres in the brain.

The third stage is *Recognition*. The pain centres are connected to the consciousness and send in pulses to create an appropriate response. The fourth and final stage of pain is *Response*. Initial response is by reflex and further response is conscious.

Once the pain centre has been stimulated, impulses are sent out, generally causing constriction of the muscles in the area, thereby creating reflex recoil. This moves the part away from any external cause. The next response is a conscious one. Movements such as shaking or gripping may be of benefit by changing the level of compression on the affected nerve endings. Whilst this almost instantaneous action is taking place, the brain is releasing endorphins, the body's natural opiates, which begin the process of pain relief by acting on the pain centres, pain gates and nerve transmission.

Pain relief is achieved by decreasing sensitivity at a local level through pain-relieving compounds from specific white blood cells and nerve fibres. The peripheral nerves and central nervous system are affected by pain-relieving chemicals.

It is important to understand that pain is not an enemy. The orthodox world has studied and engineered antipain compounds, which are of course the best-selling and most profitable of drugs. Indeed, pain relief is perhaps one of the major things that doctors can achieve for the patient. The holistic view, however, is to establish the cause of the pain and deal with that to achieve a longer lasting effect. The drug companies might prefer us to take regular painkillers for a splinter we may find in our hand, whereas a sensible physician would remove the splinter.

A recent study and publication by a pain control specialist has shown that the use of orthodox pain-suppressing drugs may actually enhance and increase the duration of pain. The hypothesis is that artificial painkilling drugs suppress the body's own painkilling response. The more drugs that are taken, the more the suppression. Chronic pain treated with drugs may relieve after an initial painful six-week withdrawal period and the individual be left with a reduced need of painkillers.

The body creates pain for three reasons:

- *Pain as a warning.* If we stick our hand near a fire, pain receptors tell us to stop. If we drink coffee and create dyspepsia through acidity, it is the body telling us not to drink coffee. Interestingly, pain is often absent in serious disease processes such as cancer, diabetes or AIDS until it is too late.

- *Pain as a repair process.* Pain initiates reflex responses. Not only does this move a body part away from the noxious stimulus but it also creates a reflex within blood vessels. A stimulated pain nerve will send an impulse to the spinal column and a reflex reaction will return an impulse to the surrounding vessels. These will dilate, allowing more blood into the area carrying more oxygen, white blood cells and nutrients for repair. Pain is associated with inflammation and inflammation is this increased blood flow which causes heat, swelling and redness. Inflammation and pain are actually healing processes and should not be inhibited unless they are interfering with the healing, which may occur if the response is too great.

- *Pain without purpose.* There are conditions where pain is no longer of use from the point of view of warning, nor does it need to continue because the repair process is already underway. Serious injuries and the late stages of a disease process do not benefit from pain. In these late diseases or injuries the consciousness of pain is incorrect. Referred pain, one that is sensed in an area that is not injured, falls into this category. The pain in a 'phantom' limb (after amputation) is an example. More commonly we may feel pain down our leg from a trapped nerve in the back, which is a referred pain acting as both a warning and a repair process but is in fact in the wrong place.

It is important not to treat pain as a problem but as a symptom. Even the orthodox world tends to avoid suppressing pain until the cause is established. Pain relief should be aimed at decreasing the sensitivity of local, peripheral or central nerve receptors, but also anything that increases sensitivity. Animal fats (which contain high levels of amino acids, caffeine and stress chemicals such as adrenaline) all sensitize the nervous system.

RECOMMENDATIONS

General Advice

- *Always establish the cause of pain. Seek medical advice and diagnostic techniques if uncertain.*
- *Examine the cause and discern whether the reason is a warning or a repair. Heed the warning and encourage the repair before initiating pain-relieving treatment.*
- *Consider structural correction through osteopathy, chiropractic or Shiatsu if the pain is due to a structural defect. Cranial, spinal, pelvic and joint malalignment is a common cause of nerve entrapment.*
- *Cranial osteopathy may be very beneficial, especially if the pain is persistent.*
- *Transcutaneous electrical nerve stimulation (TENS) is the passing of a mild electrical impulse through the nerves, which can stimulate the pain-relieving chemicals.*
- *Acupuncture may be instantly relieving and curative, as may acupressure. Specific points may be illustrated by a practitioner of acupuncture or Shiatsu and acupuncture or acupressure books.*
- *Pain is subjective and therefore techniques such as hypnotherapy, relaxation and biofeedback will benefit.*

Supplemental

- *Long-term pain may be alleviated by taking the following compounds in divided doses throughout the day at the following amounts per foot of height: eicosapentaenoic acid (300mg) and D,L-phenylalanine (300mg) and vitamin B_1 (10mg per foot of height with three meals a day for three days and then once per day only).*

Homeopathic

- *Homeopathic remedies are numerous but do not act in the same way as an orthodox or herbal painkiller. A dose of a remedy will not have an instant effect but will increase the painkilling response and help to diminish the consciousness if the pain is of no use. Homeopathic remedies encourage healing, so if a pain is warning or repairing, a remedy may actually worsen the discomfort initially. Referral to your preferred homeopathic manual will aid selection. Arnica 6 can be taken for any pain every 10min until an accurate homeopathic selection is made.*

Herbal/natural extracts

- *Acute pain may be treated with naturopathic medication but do not assume that these are necessarily free from side effects or safe. The following compounds can be used with safety topically but ingestion is best prescribed by a herbalist because the quality and quantity of any active ingredient within a herbal extract can never be certain: clove and thyme (oil or powdered extract) can be very useful on open wounds, especially gum and tooth pain, wintergreen, willow and meadowsweet all contain salicylic acid (aspirin) but there is no benefit to using this rather than the proprietary form and, for the reason mentioned above, no quantities are given here.*
- *Capsicum (in the form of hot peppers in the daily diet) and chamomile (as a strong infusion) may be beneficial for long-term pain.*

Orthodox

- *Be wary of the side effects of orthodox painkillers. Specific compounds can be reviewed in chapter 10. However, mild orthodox pain relief from aspirin, paracetemol or acetominophen can be considered if the side effects are not contraindicated.*

RESTLESSNESS

Restlessness is not a serious medical condition but most of us will struggle with the symptoms at some time in our lives. It is usually associated with boredom and when a clear correlation is apparent, the answer is to relieve the inactivity.

The difficulty is that we are often unaware of our spiritual, psychological or physical boredom and restlessness can interfere with our normal functions.

Restlessness is the chemical effect of stress neurotransmitters on the nervous system. Treatment needs to be geared towards removing excess stress chemicals and repairing any deficiencies that might be placing the nervous system under pressure.

General Advice

- *Isolate any obvious cause of a spiritual or psychological emptiness and fill it with activity, mental exercise, meditation or prayer.*
- *If there is no apparent reason for restlessness, then consider counselling or hypnotherapy to isolate a subconscious craving.*
- *Remove all neurological stimuli such as caffeine, cigarettes, excess alcohol or other drugs, all of which, directly or indirectly, will overstimulate the nervous system.*
- *If restlessness comes and goes, consider any correlation to foods eaten because food allergy may be relevant.*
- *A persistence beyond the above measures may be suggestive of a nutritional deficiency and blood and hair analysis of vitamin and mineral lack should be undertaken under the guidance of a complementary medical practitioner.*
- *Cranial osteopathy may be a temporary treatment.*

RESTLESS LEGS SYNDROME

This is a condition that is characterized by a crawling, itching and sometimes painful sensation in the legs and thighs, which is relieved by moving the legs either by shaking or walking. The condition rarely has an association with serious underlying neurological disease, although an imbalance in the central nervous system's neurochemistry is hypothesized.

Other than being an uncomfortable situation and, as it usually comes on half an hour into sleep, being an infrequent cause of insomnia, this condition is not serious.

There is certainly a relationship to stimulants, especially caffeine and other compounds that affect the nervous system, such as nicotine and alcohol. Drug withdrawal may be the cause and it is important to remember that withdrawal may not necessarily be associated with a complete cessation of use from a high level. Missing out on a nightly 'joint' when this is a regular habit may create withdrawal and withdrawal may come into effect around midday for those who drink heavily each evening. There is hereditary correlation and pregnancy may trigger the condition. This latter aspect has led to the investigation of deficiencies, and folic acid and iron are frequently found to be deficient in those who suffer. It is important to establish why these deficiencies have occurred; if there is a malabsorption syndrome, deal with that rather than just supply the supplement.

Anxiety and stress may be relevant, causing the production of chemicals that interfere with calming processes.

General Advice

- *Regular exercise, preferably in the evening, may reduce excessive stress chemical production at night.*
- *Practise a meditation technique or Qi Gong, yoga or Tai Chi.*
- *Malalignment of the spine may put pressure on nerves, and osteopathy and massage therapies may benefit.*

Nutritional

- *Consider reviewing the section on detoxifying diets if a toxin or drug is taken regularly or has recently been stopped (see **Detox diet**).*

Supplemental

- *Investigate through blood and hair analysis any mineral and vitamin deficiency and correct this through supplementation by taking three times the recommended daily dose in divided portions with food throughout the day. Pay special attention to iron, folic acid and vitamin B complex deficiencies. (Please see a nutritionist if you are pregnant.)*

Homeopathic

- *Please refer to your homeopathic manual for a suitable homeopathic remedy. There are many choices, depending upon the symptom picture.*

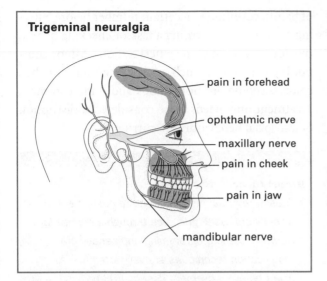

Trigeminal neuralgia

- pain in forehead
- ophthalmic nerve
- maxillary nerve
- pain in cheek
- pain in jaw
- mandibular nerve

TRIGEMINAL NEURALGIA

Trigeminal neuralgia is a sudden severe lancing pain that affects the forehead, cheek area or jaw on one side of the face. The pain is caused by irritation of the trigeminal nerve, which senses pain from three main branches that travel from each of these areas. The irritation is usually from an area of trauma at the angle of the mouth, the side of the nose or in front of the ear but may occur because of inflammation along the nerve pathway or even the presence of a tumour.

RECOMMENDATIONS

General Advice

- *A firm diagnosis needs to be established by a doctor or a neurologist and any underlying serious condition ruled out.*
- *See* **Neuralgia**.

PSYCHOLOGICAL MATTERS

AGORAPHOBIA

Literally a fear of open places or spaces, although also more commonly used to described the fear of leaving home. This condition is more common than one would expect and mostly affects women.

Mild cases can be dealt with most efficiently by homeopathy but if the condition is disrupting normal life and is unresponsive to basic treatment then counselling is recommended. Agoraphobia is commonly associated with a past event, which once examined is usually treatable.

RECOMMENDATIONS

General Advice

- *See a psychotherapist with a speciality in hypnotherapy, neurolinguistic programming or eye-movement desensitization.*
- *Avoid situations that cause the anxiety whilst you are having treatment.*

Supplemental

- *Use D,L-phenylalanine (50mg per foot of height) with each meal.*

Homeopathic

- *Review and try the homeopathic remedies Anthemis nobilis, Anarcardium and Lycopodium. These remedies should be used at potency 200, one dose each night for seven nights.*
- *In acute situations Aconite and Arsenicum album can be used at potency 6, four pills every 10min.*

ANXIETY

Anxiety like any emotion is a necessary survival factor. No anxiety means no apprehension of potential danger. Nature does not encourage this. Anxiety is not a negative emotion unless it overpowers normal function.

Anxiety can be acute or chronic: acute anxiety will occur in relation to frightening or worrying events, chronic anxiety is persistent and pathological if it has no logical foundation. Being anxious about, for instance, a loss of job or failing relationship is not wrong and would be best dealt with through counselling and some basic homeopathic remedies.

ACUTE ANXIETY

General Advice

- *Learn and practise a breathing and relaxation technique.*

Homeopathic

- *Consider the following homeopathic remedies at potency 6 every 10min: Arsenicum album or Pulsatilla for anxiety at night, Sulphur for anxiety on awakening; Aconite, Causticum or Ignatia for anxiety with fear; Aconite or Baryta carbonica for anxiety with fever. As always, it is best to review a homeopathic manual when choosing.*

Herbal/natural extracts

- *Weak, sweet tea or chamomile tea is beneficial because anxiety can be associated with low blood sugar.*

CHRONIC ANXIETY

General Advice

- *Consider counselling if the anxiety levels are altering your daily life.*
- *Relaxation or meditation techniques are essential.*
- *Alcohol can offer a temporary relief but may lead to persistent use and possible dependence in the same way that a drug such as a beta-blocker might. Avoid both.*

Nutritional

- *Avoid stimulating foods at night, especially cheese, chocolate and spices.*

Homeopathic

- *Visit a homeopath for a suitable remedy.*

COMPULSIVE OR OBSESSIVE DISORDERS

Compulsive/obsessive disorders are a group of psychological complaints characterized by repetitive actions of non-essential or useful activities. They can be looked upon as uncontrollable physical habits. The most common examples are frequent washing of hands, counting to a certain number before entering a room or performing a task or checking behind the door every time one enters a room. Minor compulsions/obsessions such as checking under the bed before sleeping are not serious and quite common. Treatment only needs to be considered if disruption or antisocial behaviour is occurring.

General Advice

- *These are not conditions that are easily treated by self-help. Seek guidance through a counsellor. Neurolinguistic programming and behavioural modification techniques are very effective, as might be eye-movement desensitization.*

Homeopathic

- *Homeopathic remedies can be utilized but need to be prescribed by a homeopath and should be used in conjunction with counselling.*

DEPRESSION

Everybody will experience depression as part of the normal cycle of emotions. Depression should not be treated except when the sadness, melancholy or dejection is unrealistic or out of proportion to the apparent cause.

If one can accept that the human being is an energy source of which some is material (body), some is mental function (mind) and the remaining part is emotion or being (spiritual), then depression must be looked at on all three levels. Depression manifests in all levels and treatment needs to be directed to correcting the imbalance.

Manifestations of depression

- Mental – increased or decreased levels of activity, an inability to sleep or an excessive desire to stay asleep, an inability to concentrate or memorize and prolonged periods of physical overactivity or inactivity.
- Spiritual – indifference to oneself or those around you, decreased ability to enjoy that which

was enjoyable, a sense of inadequacy, worthlessness and, very often, guilt, a decrease in libido, recurrent thoughts of how much better things would be if one were dead.

- Physical – weight loss or weight gain, unexplained physical weakness, persisting feelings of tiredness and lack of energy and increased or decreased appetite.

Medically speaking four or more of the above symptoms are required to be defined as depression and these have to persist for longer than a few days.

Endogenous and exogenous depression

The terms endogenous (created from within) and exogenous (caused by external influence) are really academic because they overlap to such a great extent. I do feel, however, that it helps to have a good understanding of why a depression may not be the fault of will power; also, being able to define whether a problem is endogenous or exogenous is essential in recommending treatment. Years of psychotherapy may not affect an endogenous depression, whereas the most potent drugs will not provide a cure for an allergic exogenous depression.

Endogenous depression

The causes of endogenous depression are:

- A lack of the nervous system's natural 'happy juice', such as serotonin and dopamine.
- An excess of the CNS-depressive chemicals.
- Deficiencies in the nutrients necessary for the production of 'happy juice', such as tryptophan, phenylalanine, vitamins B_6, B_3 and lecithin, to name but a few.
- Hormonal deficiencies, particularly in thyroid hormones and cortisol. Female hormonal fluctuations of oestrogen and progesterone can have profound effects on mood.
- Hypoglycaemia (low blood sugar levels), which is often associated with a diet high in refined carbohydrates.

- Seasonal affective disorder (SAD) (*see* relevant section).
- Postnatal depression created by the fluctuation of female hormones.

Exogenous depression

The causes of exogenous depression are:

- Depression created by life events, such as bereavement, job loss and relationship break up.
- Direct toxic effect from chemicals such as nicotine from cigarettes, aldehydes as the breakdown products of alcohol and the effects of most 'come downs' from recreational drugs.
- Specific doctor-prescribed drugs such as steroids, antibiotics and those drugs that may have a depressing effect on the thyroid gland or on sugar levels.
- Food allergies.
- Environmental pollutants, whether inhaled or ingested through food.
- Infections, most commonly viral but very often overlooked are fungal and parasitic infections.
- A lack of exercise, which prevents the production of the body's natural opiates – endorphins and enkephalins.

St John's Wort (Hypericum)

St John's Wort is currently an unlicensed herbal remedy in the UK and USA but in Germany it is more popular than other anti-depressants with over three million prescriptions each month. There is no doubt that it is an effective anti-depressive medication for mild to moderate depression. As the body can generally deal with herbs better than orthodox, artificial compounds, there are grounds for using this as a first line treatment. The Medicines Control Agency in the UK has suggested that this herb may interfere with other medication and should only be prescribed by a medically qualified practitioner. The following are drugs that the MCA recommends should not be taken with St John's Wort:

anti-depressants
epileptic drugs
migraine drugs
steroids
warfarin

digoxin
HIV drugs
oral contraceptive pills
theophylline tablets

It is probably wise for anyone intending to take any herbal treatment to check if there is any known adverse effect when taken with another compound.

Seasonal affective disorder (SAD)

This condition is associated with the grey clouds of the winter seasons and the shorter days and longer nights. Sunlight, in particular the ultraviolet spectrum, triggers a reduction of a hormone, melatonin, by the pineal gland and increases serotonin from this and other areas in the brain. Melatonin reduction increases female hormone activity and interferes with sleep, both of which can adversely affect mood. Serotonin is a neurotransmitter of the brain and is, effectively, 'happy juice'. A lack of these chemicals leads to mild to moderate depression. Indeed, depression is a far more common problem in the upper Northern hemisphere than closer to the equator. Perhaps the same would be found in the longer nights of the Southern hemisphere.

RECOMMENDATIONS

General Advice

- If negative feelings persist for longer than a few days and seem to be inappropriate, then discuss the matter with your preferred complementary medical practitioner.
- Further discussions with a counsellor are recommended if the feelings persist. Recourse to an orthodox medical practitioner, unless they are strongly holistic in their outlook, should be considered only as a last resort because all too often the only weapon in their armoury is drug treatment.
- Have a good look at your lifestyle and eliminate smoking, caffeine, alcohol and other drugs until the depression has eleviated. Ensure that you have a good balance between your mind/body/spirit existence. Not enough exercise, not enough time spent in meditation or prayer or indeed an excess of physical or mental activity will allow energy to flow from one level to the other, leaving deficiencies that can manifest as depression.
- Review any orthodox medication, including the oral contraceptive, which might be a depressant.
- If problems persist ask a GP to check for thyroid, cortisol and blood sugar levels. A complementary medical practitioner or GP should also check for persisting infections such as glandular fever or other such manifestations of Epstein-Barré virus or candidiasis. Chronic fatigue syndrome should be ruled out.
- Consider the possibility of postnatal or seasonal affective disorder (SAD).
- Nutritional deficiencies need to be corrected, as mentioned above, but please do not forget to drink half a pint of water per foot of height per day because chronic dehydration may manifest itself as depression.
- Encourage the production of endorphins and enkephalins through exercise.
- Regular aerobic exercise is important but daily work with Qi Gong, Tai Chi or yoga may be curative for depression.
- If seasonal affective disorder (SAD) is a possibility (and even if it is not) consider the following:

  ○ Ensure you spend time outside without glasses or contact lenses interfering with a view of blue sky or white cloud.

  ○ Consider obtaining an ultraviolet lamp. Studies suggest that a minimum of two hours exposure is necessary, but keeping the lamp within three or four feet of the desk at which you work, in the kitchen or by your favourite chair may be as beneficial.

  ○ Consider taking melatonin supplements as

directed by your GP. Doses are usually around 1mg three times a day or 3mg nightly.

Nutritional

- Avoid refined carbohydrates and any oversweet foods.
- Consider the coinciding times of depression with specific foods either by maintaining an accurate dietary journal or by having a food allergy test through blood, vega or bioresonance tests.

Supplemental

- Preferably under the guidance of your complementary medical practitioner, consider using the following supplements at high doses depending on the quality and quantity of the appetite through the depression: an essential amino acid complex that includes tryptophan (minimum 2g per day) and D,L-phenylalanine (minimum 700mg per day). (There is some controversy about the safety of tryptophan following reports of toxicity when given at high doses. Consult a knowledgeable nutritionist); vitamin B complex at up to ten times the daily recommended dose; vitamin C, folic acid and magnesium at three times the recommended daily allowance.

Homeopathic

- Homeopathic remedies at high potency (1M or above – see page 652) are potentially curative but need to be selected based on all the symptoms of depression. Consult a homeopath.

Herbal/natural extracts

- St John's Wort (Hypericum) should be considered as a first line herbal alternative to orthodox drugs, preferably with medical advice.

Orthodox

- If all else has failed, then consider the use of drug treatment. Chemicals such as Lithium carbonate are well established and, if monitored, safe enough in conditions such as manic depression.

ELECTRIC SHOCK TREATMENT (ELECTROCONVULSIVE THERAPY – ECT)

Many people are surprised to find that ECT is not only still performed but is quite common. Certain psychiatrists still hold with this as an effective treatment for severe depression that is unresponsive to drug therapy, despite the potential risks to life, long-term memory and any other brain function. Believe it or not, ECT at one time was used to change personality traits such as aggressive behaviour or suicidal tendencies. It was even used as an aversion therapy towards homosexuality. Fortunately, we have moved forward.

RECOMMENDATIONS

General Advice

- Ensure that all complementary medical avenues have been explored because orthodox medicine often overlooks the possibility of deficiencies and food allergy.

Orthodox

- Electroconvulsive therapy must only be considered when all other avenues have been exhausted.

EMOTIONS

Emotion is a normal expression of feeling and venting of any emotion is essential to long term well-being. Suppression of emotion and the consequential maintenance of high levels of adrenaline in the system may be responsible for conditions as diverse as rashes and cancer. Eastern philosophy considers emotion to create internal heat, which needs to be expressed and eventually will be.

Emotion is only a pathological matter if it is expressed out of proportion to what triggered it. It is also unwise to allow emotion to be expressed as a secondary emotion. This means that if you are unhappy about an event but then feel anger towards being unhappy, the emotion is a secondary emotion. Feelings about feelings are generally not productive and lead to inner psychological turmoil.

RECOMMENDATIONS

General Advice

- If you do not feel in control of your anger or if your anger is directed towards another emotion, organize a consultation with a psychotherapist to establish the best type of therapy.
- Learn a meditative technique and practise this daily with the yoga or Qi Gong techniques suitable for your emotional state.
- Initiate regular body work treatments, such as massage or Shiatsu, which are marvellous at dissipating unwanted emotional chemicals.

Homeopathic

- Review a homeopathic manual and use potency 200 of the remedy that most matches your emotional state nightly for ten nights.

MANIC DEPRESSION (BIPOLAR DEPRESSION)

Everybody has mood swings. Those of us who have uncontrollable changes in our behaviour pattern, from overexcitement, overactivity and sleeplessness to periods of depression, marked lethargy and apathy, are termed manic depressive or bipolar depressive.

Whilst there is a tendency for this condition to run in families, true manic depression is generally a neurochemical imbalance caused by the brain tissues either making too much or too little 'happy juice'.

Certain factors – hormonal, drug or food stimulants, hypoglycaemia or food allergy – may heighten emotions and thereby turn what would usually be regular mood swings into a type of manic depression. Pregnancy and premenstrual syndrome very commonly cause marked shifts in moods because of the sensitivity of the individual to the oestrogen and progesterone levels. This is not manic depression although some beleaguered husbands may think so!

RECOMMENDATIONS

General Advice

- If mood swings are apparent and life disturbing, discuss the matter with a psychotherapist to establish whether manic depression is a likely diagnosis. Counselling in itself may be beneficial and neurolinguistic programming may help to train an individual to recognize the early signs of either end of the emotional scale and teach control methods.
- Yeast infections in the bowel, especially Candida, may create the deficiencies that lead to bipolar depression as well as producing chemicals that enhance the condition. See **Depression** for the down side of this condition and **Hysteria** for the manic part.

Nutritional

- Eliminate alcohol, caffeine, refined foods (especially sugars), cigarettes and recreational drugs.
- Have a food allergy test performed or keep a very accurate journal listing the foods eaten and the mood felt. See if there is any isolated food or food groups that trigger either emotional state.

Supplemental

- Deficiencies in zinc, B-complex, calcium, magnesium or the active substance in lecithin known as phosphatidylcholine may all be relevant and taking four times the RDA (recommended daily allowance) may make a difference. This should be done as a trial for two weeks and if an improvement is noted the information should be taken to a complementary medical practitioner with experience in this area to analyse your diet or consider why absorption is not taking place.
- Amino acid deficiency, especially tryptophan and phenylalanine, is common.

Orthodox

- As a last resort, psychiatric administration of the drug lithium may be necessary.

STRESS

Stress is an ever-increasingly popular term invading our language and life. Medically speaking, stress is a group of chemicals known as catecholamines and steroids. The better known are adrenaline (epinephrine) and noradrenaline (norepinephrine). The body's natural steroids, cortisol being the most prominent, have a marked influence on the system and are produced in response to stress.

Stress may be psychologically induced, as common usage of the word conveys, but the chemicals are also produced through physical discomfort from overexercising, excessive tiredness and unfavourable environmental conditions (too hot or too cold). The stress chemicals may also be produced as a response to toxicity from pollution, ingestion of toxins or food allergy.

It is worth differentiating between stress and pressure. Every animal reacts better if there is a certain amount of adrenaline in the system. A challenge or an exciting prospect may produce a small amount of stress chemical, which will create a certain amount of 'drive' to perform a function. This is a good thing. In fact I would go so far as to say that without pressure we may not fare so well. Stress is an overproduction of adrenaline and other stress chemicals.

Stressors (as stress chemicals are collectively known) have evolved with us and are the principal reason why most animals survive. If other hormones had as strong an influence as stress chemicals, emotions other than fear and a need to fight would have become prominent. For example, if sex hormones exerted a stronger influence than adrenaline then our distant ancestors might have carried on making love despite the arrival of a sabre-toothed tiger. Those of our ancestors who had a stronger adrenaline response would run away. Those who did not would finish the job and probably be killed.

Natural selection has, therefore, provided us with a very sensitive anxiety response. We are no longer confronted by sabre-toothed tigers and life-threatening situations are few and far between, but we all have to face anxiety, ranging from 'where will we get our next meal?' and 'will we have a roof over our head?', to battles with our partners, bank managers and other road users! Our brain recognizes a stressful situation and tries to produce the relevant amount of adrenaline for it. Going into an unhappy job every day will produce a certain amount of adrenaline, being confronted by a masked knife-wielding foe will produce more. However, the latter event that produces a large amount of adrenaline immediately may be matched by the production of lower levels in response to lesser anxiety over a longer period of time. The long-term effects of persistent low-level stresses are well established and can cause an array of diseases and conditions, ranging from angina to ulcers. There are considered to be three stages in a stress reaction.

Initial response or alarm reaction

Faced with a dangerous situation, the level of stress hormones will rise causing two fundamental changes. Adrenaline and noradrenaline will open up blood vessels to the brain, heart, lungs and muscles, thereby encouraging oxygenation and nutrition to the organs that need to think, oxygenate and move the body. Cortisol and other steroids will flood the bloodsteam with glucose, providing energy. In combination with catecholamines, the blood supply to those organs not needed in a fight is then reduced by closing their arteries. Kidney and liver function will slow down and, more noticeably, a lack of blood to the skin will make us go pale, a lack of blood to the bladder will make us want to pass urine and a lack of blood to the bowel will make us register a need to defecate. In extreme shock we may go white, urinate and soil ourselves.

This so-called 'fight or flight' response increases the heart rate and the strength of heart contraction, increases the rate of breathing, increases sweat production (which lowers body temperature and eliminates the byproducts of metabolism that will have increased under the pressure of adrenaline) and effectively prepares us for action.

Comedown or resistance

The second stage is the comedown or resistance reaction. Here the body is no longer primed for action but is dealing with the abundance of chemicals and changes within the physiology of the body that have taken place.

Exhaustion

At some point after the resistance reaction an exhaustion phase may manifest. Under extreme stress the body may faint or even die. This is characterized by those who have noticed that helping an injured animal may initially be tolerated but by the time the animal has been placed in a box and taken to the vet it will have died. The initial fear was so great that when its life was 'spared' the resistance and exhaustion phases led to severe biochemical changes causing its death. It is rare to see this in human beings but all of us will have experienced the 'anticlimax' and exhaustion following anxious or nerve-wracking events such as exams or a first date!

The important aspect from all of this discussion is to appreciate that stress is a chemical reaction not a psychological state of mind, although the latter produces the former. Stress does not have to be manifested in sleeplessness, trauma or wide, staring eyes but can be produced without symptoms by a low persistent rate of stress chemical production. Stress creates excess energy or extra activity for the brain, heart, lungs and muscles, and exhaustion of these organs will lead to a predilection to disease. Conversely, the organs from which blood is taken may become deficient in nutrients and oxygen and may also be led to illness.

Stress management

We all undergo periods of anxiety; it is part of existing and attempting to 'better' ourselves. We,

as human beings, would not function or succeed if we were not pushed by catecholamine, cortisol and other stressors. It is important, however, to differentiate between being under pressure and being stressed. Most successful individuals, whatever their field, will achieve because of pressure. This drive should be focused on the appropriate event and not be transferred elsewhere. An employee angry with their boss should not take it out on their partner, friends or children. This act of transference is the main indicator that the drive has moved from being pressure to being stress. The stress chemicals are in abundance and are telling the body, mind and soul that it is in trouble. Trouble rarely comes in small bursts, according to our evolutionary development, and therefore a problem at work is carried through to

Aromatherapy

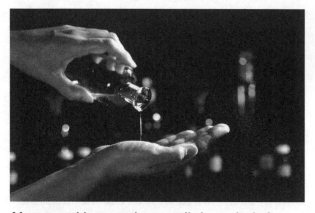

Massage with aromatherapy oils is particularly beneficial for relieving stress. The soothing effect of body work combines with the relaxing qualities of aromatherapy oils such as lavender.

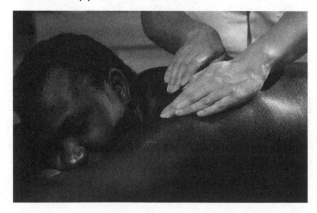

home. It is important to learn how to reduce stress chemical production and use up any excess chemicals in the bloodstream.

How to differentiate between pressure and stress is difficult. I think the answer may be simply to ask 'am I happy?' or 'can I accept this particular situation?'. If the answer is 'no' to either, then you are under stress and not pressure. If stress is present, then you run the risk of any number of conditions and diseases. It is argued by those with a strong meditative or spiritual belief that all physical ailments, except those created by age (and even that is often debated), are caused by an excess of stress chemicals.

RECOMMENDATIONS

General Advice

- *Be happy or at least at peace with the activities and emotions in your life. If you are not, sit with a counsellor and discuss the reasons.*
- *Learn a relaxation or meditation technique regardless. These produce anti-stress chemicals that will either act as a treatment or as a preventative measure. Practising for a few minutes a day is better than nothing at all, although ideally 1–2hr a day should be set aside for meditation. (I have been accused of supporting a concept of 'spiritual aerobics'!)*
- *Ensure a healthy environment both at work and home. Avoid pollution and dirt and consider the effects of radiation (see **Radiation**).*
- *Stress chemicals produce free radicals that are both damaging to cells and carcinogenic.*
- *Exercise burns up stress chemicals. Overexercising, however, may stress the body further. Set an exercise programme within your capabilities and slowly but gently increase activity. One session with a gym master or personal fitness instructor will solve your problems.*
- *Body work of any sort is beneficial. Human touch is soothing and produces chemicals that counteract stresses. Most practitioners*

are in the field because of a need or an ability to heal, and healing energy will counteract stresses.
- *Sound therapy has been researched and whether it is simply listening to music or sitting in acoustic chairs, which pass a vibration through the system, relaxation chemicals are promoted to counteract stresses.*

Nutritional

- *Consider physical causes of stress by establishing the presence of food allergies through blood tests and by avoiding these stressors.*

Supplemental

- *Take the following supplements (at the doses given per foot of height, divided throughout the day with meals) if under stress or if the diet does not have five portions of fruit and vegetables each day: beta-carotene (2mg), vitamin C (1g), vitamin E (100iu), selenium (40mg), coenzyme Q10 (5mg) and pycnogenol (grapeseed extract); maximum recommended dose on a good natural product.*
- *Supplementation with the amino acid D,L-phenylalanine, 150mg per foot of height in divided doses throughout the day. If available, tryptophan can be taken at the same dosage but, due to an unsubstantiated fear following problems because of faulty manufacture, this amino acid is no longer available as a supplement without a doctor's prescription. Tryptophan is available to non-vegetarians in meat, fish and turkey and to everyone through cottage cheese, milk, bananas, peanuts and lentils. Dried dates, interestingly, have a high proportion.*
- *Ginseng and adrenal gland extracts may be selected off the shelves and taken at twice the daily recommended dose for one week and then reduced to the recommended levels according to the packaging if an effect has been noticed within the first seven days.*

Homeopathic

- *Specific homeopathic remedies and herbal and antioxidant treatments are available but most of those that can be bought off the shelf are the wrong potency or too low in concentration to be efficacious. Stressed individuals should be under the care of a complementary medical practitioner.*

Herbal/natural extracts

- *Aromatherapy using lavender oils or other more specific extracts, depending upon the individual's personality and stress, will act as a pheromone (airborne chemical) and stimulate relaxation chemicals.*
- *Bach flower remedies chosen according to the symptoms of the individual will give benefit.*

CHAPTER 6

MIDDLE AGE AND ONWARDS

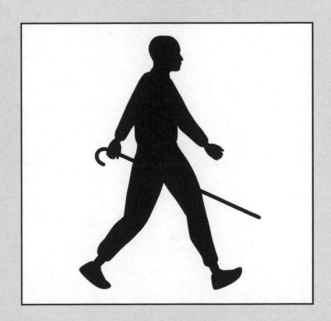

Middle Age and Onwards

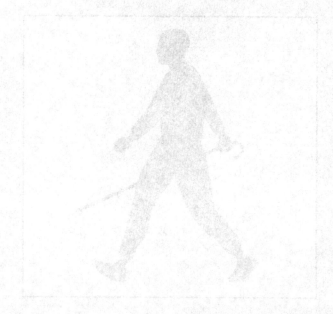

CHAPTER 6

MIDDLE AGE AND ONWARDS

I have chosen not to include a chapter in this book for old age. Complementary medical treatments are less beneficial in old age because we are reaching a time when our vital force is diminishing and repair is difficult. Treatments in old age are palliative (relieving) rather than curative.

It is better to establish health in our latter years by working on health concepts from a younger age. It is never too late to change habits and lifestyles and the advice given in this chapter will, I hope, encourage all of us to review our health at the beginning of the problems associated with ageing rather than once the damage has set in. Provided that no major damage has taken place, then the ageing process can be pleasurable, healthy and prolonged.

The process of ageing is dependent upon two factors. The first is the loss of vital force, this undeniable energy that keeps cells repairing and replicating. The second is the maintenance of good nutrition and oxygenation to all the cells in the body.

The presence of vital force is a much debated point and the Western scientific view is unlikely to agree with the Eastern philosophical view. Libraries could be dedicated to the books and journals that have been written on the principle of vital force. Proponents of meditation and mind/body energy workers would argue that it is feasible and easily possible to pull in life force from the universe to maintain health and youthfulness. Indeed, many yogis take in very little nutrition and yet maintain a very healthy lifestyle on the energy they absorb from the cosmos. This is beyond most of us in the West, who do not have a non-materialistic attitude or the time to practise the more dedicated spiritual techniques required.

A more Western orientation of ageing would be to assume that the byproducts of metabolism, the free radicals absorbed or produced, the decrease in essential hormone production and the natural process of clogging the arteries, thereby reducing the oxygen and nutrients to cells, all lead to ageing.

> **RECOMMENDATION**
>
> **General Advice**
> - *See* **Arteriosclerosis**, **Antioxidants** *and* **Free radicals**, **Stress** *and* **Meditation**. *Mastering and abiding by the rules of these areas is the simple answer to slowing the ageing process and avoiding the diseases associated with old age.*

GENERAL

ANTI-AGEING

Most of us would like to maintain throughout our lives the health that we generally take for granted up to our mid-thirties. Around this time things often start to go wrong. We can no longer work as hard and as long as we did, our memory diminishes and our ability to learn new things weakens. It takes longer for us to recover from injuries and we cannot exercise to the same degree that we once did. Our tolerance of toxins such as alcohol reduces and our recovery time from debauchery increases. Skin changes and loss of skin thickness gives outward signs of ageing and our internal organs start to diminish in their capacity. The slow process of decay is as inevitable as birth and death.

There are many factors that can be brought to bear and individual age-related conditions and diseases are discussed throughout this chapter. However, counteracting the fundamental reasons of what makes us age can influence the degree of discomfort we may have to endure in our later years. Put simply, the causes of ageing are:

1 A decrease in the blood supply to tissues.
2 A decrease in the nutrition and oxygen availability.
3 A decrease in hormones, particularly in growth hormone and others such as dehydroepiandrosterone (DHEA) that stimulates cellular growth and function.

RECOMMENDATIONS

General Advice
- *Please review the section on arteriosclerosis (atheroma), eat plenty of fresh fruit and vegetables or start early on in life taking high dose antioxidants to protect blood vessels.*
- *Maintain normal weight and exercise regularly.*

Nutritional
- *Certain scientists have suggested that eating minimal amounts of food providing all the necessary nutrition prolongs youthfulness. Full studies are still awaited on this but for the time being not eating to excess and aiming to leave the table slightly hungry may help the anti-ageing effect.*

Supplemental
- *High-dose antioxidants including vitamins A, C, E and CoQ 10. See* **Arteriosclerosis (atheroma)** *for dosages.*
- *Acetyl-L-carnitine, 500mg twice a day minimally may be beneficial against dementia.*
- *Hydergine, taken at the dosage recommended on the packaging, is an antioxidant and neurone protector that may be of benefit in age-related memory problems.*
- *Phosphatidyl serine, 500mg twice a day may improve cognition and age-related memory decline.*
- *Vitamin K as recommended on the product packaging reduces bone loss and protects against atheroma (arteriosclerosis).*

- *Carnosine, available naturally in red meat and chicken, is soon to become available in a tablet form. It mimics the protein that is found in youthful muscles and other tissues and it may be beneficial in Alzheimer's and inflammatory conditions such as arthritis.*

Herbal/natural extracts
- *Melatonin has an antioxidant and general anti-ageing property.*
- *DHEA 5mg per foot of height should be discussed with a physician or medically qualified practitioner. (Pregnenolone is another available compound that is converted into DHEA).*

Orthodox
- *Human growth hormone reduces body fat, increases muscle mass and skin thickness, but it must be prescribed by a doctor due to potential side effects.*
- *A drug piracetam claims to prevent and correct age related memory loss.*
- *The compound SAMe is still experimental. It works by preventing the breakdown of DNA, the genetic structure of human cells.*
- *Regenersen is a designer anti-ageing drug. It includes material from placenta, pancreas, testes and the amnion surrounding a foetus. The claim is that it is capable of repairing and regenerating ageing human organs by stimulating protein synthesis. Other types of RNA therapy are offered at Swiss, German and US clinics but we still await reliable studies.*

BLOOD CLOTTING AND CLOTS

The medical term for a blood clot is a *thrombus*. The formation of a thrombus is known as *thrombosis*. A thrombus differs from a clot because it forms within the cardiovascular system and is a danger because it may occlude a blood vessel or become loose and travel to a vital organ, causing obstruction at that distant site. If a thrombus moves it is known as an *embolus*.

A thrombus should form only if a blood

vessel is ruptured, which allows the blood to flow into tissues or become exposed to air thus triggering the clotting mechanism. The formation of a clot is dependent upon a cascade reaction involving 13 different chemical substances, one causing the activation of the next. The absence of one of these prevents or slows down clotting, sometimes to a fatal degree. The best-known condition is haemophilia, which is the absence of factor VIII. Factor IV is calcium and a deficiency in the availability of this mineral may influence clotting.

Hughes's syndrome (Sticky blood syndrome)

This is an autoimmune disease characterized by a tendency for blood clots to form anywhere in the body. It can be a cause of miscarriage due to clotting in the placenta, deep vein thrombosis (DVT), strokes (if the clot occurs in the brain), and it may be associated with Alzheimer's disease and multiple sclerosis.

RECOMMENDATIONS

General Advice

- *Any tendency to bruise or bleed more easily or for longer than expected should be investigated by a physician, who will perform tests for the clotting times and factors.*
- *Complementary medical work should be based on the findings. Homeopathy in particular should be considered.*
- *See* **Coronary thrombosis, Deep vein thrombosis** *and* **Pulmonary embolism** *if necessary.*

Herbal/natural extracts

- *If there is no obvious reason for a clotting deficit, consult a Chinese, Tibetan or Ayurvedic physician who will look at the problem from the view that the blood is 'too thin' and attention will be paid to correcting this through lifestyle changes, nutritional supplementation, herbal medication and acupuncture.*

DEATH AND DYING

This is a subject that could fill, and indeed has, a library of books. This short section will talk about dying rather than death, because dying is very much a part of our cycle and it is as necessary to have a 'healthy' lead up to death as it is to be healthy prior to conceiving.

Spiritually speaking, death may be considered an endpoint or a beginning. The importance is not about establishing which it is but being at peace with whichever decision you, as an individual, make. Whether you end on the right side of Jesus, in the house of Allah or reincarnate to continue your lessons, a belief is a great help in stemming the fear that is associated with dying. Indeed, one can be at rest as much with a religious belief as one can with believing that we are 'fodder for worms'. One should work towards a sense of conviction throughout life, and in doing so one will remove the fear of death.

The fear of dying is often not associated with the actual end point but more with the fear of pain and discomfort that is associated with this final act. Dying comfortably and without pain, anxiety or distress to the individual or those around is the necessary goal.

Death often arises swiftly through accident or rapid disease process, but all too often death is a process spanning over days, months or even years. Through that time the human being goes through a variety of emotions best described by Dr Elisabeth Kübler-Ross.

Denial

Initially we will deny the possibility of what we have always known to be an inevitability. However strong our conviction towards a religious or spiritual belief, the fear of the unknown will create an option for us. Do we continue to follow our lifelong belief or not? Indeed, we have had options all through our life and our mentality is not geared towards having no choice. We therefore tend to deny the possibility of this event.

Anger

Anger is due to the inevitability of death but tends to be reflected or transferred to the body, the person or those close at hand.

Bargaining

The individual will bargain with themselves, their lifestyle or their God, often as a backlash against the second stage of anger: 'Perhaps, because being upset has not worked, from now on I will be peaceful and understanding of the situation and then it may go away'.

Depression

There will come a point when the true realization occurs that this particular chapter of existence is drawing to a close and depression will set in. Regrets over actions and thoughts not realized and the feelings for those who will be left behind all come into play and create anything from mild to severe depression.

Acceptance

Most of the time, those going through the stages of dying will reach acceptance. It is a suitable end point and preferable to all the other emotional states because it invariably brings a level of calm both to the individual and to those close by.

Each stage may take a few hours to a few months to travel through and, like climbing a step ladder, we can slip or climb from one level to another but overall we generally move our way towards acceptance. There is no easy way of dealing with death in the short term, and it is perhaps better to consider dying from an early age.

It is a failing in the West that the loss of the extended family has removed most of us from being around the dying. For those who are dying there is the pleasure of having the exuberance of youth running around outside the bedroom and for those for whom death is far off it becomes less frightening when it is no longer part of the great unknown. In the West we have made death into a taboo subject, rarely discussing it in anything but morbid terms and often ending short discussions with 'I really do not want to talk about that'. Death and dying must be brought back into our social structure at an earlier age if we are to deal with this important part of our life.

RECOMMENDATIONS

General Advice

- *Start at a young age to openly discuss death and spend time with those who are dying, when possible, to experience the event.*
- *Understand the levels of denial, anger, bargaining, depression and, finally, acceptance, and relate that understanding to those around you.*
- *Constantly work on your own spiritual beliefs concerning death. By all means change your attitudes, but it is important to have a belief, whether it is considering death as a final endpoint or the start of a new life.*
- *Contend with outstanding practicalities. Deal with personalities who may find your death traumatic and also clear your own conscience by saying what needs to be said to those to whom it should be said. If possible, and should time allow, fulfil as many ambitions as possible, both practical and emotional.*
- *Discuss dying with a bereavement counsellor and ensure that you are conscious of the good and bad points of your leaving this life.*
- *Focus your attention on being comfortable and pain free. Discuss this with orthodox doctors and complementary medical practitioners because most alternative disciplines will have potentially useful techniques.*

Homeopathic

- *The homeopathic remedy Arsenicum album can be offered by homeopaths as a remedy that challenges the body when it nears death. If vital force can be redirected and be of help in comforting the individual, Arsenicum album will contribute. If the vital force is absent, the demand by Arsenicum album will not be met and the end will be smoother and less traumatic than it might otherwise be.*

Euthanasia

Although attitudes are changing throughout the world, and in certain parts of Europe and Australia medically assisted euthanasia is now legal under certain circumstances, taking one's own life is illegal. Most religions create a taboo around euthanasia and different Eastern philosophies have different views and values. Japanese society has its infamous hara-kiri, which is an accepted, expected and honoured tradition under the right circumstances. The concept of reincarnation, however, suggests that suicide or euthanasia will prevent the necessary pain, sorrow or discomfort that the soul needs to endure to avoid having to come back and learn the lesson next time round. Medically speaking it is hard, sometimes, to place the spiritual aspect above the level of physical suffering found in those who have had painful strokes, or who are struggling with neurological conditions such as motor neurone disease or multiple sclerosis or those in social circumstances that may be beyond human endurance.

RECOMMENDATIONS

General Advice

- *Always discuss thoughts of euthanasia with counsellors, and not with friends and family.*
- *Contact your National Euthanasia Society.*
- *Hunt around and you will find doctors or healthcare professionals who will be able to advise you on successful euthanasia techniques. Some may even be willing to assist, despite the legal risks. I have chosen not to include in this book the preferred and most successful technique.*

HORMONE REPLACEMENT THERAPY (HRT)

Hormone Replacment Therapy has been promoted in such a way that both the public and the medical profession assume that it is a necessary treatment course for any woman going through the menopause. However, much research since the 1960s leads to the conclusion that the use of hormones creates dangers that outweigh the claimed advantages.

The orthodox world would unhesitatingly encourage the use of hormone replacement therapy but initially alternative treatments can alleviate the problems without entailing the potential risks and side effects of HRT.

Osteoporosis and cardiovascular disease (such as heart attacks and strokes) are not the inevitable outcome of passing through the menopause, and protection against these conditions is discussed in the relevant sections of this book.

Along with vaccinations, the promotion of HRT is, in my opinion, one of the most devastating and misleading of the orthodox medical world's health guidelines. The medical profession seems to consider the menopause to be a 'deficiency disease'. It compares the lack of female hormones to that of thyroid or insulin deficiencies, which is simply not true. Four-fifths of the world's population will not have access to artificial HRT. It is ironic that this so-called 'third world' population also have strikingly lower levels of osteoporosis, heart disease, cancer and menopausal symptoms, which HRT is supposed to protect against.

Japan and Africa have negligible amounts of osteoporosis, cardiovascular disease and stroke in comparison with the West due to healthier lifestyles, nutrition and more exercise. All of these are very relevant to the disease processes that HRT supposedly helps to prevent.

Frankly and factually, the processes of ageing that the Western orthodox medical world would have us believe are due to our lack of oestrogen and progesterone are simply not reflected in those societies that have not been targeted for HRT use. Most, if not all, of the serious conditions and a majority of unpleasant symptoms are created by factors other than female hormone depletion. Nutrition, life-style and exercise are far more relevant than hormone levels.

Hormone replacement therapy is not well proven either in safety or efficacy. The pharmaceutical industry and many GPs may be unaware of scientific studies published in reputable medical journals that state that HRT has risks and is not as effective as we have thought.

Initially HRT was brought forward to remove the unwanted symptoms that the Western woman found uncomfortable. That is not to say that women from less-developed countries do not suffer similarly, but here in the West we are brought up to believe that any symptom is unnecessary and should be removed, regardless of the reason why it may be there. Most uncomfortable sensations are either a warning or a repair process and if the underlying cause is diagnosed and treated, the symptom often goes away. Unfortunately, after a few years it was found that 50 per cent of women who used HRT to alleviate menopausal symptoms stopped using the preparations because of unwanted side effects or ineffectiveness of the treatment. The pharmaceutical companies experimented with different levels of various oestrogens and progesterones and claimed that the newer preparations were far more effective. My experience and that of my senior colleagues supports latter-day studies showing that many women are still struggling with side effects, including continued periods.

The next stage was the pronouncement that HRT prevented osteoporosis. Many widely promoted studies showed that the use of artificial oestrogen prevented bone loss. Unfortunately for the HRT supporters, a large study of women in Framingham, Massachusetts is proving that shorter studies are not accurate and in fact are flawed. Only women who have been taking HRT for more than seven years show any appreciable difference in bone density and, because these women are at far greater risk of developing oestrogen-dependent cancers, the risk of more serious conditions outweighs any benefits. What is more, if women stopped their treatment after ten years, they would have the same fracture risk as the population who had not used HRT. Because most women may be advised to use HRT at around the

age of 50 years and most hip fractures (the greatest risk of osteoporosis) tend not to occur until the mid-seventies in age, one can immediately see the pointlessness of using HRT for this condition.

The industry went on to 'prove' that the use of HRT protects against coronary heart disease, stroke and raised cholesterol levels. I am afraid not. The Framingham study mentioned above suggests that the risk of heart disease is actually increased and contradicts the findings of numerous studies.

Up until 1993 the main studies supporting HRT as a protection against vascular disease were found to be markedly flawed. An example of this in one of the major trials is described in medical circles as 'selection bias'. A large group of women were divided into those who would receive HRT and those who would receive a placebo. Neither group would know what they were taking. For 'ethical' reasons all women in the group taking HRT who had any risk factors, ie health problems or genetic predispositions to diseases that were associated with oestrogen or progesterone, were eliminated but this same factor was not taken into consideration in the control group. What this meant was that those taking HRT were already at a much lower risk for cardiovascular disease than the control group. When the results came forward they were, not surprisingly, markedly in favour of HRT being a protector of women from heart attacks and strokes. The debate continues but I have yet to see any new trials that are supportive of HRT in these conditions. In fact, a recent *British Medical Journal* article showed no significant benefit from HRT in cardiovascular disease over a 10-year period.

The latest suggestion is that HRT may protect against certain bowel conditions but I think even the pharmaceutical industry is aware of this being a weak selling-point.

The risks of HRT

The availability and promotion of HRT has led to the GP neglecting or avoiding the necessary discussion about changes in our diet and the exercise we take, as well as the potentially damaging effects of smoking, alcohol and drugs. Menopause has become a trigger for GPs to prescribe either oestrogen-only preparations or the oestrogen/progesterone combinations.

To understand the risks it helps to know what the sex hormones are doing. Principally, oestrogen and progesterone stimulate cell division, especially in the inner lining of the uterus, breast tissue and ovaries. This is achieved by increasing the blood supply to these tissues by improving the strength of blood vessels and opening them up. These are exactly the reasons why people develop headaches, migraines and cramps.

The hormones also increase the clotting ability in the blood by making platelets adhere more readily and they also detrimentally raise fat levels in the blood. This combination in the slower blood flow in dilated arteries leads to blood clots, heart attacks and strokes.

Putting aside the ineffectiveness of artificial HRT, there are also the frank risks of taking these artificial chemicals. Despite discussions with gynaecologists and scientific specialists in this area, I am still very confused by what appears to me to be a simple logical argument. In the *British National Formulary*, the official publication of the Royal Pharmaceutical Society of Great Britain that lists all the drugs available, there are 27 contra-indications and 17 side effects of the use of the oral contraceptive pill. Hormone replacement therapy, made from predominantly the same chemicals, only lists seven contraindications but practically similar side effects. For some reason, when women reach the age when HRT can be prescribed, all the side effects that they may have had from the contraceptive pill a year previously are no longer a risk. Doctors, and I include myself in this, are actually told, for example, that the oral contraceptive pill should not be used in ladies with high blood pressure before menopause but at menopause this combination of artificial hormones may actually benefit hypertensives because of the 'protective' effects against heart attack and stroke. It does not make sense. I frankly find it indefensible and cannot understand why our professors persist in refusing to see the wood for the trees.

As well as the inefficiency and lack of efficacy of HRT, there are actually proven risks that each individual must take into account before embarking on a course of treatment.

Cancers

Uterine (endometrial) cancer was found to be seven times greater in women using HRT. This was at a time when oestrogen was being used without progesterone to 'oppose' it. The orthodox medical world rapidly announced that the use of progesterone negated these results but they failed to mention the continued risk of uterine cancer, which was still three times greater despite the use of progesterone.

RISK OF BREAST CANCER WITH HRT		
Years on HRT	Cases of breast cancer between ages 50 and 70	Extra breast cancer in HRT users
Never on HRT	45 per 1,000	nil
5 years	47 per 1,000	2 per 1,000
10 years	51 per 1,000	6 per 1,000
15 years	57 per 1,000	12 per 1,000

Breast cancer is also increased by the use of HRT. Studies suggesting protection by HRT are promoted by the pharmaceutical companies, contrary to the evidence of large studies showing that combination HRT (oestrogen and progesterone) increases the risk of breast cancer to four times that of non-HRT-using women if it is taken for over six years.

Certain trials have shown that oestrogens and progestogen (artificial progesterone) increase other cancers, such as cancer of the ovaries, cervix, pituitary gland, liver and the skin (melanomas).

The reason why these are not well documented

is because money is not available to put into trials that repeat negative results.

Thrombosis (blood clots), strokes and heart disease

Every doctor will advise a woman that the contraceptive pill can cause blood clots, most commonly deep vein thrombosis in the legs. Any past history or family history of blood clots, high blood pressure or obesity, history of strokes or other cardiovascular problems all contraindicate the use of oral contraceptive pills (OCP). If the OCP is known to cause problems, there is no reason to believe that because a woman ages the chemicals will alter their functions.

One of the main hypotheses supporting HRT against heart and vascular disease is the effects of HRT on reducing cholesterol. The trials, according to eminent research scientists, have all been flawed and based on the assumption that lowering cholesterol levels will alter rates of cardiovascular disease in post-menopausal women. None of this has been conclusively proven. What is more worrying is the continued promotion of these unsubstantiated studies despite the evidence of large follow-up studies showing that HRT is *not* effective in reducing cardiovascular problems and in fact may increase risks.

Osteoporosis – *see* Osteoporosis

Other side effects

Specific problems such as skin conditions, jaundice, vomiting, stitches and physiological disturbances such as depression and irritability can all be caused by HRT. One study in the UK showed that there was an increase in suicide in groups using HRT. What is more distressing is that symptoms of menopause may be worsened or initiated by HRT. I occasionally see patients who have unique symptoms such as muscular aches and pains, abdominal spasms and neurological symptoms such as dizziness and pins and needles. I cannot categorically state that these have been caused by HRT but the symptoms improve when the treatment stops.

There has been reported in one study a six-fold increase in asthma in women who use HRT.

Natural oestrogens and progesterones

There is a bandwagon rolling to support natural female hormones. These are plant derivatives that actually contain exactly the same types of sex hormones as the human body, as opposed to the artificial chemicals in HRT that only resemble ours. Natural oestrogens from plants, known as phyto-oestrogens, are much less potent than artificial hormones but the body seems to respond to them if their application is appropriate. These oestrogens are obtained from hops, fennel, celery, soya products and rhubarb, all of which can be fed comfortably into the diet. Extracts from specific plants can be obtained from healthfood shops as 'food products' because no medical claim can be made. It is interesting to note that Japanese women who have a much higher level of soya products in their diet (in addition to no red meat or saturated fat) have negligible levels of osteoporosis or heart disease.

Natural progesterone has risen in popularity on the back of the work of a doctor called John Lee in the USA. Dr Lee was unimpressed by the efficiency and effects of oestrogen and looked toward decreased progesterone as a possible cause of menopausal problems. His research and personal experience suggested, and has since shown, that a bulk of symptoms that women complain of and the diseases such as osteoporosis that are associated with ageing may be due to the lack of progesterone and not oestrogen. There is much evidence to support this. As the pharmaceutical industry cannot patent a natural compound there is no point in experimenting or studying natural progesterone and so most of Dr Lee's work has not been repeated.

Natural progesterone has been extracted from the Mexican yam (other sweet potatoes do not contain it) and needs to be administered transdermally (through the skin) because, like any complex chain, it is unlikely to survive the digestive system intact. Natural progesterone does not seem to have an effect on the hot flushes and sweats that are the main disturbing feature for most women going through the menopause, but it may have an effect on all the other symptoms. Most encouragingly, it has a profound effect on osteoporosis (*see* **Osteoporosis**).

Oestrogen-dependent tumours, most commonly found in the breast, may benefit from these phyto-oestrogens. A study in a top London hospital is currently ongoing and it would appear that these plant oestrogens may lock into oestrogen receptors, thereby preventing the stronger body hormones from exerting an effect. There may be some risk that the plant extracts will actually encourage oestrogen-sensitive tumours, but the experiments to date are encouraging. It may be that premenopausal women should use phyto-oestrogens and natural progesterones as protection factors in any oestrogen-related condition.

Foods containing phyto-oestrogens (isoflavones) include:

seaweed	soy beans and flour
tempeh	tofu
linseed (flaxseed) meal or flour	lentils
oatbran	kidney beans
oatbran	rye
hops	garlic
asparagus	pears
plums	celery
fennel	squash

Types of HRT

The oestrogens are taken as a tablet, patch, an implant or a gel. Any woman who still has her uterus (has not been subjected to a hysterectomy) must take regular progestogen (artificial progesterone), which is usually taken as a tablet. The progestogen blocks the oestrogen effect. Usually the progestogen is taken for 12 days but many women suffer the progesterone side effects, which are principally fluid retention, headaches, skin reaction such as acne and other pre-menstrual syndrome symptoms. Women who have gone through the menopause and have not had a period for at least 12 months are offered the combined preparation, which is taken continuously. These do not cause periods to occur, which is certainly a favourable option. Another option is to take an oestrogen preparation and progesterone, say, four times a year, giving a bleed every three months. This is offered to those women going through menopause who may still be having infrequent periods. I mention this for information and not as a support of their use. In fact, my views are quite the opposite.

Dosage of HRT

Hormone replacement therapy is mostly given orally or via skin patches. These may be combination pills or oestrogen with short courses of progesterone to encourage a period or offer 'protection' from the unopposed oestrogen. Implants are becoming more popular but their safety is highly questionable. For a start the ovaries, adrenal glands and fat stores (these actually make oestrogen) can all produce hormones at fluctuating rates years after the menopause. An implant delivers a set dose regardless of the amount that is made by the body naturally. This can cause overdoses, which will lead to all the risks and side effects listed above.

RECOMMENDATIONS

General Advice

- *Avoid your doctors advice, who will be encouraging the use of HRT.*
- *Work with a complementary medical practitioner if the signs and symptoms of menopause are disturbing.*
- *Obtain relevant blood tests to establish menopausal status.*

- Consider urinary protein tests and ultrasound bone densitrometry to establish a baseline for osteoporosis.
- If you are currently using or considering the use of HRT, consult a complementary medical practitioner with experience in this area.
- See **Osteoporosis**, **Stroke** and **Heart attack** to establish the alternatives to help protect against these conditions in latter years. These techniques are as useful as any positive aspects of HRT.
- Consider the use of natural hormone creams, available through specialist complementary practitioners and all doctors if they are willing to read the information and prescribe it.

Nutritional

- See **Arteriosclerosis** with regard to the better dietetic regimes and supplemental treatments to protect against cardiovascular disease.

MALE MENOPAUSE

Many men notice changes within themselves, ranging from fatigue, depression and irritability to reduced sex drive and impotence, after they get to the age of 40 years.

The term 'male menopause' has been coined but rarely is there a drop in testosterone or other male hormones (androgens) in the bloodstream. Replenishment with testosterone may increase sexual interest somewhat but most other symptoms are unaffected. It is more likely that stress combined with arteriosclerosis accounts for most of the symptoms.

RECOMMENDATIONS

General Advice

- See **Stress** and **Arteriosclerosis**.
- Increase exercise and relaxation/meditation techniques.

Nutritional

- Consider the development of food allergy and be tested.

MENOPAUSE

Menopause is the physiological cessation of menstruation, which usually occurs between years 45 and 55 of a woman's life and most commonly within two years either side of the age at which the individual's mother went through menopause. Colloquially known as 'the change' and medically termed the climacteric, this period of transition commonly lasts 2–5 years but can be noticed for up to 20 years.

Thought of as a diminution in the oestrogen levels produced by the ovaries, the menopause is actually a drop in the levels of oestrogen and the cessation of production of progesterone. Most of the symptoms of menopause are created by the loss of both progesterone and oestrogen and their effects on the blood vessels, which tend to dilate causing blood flow changes, and also on the nervous system directly. These effects cause:

- *Psychological symptoms* – mood swings, short temper, depression, anxiety, usually lowered but occasionally raised libido, and insomnia.
- *Physical symptoms* – hot flushes, sweats (especially at night), water retention, fat deposit increase, headaches, aches and pains, malaise and lethargy, and cystitis-like symptoms.
- *Physical signs* – loss of breast tissue, vaginal dryness, osteoporosis (bone thinning) and skin changes such as water retention, fat deposit increase, change in texture, wrinkling and dark 'staining'.

These symptoms and the pharmaceutical industry make the menopause sound like a disease process, which of course it is not. Many men who do not have such a dramatic drop in hormone levels will also have many of these symptoms. It is a natural change and one that has been going on since the human race began.

Seven out of ten women will have some or all of these symptoms for a short period, say up to six months, but one in two will have some or all of these symptoms for anywhere up to five years. There are in fact three stages of menopause:

- Premenopause – where periods are still regular and present but any of the above-mentioned symptoms may set in.
- Perimenopause – where the periods become irregular.
- Postmenopause – no more periods. It is fairly arbitrary as to how long a woman must go without a period but generally 6–12 months without a period would suggest that the postmenopausal stage has arrived. Periods recommencing after that are unusual and need to be reviewed by a gynaecologist.

Follicle-stimulating hormones (FSH) is the hormone produced by the pituitary glands that promotes the development of eggs in the ovary. Levels of FSH will rise in an attempt to stimulate eggs in the ovaries but if the normal cycle does not actually take place then the negative feedback mechanisms that suppress FSH production are not activated. The levels therefore remain high and can be measured scientifically to define menopause.

Other investigations that can be undertaken at the time of the menopause include saliva and blood tests for oestriol and oestradiol, the main oestrogen sub-groups. Progesterone and testosterone levels may also be informative as may the levels of dehydroepiandrosterone (DHEA), as discussed later.

A urine test can be carried out for two proteins (pyridinium and deoxypyridinium) excreted in the urine as a byproduct of bone metabolism. Raised levels of these proteins indicate increasing bone loss and preventative measures can be taken if necessary (*see* **Osteoporosis**). We can also perform ultrasound bone density scans and I recommend this at the beginning of menopause for comparison every two years. Unlike the orthodox use of X-rays of the spine and hip, these techniques are simple and harmless. Analysis of the body levels of calcium, vitamin D and toxins that may affect bone

structure, such as fluoride, can be performed through blood, cell and hair analysis. These may or may not be indicated, depending on each individual.

RECOMMENDATIONS

FOR HOT FLUSHES, SWEATS, PALPITATIONS AND HEADACHES

General Advice

- *Eliminate stimulatory foods such as alcohol, caffeine and spicy foods. Stop smoking or taking any other drugs because these will contribute to flushes and sweats.*
- *Low blood sugar (hypoglycaemia) and adrenaline will sensitize the system and make all symptoms seem worse. Learn a meditation or relaxation technique, use counselling or psychotherapy, and strictly avoid refined sugars if not eaten with other complex carbohydrates or proteins.*
- *Symptomatic relief has been shown to be obtainable through osteopathy, Shiatsu and acupuncture.*
- *Massage and especially aromatherapy may well be of benefit.*

Supplemental

- *Try vitamin B$_6$ (100mg with breakfast), vitamin E (400iu with breakfast and supper), inositol (1000mg with each meal), zinc (30mg before bed), gammalinoleic acid (1g with each meal) and calcium and magnesium (both at 200mg with each meal). If the symptoms are improved, then reduce the doses of these vitamins one at a time until you find the minimal required dosage. You may not need to take all of these.*
- *The following botanical (plant) extracts may be considered and taken in divided doses per foot of height during the day just before meals: Angelica (500mg), glycyrrhiza from liquorice (half a teaspoonful of fluid extract) and Agnus castus (0.5ml of tincture or the maximum dose of a*

capsule or pill preparation). Other herbs have been shown to be useful but should be prescribed by a herbalist.

Homeopathic
- *Review from your preferred homeopathic manual the remedies Belladonna, Lachesis, Amyl nitrate and Veratrum viride. The right remedy should be taken at potency 12 or 30 every 2hr for five days and then whenever symptoms come on.*

Herbal/natural extracts
- *Clary sage essential oil and Aloe vera essence can be used in the bath or inhaled by wafting the aroma from a bottle held three or four inches away from the nose.*
- *Aloe vera taken at night and before meals may be beneficial.*
- *The Chinese/Tibetan herb Dong quai (1g with meals) can be used, as may Siberian gingseng (50mg with each meal).*
- *Natural progesterone or oestrogen creams can be used but need to be prescribed by a specialist in this field.*

Orthodox
- *Only if symptoms are unbearable and success is not forthcoming after following the above recommendations should an individual consider using HRT.*

SENILE DEMENTIA
Senile dementia is a chronic progressive mental disease caused by a loss of brain tissue in association with ageing. There is a characteristic failing in memory (usually short and middle term) and a loss of other intellectual functions.

RECOMMENDATION

General Advice
- *See **Alzheimer's disease** for treatment options.*

THROMBOSIS – *see* Blood clots

THE HEAD AND NECK

THE EARS

DEAFNESS
Deafness or loss of hearing is a most debilitating condition. It may vary from mild loss of particular pitch or notes to a complete inability to hear sound. At whatever level, it creates social difficulties and any help that can be obtained can make a substantial difference to an individual's well-being.

Deafness is discussed in this chapter because ageing creates a certain amount of hearing loss, often within sociably acceptable levels, but of course it can occur at any age.

Acute or sudden deafness must be treated as an emergency and should be reviewed by a specialist. Deafness can be divided into two groups: conductive and neurological (perceptive).

Conductive deafness
Sound is transmitted from the external ear canal through the eardrum and the ear ossicles into the vestibular canal, which houses the ends of the auditory nerve fibres. This part of the ear can be considered the conductive part. Trauma, obstruction, infection and bone diseases such as arthritis of the ossicles can all be a cause of a loss of hearing.

Neurological (perceptive) deafness
Deafness that occurs because of damage to the neurological system may occur through trauma or infection in the vestibular canal, or neurological disease (for instance tumours such as cholesteatoma), trauma or infection along the auditory nerve to the part of the brain that registers sound. Congenital or hereditary deafness may occur because of malformation or damage to any aspect of the brain or ear.

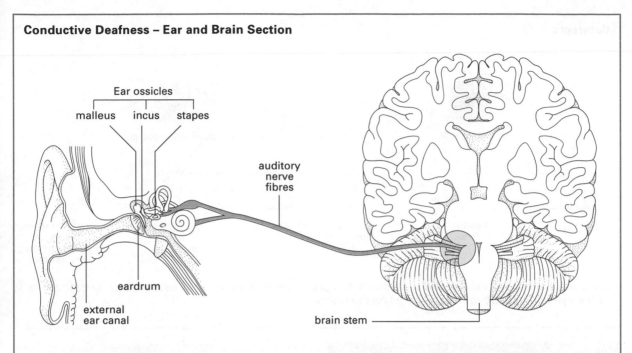

Conductive Deafness – Ear and Brain Section

Ear ossicles

malleus incus stapes

auditory
nerve
fibres

eardrum

external
ear canal

brain stem

Obstruction or infection in the external ear canal or in middle ear, containing the ear ossicles, may obstruct sound waves and prevent them from being translated into impulses in the auditory nerve fibres.

RECOMMENDATIONS

General Advice

- *Establishing the cause of deafness is paramount and any diminution in hearing should be checked by a GP, who should refer you to an ear specialist.*
- *Obstructive causes should be removed if possible. Obstruction may occur because of fluid in the middle ear (infected or not) and for treatment see* **Otitis media** *and* **'Glue' ear**.
- *Conductive deafness though damage or arthritic conditions in the ear ossicles may respond to naturopathic treatment but this needs to be specific and a visit to a homeopath and a herbalist is recommended.*
- *Do not hesitate to use hearing-aid appliances. If naturopathic treatments do not help and no surgical procedure will benefit, then the use of hearing aids can make a profound difference.*
- *If specific problems such as cholesteatoma, labyrinthitis or glue ear are the cause of deafness, please refer to the specific section in this book.*

THE EYES

CATARACTS

The lens at the front of the eye, along with the hair and nails, has no blood supply. It extracts its oxygen directly from the atmosphere to maintain its well-being. Half of all of us after the age of 65 years will struggle with opacity or clouding of the lens. The symptoms are blurred vision, seeing things through a fog, scattering of sunlight or car headlights at night and a change in your perception of colour. If the cataract is not arrested it can lead to blindness, generally repairable by surgical procedure.

Cataracts develop at varying speeds and can be associated with certain disease processes. Diabetes and malnutrition can lead to earlier and speedier development of cataracts.

Once a cataract has set in, it is difficult to remove it medically; however, the following recommendations can, and do, slow down the progress.

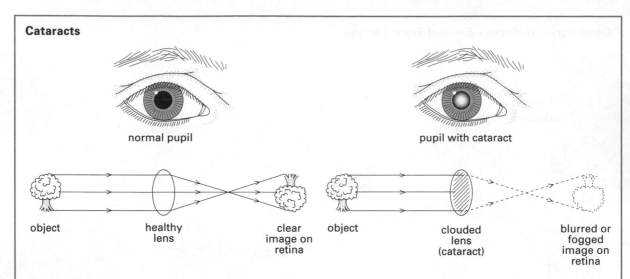

Cataracts

normal pupil

pupil with cataract

object — healthy lens — clear image on retina

object — clouded lens (cataract) — blurred or fogged image on retina

Cataracts have many causes and are a common occurrence in old age. They cause clouding of the lens in the eye and a resultant blurry image on the retina.

RECOMMENDATIONS

General Advice

- *Any problem with the eye must be checked by your GP and, if necessary, an ophthalmic specialist.*
- *With any problem of vision, learning to see rather than look can restore sight even in the blind. This sort of differentiation requires specialized training and books on Bates' eye technique and therapists should be referred to.*

Nutritional

- *Antioxidant therapy, particularly beta-carotene and vitamins C and E, helps to prevent the oxidation process and the worsening of cataracts. These can be found in yellow, orange or dark green vegetables or can be taken in specific amounts depending on your size and age. Discuss it with a complementary medical practitioner (see Arteriosclerosis).*

Homeopathic

- *The homeopathic remedy Immature cataract 200 should be taken as three doses, one each night, every two months.*
- *Once a cataract has set in, several homeopathic remedies may be indicated, depending on the symptoms, and a consultation with a homeopath is warranted.*

Herbal/natural extracts

- *There is an Ayurvedic concoction by the name of Triphalat that is available from Ayurvedic distributors. Boil a teaspoonful in a cup of water for 3min. Once cooled and strained thoroughly the eyes should be bathed using an eye bath twice a day.*

Orthodox

- *Surgical techniques are forever improving. Frequent consultations with your ophthalmic surgeon will advise you on the necessity and best times to operate. Lenses are now replaced and although they do not have the same visual acuity as your natural lens, they are generally safe and effective. See **Operations and surgery** before undergoing any surgery.*

ECTROPION

In this condition the lower eyelid loses its muscular tone and droops. This exposes the inner lining or conjunctiva, leading to dryness, discomfort and potential infection. The loss of the lower lid integrity also means that tears are not contained in the eye and tend to fall down the face.

RECOMMENDATIONS

General Advice

- *This problem usually requires surgical repair.*

Homeopathic

- *Homeopathic remedies suitable for the symptoms can be considered at potency 6, four times a day, and may be chosen from the following remedies: Borax, Mercurius, Aconite, Pulsatilla and Euphrasia.*

Herbal/natural extracts

- *Until repair is performed, use Euphrasia fluid extract in diluted form – two drops to 10ml of boiled water – and bathe the eye four times a day.*

ENTROPION

This is the converse condition to ectropion, whereby the muscles of the lower eyelid contract causing the eyelashes to press on the eyeball and conjunctiva, causing irritation and inflammation, thus allowing for infection.

RECOMMENDATIONS

General Advice

- *See **Conjunctivitis**.*

Homeopathic

- *Homeopathic remedies suitable for the symptoms can be considered at potency 6, four times a day and may be chosen from the following: Aconite, Rhus toxicodendron, Arnica and Hamamelis.*

Herbal/natural extracts

- *Euphrasia fluid extract – two drops in 10ml of boiled water – can be used as an eye bath four times a day.*

Orthodox

- *As for ectropion, the problem is usually treated surgically.*

MACULAR DEGENERATION

The macula is found at the centre of the retina at the back of the eye. It is a conglomeration of rods and cones – the nervous system's receptors for light – and is responsible for fine vision.

Macular degeneration is a medical term given when this area is damaged, usually by receiving a decreased blood supply through natural ageing, arteriosclerosis, diabetes or high blood pressure.

Other than sophisticated laser surgery, which may benefit some people with this problem, there is no orthodox treatment.

RECOMMENDATIONS

General Advice

- *A diagnosis of macular degeneration can only be made by a specialist and regular monitoring is of use to know the level of deterioration, although the individual's vision will of course be the bench-mark.*
- *See **Arteriosclerosis** and ensure that you follow the dietetic and supplementary guideline.*

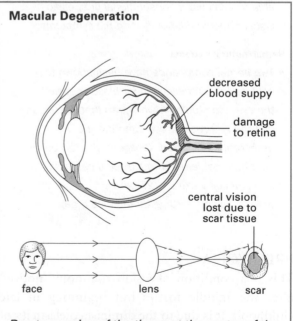

Macular Degeneration

decreased blood suppy

damage to retina

central vision lost due to scar tissue

face   lens   scar

Due to scarring of the tissue at the centre of the retina, sight loss is experienced at the centre of the field of vision.

Supplemental

- *Vitamin C (1g three times a day), vitamin E (400iu twice a day), selenium (200µg daily), beta-carotene (3mg twice a day), zinc (10mg three times a day) and pycnogenol (20mg twice a day) can all be used. These treatments should be taken for at least six months and your eye specialist will be able to tell you if deterioration has ceased.*
- *Medically qualified practitioners can offer intravenous infusions of selenium (200µg) and zinc (10mg), twice a week for one month and then weekly. This treatment is done in conjunction with taking the amino acid taurine orally, up to 1g three times a day.*
- *Lutein 2mg per foot of height may protect against harmful wavelengths and free radical damage.*
- *Zeaxanthin can also be taken at the level recommended on the product label.*

Homeopathic

- *Nutritionists may be able to advise you on the use of higher potencies and homeopaths may be able to administer constitutional or specific visual remedies depending on the symptoms.*

Herbal/natural extracts

- *Two herbal compounds have been shown to have specific predilection for blood vessels in the eye and studies have shown that these can halt the progress or even improve the deterioration in vision: Ginkgo biloba (24 per cent heterosides) – 40mg three times a day; and blueberry extract (25 per cent anthocyanidin) – 80mg three times a day.*

PRESBYOPIA

This is a condition of vision commonly noticed after the middle forties but beginning in late childhood. It is due to the diminished elasticity of the lens so that the individual has difficulty in focusing on near objects and in reading fine print.

The condition is the same as hypermetropia (long-sightedness) but caused for a different reason.

RECOMMENDATION

General Advice

- *See **Myopia and hypermetropia**.*

PTERYGIUM

Pterygium is a growth of tissue from the white of the eye (sclera) that grows across the cornea.

This overgrowth is considered to be caused by excessive exposure to sunlight, but an association with some other factor is probably necessary because most people do not develop this problem even if they are in the sunshine. Mineral deficiencies, especially zinc, may be relevant.

RECOMMENDATIONS

General Advice

- *Mineral analysis and correction of any deficiencies may halt the progress.*
- *Dark glasses should be worn in extremes of sunlight by those who have a tendency to develop this condition.*

Orthodox

- *Surgical removal is a simple procedure for an ophthalmic surgeon.*

PTOSIS

A ptosis is a prolapse or 'falling down' of an organ or part of an organ. It is generally applied to the drooping of the upper eyelid. This usually occurs because of damage or inflammation to the nerve (part of the third cranial nerve – the oculomotor nerve). In one particular condition known as Horner's syndrome, the eyelid droops, the eye appears sunken and the pupil constricts.

Damage to the neuromuscular junction in rare conditions such as myasthenia gravis needs to be considered, although ptosis may simply be a result of ageing.

General Advice

- *Ayurvedic facial massage techniques may benefit the condition.*
- *Acupuncture may have a profound effect. The topmost acupuncture point for the bladder rests by the eyelid and bladder energy weakness may be responsible.*
- *See **Nerve injury**.*

THE MOUTH

RECEDING GUMS

Receding gums, if left unattended, will lead to the loss of teeth and persistent discomfort and visits to the dentist to deal with infection. Care of the gums is essential from an early age to avoid this happening as we age and go through years of bacterial attack on these very exposed tissues.

General Advice

- *See **Gums, care of**.*
- *Dental cleaning on a daily basis with a good toothbrush action as well as a three-monthly visit to the dental hygienist is recommended.*

Nutritional

- *The avoidance of refined sweet foods is extremely important.*
- *Other nutrients are essential for good healthy gums and should be obtained by eating at least five portions of fruit and vegetables per day. The chewing of fibre is also a relevant factor because it encourages blood flow and thereby oxygen and nutrients reach the gums.*

Supplemental

- *Vitamin C (500mg per foot of height in divided doses during the day with food) and zinc (5mg per foot of height before bed) are relevant supplements.*

THE CHEST

ANGINA

Angina is the medical term given for pain caused by lack of oxygen to a part of the body. It is most commonly associated with pains in the chest created by a lack of oxygen to the heart muscle. This oxygen deprivation is generally caused by Arteriosclerosis forming in the cardiac blood vessels but may be caused by spasm in these arteries or damaged cardiac muscle. The chest pain of angina is generally described as a grip in the centre of the chest, occasionally associated with radiation to the back, up to the neck and jaw and down the left arm. Angina is most commonly associated with exertion and can come on with walking, climbing stairs and even love-making. More rigorous exercise will of course initiate discomfort as well. There is often an associated shortness of breath.

Chest pains that are non-responsive to resting or experienced whilst sitting or lying down are termed *unstable angina* and require immediate attention. Another form of angina known as *Prinzmetal* angina is created by constriction of the coronary vessels with or without underlying atheroma changes.

General Advice

- *Every chest pain that is not easily relieved or that recurs must be attended to by an orthodox doctor.*
- *In the case of cardiac problems it is better to be treated by a medically qualified complementary practitioner or with your cardiologist or GP in close attention. Do not stop taking cardiac drugs without medical support.*
- *Angina is most often created by blockage to the heart arteries (see **Arteriosclerosis** and **Cholesterol**).*
- *Obtain advice from a nutritionist, herbalist and homeopath because all can give sound judgements and offer good treatments.*

- *Exercise to just before the point of discomfort is encouraged but yoga and Qi Gong are the preferred methods of activity. Walking and swimming are mandatory.*
- *To reiterate, I do not recommend self-medication other than antioxidants for cardiac conditions.*

Nutritional

- *Consider the Ornish or Pritikin diets (see chapter 7).*

Supplemental

- *Use antioxidants (see **Arteriosclerosis** and **Antioxidants**).*

Orthodox

- *Once angina has been diagnosed, medications will be recommended by the orthodox practitioner ranging from glycerine trinitrate (GTN) placed under the tongue or administered as a spray to more aggressive cardiac drugs. Take the treatments and then obtain curative advice from a complementary medical practitioner.*
- *The orthodox world will offer surgery of some sort if the condition is not controlled by drugs. Be very wary and please read the section below on coronary artery bypass procedures.*

Coronary artery bypass procedures

If the coronary arteries are blocked by atheroma and drugs are failing to open the arteries enough to allow a sufficient blood flow, then the orthodox world is left with no option other than some form of surgical procedure. There are two types.

Angioplasty

This literally means plastic surgery of injured or diseased blood vessels but is now in common use for the technique that inflates a balloon within the occluded artery. The specialist inserts a long tube into the femoral artery in the groin and feeds it up through the aorta and into the coronary (heart) blood vessels with the use of specialized X-ray equipment. Once in place, the balloon at the tip of this tube is inflated and stretches the occluded artery wall, breaking down the atheroma and, hopefully, removing the occlusion.

There are dangers in this procedure because the balloon may rupture the vessels, so the technique is done only in specialized units. A cardiac surgeon and emergency operating theatre must be immediately on hand. The procedure remains controversial because long-term studies and data suggest that the technique is less safe and no more efficient than coronary artery bypass grafting.

Coronary artery bypass grafting (CABG)

Until recently CABG has been considered the most beneficial of complex surgery. A recent report in *Heart*, one of the top medical journals, has shown that CABG is not all that successful in the long term. The heart is exposed by a cardiac surgeon, who finds the occluded vessel and literally bypasses the blockage using a short piece of the patient's own vein (taken from the leg). The procedure is risky but undoubtedly has a profoundly successful effect in the short term. Sadly, it would appear that the procedure does not lead to a longer length of life in the majority of cases.

RECOMMENDATIONS

General Advice

- *Consider all alternative possibilities, both orthodox and complementary, before considering any form of surgery.*
- *The orthodox world is quick to condemn chelation therapy (see below) but small studies are suggestive of it being a suitable alternative to the not-so-successful surgical techniques.*
- *See **Operations and surgery**.*

Chelation therapy

Chelation is a word derived from *Chela*, which is Greek for a crab or a lobster's claw. It illustrates the way certain compounds may interact with others, forming a bond. It is used in medicine to describe compounds that bind toxic compounds, especially heavy metals and the cholesterol deposits found in arteries and known as atheroma.

Medical chelation uses a compound called ethylene-diamine-tetraacetic acid (EDTA). Chelation has been used to treat atherosclerosis, high blood pressure, angina, occlusive vascular disease, porphyria, rheumatoid arthritis and cancer. There is good scientific reasoning and research to show how EDTA may work, but controversy still exists. I suspect that this controversy is due to the potential for the use of EDTA in many conditions that dominate and are vastly beneficial to the pharmaceutical industry. If EDTA was proven to be an effective treatment for the conditions that I have mentioned above, billions of dollars of profit would be wiped out. The compound EDTA cannot be patented, so the necessary research has come to a grinding halt.

RECOMMENDATIONS

General Advice

- *The use of chelation therapy in any of the above-mentioned conditions should be considered.*
- *Chelation/EDTA therapy must be used before coronary artery surgery is considered, in my opinion.*
- *Ensure that the provider of chelation therapy is a fully qualified doctor or has had many years of experience in this treatment. Specific tests must be made on liver and kidney function throughout the treatment course because there is evidence of EDTA being toxic.*

ASTHMA IN POSTMENOPAUSE

Asthma and its treatments are discussed earlier. However, it is worth noting that the use of hormone replacement therapy (HRT) has been shown to increase the possibility of asthma attacks in postmenopausal women.

RECOMMENDATIONS

General Advice

- *If you have started on HRT and suspect the beginnings or notice a worsening of current asthma, consider stopping HRT.*
- *See* **Hormone replacement therapy**.

CHRONIC BRONCHITIS

Chronic bronchitis is defined by having a minimum of three months' continual green, or at least infected, production from the lungs via a cough. As we age, our cough may not be strong enough to remove the infection and physiotherapy may be required to help bring up the product. Chronic bronchitis is more frequent in smokers and people who have spent their lives in polluted areas. It is caused by infection setting in when the little hairs that usually remove bacteria from the lungs (called cilia) have been destroyed over the years.

RECOMMENDATIONS

General Advice

- *See* **Bronchitis**.
- *Place yourself under the care of a medically qualified complementary practitioner.*
- *Regular visits to a physiotherapist will help to clear the chest through the technique of chest-clapping.*

Nutritional

- *If there are good and bad days, note your diet accurately for two weeks to see if you have any obvious mucus-producing foods in your diet. If you see any obvious associations, avoid these foods.*

Supplemental

- *Beta-carotene (2mg with each meal), zinc (10mg at night) and vitamin C (500mg with each meal) can be taken but discuss higher doses with your complementary practitioner.*

Homeopathic

- *Homeopathic remedies are essential. They need*

to be chosen depending on your constitution and symptoms.

Herbal/natural extracts

- *Inhalations of lavender essential oil (five drops in a bowl of water, four times a day) can be very relieving. Eucalyptus oil and Olbas oils can be used but should not be used in conjunction with homeopathic remedies.*
- *Ayurvedic, Chinese and Tibetan practitioners have a selection of herbs that can ease breathing problems and they will use chest-cupping (a technique of removing congestion from the lungs by applying a vacuum to the chest wall).*

EMPHYSEMA

Emphysema is the medical term for the enlargement of the air spaces in the lungs caused by destruction to the tissue of the lung walls, known as the alveoli.

This loss of lung tissue means that less oxygen can be absorbed and carbon dioxide is stored in these enlarged spaces causing breathlessness and a characteristic enlarging of the chest usually known as barrel-chest.

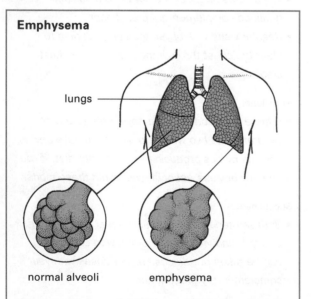

Emphysema

lungs

normal alveoli   emphysema

The breakdown of the lung walls in the alveoli, the small air sacs in the lungs, results in fewer larger alveoli and a subsequent loss of breath.

A certain amount of emphysema will develop in all of us as we age and our body loses the ability to replace destroyed lung tissue, but very often emphysema is brought on at an earlier age and to distressing levels by smoking and recurrent infections in people with chronic bronchitis or even poorly treated asthma.

Once lung tissue has been destroyed it is unlikely that the body will be able to replace it, so spotting emphysema early and preventing its progression is the best treatment.

RECOMMENDATIONS

General Advice

- *Any persisting shortness of breath should be reviewed by a doctor.*
- *Stop smoking and remove the patient from smoky, polluted or dusty environments.*
- *Breathing exercises from Buteyko, yoga or Qi Gong should be taught and utilized daily to encourage energy flow into the chest as well as oxygen intake and carbon dioxide removal.*
- *In advanced emphysema, acupuncture may be of some benefit.*
- *Cannabis has been linked to a worsening of emphysema.*

Supplemental

- *The following vitamins should be taken at the given doses per foot of height to encourage membrane stability and protect against infection: beta-carotene (2mg), vitamin E (20iu), vitamin C (500mg) and zinc (5mg). All should be taken in divided doses during the day except for zinc, which should be taken as one dose before sleep.*

Homeopathic

- *Any individual who may have lung damage by particle intake should be given the homeopathic remedy Pothos foetidus 200, one dose a day for five days.*

Orthodox

- *If emphysema is suggested, either on clinical*

examination or by chest X-ray, treatment should be initiated immediately.

- The use of oxygen delivered by mask or nostril prongs can be organized by your GP at home.

EMPYEMA

Empyema is the medical term for the presence of pus in a cavity or body space. It is most commonly referred to in association with pus in the lung cavity and is usually a secondary event following a severe chest infection, pneumonia or pleurisy (infection or inflammation of the external lining of the lungs).

RECOMMENDATIONS

General Advice

- Once the problem has been dealt with from the acute emergency angle, then discussion with a complementary medical practitioner can be considered.

Supplemental

- If antibiotics are used take high doses of Lactobacillus acidophillus concurrently or the equivalent – around 2 billion organisms – before each meal.

Homeopathic

- Homeopathic remedies can be used on the basis of the symptoms but specifically Hepar sulphuris calcarium 6, which is a remedy renowned for removing trapped pus or abscesses from the system. Take it every 2hr regardless of any other medical intervention – it may work by itself.

Orthodox

- Pus in any part of the body is a serious condition that requires an orthodox assessment and the possible use of antibiotics. There may be a need for surgical intervention to drain the infection from the lung cavity.

PNEUMONIA

Pneumonia is a severe chest infection that has developed to involve the lung tissue and air sacs (known as the alveoli) as opposed to just the bronchial tree as in bronchitis. The symptoms are a persistent cough with (more commonly) or without the production of colourful sputum, shortness of breath and shallow breathing, fever, rigors (shaking) and, if the lining of the lung is affected, pain from pleurisy. Chest X-ray will show patchy white cloud-like appearances and a stethoscope will reveal absent breath sounds if the congestion is marked or crackles and wheezes in the area of infiltration.

Pneumonia, like bronchitis, is most common in smokers and commonly in individuals whose immune system is weak. The common causes are viral and bacterial, but noxious gases, fungal infections and parasites may all trigger pneumonia. Pneumonia is particularly risky in the elderly because of the marked reduction in oxygen absorption. It is the fifth leading cause of death in the Western world.

RECOMMENDATIONS

General Advice

- See **Bronchitis**. Medical advice should be sought swiftly if pneumonia is suspected. The vitamin supplement dosages are the same as for bronchitis.
- An acute pneumonia in the immunocompromised, the very young or elderly should be treated with antibiotics after a sputum sample has been taken if the following alternative options do not seem to be benefiting within 24–36hr.
- Bed rest is recommended because exertion will increase oxygen demand.
- Increase water intake to dilute down mucus and allow easier removal from the lungs.
- Osteopathy will open the inevitable contraction of the chest wall muscles.
- Acupuncture can be immediately relieving.
- Eastern physicians may use a technique called cupping, which is a vacuum technique placed around the chest and back to pull blood to the surface.

Nutritional

- *Reduce refined sugar intake because it promotes bacterial growth.*

Herbal/natural extracts

- *Encourage expectoration by using inhalations of Lavender, Olbas and Lobelia. Their fluid extracts should be dropped into steaming water and inhaled.*
- *Seven drops of Lobelia with seven drops of liquorice in a cup of warm water should be taken four times a day by an adult and may be used by a child but needs to be taken in half dosage under the age of 14 years.*
- *Echinacea or Hydrastis (Golden Seal) can be taken in a powdered form at two times the recommended dosage on a proprietary medicine.*

PSITTACOSIS

Psittacosis is a chest infection that can often develop into pneumonia but is usually acquired by human beings from birds, particularly budgerigars, parrots and pigeons. Other pets and farmyard fowl may also spread this condition, which is also known as parrot fever. It is caused by a parasite similar to *Chlamydia* that can cause venereal disease.

The infection is found in the droppings of the birds, and cleaning of bird cages and hen-houses is common sources of infection. The condition is not confined to middle-aged people, but the elderly, who frequently keep pets, are more prone because of their diminishing immune capabilities. Young children and professionals in contact with birds may have more exposure but a better defence.

RECOMMENDATIONS

General Advice

- *Wear a mask when cleaning bird-soiled areas.*
- *See **Chest infection** and **Pneumonia**.*

THE DIGESTIVE SYSTEM

DIVERTICULAR DISEASE
Diverticulosis and diverticulitis

The colon or large intestine has a muscular layer running along its length and bands of muscle that circumvent it. In combination, these muscles contract to form peristaltic waves that push the faeces onwards towards the rectum before expulsion.

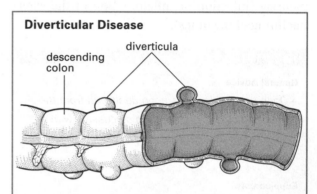

Diverticular Disease

descending colon

diverticula

Weakness in the intestinal muscles causes diverticular, small bulges in the intestinal lining to protrude. This may lead to inflammation and the discomfort associated with diverticulosis.

A tendency to weakness along the muscle wall, either hereditary or due to a prolonged low-fibre diet which does not allow the bowel to exercise its muscle and keep it firm, lets small pouches of the mucosal lining to protrude through the muscular layer in a form of herniation.

This condition may be symptomless or cause mild discomfort. If faeces get trapped in the diverticula it will cause swelling and inflammation, which in turn can lead to infection. When this occurs the condition is known as diverticulitis.

Diverticulosis may need no attention but diverticulitis, which is characterized by much stronger cramping pains, tenderness on palpation, a tendency to alternate between diarrhoea and constipation and, rarely, bleeding, needs to be dealt with effectively. Prolonged and untreated diverticulitis can lead to colon abscesses with the risk of perforation and peritonitis. These are serious and potentially fatal conditions. A fever associated with these symptoms should sound alarm bells because it is probable that infection has set in.

RECOMMENDATIONS

General Advice

- *Establishing the diagnosis of any abdominal pain should be done by a GP. A suspicion of diverticulosis or diverticulitis may lead to further investigations, such as ultrasound, barium enemas and colonoscopy. As always, whatever precautions can be used to protect against investigation should be reviewed in the relevant section, but diagnosis is important when treating abdominal conditions.*
- *Diverticulosis/itis is often associated with dehydration and adequate fluid intake is essential.*

Nutritional

- *Discuss your diet with a nutritionist, paying special attention to increasing fibre. The orthodox world is quick to encourage the use of bran or other specially extracted fibre but this tends to bind salts and electrolytes such as calcium and magnesium that are necessary for strengthening bowel muscle and is therefore not as effective as natural fibre from fruit and vegetables.*
- *The juice of two carrots, two celery stalks and three ounces of cabbage made up to half a pint of fluid with water should be taken after breakfast.*

Supplemental

- *Ensure the use of a good Acidophilus or other yoghurt-based bacterial combination taken with each meal. Correction of any abnormal bowel flora can be rapidly beneficial.*

Homeopathic

- *Homeopathic and herbal medicine can be used based on the symptoms but are best prescribed by specialists in the field.*

Herbal/natural extracts

- *Avoid any herbal treatments that may encourage bowel motivity because this may worsen symptoms.*

THE UROGENITAL SYSTEM

ATROPHIC VAGINA (DRYNESS)

As women pass through the menopause the oestrogen/progesterone effect on the cells that line the vagina is diminished and the mucus secretion disappears. This leads to a dryness that can be both irritating and painful on intercourse.

Certain products that contain natural oestogens can be beneficial, as well as supplements and topical applications.

RECOMMENDATIONS

General Advice

- *Non-medicated lubricants are preferred to oestrogen creams if they are effective. If not, use pharmaceutical ointments. They do not seem to be particularly harmful. Calendula-containing oil-based creams are preferable.*

Nutritional

- *Increase your intake of soya products, including soya milk (up to one pint per day), tofu, fennel, celery, ginseng, alfalfa, liquorice and aniseed. When it is in season, eat rhubarb.*
- *Hops are an excellent source of phyto-oestrogens and can be taken as real ale or as supplements.*

Supplemental

- *Vitamin B_6 (50mg) can be taken with breakfast and lunch.*

Herbal/natural extracts

- *A persisting problem can be dealt with by using natural oestrogen extracts topically and this needs to be discussed with your complementary medical practitioner.*

Orthodox

- *The use of hormone replacement therapy can be a last resort for unrelenting conditions (see* **Hormone replacement therapy***).*

ERECTION DIFFICULTIES

Erection problems in middle age and upwards are due predominantly to poor control of the blood circulation, either through damage to the blood vessels or through prostate enlargement causing pressure on the nerves or the blood vessels (*see* **Prostatism and prostate enlargement**). Other potential treatments for erection difficulties are discussed in chapter 4 (*see* **Erection failure**).

INCONTINENCE

Incontinence is very much an age-related condition. As a child, incontinence is a matter of training and is to some degree anxiety-related, but with older age it is predominantly due to weakening muscle control. Prolapse of the uterus or the bladder makes things worse. Incontinence can occur following pregnancy and a condition known as stress incontinence defines the loss of urine with increased intra-abdominal pressure, such as coughing and sneezing, in association with a weakened bladder valve.

Incontinence is associated with the weakening of muscles that act as valves; treatment is aimed at strengthening these muscles through exercise,

naturopathic medicines and, if other measures fail, surgery. Certain drugs can be used to relax the bladder muscle-wall contraction and thereby reduce the pressure but this is making no attempt at curing the underlying weakness, is temporary at best and more often than not is pointless.

Incontinence – an inability to hold the urine – may be created by urethra or bladder infections (cystitis) and is temporary. Malalignment of the lumbar or sacral vertebrae may put pressure on the central nervous system (CNS) and the part that controls the bladder and its valves.

Incontinence needs to be differentiated from urgency. In urgency there is a need and sometimes uncontrolled desire to pass urine, which may lead to incontinence. This can occur because of a problem with the bladder muscle (detrusor) but is more commonly found with mild inflammations following intercourse or with infections of the urethra or bladder.

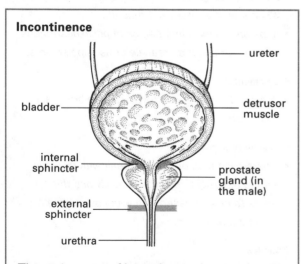

Incontinence

ureter

bladder

detrusor muscle

internal sphincter

prostate gland (in the male)

external sphincter

urethra

The main cause of incontinence is a weakness of the sphincter muscles which act as valves to the bladder. Infections of the urinary system may also be a contributory factor.

RECOMMENDATIONS

General Advice

- *Take a first morning urine sample to your GP or laboratory to ensure that there is no infection and that therefore the problem is temporary.*
- *Consult a yoga practitioner for specific pelvic floor exercises.*
- *Avoid drinking large amounts of water or fluid at any one time and get into the habit of passing urine regularly, regardless of any urgency.*
- *External pads are a social and hygienic requirement. Ensure the use of a Calendula-based cream and unmedicated talcum powder to protect the surrounding skin from irritation.*
- *Hypnotherapy and biofeedback techniques can affect mental control over the external pelvic muscles that control urine release.*
- *Acupuncture may be of benefit.*
- *Osteopathic techniques may relieve the problem if a neurological cause is suspected. Osteopathy is particularly effective during pregnancy.*

Homeopathic

- *Homeopathic remedies have been cited in the past as being helpful in incontinence although in my experience remedies by themselves have not been effective. The choice should be made by a qualified homeopath, who would need to consider the constitution in association with the symptoms.*

PROLAPSE

Uterine prolapse is found most frequently in women who have had many pregnancies and in an increased number of women in the West whose pelvic floor muscles are not well exercised.

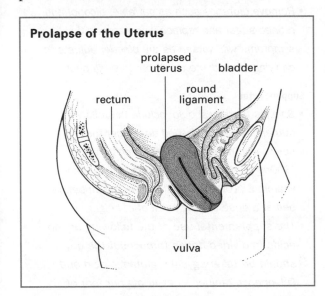

Prolapse of the Uterus

prolapsed uterus · bladder · round ligament · rectum · vulva

Prolapse occurs because the ligaments around the uterus that hold it in place become stretched and the muscles involved in supporting the uterus become weak. The outcome is that the uterus falls through the vaginal cavity.

The size and symptoms of this condition vary from an increased frequency and desire to urinate because the uterus is pushing on the bladder, to uncomfortable intercourse or actually visualizing the cervix at the entrance of the vagina. In severe and untreated cases the whole uterus may fall out and is often manually replaced by the patient.

PROSTATE

The prostate is an organ that surrounds the neck of the bladder and the beginning of the urethra in the male. It is composed of muscular and glandular tissue surrounded by a distinct capsule. Its function is to act as an involuntary valve to the urinary outlet and also to provide 40 per cent of the fluid (or semen) in which sperm receive nutrition.

The prostate is the seat of the lowest point of energy in the male in most Eastern philosophies

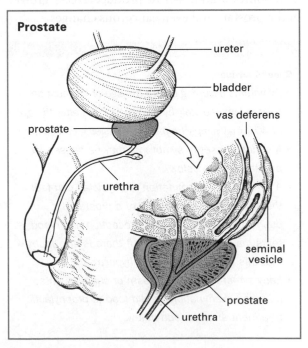

Prostate

ureter · bladder · vas deferens · prostate · urethra · seminal vesicle · prostate · urethra

and therefore has a central role in the provision of energy to the system. A block or weakness in energy flow will lead to prostate disease.

Prostatism and prostate enlargement (hypertrophy)

This condition is characterized by a difficulty in passing water, frequency of urination, excessive dribbling after urination, as well as a frequent desire to pass urine. The symptoms are created by prostatic enlargement and will occur to some degree in all men over the age of 40 years. In approximately 10 per cent of cases over the age of 70 years the enlargement is so disturbing that treatment is necessary.

Prostate enlargement is primarily caused as a natural result of continually using a muscle for many years, but in some people an excess of a hormone known as DHT (dihydrotestosterone), which has a testosterone or masculine effect on the system, is produced in excess. This actually causes cells in the prostate to multiply. A deficiency in zinc and essential fatty acids is known to be involved in those who produce too much. Excess cholesterol is broken down and these metabolites are known to produce excess growth in the prostate and even cancerous changes.

RECOMMENDATIONS

General Advice

- *Symptoms occurring before the age of 40 must be checked immediately by a physician, but after the age of 40 it may simply be part of the ageing process.*
- *A sudden onset of symptoms may be caused by prostatitis (see below).*
- *A yearly rectal examination (a physician can feel the shape, size and texture of a prostate by pushing forward) is a wise precaution and blood tests may be recommended if there is any doubt that this condition is benign hypertrophy.*
- *Early symptoms of prostatism or changes noted following examination should lead to prophylactic treatment as described below.*

Nutritional

- *Increase zinc-containing foods such as meat, liver, seafood (especially oysters), wholegrain wheat, pumpkin seeds and eggs. Organic foods are best because trace metals in agricultural chemicals may remove zinc. Certain pesticides actually increase the levels of DHT and it may be these that are responsible for the ever-increasing numbers of prostatic enlargement that we are finding nowadays. Cholesterol foods must be kept to a minimum and high cholesterol levels should be actively reduced.*
- *Increase oily fish intake to at least three times a week by eating salmon, herring, mackerel, etc.*
- *Remove diuretics such as caffeine, alcohol and refined sugar and replace with water. Initially symptoms will worsen as the bladder adjusts to carrying more dilute urine, but this will pass.*

Supplemental

- *Specific therapy should include the following nutrients taken in divided doses per foot of height with meals: eicosapentaenoic acid (300mg), linseed oil (half a teaspoonful) and vitamin E (100iu). Zinc should be taken before bed at a dose of 5mg per foot of height.*
- *The supplemental use of the following amino acids in divided doses throughout the day should be taken: gycine, glutamic acid and D,L-phenylalanine, all at 40mg per foot of height.*

Herbal/natural extracts

- *Try the herb Saw Palmetto (20mg per foot of height in divided doses twice a day) and a herb called Pygeum africanum (10mg per foot of height in divided doses twice a day). Ginseng taken as a dried root (2g per foot of height) may have a profound effect. All of these doses should be reduced as improvement occurs.*
- *The compound Lycopene and soya proteins may be effective in dealing with prostatism as they have a strong effect in prostatitis.*

Orthodox

- *The orthodox world will consider drugs known as Alpha-blockers or drugs that inhibit testosterone production since these can chemically reduce the size of the prostate. Surgery known as trans-urethral section of the prostate (TURP) is now undertaken using sophisticated equipment but can leave the individual impotent. Use these only if the alternatives do not work.*

Prostatitis

The prostate can develop inflammation through infection tracking up the urethra, through trauma or excessive sexual activity. The symptoms are that of prostatism and/or severe continual pain, often worse on passing urine. The discomfort may appear anywhere from the tip of the penis to the kidney area in the back, but most often can be pinpointed in the area between the scrotal sac and the anus.

AMERICAN UROLOGICAL ASSOCIATION SYMPTOM INDEX

Questions to be answered

AUA symptom score
(circle one number on each line)

Over the past month, how often have you had a sensation of not emptying your bladder completely after you have finished urinating?	0	1	2	3	4	5
Over the past month, how often have you had to urinate again less than 2hr after you finished urinating?	0	1	2	3	4	5
Over the past month, how often did you find that you stopped and started again several times when you urinated?	0	1	2	3	4	5
Over the past month how difficult have you found it to postpone urination?	0	1	2	3	4	5
Over the past month, how often have you had a weak urinary strain?	0	1	2	3	4	5
Over the past month, how many times have you had to push or strain to begin urination?	0	1	2	3	4	5
Over the past month, how many times did you most typically get up to urinate from the time you went to bed at night until the time you got up in the morning?	0	1	2	3	4	5
Sum of 7 circled numbers (AUA symptom score)	0x	1x	2x	3x	4x	5x

(score: 7 or less = mild symptoms; 8–19 = moderate; more than 20 = severe)

General Advice

- *Diagnosis should be made by a physician's examination. The prostate will be extremely painful if pushed.*
- *Urine and semen samples should be taken for accurate diagnosis of the infection in case an antibiotic is required. These should only be considered after alternative methods have failed because long courses are often required.*
- *Sit in a bath of comfortably hot water up to hip level. Using the bath's shower-head, apply 30sec bursts of cold water to the perineal (that part between the scrotum and the anus) area, repeating the process ten times and remembering to heat up the bath water in-between.*
- *Please note that these recommendations may need to be taken for up to three months to avoid recurrent or chronic prostatitis.*

Supplemental

- *Please follow the supplemental advice given for prostatism (see **Prostatism**).*
- *Vitamin C (1g per foot of height taken in divided doses with food throughout the day) should be added to those supplements advised in the section on prostatism.*
- *Ginseng (2g per foot of height in divided doses with meals throughout the day) may be beneficial.*

Homeopathic

- *The homeopathic remedy Sabal serrulata, taken at potency 30 four times a day until a more suitable remedy is selected by a homeopath, may be curative.*

Herbal/natural extracts

- *Echinacea and Hydrastis (Golden Seal) used at three times the quantity recommended on a proprietary preparation should be administered.*

Prostate cancer

Cancer of the prostate is an increasingly common problem. It is possible that the increased incidence is due to better techniques of discovering cancer which is performed through a blood test for a chemical released from inflamed or cancerous prostate cells called prostate specific antigen (PSA). This blood test is often done on routine screens and whenever somebody complains of prostatism. Confirmation can be made through ultrasound and biopsy.

There is strong evidence, however, that many men develop prostate cancer and have no problems with it. Although it can be aggressive and spread to the bones and other parts of the body there is a suggestion that many do not.

Each year 20,000 men are diagnosed in the UK with prostate cancer. There has been a marked increase in this condition and if the trend continues there will be nearly a 50 per cent increase in that number by the year 2021. It is accepted that many men will develop prostate cancer but have no problems with it, and that the increased reported incidence may be accounted for by better techniques of diagnosis rather than a true increase in this cancer. However, 9,500 men will die of prostate cancer each year in the UK, so the condition has to be taken seriously.

Prostate cancer tends to be a slow-growing tumour and may be in place several years prior to symptoms appearing. Prostate cancer cells can travel to local lymph glands and in particular tend to settle in bone. This makes prostate cancer a potentially painful condition and pain is often the primary symptom before anything such as urinary symptoms are apparent.

Prostate cancer is rare before the age of 40 and there is a slightly higher incidence if the condition is in the family. Symptoms of localized prostate cancer are similar to those of prostatism, specifically frequent urination, weakened urinary stream, hesitancy when starting to urinate, pain or burning on urination and/or ejaculation, leaking or dribbling of urine after completion and a feeling of incomplete emptying of the bladder.

Diagnosis is partially made by rectal examination by the experienced finger of a doctor and this is generally supported by a blood test for prostate specific antigen (PSA). Suspicion is aroused if the PSA is raised (although it can be raised in inflammatory processes such as infection in the prostate) and further investigations are carried out using ultrasound or, possibly, a biopsy.

RECOMMENDATIONS

General Advice

- See **Cancer**.
- Discuss matters fully with an orthodox specialist in this field and question the need to do anything.
- Regardless of there being symptoms, follow the supplemental recommendations under **Prostatism** and **Prostate enlargement**.
- People with prostate cancer should not use the natural arthritis treatment Chondroitin sulphate because it forms a complex with a protein called Versican found in joint cartilage. Prostate cancer cells also produce Versican and when this complex is formed it seems to help the cancer travel around the body more swiftly.
- See **Cancer**.

Nutritional

- Research from the University of California has shown that a low fat, high fibre diet combined with regular exercise may slow the growth of prostate cancer cells by up to 30 per cent. It is thought that this diet can affect hormones and other growth factors that influence prostate cancer cell growth.

Herbal/natural extracts

- Considerable research is going on concerning natural oestrogen extract, especially from red clover, and its efficacy with prostatic disease. Although no conclusive studies have yet been published, there is evidence that it may be beneficial in the prevention of prostate cancer. If this is the case, the use of 160mg daily is a minimum dose.

Orthodox

- Radical prostatectomy (removal of the whole prostate gland) is a most common treatment for early stage prostate cancer. There is a 58 per cent risk of impotence and approximately 8 per cent risk of urinary incontinence. External beam radiotherapy is given as a series of treatments for up to eight weeks. Risk of impotence runs as high as 30 per cent and incontinence at around 3 per cent. Radiotherapy itself carries other problems.
- Brachytherapy (radioactive seed implants) has been available in the USA for over a decade and is now becoming more popular in the UK and Europe. It offers the hope of a minimally invasive, cost effective procedure with a survival rate comparable with that of surgery. There are fewer side effects. Always ask about the availability of this technique.
- Hormone therapy treats prostate cancer by blocking testosterone as this enhances prostate cancer growth. This is a therapy considered if the tumour cells have spread to other parts of the body.

RETENTION OF URINE – *see* **Urination** *and* **Prostatism**

UTERINE CANCER (ENDOMETRIAL CANCER)

Uterine cancer usually presents as an unexplained bleed from the vagina but can be a difficult cancer to diagnose since it may produce no symptoms until late in its growth. Like any cancer, it needs to be under the direct care of specialists in both orthodox and alternative medicine (*see* **Cancer**).

Cancer of the uterus occurs most frequently in women who have not been pregnant (nulliparous) and we know of a sixfold increase in uterine cancers in women using HRT for more than seven years. Individuals falling into either of these categories must be checked regularly by a doctor using ultrasound, specific blood tests (if available) and complementary blood tests such as the Humoral Pathological Laboratory Test or Vega/bioresonance.

A regular visit should be made to a complementary medical practitioner who uses pulse, iridology or other alternative diagnostic techniques to spot the problem before it sets in.

RECOMMENDATIONS

General Advice

- *See* **Cancer**.
- *Do not ignore any bleed or discomfort in the lower pelvis or vagina. Obtain advice from orthodox and complementary medical practitioners.*

Orthodox

- *Provided that the underlying cause of the development of a cancer is dealt with, operative procedures are often necessary and curative. In the case of a cancer of the uterus spotted early, hysterectomy may be curative and considered appropriately.*

STRUCTURAL MATTERS

ACHES AND PAINS

Aches and pains in middle age may be associated with arthritis (*see* **Arthritis**). Unlike with the aches and pains in younger years, those of middle age and upwards are usually due to underuse and previous injury.

RECOMMENDATIONS

General Advice

- *Ensure good rehydration – an intake of at least one litre per day.*
- *Qi Gong and yoga keep the muscles stretched and active and should be used in conjunction with regular exercise such as swimming or walking.*

Nutritional

- *Calcium, magnesium and copper found in deep-green leafy vegetables, root vegetables, meat, fish and chicken must all be taken regularly to supply these minerals.*

Supplemental

- *A multimineral supplement is useful if taken at twice the recommended dosage.*

ARTHRITIS

Arthritis is the medical term for inflammation of a joint. Arthritis is divided into *acute* and *chronic*, depending on the longevity of the discomfort. Pain may be a dull ache or a sharp and severe pain. The joints may be inflamed and deformed or show no external changes at all.

Rheumatoid arthritis and *osteoarthritis* are the most common forms. Rheumatoid arthritis is an autoimmune disease whereby the body attacks its own joints. It is uncertain why this happens but the possibilities are discussed in the section on autoimmune disease (*see* **Autoimmune disease**). Osteoarthritis is an ageing process created

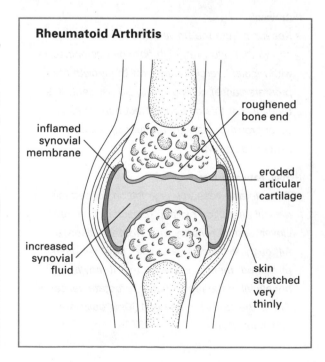

Rheumatoid Arthritis

inflamed synovial membrane

increased synovial fluid

roughened bone end

eroded articular cartilage

skin stretched very thinly

simply by wear and tear on joints. Individuals who have sporting and active lives often struggle with osteoarthritis more so than those who are sedentary because of repeated small injuries to the joints. It is worth noting that studies have shown that smoking worsens arthritis. Another study has shown less arthritis in women who wear gold.

Acute arthritis

Acute arthritic conditions are triggered by infections such as viruses, bacteria and other parasites but certain drugs and, of course, injuries can all cause an acute attack.

There is a frequent association between inflammation of joints and problems in the bowel. There is evidence that mild inflammation in the gut may cause an increased permeability of undigested food molecules through the bowel wall into the bloodstream. It is thought that this leaky gut syndrome may cause the body to trigger an autoimmune response. The body recognizes a protein sequence in an absorbed food and, if it resembles a protein sequence in the joints, antibodies are formed that attack both. This so-called 'molecular mimicry' may explain many aspects of autoimmune disease. *See* **Leaky gut syndrome**.

RECOMMENDATIONS

General Advice

- *Ice wrapped in a flannel applied to the joint reduces the inflammation temporarily without influencing the healing ability of the body. If ice does not ease the discomfort, try a heated application instead.*
- *As a general rule, rest the joint until improvement is certain.*
- *Persisting discomfort in a joint should be reviewed by a complementary practitioner with knowledge of osteopathy, chiropractic and especially acupuncture, which can be instantly relieving.*

Herbal/natural extracts

- *Homeopathic remedies such as Arnica if the joint is better for resting or Rhus toxicodendron if the joint is better for motion and warm applications should be used.*
- *Application of an Arnica cream several times a day can be beneficial.*

Orthodox

- *Avoid anti-inflammatories and cortisone injections because these will remove the pain but allow movement, which in turn can increase the damage. Anti-inflammatory treatment can also prevent healing from taking place.*
- *Painkillers with low anti-inflammatory effect, such as paracetamol and acetominophen, may be used to take down the pain. If this and the naturopathic recommendations are not working, then consider using anti-inflammatories.*

Chronic arthritis

This is a persistence of pain in a joint or joints. The causes can be loosely divided into: persistence of injury or infection, rheumatoid arthritis, other autoimmune diseases, and osteoarthritis.

Pay special attention to the possibility of food allergies, which should be tested for in all cases of arthritis.

Osteoarthritis is the progressive decay of joints that is associated with overuse and ageing. All joints will have some evidence of osteoarthritis as we age and all joints will show some stiffness. Treatment can be useful at all stages of arthritis from stiffness to pain.

RECOMMENDATIONS

FOR ALL CHRONIC ARTHRITIS

General Advice

- *Copper bracelets may be effective but only if the level of copper is normal in the body. Each individual has his/her own normal copper level* so a copper bracelet needs to be used with copper supplements to be effective.

- Wear gold next to the skin in the form of jewellery, such as a wedding ring.
- Reflexology, especially in conjunction with massage, is beneficial.
- Yoga and Qi Gong are of long-term benefit.
- Tai Chi has been shown to improve arthritis, especially in the winter months.
- Writing about stressful events can reduce the overall disease activity of rheumatoid arthritis. As this has been proven it would suggest that counselling or psychotherapy is likely to help.

Nutritional

- Chicken cartilage is a Russian treatment. The cartilage from a chicken carcass should be eaten once a day. This includes the mobile part of the breast bone and the cartilage of the wing and leg joints. There is currently no preparation of this and a friendly butcher or chicken farmer needs to be approached.
- The juice of an avocado daily or eaten whole may be protective.

Supplemental

- Take selenium (100µg twice a day), vitamin C (1g three times a day), vitamin E (200mg twice a day) and evening primrose oil (2g with each meal). These can all be reduced as improvement is forthcoming.
- Vitamin B_5 and vitamin B_3 (both at 25mg per day) can be taken but not at night.
- Test for hydrochloric acid production in the stomach and, if low, supplement with hydrochloric acid tablets.
- Carnosine, taken at the dosage recommended on the packaging, may have an anti-inflammatory effect and be beneficial in arthritis.

Homeopathic

- Homeopathy is undoubtedly useful and the choice of remedy should be made on the symptoms of the arthritis. A homeopathic prescriber is best utilized but attention can be paid to the remedies Rhus toxicodendron, Bryonia, Apis and Pulsatilla.

Herbal/natural extracts

- Six drops of rosemary and chamomile essential oils can be added to a bath or can be applied directly if mixed into almond oil. Sesame oil can be effective by itself when rubbed in and may be even more effective if the oil is slightly heated with cayenne or ginger.
- Green-lipped muscle extract, 100mg twice daily.
- Glucosamine sulphate, 500mg taken with each meal.
- Chondroitin sulphate, 500mg with each meal. Do not use chondroitin if there is any possibility of having prostate cancer.
- Methyl-sulphonylmethane (MSM) a potent antioxidant and high sulphur-containing compound has been shown to be beneficial in arthritis.

Orthodox

- Aspirins, NSAIDs and steroids are first-line orthodox treatments and should be left until last because of the high incidence of side effects.
- A new form of anti-inflammatory known as COX-2 inhibitors are likely to become first choice as they have fewer gastrointestinal side effects than aspirin and NSAIDs.
- Regenersen is an anti-ageing 'designer drug' that is extracted from placenta, pancreas, testes and other tissues and may stimulate protein biosynthesis in degenerative conditions.

Rheumatoid arthritis

This is a chronic disease of unknown origin in which symptoms and inflammatory changes occur in the body's connective tissues, predominantly in the joints and related structures. The symptoms, as in any arthritic condition, are of pain, limitation of motion and joint deformities.

FOR RHEUMATOID AND AUTOIMMUNE ARTHRITIS OR OSTEOARTHRITIS SHOWING JOINT DESTRUCTION

General Advice

- *Use the recommendations opposite.*
- *Avoid all tobacco, which is a solanum.*
- *I have noticed that tea may exacerbate arthritic conditions and should be avoided for three or four weeks and reintroduced as an experiment if an improvement has been noted. If the discomfort returns, then tea may be a culprit.*
- *A six-day water-only fast has shown efficacy in acute arthritis affecting chronic sufferers. This should be done under complementary medical supervision.*
- *Smokers, especially those smoking more than twenty cigarettes a day, have a much higher risk of rheumatoid arthritis and so they should stop smoking.*

Nutritional

- *Avoid members of the solanum plant family, specifically potatoes, peppers and tomatoes.*
- *If improvement is not forthcoming, avoid wheat, corn and animal proteins (including cheese, milk and eggs) and consider food allergy testing.*

Supplemental

- *Glucosamine sulphate (500mg) can be taken with each meal. Chondrotin (500mg) may be used as well.*

Herbal/natural extracts

- *Green tea has been shown to improve symptoms.*
- *Methyl-sulphonylmethane (MSM) a potent antioxidant and high sulphur-containing compound has been shown to be beneficial in arthritis.*

Orthodox

- *Orthodox treatment is not curative. All drugs are geared towards relieving the pain but not helping to improve the structure of the joint. They should*

be used only as a last resort.
- *Under medical supervision only, use 10g of fish oil per day. Patients and their clinicians must be aware of a slightly increased risk of brain haemorrhages and the white blood cell count must be monitored. This treatment should only be encouraged in very severe and non-relenting arthritis.*
- *If the above do not show improvements, then surgery may be considered as an option for large joints.*

BUERGER'S DISEASE AND INTERMITTENT CLAUDICATION

Named after an American physician, this disease process of aggressive arterial occlusion is found at any age, although more common in middle age, and is associated with smoking. Arteriosclerosis (*see* **Arteriosclerosis**) with associated inflammation, especially in the arteries of the lower limb, causes severe pain that is worse on walking. This is known as *intermittent claudication*, which may occur in non-smokers. The occlusion of arteries can be so severe that the outcome, especially in those who continue to smoke, is often amputation. The occlusion can occur in arteries other than in the leg and more serious operations may be required if occlusions occur in the bowel.

General Advice

- *Stop smoking (see **Smoking** and **Cigarettes**).*
- *See **Arteriosclerosis**.*
- *See an acupuncturist and obtain electro-acupuncture in preference.*
- *Regular massage can be most beneficial.*

Herbal/natural extracts

- *Ginkgo biloba extract, 120mg daily, is beneficial and can increase pain-free walking distance markedly.*
- *Padma 28 – a multi-compound herbal formula, taken at the recommended doses on the product*

label may show beneficial signs within four weeks. Carry on for at least six months if treatment is effective. No side effects or other drug interactions have been noted to date but the doses should be taken with food to avoid potential mild stomach discomfort.

CIRCULATION

As we age the body has a tendency to clog up its arteries with depositions of cholesterol and other unavoidable chemicals. This reaction, created by the body's own defence system, is discussed in the section on arteriosclerosis (*see* **Arteriosclerosis**) and is aided and abetted by mast cells, which are specialized white blood cells that collect unwanted molecules such as cholesterol and free radicals and then bind to the nearest surface, taking the dangerous compounds out of the circulation. This process is inevitable and necessary for the well-being of delicate organs such as the brain.

Care of the circulation should start at an early age with the avoidance of cholesterol-containing foods, and with daily exercise, good breathing techniques and proper nutrition full of anti-oxidants. Unfortunately this advice is not well heeded and the ravages and difficulties occur in our latter years.

RECOMMENDATIONS

General Advice
- See **Arteriosclerosis**.
- At the first sign of circulatory difficulties, use common sense by wearing hats, gloves and warm footwear.
- Internal circulatory difficulties such as the clogging of the heart arteries may not be noticeable until a very late stage. If symptoms occur, please refer to the relevant section in this book and contact your complementary medical practitioner immediately.
- It is never too late to exercise, and yoga, Qi Gong and Tai Chi are the best forms.

Herbal/natural extracts
- Cayenne capsules or a level teaspoonful of turmeric in a cup of heated milk, three times a day may help peripheral circulation in those who have cold hands and feet.
- Padma 28 – a multi-compound herbal formula, taken at the recommended doses on the product label may show beneficial signs within four weeks. Carry on for at least six months if treatment is effective. No side effects or other drug interactions have been noted to date but the doses should be taken with food to avoid potential mild stomach discomfort.

Aneurysm

Aneurysm is the term given to an artery that loses its integrity from a source other than an injury. Broadly speaking, an aneurysm can be a weakness within the arterial wall or 'dissecting', where the inner lining of the artery ruptures but the outer lining holds, causing a swelling in the arterial wall.

ANEURYSMS – Common and Dissecting

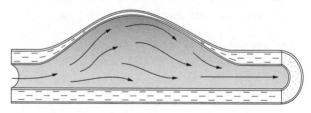

A

A shows a common aneurysm where the middle wall of the artery is weakened.

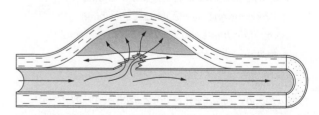

B

In B, a dissecting aneurysm, the inner wall is torn, allowing blood to flow through.

If not surgically treated, aneurysms can be fatal when they occur in arteries in the brain, other vital organs or the aorta (the main vessel from the heart). Sudden abdominal or chest pain, a sledge hammer-like blow to the head, sudden blindness or neurological symptoms (paralysis, pain) must all be treated as an emergency and reviewed by a surgeon.

RECOMMENDATIONS

General Advice

- *Aneurysms are difficult to diagnose and any sudden pain should be seen by a medical practitioner.*
- *There is no complementary treatment other than support for pre- and post-operative care.*

Homeopathic

- *On your way to hospital or awaiting the doctor's arrival, use Aconite 6, 12, or 30, one dose every 10min.*

DUPUYTREN'S CONTRACTURE

This condition, named after the French surgeon who put it into the medical books at the turn of the 19th century, is a painless contracture of tendon or tendons in the palm of the hand. This causes the fingers to curl inwards and creates an inability to fully extend them. It occurs most commonly in the third and fourth fingers, chiefly in adult males, and there is no known cause as far as Western medicine is concerned. The acupuncture energy meridians point out that the tendons most commonly affected are those of the heart, pericardium or sexual function and the triple heater (triple burner). These meridians or energy channels are most affected by heat, such as created by excess adrenaline or stress and by smoking (inhaling smoke at around 250°C) and by emotional upsets. As Dupuytren's contracture can often take years to form, I have often found it to be associated with long-standing suppression of emotion in smokers.

RECOMMENDATIONS

General Advice

- *In the early stages, assessment and change of emotional deficiencies may stop the progress.*
- *Gentle massage three times a day with Arnica creams may prevent further deterioration and may even alleviate the problem.*
- *Osteopathic, chiropractic, acupuncture and Shiatsu techniques may all stretch the tendon and prevent worsening, if not actually improve the situation.*

Orthodox

- *If the fingers are becoming useless then an operative procedure, best performed by plastic surgeons or orthopaedic surgeons who specialize in hands, is an effective technique that may solve the problem for several years, but it can recur.*

Dupuytren's Contracture

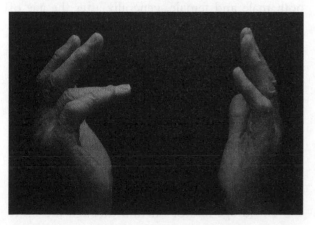

FRACTURES AND BROKEN BONES – *see* Fractures

Bones in the elderly often heal more slowly and it is very important to maintain a calcium and magnesium intake along with the remedies *Calcarea phosphorica* and *Symphytum* as mentioned in chapter 4.

Bones heal better if they are active, and gentle exercises as taught by Alexander Technicians or yoga teachers are very important to prevent arthritis setting in rapidly. The possibility of osteoporosis must be excluded (*see* **Osteoporsis**) and healing time will be improved.

Hands-on healing can be most beneficial in this age group.

MYASTHENIA GRAVIS

This is a disorder characterized by a fluctuant weakness of certain voluntary muscles. Those muscles most commonly affected are found in the face and neck and this condition tends to affect women twice as commonly as men and it tends to form in older people. Hyperthyroidism, thymus gland problems or cancer may be associated with the condition and need to be ruled out by a physician.

The problem occurs because of an autoimmune (body attacking itself) attack on certain receptors in the muscles, which prevents the nerves from transmitting their orders.

RECOMMENDATIONS

General Advice
- *See* **Nerve injury** *and use the supplements recommended there; see* **Autoimmune disease**.
- *Acupuncture may be beneficial.*
- *The drugs used in MG are immunosuppressive. Taking the following naturopathic advice will offer some protection.*

Supplemental
- *Take high dose antioxidants (see those listed for* **Arteriosclerosis***).*

Homeopathic
- *Homeopathic constitutional remedies may be chosen by an experienced homeopathic practitioner. The remedies Natrum muriaticum and Silica may be of marked benefit.*

Herbal/natural extracts
- *Tibetan medicine, much geared towards energy flow through the nervous system, may have some answers.*
- *Provided there is no suggestion of interaction with other drugs being taken, consider Echinacea at doses recommended on the packaging for three-week bursts and two weeks off in between.*

Orthodox
- *There are a variety of drugs available to help the various symptoms but they may increase the risk of infection as most reduce the immune system function.*

OSTEOARTHRITIS

Osteoarthritis is the term given for the age-related loss of cartilage and subsequent bone damage to the ends or joint aspects of bones. The condition is due to wear and tear and may therefore come on before the usual onset at the age of 60 years, particularly in athletes or in the persistently overweight.

RECOMMENDATION

General Advice
- *See* **Arthritis**.

OSTEOPOROSIS

Osteoporosis is the decrease in bone tissue leading to structural weakness and increased risk of fracture. The bones that are most commonly affected are the spine, hips and the ribs.

Symptoms are usually absent until osteoporosis is severe, when backaches or structural changes such as a decrease in height or 'hunchback' deformities occur. Spontaneous fractures, or breakage following minor accidents, are the result of osteoporosis.

The density of bone will decline in all of us, both male and female, generally after the age of about 40. This is partially because of a decrease in exercise, which maintains bone integrity, but also because of the loss of oestrogen levels in women and of calcitonin – a calcium-level-controlling hormone made in the thyroid glands – in both sexes. Decreasing levels of stomach acid, and skin and bowel membrane changes all lead to diminished blood levels of calcium, magnesium, boron and vitamin D, all of which are essential to the production of bone. A diet too high in protein can encourage loss of calcium through the urine and is probably one of the major causes of the condition in the Western world. Other dietary factors are undoubtedly relevant, as is borne out by the fact that osteoporosis is very much a condition affecting the West, as opposed to in Africa and Japan where the incidence is negligible. The ageing process is by far the most common cause of osteoporosis but other conditions must be ruled out before age-related osteoporosis is treated.

Alcohol, steroids and a few prescribed drugs can all cause osteoporotic conditions. Paralysis or other causes of decreased movement, such as arthritis, lung or heart disease, will also reduce bone density. Certain congenital conditions, malnutrition and a variety of glandular (endocrine) diseases can all cause osteoporosis.

Postmenopausal osteoporosis is not, as the pharmaceutical industry would have us believe, solely created by a diminution in oestrogen. In fact oestrogen has a very small role to play in maintaining bone density, whereas other hormones such as progesterone and dehydroepiandrosterone (DHEA) actually help build bone. Several trials show categorically that weight-bearing exercise is as beneficial, if not more so, as oestrogen replacement. This is borne out by the fact that the risk of fracture in a male is equal to that of a female after the age of 70. A good diet containing all the necessary supplements is also essential.

Most of us make the assumption that bone density is governed by the levels of calcium, and to an extent this is true. However, calcium is trapped in the bone on a network or matrix of protein fibres. Osteoporosis is as much due to a deficiency in this matrix as it is due to mineral deficiency. Interestingly, high animal protein diets have an adverse effect whereas vegetarian diets, which are heavy on vegetable protein, seem to be protective.

One important factor has come to light recently. It appears that osteoporosis is more profound in individuals who underwent malnutrition before the age of the menarche (start of the periods). It would appear that the foundation of bone density is laid at this early age. This has led to the suggestion that cow's milk is a must for children. This is incorrect since milk is not a good dietary source of *absorbable calcium* and is a food that many humans are actually allergic to (*see* **Milk**).

Investigations

The orthodox medical world is quick to promote the use of X-ray investigations of the spine and hip to measure bone density. Whilst the levels of radiation are low, bear in mind that three per cent of the population carry a gene that is sensitive to radiation and may become cancerous. There may be times when X-rays are necessary but as a routine screen, non-invasive and simple tests are available.

Urine

Urine testing for two proteins called pyridinium and deoxypyridinium – principal proteins involved in the bone matrix that trap the calcium – should be carried out because an increase in levels of these proteins may suggest an osteoporotic tendency.

Ultrasound

An ultrasound of the heel bone (calcaneus) has been shown in comparative studies to be as effective as radiological (X-ray) investigation. Ultrasound is harmless (unless used excessively in pregnancy) and is therefore preferable.

Other tests

Minerals as trace elements can be analysed by a simple blood and hair analysis and deficiencies of calcium, magnesium, zinc, copper, silicon and boron can be established, all of which are known to be integral in the formation of strong bones. Orthodox sources may suggest that increasing these minerals in the diet will have no effect and they are absolutely right if one takes an artificial form of any of these and gives it to an individual without the others. Many trials have

Densitometry – Scan of Spine

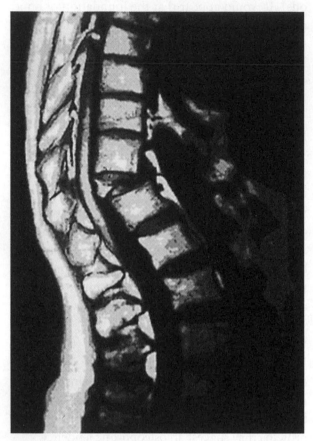

Densitometry scan of a normal lumbar spine. This technique measures the density of the bone and is used in the assessment of osteoporosis.

shown that natural forms of mineral supplementation, especially those in a combined (chelated) form, will be absorbed rapidly not only in the bloodstream but also effectively into the bones themselves.

Vitamins B$_6$, C, D and K are all essential for bone growth and stability. These levels can be tested in the blood. The absorptive capacity of these and all the necessary minerals and proteins is dependent on an intact bowel. Low stomach acid, poor pancreatic function (*see* **Gastrograms** and **Pancreatic Exocrine Tests**) and bowel bacterial integrity are all very important.

Bowel conditions such as coeliac disease or the less severe gluten (a wheat protein) sensitivity, Crohn's and other inflammatory conditions, and

the leaky gut syndrome must all be considered as possible causes of osteoporosis. These may all be tested for.

The levels of phosphorus and its derivative phosphate are balanced in the bloodstream by the kidneys. Phosphorus encourages the kidneys to eliminate calcium. Phosphates are found in most foods but especially in carbonated drinks and meat products. Is there a correlation, I wonder, between the high incidence of osteoporosis in developed countries and their intake of fizzy drinks and burgers?

There is much press at this time discussing the use of natural progesterone (extracted from the Mexican yam). Dr Lee, a gynaecologist from the USA, has spent over a decade studying the effects of progesterone on osteoporosis and other menopausal problems. His conclusions are that progesterone, not oestrogen, is more effective in maintaining bone density. His work needs more study but theoretically he is correct. The use of natural progesterone is becoming more popular and studies over the next few years should help to decide if this is a preferred method of maintaining bone density and avoiding osteoporosis.

RECOMMENDATIONS

General Advice

- *Increase weight-bearing exercise. Thirty to forty minutes of walking each day is a minimum for those with osteoporosis but 20min of work in a gym or as a racket sport three or four times a week is good for maintenance.*

- *Blood and hair analysis for mineral deficiencies, phosphorus, fluoride and strontium toxicity and calcitonin should be taken as the baseline and monitored on a yearly basis or treated as required. Please note that strontium, whilst toxic in excess, is necessary for good bone strength and deficiencies should be remedied.*

Nutritional

- *Prevention is the best form of cure. Ensure,*

OSTEOPOROSIS PROFILE

Reference: DJ1J ASSB C90
Patient: Mrs Jo Public
Doctor: Dr Mustafa Consult

Age: 72
Sex: Female
Date: 10/02/91

SERUM:	Result	Units	Reference Range
Alkaline phosphatase:			
Total	= 109	units	40 – 190
Bone	= 24	units	35 – 90
Tartrate resistant acid phosphatase	= 2.6	units	1.5 – 4.3
Inorganic phosphorus	= 0.93	mmol/l	0.8 – 1.4
Calcium	= 2.46	mmol/l	2.25 – 2.75
Copper	= 22.0	µmol/l	12.5 – 25.0
Manganese	= 14	nmol/l	9 – 25
Vitamin C	= 1.1	mg/dl	0.4 – 2.0
WHITE CELL:			
Zinc	= 5.7	µg/10–6	5.4 – 8.2
RED CELL:			
Magnesium	= 2.03	mmol/l	2.8 – 3.00
24 HOUR URINE:			
Volume	= 1900	ml	
Phosphorus	= 38	mmol/24 hours	15 – 45
Calcium	= 3.1	mmol/24 hours	2.5 – 7.5
Zinc	= 3.70	µg/24 hours	220 – 590
Hydroxyproline	= 11.00	mg/24 hours	up to 13

These tests include essential nutrients of known importance in the development and maintenance of bone. Changes in the excretion of calcium and phosphorus occur in some types of bone disease and increased urinary zinc and hydroxyproline are found in osteoporosis. Recent research demonstrates changes in bone alkaline phosphatase levels in osteoporotic women.

This profile does not replace the measurement of bone density.

Comments on Results
There is a reduction in bone formation (low bone ALP) with a normal resorption rate (normal TRAP). This is consistent with mild bone loss.

especially in children, a good source of calcium and other relevant minerals. Soya, fish, nuts and deep-green vegetables such as spinach, collard greens and broccoli are all excellent sources. Milk and milk products such as cheese are not necessarily a good source although yoghurt is excellent.

- Increase proteins from vegetables rather than animals and if osteoporosis is noted, switch to a predominantly vegetarian diet.

- Meat products are particularly high in phosphorus, which increases calcium excretion and should therefore be reduced. Carbonated drinks contain a marked level of phosphates and must be avoided.

- Avoid excesses of protein, alcohol, tobacco and caffeine. Specific osteoporosis formulae are available, all of which combine the necessary co-factors needed for good calcium absorption. A nutritionist would recommend particular brands.

Supplemental

- Ensure an adequate intake (around 1,000–1,500mg) of calcium each day from the sources listed in chapter 7 (see **Calcium**) rather than milk.

- Remember that calcium is directly linked to vitamin D and up to 200iu should be taken on a daily basis if there is any sign of bone thinning. Higher doses may be necessary via your complementary practitioner.

- Supplementation of the following may be beneficial but it is best to check your levels before self-prescribing. Overdosing is not possible on the recommended dosages but the supplementation is not necessary if levels are not proven to be deficient. The following supplements should be considered and taken in divided doses per foot of height throughout the day: calcium (150mg), magnesium (150mg), copper (500µg), manganese (4mg), silicone (200µg), boron (500µg) and zinc (500mg before bed).

- The following vitamin supplements should be taken in divided doses per foot of height with food throughout the day: vitamin B_6 (10mg), folic acid (50µg), vitamin D (100iu) and phylloquinone (vitamin K_1) (200µg).

- Plant oestrogens (phyto-oestrogens), natural progesterone and specific herbal treatments should be considered in osteoporosis but prescribed by a complementary medical practitioner.

Orthodox

- Your GP will recommend calcium and vitamin D supplementation followed by a choice of drugs that are reasonably well-tolerated but have a few adverse effects. This group, known as bisphosphonates, would be recommended initially but your GP will also discuss HRT (see **Hormone replacement therapy**).

- A moderately recent development is Selective Oestrogens Receptor Modulators (SERMs). These have been developed with the aim of maximizing the benefits of oestrogenic action in the bones, avoiding hormone replacement effects elsewhere. (see **SERMs**).

- Use of DHEA (dehydroepiandrosterone) may be prescribed under medical supervision along with natural progesterone creams to increase bone density.

POLYMYALGIA RHEUMATICA (PMR)

This condition describes an inflammatory process that affects the muscles. It is characterized by stiffness, pain and limitation of movement of the hips and shoulders in particular. General malaise, weight loss, night sweats and fevers may also be associated. The condition is often association with inflammation of blood vessels.

Arterial inflammation may be found in 50 per cent of cases and if left untreated can develop into neurological problems if it affects the arteries in the nervous system or brain. This may include blindness or stroke. Polymyalgia rheumatica is considered an autoimmune disease – one where the body's immune system attacks itself. This generally occurs after a prolonged subclinical allergy, usually a food intolerance or an incorrect response to a viral, bacterial or other infection. A full constitutional view, taking into account the well-being of the individual from birth onwards, is necessary to speed up the process of repair and prevent further autoimmune disease settling in. The Eastern philosophies would look upon this particular condition as being a stagnation of energy (Qi) and excess heat in the blood.

RECOMMENDATIONS

General Advice
- *Any unexplained loss of power or pain that persists must be reviewed by a doctor.*
- *Investigations will show a raised ESR (a test for the sedimentation rate of red blood cells) and other changes.*
- *The condition is an autoimmune syndrome (see* **Autoimmune disease***).*
- *Yoga and Qi Gong, acupuncture and massage will all help the muscle groups and help move the stagnant Qi.*

Nutritional
- *Allergy testing is essential and correction of diet aimed at removing allergens and heat-creating foods such as caffeine, alcohol, spicy foods and refined foods must be adhered to strictly.*

Herbal/natural extracts
- *Plant extracts that include steroids are used by experienced herbalists and Chinese-trained physicians, but the quantity is variable depending upon the distilling process from each plant and, although available, I think in PMR with arterial involvement conventional drugs should be used.*
- *In cases where arterial involvement is not present, herbal treatment under the guidance of an expert may be beneficial and should be continued until the patient has been symptom-free for at least three months. A trial period*

without treatment may allow symptoms to return, in which case the treatment should be recommenced for at least another three months.

Orthodox
- *If there is any evidence of inflammation of the arteries (as diagnosed by a physician) then steroids should be used.*

THE SKIN

LEG ULCERS (VARICOSE ULCERS)

If a mottled appearance occurs (frequently just above the bony parts of the ankle) and, commonly following a gentle knock, the skin breaks down and does not heal well, the likelihood is this is a varicose ulcer (commonly termed a leg ulcer).

Leg ulcers in middle age and onwards are generally caused by poor circulation secondary to varicose veins. The poor return of blood, due to a diminution of the effect of the valves in the leg veins, causes stagnation and tension in the tissues of the lower leg. Without a good blood flow, oxygen does not readily reach the tissues, the toxins from normal metabolism are not removed, and oxygen and nutrients are not brought into the area. (*See* **Varicose veins**.)

Other causes include localized infection following insect bites, and similar ulcers can form on the legs of diabetics.

RECOMMENDATIONS

General Advice
- *Always obtain a medical opinion for any long-term injury.*
- *Keep the area as clean as possible.*
- *Keep the area covered if you are mobile but exposed to clean air unless otherwise directed by a practitioner.*

Nutritional

- *Ensure good fruit and vegetable intake. Eat five portions daily and increase the intake of blueberries, bilberries and other berries, and cherries.*

Supplemental

- *Beta-carotene 2mg per foot of height in divided doses through the day.*
- *Vitamin E 100iu per foot of height in divided doses through the day.*
- *Linseed oil 200mg per foot of height in divided doses through the day.*
- *Anthocyanidin 150mg per foot of height in divided doses through the day.*
- *Rutin 300mg per foot of height in divided doses through the day taken with food.*

Homeopathic

- *The following can be taken at potency 30, three times a day:*
- *Hamamelis as a starting remedy.*
- *Mercurius solubilis or Hepar sulphuris if the wound is infected.*
- *Silica if particularly long-standing or recurring.*

Herbal/natural extracts

- *Apply Manuka honey twice a day.*
- *Clean the area with witch hazel and calendula lotions.*

Orthodox

- *Pressure bandaging, with or without support stockings, and frequent antiseptic dressing are generally applied by a practice or district nurse.*
- *Artificial skin sprays can now be applied.*
- *Skin grafting is a last surgical option and will be necessary after attempts to repair the venous problem.*

THREAD VEINS (SPIDER VEINS)

These thin spindly veins show up under the surface of the skin on the calves and thighs of women more often then in men. About 50 per cent of women will develop these unsightly yet harmless lesions. They more commonly arrive with age but are often noticed in pregnancy. Thirty per cent of these thread veins arise because of weak valves in the deeper vein (*see* **Varicose veins**) but the other 70 per cent are due to backpressure. The more blue, purple or deep red the veins are, the deeper they tend to lie and treatment is best achieved by a technique called microsclerotherapy. This technique involves an injection of sclerosing solution and this causes the veins to collapse and stick together, thereby not allowing any further blood flow. These deeper thread veins make up about 90 per cent of the problem. The remaining 10 per cent are generally bright red veins lying closer to the surface. These tend to be treatable using a laser technique.

RECOMMENDATIONS

General Advice

- *See a specialist. Undergo a Doppler ultrasound to test whether the deep vein valves are functional or not and accept treatment accordingly.*
- *See* **Varicose veins** *for further naturopathic options.*

Orthodox

- *The techniques described in the text above may be required if skin creams provided by specialists do not do the trick.*

THE NERVOUS SYSTEM

MOTOR NEURONE DISEASE

This condition – which is medically known as progressive spinal muscular atrophy – is a progressive wasting of individual muscles or groups of muscles due to the degeneration of nerve cells and pathways affecting the spinal column and parts of the brain that control muscle movement. It is a particularly distressing disorder because it slowly and relentlessly diminishes an individual's ability to move, swallow and communicate but leaves the thought process, awareness and pain receptors intact.

The condition, which can strike at any age, usually occurs after the age of 50 years and can progress to an incapacitating level within two years but it may take up to 15 years to reach its end point. Usually individuals will die from infection because of an inability to breathe properly, allowing bacteria to settle into the lungs. The cough and gag reflexes eventually disappear.

There may be a genetic factor but an infective or toxic cause is most likely. The condition has been known to be triggered by deficiencies in vitamins, specifically vitamins B_{12}, B_6 and E.

I do not recommend self-help in this condition because aggressive treatment is best suited and a course should be set and monitored by an experienced medical practitioner.

More so than with other neurological conditions, a philosophical attitude must be taken and I believe the question needs to be asked: 'what lessons can be learnt on a spiritual or karmic level by being struck with a condition that slowly moves an individual to a position of total dependence?' More so than many conditions, the question of euthanasia arises in patients who have this condition and full and frank discussions must be undertaken on a spiritual level as soon as motor neurone disease is diagnosed.

RECOMMENDATIONS

General Advice
- *Yoga and Qi Gong training, along with the Alexander Technique, may maintain neurological and muscular control for longer.*
- *Specialized Ayurvedic and Tibetan massage techniques such as Marma and neurotherapy must be undertaken.*

Nutritional
- *Assessment of digestive capabilities, both stomach acid and pancreatic enzyme production, must be assessed.*

Supplemental
- *Deficiencies of vitamins and amino acids (the breakdown products of proteins) must be plugged.*

Homeopathic
- *A homeopathic consultation with an expert is essential.*

Herbal/natural extracts
- *A herbalist should assess the possible benefits from herbal medicines, especially alfalfa, broom and mushroom or toadstool derivatives.*
- *Tibetan medicine, based considerably on energy flow through neurological pathways, may have some answers.*

Orthodox
- *A full blood and hair analysis for deficiencies in vitamins, nutrients and amino acids and toxicity from heavy metals and agrochemicals (including pesticides) must be undertaken.*

PARKINSON'S DISEASE

Parkinson was an English physician in the 18th century. He described a clinical state that has taken on his name. Parkinson's disease is characterized by an expressionless face, infrequency of blinking, a poverty and slowness of voluntary movement, rigidity of muscles with a rhythmic 3–4 per second tremor that is more pronounced at rest, a stooped posture and a wide-legged walking stance. This latter symptom is caused by a loss of the normal postural reflexes. The condition is characterized by a shuffling walk and the initiation and cessation of movements are impeded. Crossing a road may, in extreme cases, be difficult because timing is important and being able to stop is difficult. Memory loss and an inability to concentrate are prominent symptoms.

Parkinson's disease may occur in middle or later life due to the degeneration of cells in the brain that produce a chemical called dopamine. Dopamine has a pronounced effect on the control of muscles and posture. Parkinson's disease may occur as a sequel to encephalitis or poisoning from certain drugs.

Aluminium has been cited as a potential cause of the destruction of that part of the brain that produces dopamine. Other chemicals, including pesticides, are suspected but yet to be proven as causative agents. Most chemicals are destroyed in the liver and so Parkinson's disease may be a consequence of liver weakness or deficiencies in antioxidants, which are also responsible for the breakdown of toxic compounds. Nutritional deficiencies may lead to a reduction in dopamine so long-term poor diet may be a trigger to the condition.

RECOMMENDATIONS

General Advice

- *Any neurological symptoms that persist must be reviewed by a specialist and a firm diagnosis made.*
- *Consult with a complementary specialist with experience in the field for measures of toxicity, nutritional deficiencies and liver function. These need to be corrected.*
- *Bioresonance techniques may be beneficial in helping to illustrate any underlying cause of the destruction of dopamine-producing brain cells.*
- *Cranial osteopathy, osteopathy, polarity therapy, yoga and Qi Gong may all have a beneficial effect on reducing the symptoms and delaying the progression of the disease.*
- *Marma massage and neurotherapy, both Ayurvedic disciplines, can be beneficial.*

Supplemental

- *Particular attention should be paid to blood cell copper levels and this should be corrected by taking an absorbable copper supplement at a level of 1mg per foot of height.*
- *The amino acid tyrosine should be taken (400mg per foot of height) in divided doses throughout the day. L-Methionine is another amino acid that should be taken at a level of 1g per foot of height.*
- *High-dose antioxidants should be considered if there is any level of toxicity.*

Homeopathic

- *Any specific toxins that may be isolated should be treated by their homeopathic equivalent at a potency of 30, twice a day for one month, and the levels re-measured. If there is no diminution, then repeat using potency 200 twice a day for two weeks.*

Herbal/natural extracts

- *If the disease is progressing, Tibetan medicine should be employed under the care of a Tibetan-trained physician.*

Orthodox

- *Orthodox drugs are geared towards correcting the loss of dopamine (see **Anti-Parkinson's drugs**). These drugs seem to lose their effect after a few years and are therefore not started by most neurologists until the disease process is inhibiting normal function. The alternative treatments above should be tried as soon as possible and orthodox treatment delayed as long as possible.*
- *We watch with interest the outcome of trials of implanting dopamine-producing cells from pigs into brain tissue and the use of electric implants that stimulate the cells that make dopamine.*

STROKE (CEREBROVASCULAR ACCIDENT, CVA)

A stroke denotes the onset of a neurological deficit, most frequently the paralysis of one side of the body with or without an effect on the contralateral side of the face. This weakness may develop within minutes and is usually associated with an arterial problem or may develop over a much longer period of time, even months, which may be indicative of a disease process, most commonly a tumour. Ninety-five per cent of strokes are caused by a lack of oxygen due to a blood vessel in the brain being blocked by a clot, closing up because of atheroma or, rarely, going into spasm through some neurological or chemical influence. Atheroma may also cause a fragility in the blood vessel, which leaks causing a haemorrhage that then clots and obstructs blood flow beyond that point.

Thus, most strokes are cerebrovascular accidents, either haemorrhagic (caused by bleeding) or infarctions (caused by blockage). A stroke is further classified by considering whether the event is completed or still evolving. Finally, in categorizing stroke, the type and severity of the neurological problems will give a clue as to where the arterial damage occurred. This is mostly of diagnostic value because the treatment is the same and based entirely upon the deficit.

Any condition that can lead to vascular damage will predispose to a stroke. High blood pressure may burst the small vessels in the brain, although the mechanism to protect brain blood pressure is one of the most evolved mechanisms in the human being. Atheroma and the eventual clogging up of the arteries, with the increased tendency for a clot to form in such blood vessels, is much more likely to cause a stroke, and small emboli (clots from other parts of the body) may fire off atheroma plaques in other vessels or come from diseased heart valves to occlude the arteries. Preventing any of these factors is the primary concern in fighting stroke and even if a stroke has taken place, active therapy against these conditions may prevent a worsening or a recurrence of the problem.

Stroke is the third most common cause of death in the Western world, behind heart disease and cancer. It is, however, the commonest cause of severe chronic disability and happens to two out of every 1000 people each year. Three-quarters of this number are over the age of 65 and the event is twice as common in Blacks as it is in Whites. It is worth looking at these figures because conditions such as hypertension are actively fought regardless of the risks of side effects of these drugs. Very simply, and not absolutely accurately, these figures suggest that 1 in 500 adults at the age of 65 or more will have a stroke. We are told that if one has hypertension the risk is six times greater, which brings the risk to one in 83 people. Whilst this is a marked increase, the chances are still 82:1 that an individual with high blood pressure will *not* have a stroke. I mention this simply because so many people are frightened by their high blood pressure because of the risk of stroke, but the chances are still low even if the problem is not treated. More people on antihypertensive drugs will end up having a stroke than those who do not use such drugs, but this matter is discussed more fully in the section on hypertension (*see* **Hypertension**).

Prevention is the key word in stroke because full recovery from neurological deficit is rarely possible. Most individuals who have anything other than a major stroke will have some degree of recovery. If the correct treatment is undertaken, an indication of the repair process can be gleaned at about three months when 90 per cent of lost abilities will have returned.

Immediate first aid and orthodox emergency medicine reduce the risk of death and a knowledge of cardiopulmonary resuscitation is always advisable because a stroke may affect breathing and cardiac response.

RECOMMENDATIONS

General Advice

- *Avoidance by correct control of atheroma and hypertension at an early age is the best form of treatment (see* **Atherosclerosis** *and* **Hypertension***).*

- *Full assessment by a neurological specialist is mandatory and push the point to discover whether the stroke is caused by a haemorrhage or an occlusion (or both). Treatment varies depending upon the cause.*

- *Physiotherapy is an integral part of rehabilitation but all forms of Eastern medicine, principally Chinese, Tibetan or Ayurvedic in origin, have physical, acupuncture and herbal treatments that have been used for thousands of years with great effect. Do not ignore Western therapy techniques but use them in conjunction with an experienced Eastern medical practitioner.*

Nutritional

• *Consider the macrobiotic diet (see chapter 7).*

Herbal/natural extracts

• *Herbal treatments such as Ginkgo biloba are frequently recommended, but increasing blood flow in the brain of those who may have a tendency to haemorrhagic strokes is unwise.*

Orthodox

• *Treatment of a stroke is dependent upon the cause. There is strong recommendation for the use of prophylactic aspirin because this prevents clotting but of course will make the situation worse if the stroke is caused by a haemorrhage. Many people are mistakenly taking aspirin because they have heard that it reduces the risk of stroke but it may do the opposite.*

• *Stop taking the oral contraceptive pill if you are at risk or have a family history of cardiovascular disease or stroke. The pill increases the risk of blood clots.*

TRANSIENT ISCHAEMIC ATTACKS

A transient ischaemic attack is a temporary neurological deficit, usually comprising a dimming of vision, a lack of power or movement on one side of the body, numbness, dizziness and difficulty in speaking that usually lasts 10 minutes or less but may last as long as 24 hours. These attacks are usually related to a temporary blockage in a blood vessel in the brain caused either by spasm of an already atherosclerotic vessel or by an embolism (travelling blood clot or other matter). The longer the attack, the more probable the effect was caused by an embolism.

Recovery is usually complete but transient ischaemic attacks usually recur and may be a warning of an impending stroke. Recommendations for treatment are as for **Stroke** but also *see* **Atherosclerosis**.

TREMOR AND TREMBLING

A tremor is a regular rhythmic oscillation of a part of the body caused by alternate contractions of muscles either side of a joint. Trembling is simply an exacerbation of a tremor affecting a larger part of the system, such as an arm or leg.

Anything that affects the nerves or the neuromuscular junction will potentially cause a tremor and the most common causes are the toxic effect from alcohol withdrawal (delirium tremens), caffeine or other stimulatory drugs such as amphetamines or cocaine. An excess of thyroxine or adrenaline (such as in extreme nervousness) may cause such problems and may indicate underlying conditions such as hyperthyroidism or adrenal tumours. Other symptoms such as sweating and weight loss are usually associated.

Neurological diseases such as Parkinson's disease, which can cause a tremor when resting, or stroke, which may affect the coordination centres, can be differentiated by causing an unintentional (one that does not disappear on intentional movement such as picking up a pen) tremor. Fevers may trigger trembling or tremors because the body uses muscular movements to increase its temperature to kill off the bugs.

A twitch is the involuntary contraction of a single muscle group and is usually an indication of an entrapped nerve or peripheral neurological damage. A twitch is known medically as a fasciculation and may be an indication of more serious neurological conditions, such as motor neurone disease.

RECOMMENDATIONS

General Advice

• *Any shake that is not associated with an obvious cause such as nervousness, excess drug intake or withdrawal should be reviewed by a doctor for a firm diagnosis.*

• *Treatment should depend upon the underlying cause and reference should be made to the relevant section in this book.*

Homeopathic

• *The homeopathic remedy Agaricus muscarius may*

be taken at potency 30 four times a day until a diagnosis is made. Trembling due to nervousness may benefit from Ignatia 6 taken every 15min or Argentum nitricum may be used instead.

PSYCHOLOGICAL MATTERS

ALZHEIMER'S DISEASE AND SENILE DEMENTIA

Alzheimer's disease is the process of premature senile dementia. Treatment for both of these conditions is similar.

The principal cause of dementia is reduced blood flow through clogged arteries, preventing oxygen and nutrients from reaching brain tissue. Viruses, environmental toxins such as aluminium, and underusage of mental faculties are other causative factors. There is also a genetic predisposition to early dementia.

Tomograph of brain – Alzheimer's disease

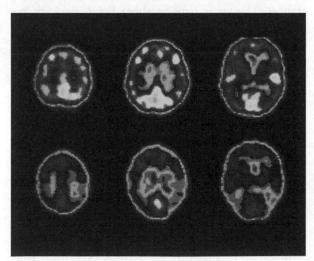

Tomograph scans of a normal brain (top row) and that of an Alzheimer's patient (bottom row). The brighter colours in the normal brain show higher brain activity.

RECOMMENDATIONS

General Advice

- Conversation and debate are essential stimulants. Crossword puzzles, listening to the radio and reading educational books also help. Television and non-stimulating reading are arguably part of the cause of the increasing levels of dementia.
- It is worth noting that dementia is not necessarily so much a problem for the patient as for the relatives. If your life is affected by another with dementia, seek support from a group or counsellor.
- Craniosacral osteopathy can increase blood flow to the brain and be of great benefit.
- Alzheimer patients absorb more dietary aluminium, so those with a family history of dementia should actively avoid contact with aluminium in containers or cooking vessels. Beware the inner lining of cartons in particular.

Nutritional

- Proper concern towards keeping cholesterol levels low and reducing arteriosclerosis/atheroma is essential (see **Arteriosclerosis**).
- Daily intake of antioxidants (see **Antioxidants**) is necessary either through diet or supplementation. Vitamin C in particular has been shown through trials to benefit cognition in Alzheimer's disease – take 1g with each meal.

Supplemental

- Acetyl-L-carnitine 500mg twice a day increased every two weeks up to a total of 3gm in divided doses per day if required.
- Hydergine, an antioxidant and neurone protector that may be beneficial in memory problems. Please take the recommended dose on the packaging.
- Phosphatidyl serine 500mg twice a day increasing to up to 3gm per day in divided doses if required.
- Carnosine, follow the directions on the product label.

Herbal/natural extracts

- *Ginkgo biloba – the standard dose is 40mg with each meal – has shown some benefit, and also several Ayurvedic and Tibetan herbal mixtures best prescribed by specialists in those fields.*
- *DHEA 500mg daily increasing under medical supervision if required.*
- *A compound called Vinpocetine, derived from the lesser periwinkle plant, taken at dosages recommended on the packaging works by increasing blood flow to the brain, increasing efficiency of oxygen uptake into the brain tissue cells and improving neurological metabolism.*
- *Hormone replacement and especially oestrogen has been shown to be beneficial. Studies show its best protection is against Alzheimer's disease in women under the age of 65. Therefore, natural oestrogens from plant sources may be equally beneficial without carrying the potential side effect risk.*
- *Ginseng has been shown to sharpen the memory. A combination of this with gingko has an even more powerful effect.*

Orthodox

- *Piracetam, taken as recommended on the product label.*
- *See the comment about HRT in the herbal/natural extracts section above.*

ANNIVERSARY REACTION

Anniversary reaction can occur at any age but is more common as we pass through middle age into our advanced years. Anniversary reaction is, as it suggests, a sadness, anxiety or depression that occurs on the anniversary of a shock.

It is usual for all of us to have some memory of unhappy events brought back to us by reaching a certain date. Severe depression can occur, however, which needs treating.

RECOMMENDATIONS

General Advice

- *Counselling, preferably with a bereavement counsellor, is nearly always beneficial.*

Homeopathic

- *Homeopathic remedies are excellent in this area but need to be given at high potency and after full consultation with a homeopath.*

BEREAVEMENT AND GRIEF

Generally speaking we will all have to undergo a grief reaction from the loss of a loved one. Bereavement is an inevitability as we progress to our latter years. I discuss bereavement in this chapter because, beyond all other ailments that we contend with as we age, the loss of our loved ones and friends is a deep pain that is unresponsive to medicine.

The grief associated with the death of those close to us generally follows a typical pattern. We all suffer the emotions and feelings of denial, anger, compromise, depression and acceptance.

The length of time that we go through each of these emotions varies depending on the circumstances. Denial is usually short-lived, perhaps no more than a few days, whereas anger either towards those who the individual feels are to blame for the death or self-guilt because the individual did not do enough to prevent the death, can last for years. The depression may be mild and short-lived or deeply ingrained and persistent. Suicidal thoughts and possibly even attempts may occur.

Everyone will have their own way of dealing with bereavement but most people will have memories and reactions that can recur possibly for the rest of their lives. The so-called 'anniversary reaction' is a sense of emotion that occurs on or around the anniversary of the death (*see* **Anniversary reaction** and **Death and dying**).

General Advice

- *Turn to friends and family. There is no shame in venting emotions.*
- *If close support is not available or not helping, then consult your GP or complementary therapist and have a session with a bereavement counsellor. It may be necessary to attend for a few sessions.*
- *Physical body work such as massage using selected aromatherapy oils can be most beneficial.*

Homeopathic

- *Immediately on hearing bad news, use the remedy Arnica 200, one dose every 4hr. If a sense of fear or 'what is going to happen to me now' is the initial reaction, use Aconite 200 at the same dosage. Once the initial shock has subsided use Ignatia 200, one dose on waking and one dose on retiring. If physical symptoms manifest, such as skin rashes, indigestion and flu-like symptoms then use Natrum muriaticum 200, one dose three times a day for one week.*

Herbal/natural extracts

- *The Bach flower remedies can be used to great benefit: Elm and Larch for those who do not know what to do; Pine if guilt is the overwhelming emotion; Sweet chestnut and Star of Bethlehem if desolation and suppressed emotions are present.*

CONFUSION

Confusion in the elderly is often due to the natural process of brain tissue diminution (*see* **Alzheimer's disease** *and* **Senile dementia**).

Confusion can, however, be caused by metabolic changes such as an inability to control sugar levels, poor nutrition, fevers and illnesses such as coughs, colds and flus and drug reactions such as those found by people taking sleeping pills or antidepressants. Other drugs such as antibiotics can cause confused states.

General Advice

- *Rule out any infectious or drug cause by visiting your GP.*
- *Encourage adequate oxygenation of the brain by using a breathing technique best taught by a yoga or meditation teacher.*
- *If the problems persist, consult a naturopath or homeopath (see* **Alzheimer's disease** *and* **Senile dementia***).*

Nutritional

- *Ensure good nutritional input by balancing the diet or visiting a nutritionist or dietician. Please consider using the macrobiotic diet (see chapter 7).*

MEMORY LOSS OR IMPAIRMENT

The formation of memory is a complex matter involving input and recollection processes dependent on brain chemicals (neurotransmitters) and pathways being intact.

As can be seen by the diagram (below), it is important to isolate the area where the memory problem lies. Difficulty in the input, ie the senses of sight, hearing, touch, smell and taste, can lead to incorrect assessment. Once the brain has

Memory Loss Diagram

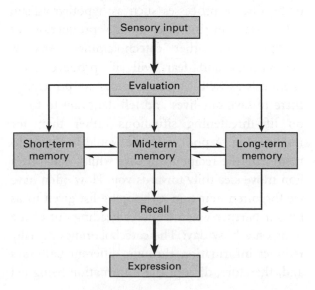

551

assessed the situation, it will decide whether to store the event in short-, medium- or long-term memory stores; for example, the brain will register the colour of a tie that somebody was wearing at a meeting. This is not considered to be an important factor in survival and therefore will probably be stored in short-term memory. After a while the chemicals that have been formed and stored in one part of the brain will be broken down and that memory will be erased. Medium-term memory will register, say, the directions to a party but if the venue is unlikely to be visited again this too will be erased. Long-term memory will have neurotransmitters and pathways formed for important matters or those laid down in youth when the brain is at its most receptive. As the diagram shows, short-term can pass into medium-term, which in turn can be logged into long-term memory.

Recall from any memory centre is an important part of memory function and then the ability to express it finalizes the pathway. How often do we all sit there complaining that we know the answer but just cannot bring it to mind?

Any condition that interferes with the pathways, the formation of neurotransmitters or the actual parts of the brain that retain facts and events, can cause an impairment or loss of memory.

Fatigue, whether caused by overdoing things or by disease processes such as hypothyroidism, will create an increase in the production of adrenaline or other catecholamines. Anxiety, nervousness and fear will all produce these chemicals as well. Catecholamines are principally there to save our lives and tell the brain to focus on life-threatening situations rather than for memorizing. A poor example would be trying to memorize the recipe for a cake whilst watching a lion move stealthily towards you. How often have we forgotten items on a shopping list given to us by our partner when we were heading out of the door on a busy day? The catecholamines actually redirect information through different pathways and, therefore, disrupt the information being fed into the memory centres. Hypoglycaemia (low blood sugar) can have the same effect by increasing stress chemicals but also diminishes the function of the brain, which exists only on its supply of glucose.

Toxins such as alcohol, drugs of abuse, smoking, agrochemicals (including pesticides) and specific foods to which individuals may be allergic can all put chemicals in the system that interfere with both the production of neurotransmitters and the pathways.

Damage to the brain or the pathways through trauma, stroke or tumour may affect memory. Decreasing the amount of brain tissue, as in Alzheimer's disease or senile dementia, and decreased oxygenation and nutritional supply by a narrowing of the arteries (atheroma) will all interfere with memory by destruction of tissue or nerve pathways. A recent study has postulated that low dose HRT may be beneficial to women who are at a high risk of memory decline (those with a family history of dementia). If this proves to be the case, then the use of plant extract phytoestrogens may be beneficial (*see* **Natural oestrogens**).

RECOMMENDATIONS

General Advice

- *Blood and hair analysis for the detection of deficiencies and heavy metal toxicity should be undertaken. Lead, aluminium and mercury may all be culprits in memory loss.*
- *Relaxation techniques and counselling, if necessary, should be considered in stressed individuals.*
- *Exercising the brain through intellectual reading, crosswords, debate and puzzles is essential, especially in older age.*
- *Ensure that hypoglycaemia is not an issue (see* **Hypoglycaemia***).*
- *Avoid smoking, excess alcohol and drug abuse. All drugs will create potentially long-term damage to neurotransmitter production and pathways.*

- Temporary memory loss is most commonly caused by poor concentration or toxic intake such as alcohol. No treatment is necessary but caution is advised on intake and stress levels.
- Memory loss or impairment that is persistent needs to be assessed by a specialist to isolate the cause. Special memory tests and CT scans of the brain may be employed. Remember that orthodox neurologists may not consider agrochemicals, food allergy or low blood sugar as a cause of memory loss.

Supplemental

- Deficiencies in proteins, zinc, vitamin B_{12}, folic acid and lecithin are common in the elderly, the stressed or the unwell who have decreased appetites. Deficiencies in fat intake caused by strict and incorrect dieting may also create a problem. Deficiencies should be measured and corrected.

- Vitamin E and C supplements may help maintain mental function, especially in older people.

Homeopathic

- Homeopathic remedies may be of benefit. High-potency Plumbum (lead), Mercurius and Alumina may all be beneficial if heavy metal poisoning is found to exist. The homeopathic remedies Anarcardium and Sulphur may be useful at potency 200 taken daily for five days if the ability to remember names and words is a problem.

Herbal/natural extracts

- Gingko bilboa significantly improves concentration and Ginseng can sharpen up the memory. They can be used individually or taken in combination. Extracts vary in concentration so take the maximum dose recommended on the packaging.
- Consider taking a daily recommended dosage of a phytoestrogen supplement or increasing foods in the diet that contain these compounds.

PART TWO

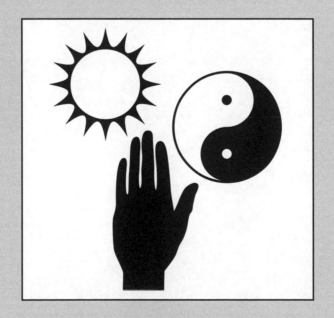

NUTRITION

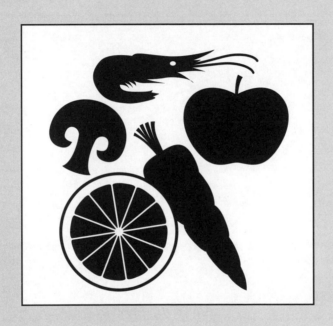

Chapter 7

Nutrition

Introduction

There is a plethora of books on nutrition lining the shelves of every bookshop and healthfood shop. They all have their merits and failings and I would not presume to comment on the expertise of my colleagues and their interpretation of a healthy diet.

I do feel, however, that there is no set diet that is good for everyone. To suggest that Eskimos, who spend their lives eating blubber, would fare well on a macrobiotic diet, or New Guinea tribesmen, whose diet differs markedly from that of Parisians, would do well to change their habits would be incorrect. Trial and error is principally the best way to isolate your preferred dietetic regime.

This short chapter cannot encompass a fraction of the knowledge we have about nutrition but attempts to point out some essentials and the basics of which an individual should have a grasp. Sadly, despite the brevity of this section, it magnifies a thousand-fold the instructions that the average doctor is given on nutrition through their medical training. Diet is not only about calorific input and output, nor about balance of nutrition. It is to do with these factors plus an understanding of the vital force imparted from foods, the spiritual and psychological connection with nutrition and the need to return to instinct when choosing and preparing food.

The Eastern philosophies consider all food to have a variety of energies, some more prominent than others. All foods have a balance of masculine and/or feminine energy or a mixture of both. Foods contain different categories and states of our universe, specifically space, air, fire or heat, earth, wood, metal and water. Food is sweet, bitter, sour, salty or spicy and may be hot, warm or cold.

The choice of food should be based on the requirements of an individual at any time in relation to the balance of all these energies. It is not hard to do and if left to instinct the body, when healthy, will automatically balance and absorb its requirements.

RECOMMENDATIONS

General Advice

- *When choosing the diet, put aside the orthodox concept until later and focus on the energy requirements.*
- *Keep in touch with your instincts. Eat what you feel like eating but ignore unhealthy cravings. If the desire is for a piece of chocolate then the body is suggesting a desire for sweetness and energy – have some fruit. If the craving is for pasta, make it wholegrain.*
- *Balance temperatures. On a hot sunny day enjoy a salad; in the depths of winter prepare hot soups. The rule of thumb is that raw and steamed are cooling; stewed, baked and stir-fried are warming and deep-fried, roasted, grilled and barbecued are heating. (Barbecues in the summer? An occasional aberration is an enjoyable cheat!)*
- *Balance raw and cooked foods, depending upon the amount of environmental heat. Even a hot summer's day requires some heating foods, but a predominantly raw diet is best. Predominant is the operative word.*
- *Try to balance all flavours throughout the day or even at each meal. The salt of a fish can be balanced by the sour of the lemon. The spice of an Indian meal is often counteracted by the bitter of aniseed from seeds at the end.*

PSYCHOLOGICAL AND ENERGETIC CONSIDERATIONS TOWARDS FOOD

All holistic practitioners consider there to be a mind–body connection. The energy of one directly influences the energy of another. Science is beginning to pick up on energy wavelengths that may affect the nervous system and therefore influence both the mind and the body. Energy is provided through the sun, the air we breathe and, of course, the food we eat. Our psychological attitude toward our food is (both theoretically and in my experience) relevant to the benefit we derive from our nutrition.

RECOMMENDATIONS

General Advice

- *The kitchen. The place of preparation must be comfortable, convenient and happy. It generally is, and it is not coincidental that people migrate into the kitchen at parties. Very often family gatherings are only found around food and ensuring a clean, hygienic, bright and airy kitchen is an essential prerequisite to deriving the most from nutrition.*
- *Putting aside time to eat. All day we expend energy, and like a car we occasionally need to stop to refuel. Short, rushed meals are equivalent to putting small amounts of petrol in the tank – the car will only run for a short period. The longer we spend eating, the more benefit we derive. Unlike the car analogy, it is not about quantity but about the time spent in a mental and physical state of absorption rather than usage. Set aside time in the day to eat with no disturbance allowed.*
- *The Chinese state that 'the stomach has no teeth'. Chew food well and lessen the work of the digestive system.*
- *The Chinese believe that we should work slightly cold and slightly hungry. Ingesting too much food overburdens the system and requires energy to*

process all the matter. Eastern philosophies describe it as creating stagnation and as we return to our daily function after a meal our energy is split between function and digestion.
- *Feed the body appropriately for its requirements. A big breakfast for a busy day, a lighter lunch because half the day is done and a light supper because we are about to rest.*
- *Believe in the concept of energy within food. Eat foods with vital force. Organic food from the environment imparts energy from that part of the world in which you live. Preserved food is food contaminated with chemicals or radiation that kill bacteria. These kill life. These kill energy in food. Avoid anything with preservatives, additives or foods that have been 'nuked' by microwave. Remember that all foods that are on the shelves of our supermarkets may have been irradiated as part of the food industry's attempt to prolong the 'sell by' date. As a general rule avoid anything that has a 'sell by' date longer than the time that you would keep that product in the fridge if you had prepared it yourself.*

PREPARATION OF FOOD

Many so-called primitive races who have maintained contact with their spiritual past consider all foods to have an energy. A hunter will apologize and pray to the victim of the arrow or spear. The circle of life so popularized by wildlife programmes is taken to its spiritual conclusion by such predators. This attitude is not easily transferable into modern Western culture because the killing of our animals is now done at arm's length by a third party. The availability of our fruit and vegetables is also limited by our busy schedules and lack of space. In an ideal world we would all eat the produce from the soil upon which we live because the balance of nature provides what we need, depending upon our environment. According to Eastern philosophies, honey produced in sunny countries such as Australia will contain more fire or *pitta* energy than the honey manufactured by the bees of the cooler climate of, say, England. And within England the pollens that the bees eat in Surrey are different from those in Lancashire and our immune system is geared towards those in our own atmosphere and will therefore deal with the honey from our region better than from elsewhere. Hot climates produce foods suitable for the digestion of humans adapted to heat, to such an extent that chillis are eaten in hot climates and cucumbers more so in cold climates. These balance the external and internal (body) heat when extremes exist. As seasons change, so does our instinctive input. Soups and stews fill our table through the winter months, providing heat to balance the cold, and salads and fruits become more prominent to counteract our hot summers.

If allowed to eat by instinct and not by time constraints and availability, the human body would set its own pattern. The food eaten should be chosen and prepared by instinct and with respect. Eastern philosophies remind us of the interchange between different life forces and that the lion at the top of the food chain will eventually be the food for the grass.

RECOMMENDATIONS

General Advice
- *Food should be selected by instinct, smell and on how it looks. Over- or under-ripe foods should be avoided.*
- *Once obtained, food should be stored correctly and as soon as possible.*
- *The area where food is prepared should be clean and comfortable. A kitchen where the cook is unhappy will create an energy that passes into the food and those who eat it.*
- *The water supply to clean and prepare food should be as purified as possible by the use of filters (see **Water**).*

- *In a family, touching the food should be encouraged, but the hands should be cleaned with non-medicated soap prior to commencing.*

EATING

Eating is not just about obtaining calories. It is about energy and about communication. The wonderful phrase 'table culture' was introduced to me recently and is something that many parts of the world excel in whilst others substantially lack.

The fast food and TV-dinner concept is removing a very important time of 'herd communication'. Children learn manners and improve their vocabulary and grammar around a table and bonding is much increased at meal times. It is worth remembering that the human body derives pleasure from both input and output. The time spent eating and drinking should be maximized (and to balance the paragraph, elimination should be allowed to take as long as is required).

All the senses should be brought into play whenever possible. The sight of well-prepared food is stimulatory to the gastric juices, as are the smells. Texture is dependent upon good cooking, which in turn is dependent upon experience and patience. Taste, whilst the sense that most associate with food, is actually the last to come into play.

If any one of the senses is not pleased by a particular food, then that food should be avoided.

RECOMMENDATIONS

General Advice
- *Spend time with your food. Make it a time of worship because you are only what goes into you and your nutrition is a major part of that.*
- *Ensure cleanliness of food, preparation surfaces, utensils and especially hands.*
- *A pleasant environment for the preparation and eating of meals. Home-makers may spend much of their lives in the kitchen and, therefore, a*

corresponding amount of energy should go into making it a homely and comfortable place.

HIGH-FIBRE INTAKE

The variety of food groups and types of nutrients are discussed in various parts of this chapter, but perhaps most important, because it is frequently overlooked, is the necessity for a high fibre intake.

High-fibre foods are principally those that are difficult to digest because of their cellulose content. The human gut is not adept at breaking down cellulose and so this compound, found in most plants, remains in the gut and acts as a cleanser and detoxifier. Cellulose acts as a sponge, absorbing many compounds but particularly excess fats and cholesterol. The 'roughage' acts much like a pipe-cleaner and scrapes adhesive debris off the bowel wall. This is extremely important in the colon, where waste products and toxins are stored.

Fibre gives bulk to the faeces, which allows the muscle wall of the colon (large intestine) to maintain its strength. This encourages the fast removal of waste products and oxygenation to the bowel itself, considerably reducing the risk of disease.

Fibre will swell in the presence of fluids and can be a very useful appetite suppressant with no side effects. Pumpkin and sunflower seeds are an extremely useful aspect of any weight reduction programme, supplying fibre that swells in the stomach to give an impression of fullness. Fibre-containing foods are simply: vegetables, fruit, wholegrains, nuts and seeds.

DESIGNING AN IDEAL DIET

There are thousands of books declaring the ideal diet. Frankly there is no such thing because everybody is different and will have their own vision of ideal. Attitudes and body types vary to such an extent that what is good for one person may not necessarily be healthy for another. To persuade an Eskimo that a high-fibre, vegetarian diet is liable to be his best bet when an Eskimo might never actually see a vegetable is as pointless as advising the heavily meat-eating Argentines to exist on a vegan diet.

The Eskimos are an extreme example of the adaptability of the human race. Most races should gear their dietetics around individual instincts and the produce of their environment. Our instincts are suppressed by unnatural, 'man-made' produce such as refined sugars. A carrot is sweet but how many of us remember that? Spend five days away from any refined sweetness and that quality of the carrot will return. Put a piece of chocolate into an infant's mouth and watch its rejection. By the age of two years, however, the hidden sugars in many processed foods will have changed this natural instinct.

ESTABLISHING YOUR IDEAL BALANCE

The preceding tips now have to be balanced with more orthodox advice.

Principally, a diet has to be balanced between carbohydrates, proteins and fats. Nutrients are

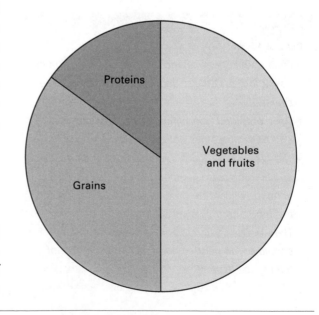

absorbed from all of these groups and an understanding of which type of food falls into which group is essential. Ideally we should have our diet made up as follows.

- Vegetables and fruits should make up 50 per cent of the diet.
- Grains should make up 35 per cent of the diet.
- Proteins should make up 15 per cent of the diet.

More simply, half of our diet should be fruit and vegetables and we should eat twice as much grain as protein. There, that saves you reading any more books on nutrition! The following are just details!

Vegetables and fruits

Balance is the order of the day but it is best to eat one type of fruit at any sitting. Vegetables may be mixed. Vary vegetables by their colour, having deep green, light green, yellow, white and red vegetables in a 5:4:3:2:1 ratio over a seven-day period. (White vegetables refer to potatoes. Yams and sweet potatoes are in-between the yellow and white groups.)

Fruits should generally be raw, although an occasional apple pie or stewed prune is enjoyable and nutritious. Vegetables should be a 50:50 mix of cooked or raw. Lightly steamed and/or stir-fried vegetables can be considered a mix of both.

Grains

Wholegrains include wheat, oats, barley, rye, corn, brown or wild rice and the myriad of lesser known but equally available complex carbohydrates such as millet, buckwheat and spelt. Potatoes and other starchy vegetables partially fall into this group.

Proteins

Many people are under the impression that meat, fowl and fish are the best sources of protein. Whilst they certainly are a good source, animal protein is harder to break down, digest and absorb than vegetable proteins. Beans, lentils, soya products and nuts are all high-protein foods. Animal products such as yoghurt and cheeses fall halfway between the two as far as ease of absorption is concerned.

Water

Most diet and nutrition books frequently make mention of water but none, I feel, emphasize that without good hydration all other advice becomes pointless. No biochemical process works without water and therefore the balancing of nutrition is futile unless good hydration is obtained and maintained.

The minimum requirement is half a pint per foot of height and additional water must be taken in for any excess sweating, caffeine or alcohol intake and the ingestion of anything artificially sweet. (*See* **Water** at the end of this chapter.)

The ideal balance

The type of food may vary but the balance should remain within narrow guidelines. Any dietetic regime should be based around: 60–70 per cent complex carbohydrates; 20–25 per cent protein; 10–15 per cent fat.

All the food groups should be as free from additives and preservatives as possible and eaten as fresh as is feasible. Each food group contains

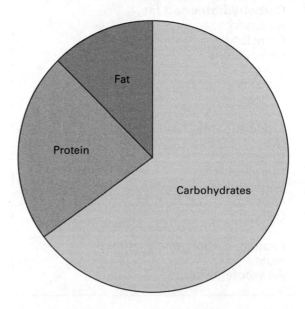

Food Groups

Predominantly protein
Poultry (skin removed)
White fish (skin removed)
Shellfish
Eggs
Low-fat yoghurt
Low-fat dairy produce

Protein and fat
Red meat
Pig meat
Cheese
Yoghurt
Milk
Cream
Ice cream
Oily fish
Fish with skin

Protein with carbohydrate
Soya
Lentils
Beans
Seeds

Predominantly carbohydrate
All refined grains
Potatoes
Fruits
Most vegetables
Sugars, including honey and maple syrup
Herbs

Carbohydrates and fat
Avocado
French fries
Crisps/chips
Cakes
Biscuits
Sauces

Predominantly fat
Oils
Butter
Margarines
Vegetable-oil spreads
Lard
Dripping

Protein, carbohydrate and fats
Nuts
All wholegrains

specific nutrients and all the vitamins, minerals and trace elements must be taken in regularly. They contain good – and bad – quality nutrients and the lists below clarify the contents. It is very important to note that many foods combine different groups. For example, cheese contains both fat and protein, lentils contain protein and carbohydrate, avocados contain carbohydrate and fats. All of these have a variety of different nutrients and none are particularly good or bad provided that they are taken in moderation and in balance.

This term 'imbalance' keeps coming up in both holistic medicine and health maintenance. If nature provided us with simple foods neatly categorized we would probably not have any problems but nature is not black and white; there is a lot of grey. Foods are rarely only protein or only carbohydrate and it is important to understand what we are eating. The shortlist opposite gives a rough guide to the balance existing within major foods and I hope it will be a simple list from which to create an individually suitable diet plan.

Using the previous chart and without becoming in any way obsessive, try to balance all meals according to the $65:22\frac{1}{2}:12\frac{1}{2}$ ratio mentioned above. Failing to do so at each meal can be corrected on a daily basis. For example: a heavily protein-biased breakfast of eggs and bacon can be counterbalanced by a vegetable or fruit lunch and a baked potato supper. A toast and honey breakfast with a fruit lunch would entitle the diner to a slightly more protein-orientated supper such as fish and vegetables.

Maintaining a balance is extremely important. It is incorrect to assume that removing fats is the best way to lose weight because many essential vitamins and fatty acids will soon become deficient and craving will set in, leading to an eventual overwhelming desire to eat what is missing. Similarly, the concept that red meat is 'bad' for you can lead to deficiencies in amino acids if a correct balance of other protein-containing foods is not allowed to redress the situation.

TOXINS AND FOODS LACKING QI

Foods that inevitably contain toxins or foods lacking in vital force or Qi (*see* **Weight loss**) are:

- Fried foods.
- Foods containing refined sugars, such as chocolates and sweets.
- Jams, marmalades and preserves with added white sugar.
- Foods made from refined flour, including white bread.
- Non-organic meat and pig products in general (pigs are mostly fed on waste from human tables).
- Caffeine-containing compounds (coffee, strong tea, chocolate and many carbonated drinks), squashes and most preprepared juices (most contain extra sugar regardless of the labelling because manufacturers are allowed to replace an estimated amount of sugar that may be lost in the manufacturing process – *see* **Fruit juice**).
- Any smoked food where the fumes come from a chemically treated charcoal.
- Any alcohol product.
- Any products with added salt.
- High-fat foods such as pizzas, burgers, French fries.
- Mass-produced eggs or poultry.
- Any food with additives or preservatives.
- Any tinned foods and any coloured or flavoured foods.

This advice is not about being overzealous, it is about avoiding foods that are known to cause illness and disease. I am now amazed at the lack of nutritional knowledge I had, despite a medical training and a wise father with an interest in the subject. It is the same for most of the people I meet. This is by no means our fault. Responsibility must lie in the poor level of education and high level of promotion by the food industry.

Eating healthily is not encouraged and not made easy. There are few organic butchers and vegetable suppliers and those that exist have to have expensive products to make ends meet.

Water is an extremely important part of diet. I discuss water further in its own section so it suffices here to say:

- Ensure a purified water source for drinking and the preparing of food.
- Drink at least half a pint per foot of height in divided doses throughout the day.
- Remember that fluids other than water, such as juices and infusions, are *not* water. These can be taken in addition but not *instead* of plain and simple water.

COOKING UTENSILS

The type and cleanliness of cooking utensils is of paramount importance in protecting one's nutrition. Not only will food remnants on cooking utensils encourage the growth of bacteria, but also the ingestion of chemicals from washing-up liquids may be harmful.

All detergents have been known for a long time to be potentially carcinogenic but little is said or done to encourage adequate rinsing. A happy balance needs to be struck between the right amount of cleansing solution to rid the utensils of food debris and a thorough rinsing. Most machine washes are adequate but the addition of a 'rinse' compound to make utensils more shiny should be discouraged.

Avoid using pans that contribute chemicals to the water or fats in cooking. Aluminium is the most notorious and may be cited in neurological conditions. Avoid cooking in tin cans, as is often seen on camp sites. Stainless steel is a safe material. Non-stick surfaces are safe provided they stay in the pan. Change such utensils regularly and immediately if any chip or wear and tear is noticed.

YIN AND YANG FOODS

Put simply, the Yin is the fluid of the body, which acts as our fuel reserve and lubricant within the system. The Yang is the heat or fire within the system. Whilst Yin is the fuel, the Yang is the spark that ignites it.

Most conditions of ill-health are created by an excess or deficiency in one or the other. A common sense assessment of the disease process can give clues as to the dietary requirements based on Yin and Yang. While all foods contain Yin or Yang, many have a balance and are not considered either one or the other predominantly. Below are a list of foods that can be used to aid a speedier recovery.

Yin foods

Yin foods tend to be sweet and cooling. They create dampness, such as milk products that produce mucus, and are principally foods with a variety of nutrition within their substance. Yin foods include:

- Most fruits, especially apple, pineapple, citrus fruits, pears and watermelon.
- Eggs, oysters, rabbit, duck and pork.
- Tofu, yam, tomatoes, asparagus, kidney beans and peas.
- Milk and cheese.
- Honey (an excellent method of supplying Yin).

Yang foods

Principally these foods are warming. They are foods that benefit from cooking and are pungent, strongly flavoured foods. Herbs and spices are generally Yang. Yang foods include:

- Most herbs and spices but particularly ginger and garlic.
- Lamb, lobster and shrimp.
- Nuts, especially the chestnut and walnut.
- Offal such as kidney.
- Clove and nutmeg (these have particularly powerful Yang effects).

SPECIFIC DIETS

ANTI-*CANDIDA* (ANTI-YEAST) DIET

I am not a great supporter of the anti-*Candida* diet. Generally yeast overgrowth in the bowel occurs because of a diminution in the bowel's normal flora due to poor diet and the injudicious use of antibiotics and the unintentional ingestion of antibiotics through meat products that have been processed and include antibiotics within their fibres.

Recommendations against *Candida* include long periods of abstinence (I have read suggestions ranging from three months to a year) from sugars and yeast-containing foods, which principally rules out bread and beer, fruits, milk, cheese, alcohol and many condiments, such as caffeine, ice cream, lentils, pumpkin, potato and peas.

It is ridiculous.

For those of us who may have the time to prepare steamed vegetables and limit our diet to one that avoids most convenience foods the concept is okay, even if it may deny any 'naughty' treats, but I sense that most people cannot function like this.

It is better to reduce substantially the foods that particularly stimulate yeast growth, such as refined sugars, caffeine and high-fat foods, and perhaps cut down on yeast products such as leavened bread and mushrooms (which, apparently, encourages yeast growth) and at the same time use an anti-*Candida* therapy.

Trying to kill *Candida* with potent drugs can lead to the growth of resistant strains but inhibiting their multiplication will result in their dying off from old age and not being replaced. There is less risk of resistance developing and the outcome within three months (the general life-span of a yeast cell) is similar to a vigorous and restrictive dietary existence. Details are discussed in the section on *Candida* (see *Candida*).

Yeast-supporting foods to avoid, but not necessarily to exclude, are as follows:

Bread (unless yeast-free)	Dry fruits
Cow's milk products	Grapes
Mushrooms	Vinegar
Tomatoes	Salt
Wine/champagne	Caffeine
Apples	White sugar
Pears	Artificial sweeteners

If treatment and moderate dietary restrictions do not work then an anti-yeast/anti-gut fermentation diet is probably required. The one designed and recommended by Dr Harald Gaier, a leading naturopath in the UK, is a useful guide. My thanks go to him for permission to reprint this.

Get into the habit of reading labels. It is really surprising how many products contain sugar in various forms (dextrose, glucose, maltose, commercial fructose, etc) and monosodium glutamate (MSG). Omit foods to which you react badly.

GUT FERMENTATION DIET

Allowed	Not Allowed
The following made only from goat's or ewe's milk: yoghurt, cottage cheese and other cheese, and tofu (made from soya); Rice Dream, or soya milk.	Cow's milk products, such as whey, curds, butter, yoghurt, cheese, sour cream, cream, ice cream, buttermilk, sour milk, and margarine except that of pure vegetable origin.
Meat, poultry, seafood, crustaceans and fish. Eggs (chicken, duck or goose).	Yeast and yeast-like substances (mushrooms, fungi), dried fruits, malted products, commercial fruit drinks, citric acid, tinned tomato products, monosodium glutamate (MSG), quorn, vinegar, pickles, condiment sauces, etc.
Artificial sweeteners, such as saccharin, Nutrasweet, cyclamate, aspartame and lactose (it cannot ferment).	All sugars (honey, maple syrup, molasses, treacle, commercially-prepared dextrose, maltose, glucose, sucrose, fructose, sorbitol, etc.)
Mainly tropical fruit, such as mango, melon, paw-paw (papaya), pineapple, avocado pear, star fruit, kiwi (unless there is an adverse reaction). Also most berries (but not strawberries). Figs, lychees, cactus fruits, and dates.	Citrus fruits, bananas, apples, pears, quince, strawberries, crab apples, cape gooseberries, grapes, and all deciduous fruit (such as cherries, apricots, peaches, plums and nectarines).
Vegetables, fresh or cooked (in filtered water if possible), except mushrooms. So, potato, onion, garlic, legumes (pulses) and fresh culinary herbs are allowed.	All fruit and vegetables showing bruising or mould.
Nuts: almonds, cashews, pine nuts (unless there is an adverse reaction), but no other kind. Seeds: sesame, pumpkin. Oils: maize (corn) or olive.	All peanuts, pistachio nuts, Brazil nuts, macadamia nuts, pecan nuts, walnuts, hazelnuts (filbert nuts). Sunflower seeds or oil.
Drinks: coffee, milk (goats', ewes'), soya milk, rooibosch tea, spirits such as vodka and gin (a little), mineral water, sugar-free fizzy drinks. Infusions of mint, rosehip, chamomile, etc.	Ordinary tea, spices and dried culinary herbs. Fermented beverages (alcoholic and non-alcoholic) such as beer, cider, wine, champagne, ginger beer or ale.
Grains: rice, maize, millet, quinoa, tapioca, and sorghum.	All foods containing wheat, rye, barley (malt), buckwheat, oats (most soya sauces contain wheat).
Tapioca bread, white or brown rice bread, rice cakes.	Cocoa or chocolate in any form. Soda bread.
Kallo rice cereal, Lima corn flakes or other malt-free corn flakes.	Malted corn flakes (such as Kellogg's).
Polenta, wheat-free corn pasta, rice noodles, Australian shell pasta (that is wheat-free), rye, barley, and oats.	Normal pasta and semolina.
Gram flour, rice flour, maize (corn) flour, and the flours of sorghum, quinoa, millet, tapioca, and soya beans.	Flours of wheat, rye, barley, oats, and buckwheat.
Filtered or mineral water for cooking is preferable.	

Sample breakfast items

Eggs, bacon, tomatoes, ham, permitted cheese, grilled potato waffles, Lima corn flakes, tropical fruit salad, permitted yoghurt (if absolutely necessary, an artificial sweetener may be used).

Other meals

Depending on how acceptable your palate finds untoasted tapioca or white rice bread, sandwiches made with either of these. Failing that, buy a robust lettuce (cos or iceberg) and use the leaves as 'sandwich covers' – wrap them around poultry or meat slices. Use celery in the same way – the middle can be filled with, say, goat's cheese – or it can be chopped with raw vegetables such as carrot, tomato, cucumber, bell peppers, French beans, and cashews, and taken for lunch in a plastic-lidded container. Salads can be boring, so dress them with maize or olive oil and a little squeezed lemon. Use permitted yoghurt (live), and add flavourings, such as mashed Camembert (if made of ewe's milk), goat's cheese, cucumber, and pesto (made from basil – but check the label to make sure it does not contain disallowed substances).

THE BUDWIG DIET

This is a specific anti-cancer diet designed by Dr Budwig to contain several anticancer nutrients.

The basic mixture consists of one tablespoonful of pure virgin cold-pressed unprocessed linseed oil (flaxseed oil) and half to one cup of low-fat cottage cheese. This combination of fatty acids and sulphur-rich protein can be taken alone or as a mixture. Add natural flavouring or other food ingredients to suit you own taste. Eat this mixture three times a day.

The recommended diet

- Fresh fruits – three or four medium-sized portions daily.
- Fresh vegetables – four to six cups. Several tablespoonsful of linseeds and/or two tablespoonsful of the oil can be used in the salad dressing or on the vegetables; be sure to include cabbage, broccoli and maitake mushrooms.
- Unprocessed wholegrain breads and cereals – 3–4 cups or portions.
- Fresh fish – 4–8oz. An excellent source of omega-3 fatty acids is rainbow trout (preferably the coldwater variety).
- Fresh meat and poultry – organic (without hormones), low-fat and animals that have been fed food without pesticides or antibiotics.
- Liquids – bottled water or water purified by reverse osmosis. Two litres a day are recommended but do not worry if this is not manageable. Place one glass of your favourite juice in a litre bottle and fill the remainder with water. It is a cheat but makes drinking easier.
- Fresh fruit juices – citrus fruit should not be taken within several hours of the linseed oil/cottage cheese mixture.

Eating any processed oils will counteract everything you are trying to do. They should be treated as poison, as should all fried foods. Eliminate as much sugar as possible from the diet. Remember that honey is primarily sugar and prepared foods must be devoid of all artificial preservatives or chemical additives. Artificial sweeteners are absolutely forbidden.

THE DETOX DIET

All water should be bottled or filtered, preferably by reverse osmosis (*see* **Water**). If you are hungry during the day, please have some of the pumpkin and sunflower seeds usually reserved for the end of the afternoon.

Choose your favourite herbal teas and try to drink between one and two pints per day but not within half an hour of any meal.

Day 1

Between waking and breakfast
One pint of water

Breakfast
Up to one to two pounds of washed grapes

Between breakfast and lunch
One pint of water

Lunch
Any steamed vegetable, but only one type

Between lunch and late afternoon
One pint of water

Late afternoon
A handful of mixed pumpkin and sunflower seeds

Between late afternoon and supper
One pint of water

Supper
Four ounces of bran or rolled oats with two teaspoonsful of lemon juice and apple juice/water mix for moisture, preferably soaked all day

Day 2

Between waking and breakfast
One pint of filtered or bottled water (water to be taken between meals as on day 1)

Breakfast
Two mangos, pawpaws or other 'exotic' fruit

Lunch
Any steamed vegetable but only one type

Supper
Up to one to two pounds of potatoes (only pepper may be added, although the potatoes may be had in any form but with no butter)

Day 3
Water to be taken as on day 1

Breakfast
Up to two grapefruits

Lunch
Any steamed vegetables, but only one type

Supper
Eight ounces of live yoghurt with one type of fruit and two teaspoonsful of honey (two tablespoons of an unsweetened oat cereal may be added)

GERSON DIET

The Gerson diet is part of a regime that includes coffee enemas, iodine and potassium supplements and the preparation of vegetable and fruit juices. This diet is low in fat, low in animal protein, high in complex carbohydrates and contains large amounts of organic fruits, vegetables and wholegrains. Salt is excluded and foods higher in potassium are increased.

Thyroid supplements may also be administered and initially raw liver juice was prescribed but this has been withdrawn because of bacterial growth within the substance.

Max Gerson, a physician born in Germany but who emigrated to the USA, discovered this treatment because he was using sililca techniques for dealing with tuberculosis. It is difficult to come up to the rigorous scientific standards when using a dietetic technique because other therapies may be in use at the same time. However, both the National Cancer Institute in America and a study published in the *Lancet* accepted that this required further study and may be 'a way forward' in cancer care. There is currently a retrospective study of more than 5,400 patients under way, which we hope will bring forward some answers.

The Gerson therapy is undoubtedly of benefit to confidence and mood, general well-being, faster healing after operative procedures and reduction of pain.

THE HAY DIET

Dr Hay devised this concept in the 1920s. He hypothesized that because the human race developed as both hunters and gatherers, it was unlikely that we would eat both animal protein and carbohydrates at the same time. He further suggested that the stomach and digestive tract were therefore geared towards digesting one type of food at a time.

Food combining, better termed as food non-combining, regimes have developed from his hypothesis.

Quite simply, protein foods, including soya and lentils, should be eaten separately from carbohydrates such as rice, potatoes and wheat. Vegetables may be mixed with either group but fruit needs to be separated from other foods by at least one hour.

The reasoning is simple. Protein requires longer to digest and is, therefore, held in the stomach in the presence of acid for a longer period than other food groups. Keeping starch in the stomach for too long causes much higher liquefaction of the carbohydrate into glucose which will then be absorbed at a much more rapid rate once it enters the small intestine. This in turn causes a much greater insulin production which leads to a reflex hypoglycaemic state causing tiredness amongst many other biochemical changes. The increased availability of glucose can also encourage yeast growth within the intestine along with its inherent problems.

Vegetables are carbohydrates. Fruit, with its high content of fructose (fruit sugar), will actually ferment in an acid environment and the alcohols produced can affect the body directly and also enhance the growth of yeasts through the rest of the bowel. It should therefore be eaten separately to ensure quick passage through the acid of the stomach.

Many books have been written on the subject but in principle the preceding rules should be followed and an attempt should be made to have one protein meal, one starch meal and one purely vegetarian or fruit meal a day. The fruit/vegetable meal encourages alkalinity and this diet can therefore be used very effectively as a Detox regime. For the best benefit, have two days per week purely on fruit and vegetables.

HYPOGLYCAEMIA – *see* Hypoglycaemia

Allowables

- Vegetables – any
- Fruits – any, but with exceptions below
- Juices – any unsweetened cranberry or vegetable juice is allowable (fresh/squeezed fruit juices)
- Beverages – herb teas, decaffeinated coffee and coffee substitutes (once on the road to recovery, you may sweeten your drinks with honey if desired. Remember, use honey only in mild cases or after the initial programme is relaxed)
- Desserts – fruit, unsweetened yoghurt or carob-sweetened snacks

Food and drinks to avoid

- Alcoholic and soft drinks, such as club soda, dry ginger ale, whiskey and liquors
- Sugar, chocolate, candy and other sweets, such as cakes, pies, pastries, sweet custards, puddings and ice cream
- Caffeine: ordinary coffee, strongly brewed tea and beverages containing caffeine
- Decaffeinated drinks
- Grapes, raisins, plums, figs, dates and bananas (all high in sugar)

Hypoglycaemia Diet

Upon arising

A small bowl of yoghurt or half a grapefruit

Breakfast

One egg and half a slice of bread only (it may be toasted) with herb tea

Two hours after breakfast

A snack of two handfuls of either raw nuts or a mix of sunflower and pumpkin seeds

Lunch

- Salad (large serving of lettuce, tomato, vinegar and oil dressing)
- Vegetables if desired
- Slice of bread or toast with butter
- Dessert – *see* below list of allowable foods
- Beverage

Two hours after lunch

As after breakfast or two pieces of fruit

Two hours before dinner

A light snack of raw nuts, cheese, celery or other vegetables stuffed with cheese

Dinner

- Soup, if desired (not thickened with flour)
- Vegetables
- Liberal portion of meat, fish or poultry
- Beverage

Two hours after dinner

Dessert – *see* allowables listed below

Every 2 hours until bed-time

A small handful of nuts or fruit

- Doughnuts, jams, jellies and marmalades (all high in sugar)
- Wines, cordials, cocktails and beers (the alcohol content is high in carbohydrate)

MACROBIOTIC DIET

The Macrobiotic Diet was created by a Japanese teacher who wrote under the name of Georges Ohsawa. He integrated Eastern and Western cultures and created a ten-stage diet, designated from −3 to +7. The −3 Diet consists of 10 per cent each of cereal or grains and soups, 30 per cent each of vegetables and animal products, 15 per cent salads and fruits, 5 per cent 'desserts' and very little to drink. As the number climbs, the diet changes and at the +3 stage the individual is on 10 per cent soups, 30 per cent vegetables and 60 per cent cereals. I believe that it is necessary to sit with a macrobiotic nutritionist or have a patient attitude towards a good book to appreciate fully the holistic sense of macrobiotic dieting.

Studies have been made on macrobiotic diets with regard to blood pressure, cholesterol levels and oestrogen metabolism. Most studies have been made in either treatment or prevention of chronic disease, although the success of the macrobiotic diet on blood pressure and cholesterol supports its use in conditions associated with these components.

RECOMMENDATIONS

General Advice
- *This is undoubtedly a safe and healthy diet.*
- *Special attention to this regime should be considered by those with high blood pressure or raised cholesterol levels, those with family histories of strokes or heart disease and smokers.*

ORNISH DIET

The Ornish diet was developed by Dean Ornish, a doctor from San Francisco. This diet is strictly vegetarian, allowing no meat or animal protein except for the whites of eggs. The aim is to provide less than 2,000 calories a day, mostly from carbohydrates with less than 10 per cent coming from fat.

This diet is encouraged for those with cardiovascular disease, particularly angina (heart pain), raised cholesterol and arterial occlusion. Studies for such conditions have proven successful under rigorous scientific standards.

PRITIKIN DIET

Named after Nathan Pritikin, this is a vegetarian, high-complex carbohydrate and fibre diet that is specifically low in cholesterol and fat. It is prescribed in association with 45 minutes of daily walking.

It is possible to obtain books on this diet, although the Pritikin Centre in California recommends that a patient attends a 26-day programme to adjust to their new type of living.

Good scientifically based studies showed that this diet was of great benefit in patients with cardiovascular problems and can be considered of use in non-insulin-dependent diabetes provided that it is initiated early on in the diagnosis.

VEGAN DIET

A vegan is a vegetarian who excludes all protein and other products of an animal origin. There is an ongoing debate as to whether or not a human being should eat meat. We have digestive enzymes capable of dealing with animal protein and incisor teeth may be relevant to the kill. One may argue that these teeth are only for defence and that the protein-digesting enzymes are designed for vegetable proteins, so it is hard to pin down exactly what nature intended. The fact of the matter is that the human being has developed into an omnivore (subsistence on a wide variety of food). Anthropologists point out that the human being is extremely adaptable and, for example, the Eskimo who may never see a vegetable is capable of surviving on meat alone whereas many populations are principally vegetarian.

Being vegan is an extremely intricate art and requires a good knowledge of how to obtain adequate amounts of protein from vegetable sources. Many vitamins, such as vitamin B_{12}, are found predominantly in animal products and deficiencies are common in uneducated vegans. It may take several years but eventually most vegans will fall into deficiencies if they don't take supplements.

As a cleansing process, vegan diets are extremely useful. Provided that specific allergy is not noted to gluten or other proteins found in grains, vegan diets are inevitably healthy if taken for a short period of time. Six weeks, I believe, is a maximum without at least a 10-day break of animal product intake.

The choice of becoming an educated vegan is up to an individual but I think that it is more suited to those who have a smaller bone and muscle structure such as the Asian race.

RECOMMENDATIONS

General Advice

- *Avoid the long-term regime of a vegan diet as a general rule.*
- *Ensure that adequate vegetarian protein is ingested. Beans, pulses, lentils and tofu must be taken in sufficient quantities on a daily basis.*
- *Smaller bone and muscle mass may predispose to a better tolerance of a low-protein diet.*
- *Discussion with a nutritionist or strict adherence to a vegan guideline book is necessary and beyond the scope of this book.*
- *Every six months have a blood and hair analysis to establish vitamin and mineral status.*

SPECIFIC FOODS AND NUTRIENTS

There is a lot of disinformation put out by various groups whose motivation is the profit factor.

I think it necessary to make mention of some of the more common and possibly dangerous pieces of advice that are fed to us by 'the powers that be' through the media. The following covers some of the most commonly asked questions and misunderstood foods within the common diet.

ACID/ALKALINE FOODS

The body works at a pH (the measurement of acid/alkaline levels) of 7.35–7.45. Any movement outside this range is strongly resisted by the body, specifically the kidneys and lungs, which battles to correct the balance by breathing faster or eliminating hydrogen and other charged particles through the urine. A food is not judged to be alkaline by its own pH but by the effect that it has on the body.

Acid-forming foods	Alkaline-forming foods
Animal protein	Most vegetables
Most grains	Most fruits
Most nuts	Salty fish
Plant seeds	Soya
Sugar	Almonds and Brazil nuts
Honey	Millet and buckwheat
Coffee	
Dairy products	
Most berries and tomatoes	

A common misconception is that milk is alkaline. If it is unpasteurized it has a neutral quality but generally the actual alkalinity in the milk itself causes the stomach to produce more acid and therefore acidifies the system.

Acid production is dependent upon the quantity eaten: the less we fill ourselves, the less acidic we are. Not mixing foods, as in the Hay diet or other food-combining disciplines, generally moves food out of the stomach quicker, thereby reducing acid production and creating a tendency towards alkalinity.

ACIDOPHILUS

Acidophilus is the best-known yoghurt bacteria, although there are many other types, including *Probifidus* and *Bifidus*. These bacteria encourage and promote the growth of the human bowel flora, in particular, *Escherichia coli*. There are bad *E. coli* and if an infection of one of these is found then acidophilus and its cousins should not be taken.

There are many different strains on the market, some found in yoghurt, others in powder or capsules. I currently recommend a French brand *Lactibiane* which reconstitutes from a dehydrated form when mixed with water and which, when drunk, decreases the stomach acidity, allowing the acidophilus to reach the intestine. Other brands must be in acid-resistant capsules. Not much gets past the high acid levels in the stomach, which is a good thing and one that nature intended. Acidophilus is no different, although slightly more resistant, than other organisms. Small amounts of acidophilus will escape into the alkaline intestine if enough yoghurt or powdered acidophilus is ingested but I doubt that these will have any profound effect on the colon 30 feet away where the bulk of *E. coli* lives. Where possible, take the compound with or after a meal in an attempt to avoid the abundant acid.

ALCOHOL

Alcohol is fun. It is not nutritious and is probably harmful if taken in excess and any suggestions that it may actually be protective of conditions such as atheroma or atherosclerosis are probably true but the risks overrule the benefits. In any case, it is probably not the alcohol that is protecting, it is the nutrients taken in coincidentally.

It is hard to define a safe level of alcohol but as a rule of thumb if you do not feel the effects psychologically then the body is probably dealing with the amount you have taken. Unfortunately, this rule of thumb diminishes in accuracy if you constantly drink enough to get drunk and then find yourself needing more. Here, the body is simply becoming tolerant. For those not addicted, a method by which a safe level can be assessed is to not drink alcohol for approximately three weeks, eat a light meal and drink a small amount of alcohol 10 minutes later. Repeat this every 10 minutes and as soon as you feel relaxed or merry then that is your limit. One or two drinks is usually found to be the level. Once this is established, that amount of alcohol in a day is not likely to do you any harm whatsoever.

If you wish to exceed your tolerance level, bear in mind that it takes the liver approximately two days to recover from the insult of being tipsy or drunk. Try to give the liver that amount of time between alcohol binges and never drink to a point where your coordination is clearly embarrassing. Regardless of how you feel, coordination is insulted by anything over your personal tolerance level, as established from the technique above, and no important manual tasks should be undertaken. Driving is an important manual task! Our body cannot deal with an impact at any speed above that of a walk without some damage occurring. Driving, even at 30mph, is well beyond the body's capability to deal with should it suffer an impact, and consequently driving at any speed is a life-threatening condition. Do not drink and drive.

ANTIOXIDANTS AND FREE RADICALS

Free radicals are negatively charged particles that are known to affect the genetic strands within the cells, triggering a potentially cancerous change. These negative ions also damage cell surfaces in blood vessels thereby encouraging clot formation, which in turn attracts calcium and cholesterol to form obstructive plaques.

Antioxidants (incidentally, nothing at all to do with oxygenating of a molecule or cell) bind with free radicals and remove their danger. The antioxidants are vitamins A, C and E, selenium, grapeseed extract, coenzyme Q10 and, to a lesser extent, zinc. Many different plant extracts contain some or all of these components and therefore have antioxidant activity and we are constantly being advised by our nutritional scientists of newer and stronger antioxidant compounds.

Free radicals are found in animal products, fried foods and any fat exposed to heat, oxygen and light. Barbecued and smoked products are particularly full of free radicals. Anything smoked, including tobacco and engine fuels, provides free radicals.

Five portions of fresh fruit and vegetables will protect the average adult provided that excessive free radical intake is not encouraged, otherwise daily supplementation from as early an age as possible is recommended.

ARTIFICIAL SWEETENERS

When artificial sweeteners were first developed in the 1950s the compounds, known as cyclamates, were found to be linked to cancer. These were replaced by saccharin, which petered out due to similar fears. These were replaced by a compound called aspartame, which is made from the amino acid phenylalanine, another amino acid and an alcohol. Phenylalanine is the precursor to serotonin, one of the body's natural calmers, and an increased production of this due to extra availability of its precursor leads to a diminution in other relaxation neurotransmitters, such as dopamine. This can have mild effects on the nervous system, which may or may not be noticed. The alcohol may actually cause a hangover effect and it is known that large amounts of aspartame can even cause seizures. This compound may also be considered as foreign matter and set up an immune response or food allergy. Rashes and itching are not uncommon. Might it even be responsible for the increase in asthma that is being seen in the West? I think it might.

Insulin levels are principally governed by the levels of sugar in the system. There is a possibility that aspartame, which is over a thousand times sweeter than sugar, molecule for molecule, may trigger insulin production via a reflex caused by recognition of sweetness by the taste buds. Do not use artificial sweeteners as a general rule.

BEVERAGES AND DRINKS

Water, and water alone, is what the body utilizes in the form of fluids. The body knows exactly what to do with water and can place it in the right compartments (cells, tissues or blood vessels) swiftly and easily. Anything mixed with the water has to be separated and this requires energy, which in turn utilizes water, thereby decreasing the availability for the rest of the body. Very dilute fruit juices and herbal teas may not cause the body too much trouble, but anything sweet, caffeine- or alcohol-filled or flavoured artificially requires processing, which is a strain on the system.

Milk is discussed as a separate entity later on in this chapter (*see* **Milk**) but is a wholly inadequate method of obtaining hydration (*see* **Dehydration**).

These facts do not mean that enjoyable flavours cannot be imbibed. Select and enjoy from a vast number of herbal teas and fresh fruit and vegetable juices with the knowledge that they will have cleansing and nutritious effects, but do not assume that they will substitute for water.

Artificial drinks such as colas, squashes and carbonated, highly artificially sugared drinks are not just not good for you but they are actually *harmful*. They dehydrate, put pressure on the biochemistry and organs in the body and stimulate the nervous system. The same can be said for caffeine and alcohol but multiply the damage by ten. If you are going to enjoy these 'sins', match every glassful with at least the same amount of water, preferably half an hour before or after imbibing.

BOWEL FLORA

As soon as we are born, we start to swallow bacteria from our environment. We pick up flora as we travel down the vaginal vault from the uterus and continue to pick up bugs from the inevitable kisses and close contact with parents, relations and friends. Breast-feeding also passes bacteria into the system. Those that require oxygen tend not to survive within the intestine but the outcome is the development of 10^{14} anaerobic bacteria per square centimetre of bowel content. Less live in the stomach and the upper part of the small intestine, but the numbers increase the lower we go.

These flora are essential for the breakdown of indigestible foods, the release of nutrients from plant cells and the provision, as biproducts of their own metabolism, of vitamins and trace elements. Our body is very dependent upon bowel bacteria for the production of vitamin B_{12}, for example.

The majority of these bowel flora are *Bifidolactobacillus*. *Eschericha coli* (abbreviated to E coli), and *streptococci* strains make up the rest, with a smaller fluctuating group known as enterobacteria. Within the bowel, these bugs are of great use but outside they can be dangerous since they multiply rapidly and may produce a considerable amount of toxin which is harmlesss within the bowel but potentially harmful elsewhere. There are thousands of different strains, only a few of which are particularly harmful.

Maintenance of healthy bowel flora is a prerequisite of health and many conditions from allergies and all their associated conditions (such as eczema, asthma and hay fever) and arthritis to chronic conditions such as cancer may be associated with poor bowel function which, in turn, is caused by or creates gut 'dysbiosis'. This term indicates incorrect function or proliferation of the wrong sort of bowel flora.

Conditions such as irritable bowel syndrome and the 'leaky gut syndrome' are, in my opinion, invariably linked with gut dysbiosis and more chronic conditions such as Crohn's and ulcerative colitis may also be related.

Living within the confines of the gut is a myriad of yeasts, fungi and other parasites that are kept at bay through what is known as competitive inhibition. There is only a certain amount of food available and if the bowel flora is in abundance and healthy it eats most of the nutrition available. This means that the 'bad bugs' have a limited food supply and cannot, therefore, multiply at any great rate. If the bowel bacteria are insulted, their competitive edge diminishes and yeasts such as *Candida* can flourish. The ingestion of antibiotics from doctor's prescriptions or inadvertently through foods (particularly processed meats),

THE FAMILY ENCYCLOPEDIA OF HEALTH

nitrates and other food additives and the preservatives we have in our foods all kill off the bowel bacteria but do not affect the yeasts and fungi.

A normal balanced diet should not challenge the bowel flora but the regular use of yoghurt bacteria in supplemental form is strongly advised when the Western diet is the predominant intake (see **Antibiotics** *and* **Acidophillus**) because these encourage the 'good bacteria'.

CAFFEINE

Caffeine is a marked stimulator of the nervous system and is found in abundance in coffee, tea, soft drinks, chocolate and other cocoa products and a myriad of over-the-counter drugs used for anything from the common cold to stomach upsets.

Initially caffeine's stimulation of the nervous system gives a 'buzz' of increasing energy, concentration and a sense of euphoria. Caffeine is, at the end of the day, an adrenaline-like compound. Caffeine's effect is to raise blood sugar levels, giving a short-term supply of available energy.

Decaffeinated coffee is rarely completely free of caffeine and the chemicals used to remove the compound may themselves be stimulating and are potentially carcinogenic (cancer-causing). It is also worth remembering that most coffee-making countries will be treating their coffee plants with pesticides and insecticides, and these are going to be fed into your system as well.

Coffee causes cancer? I am afraid so. There are associations between caffeine and cancer of the pancreas, prostate and bladder. It is also known that caffeine may be associated with miscarriage, diabetes, hypertension and I hypothesize that it may create a food allergy state leading to asthma, eczema and hay fever. In fact, I place caffeine at the top of the list of health hazards, even above smoking and the eating of refined foods.

Give it up absolutely and totally. There is no benefit in it whatsoever. If you find the thought of actual withdrawal difficult, then you are addicted and the long-term effects of any addiction are going to be detrimental to your well-being. Ask

for help with the same determination that a heroin addict might should he choose to withdraw from his drug.

CALCIUM

Calcium is found throughout the body, either as a structural or biochemical necessity. Calcium is the main component of teeth and bones and is the reason that muscles can contract. It is very difficult to be calcium deficient because it is spread throughout the foods we eat. It is a fallacy to assume that milk is an essential aspect of calcium intake or that a lack of milk will create calcium deficiency problems such as osteoporosis. In fact, the majority of the world's population does not consume milk products, and is intolerant or unable to utilize the calcium in milk. The incidence of osteoporosis (thin bones) is highest in countries that consume the most milk (see **Osteoporosis**).

Calcium is found in abundance and in an easily absorbable form in sesame seeds, kelp, almonds, meat, poultry, fish, especially salmon and most deep-green vegetables. These foods should be used regularly, especially in young children and teenage girls, the latter of whom will benefit from reduced osteoporosis if their calcium levels are high when the bones are forming.

CARBOHYDRATES

A carbohydrate is an organic substance containing carbon, hydrogen and oxygen. That tells us nothing unless we happen to have done a degree in chemistry! Put simply, sugar molecules such as glucose are built up into chains and at some arbitrary point, when five or six carbon atoms are present, a carbohydrate is formed. As these chains get bigger, compounds such as cellulose are formed and around these the addition of proteins and nutrients attach and we have plants. Change the molecular configuration slightly and add in one or two other compounds and starch is born. Carbohydrates encompass plants and their products, such as potatoes, berries, fruits and anything sweet. We should derive up to 70 per cent of our energy from carbohydrates, the remainder coming from protein (20 per cent) and fats (10 per cent).

CHOLESTEROL

Studies over the last 30 years have shown cholesterol to be a danger if it is found in excess. There are several types of cholesterol. The three better known are high-density lipoproteins (HDL), low-density lipoproteins (LDL) and very-low-density lipoproteins (VLDL). The LDL, VLDL and another fat-containing protein called apolipoprotein attach to damaged areas within arteries to help them repair (and they also carry fats to the tissues). Unfortunately this process has a poor control mechanism and the over-repair process causes plaques to form, which eventually clog up the artery. The HDL acts by blocking LDL action and takes fats to the liver for processing. Putting it simply, HDL is 'good' cholesterol and LDL is 'bad'. Doctors will look at the total cholesterol: HDL/LDL ratio and the risk ratio is discussed below.

Raised cholesterol and tryglyceride levels have been brought to prominence because of the discovery of lipid (fat)-narrowing agents, which were a sellable and patentable drug regime. There is no doubt that raised cholesterol levels will increase the chances of heart attacks and strokes but what the orthodox medical world neglects to tell the patient is that the risk of the use of these drugs may outweigh the benefits. The drugs have many serious side effects, including a propensity to severe depression, thereby increasing the risk of suicide. Some of the lipid-lowering agents also inhibit the production of certain essential heart nutrients, such as co-enzyme Q10. Cholesterol is required for the cell membrane of nearly all tissues in the body and is also required for the production of adrenal hormones, which govern our stress and water balance, for coating our nerves to allow correct conduction and for all our sex hormones. Admittedly the level at which treatment is recommended for raised cholesterol

has been rising, but the dangers of cholesterol need to be put into context with other factors that encourage cardiovascular disease, such as smoking, the oral contraceptive pill, poor exercise and diet.

Raised cholesterol by itself does not suggest danger because the amount of the protective HDL is the relevant factor. A term known as the 'risk ratio' is calculated by dividing the total cholesterol level by the HDL level. If the figure is above 5 for a man and above 4.4 for a woman, then the cholesterol levels are relevant to health. If below these figures, the levels are not relevant. For example, a total cholesterol level of 6mmol/l with an HDL level of 2mmol/l gives a risk ratio of three despite the cholesterol level being above 5.2mmol/l, which is a typical 'upper level' of normal (*see* **Atheroma**).

Cholesterol needs only to be considered dangerous when other factors are considered, such as deficiencies in certain vitamins, minerals and amino acids, all of which are mentioned below in the recommendations. An excess of cholesterol in the diet is occasionally relevant although most cholesterol is made by the liver at the body's request. The following foods should be reduced, not only because of cholesterol but also because they can form free radicals, which are, probably, much more involved in arteriosclerosis, heart attacks and strokes.

High-cholesterol foods

- Red meats
- Offal – especially kidney and liver
- Cheese
- Cow produce (except specially prepared low-fat)
- Prawns and shrimps
- Pork

Those who have read about the evils of cholesterol may be surprised to see that eggs and avocado are not included in this list. Eggs, whilst having a high cholesterol content in the yolk, actually promote a rise in HDL and, in any case, a combination of cholesterol with the lecithin in the white of the egg whilst digestion takes place in the acid environment of the stomach causes the cholesterol to bind with the lecithin and not be easily absorbed. Avocados actually contain no cholesterol. They are a high-fat food and are not useful if triglyceride levels are high or someone is trying to lose weight but a small avocado will not be harmful in comparison to, say, a slice of bacon.

So, in a nutshell, cholesterol and other lipids are not the dangers that the orthodox medical world say they are. The real problem lies in deficiencies and other factors that damage blood vessels and high levels of LDL may enhance the problem.

RECOMMENDATIONS

General Advice

- *A regular check on cholesterol levels is advisable but please put it into context with the co-risk factors mentioned below.*
- *Avoid smoking, caffeine, stress, oral contraceptives, refined sugar, pollutants and additives.*
- *Those with a family history of heart disease, atherosclerosis or strokes should consult with a complementary medical practitioner and special attention should be paid to levels of copper, chromium and magnesium, a low level of which will predispose to problems.*
- *The body will create more cholesterol to wrap around cells to hold in water if an individual is dehydrated. Ensure that adequate amounts of water are drunk each day (see **Dehydration**).*
- *Increased liver activity from an input of toxins or an excess of stress (the liver has to work harder to break down excess adrenaline) should be avoided. The faster the liver works, the more cholesterol it makes.*
- *Not only because it can reduce cholesterol levels but also because of its protective factor from the damage that cholesterol may cause with other co-factors – reduce your stress by changing lifestyle or meditating.*

Nutritional

- *Consider the Ornish or Pritikin diet.*
- *Consider using the macrobiotic diet.*
- *Ensure that the diet is rich in vitamin C, niacin (vitamin B$_3$), vitamin E and the omega 3 and omega 6 essential oils. This can be done by enjoying mackerel, herring, salmon or halibut three times a week. Vegetarians should consider taking supplements of these oils. Three to five portions of fruit or vegetable each day will cover the vitamins.*
- *Avoid the high-cholesterol foods listed in the text above, which may increase cholesterol levels.*

Supplemental

- *If cholesterol levels are raised and reduction in dietary sources has proved inefficient at bringing the levels down, then consider taking the following supplements in divided doses per foot of height three times a day with food: vitamin C (1g), vitamin B$_3$ (niacin, 20mg), vitamin E (150iu), copper (500µg), magnesium (100mg), chromium (50mg), L-carnitine (150mg) and N-acetylcysteine (250mg). This all gets a bit complicated and it might be simpler to discuss the matter with a complementary medical practitioner. More simply, take garlic capsules (200mg per foot of height per day divided into three doses with food).*

FASTING

Fasting is becoming an increasingly popular activity which can range from a total fast where nothing passes the lips to a variety of semi-fasts ranging from an intake of water and fruit juices to fruits and vegetables.

The benefits of a fast are manifold. Time without imbibing allows the mouth a period of time to cleanse through the mouth's natural saliva, which contains many antibodies and cleansing chemicals. The parietal cells of the stomach (which produce hydrochloric acid), the pancreas, liver and gallbladder are allowed a rest from the production of their digestive juices. The bowel muscle wall will not contract as frequently and the colon will be given some time to evacuate the faeces that can build up and adhere to the large intestinal wall.

The liver, the chemical factory of the body, can spend time on cleaning the blood rather than digesting new foods and the kidney can filter out some of the longer lasting toxins in the system. The fat stores that contain some of the body's toxins that may have been stored there to avoid circulating them will discharge some of these toxins into the bloodstream and be dealt with better by the less-pressured liver and kidneys.

The islets of Langerhans, which produce insulin in the pancreas, will also have a rest. So, all in all, a body should benefit from some time away from food consumption. However, like all good things, there is often a reverse side. A total fast excludes all food but must include water at a level of one pint per foot of height per day. Water-restricted fasts must be followed only under the supervision of an experienced naturopathic physician and are only beneficial in certain treatment protocols.

I am not a great supporter of total fasts because I think that the cleansing effect can be achieved without starving the body. I prefer semi-fast diets and recommend the one below as a general guideline.

There is no set fasting technique that suits everybody. Individuals with any tendency to hypoglycaemia (low blood sugar) will not benefit from a complete fast. Others, who lack nutrients, may have malabsorption syndromes or chronic debilitating diseases such as cancer or AIDS may, in fact, make their situation worse with a complete fast.

The Eastern philosophies view each individual as having too much or too little air, water, earth, wood or metal, and therefore a fast for someone deficient in any of these humours may, once again, be detrimental.

RECOMMENDATIONS

General Advice

- *Except under expert advice, any fast must include a suitable amount of water intake.*

- *Specific semi-fasts may be tried on a trial and error basis over a 24-hr period. If the individual feels better, then a second day may be even more beneficial. Do not fast for more than 48hr unless advised by an expert.*

A semi-fast diet

A short time on a semi-fast diet may help you feel generally better and it can be a great pick-me-up if you are chronically tired. It is better to start the diet on a day when you do not have to exert yourself physically.

Day 1

Drink freshly squeezed or pressed fruit and/or vegetable juice at approximately four-hourly intervals. Quench your thirst with mineral water or herb tea, and make sure you drink at least two litres (four pints) of fluid during the day. Some suggested juices are apple, orange, grape, pineapple, grapefruit, blackcurrant, mango, cranberry, carrot, beetroot and celery.

Day 2

As for Day 1 but add up to one pound of grapes and three bananas. Only eat as much as you want.

Day 3

Add raw and lightly cooked vegetables and any other fruit to anything you want from the previous days.

Day 4

Anything you want from previous days and add wholegrain cereals, nuts and seeds.

Day 5

As for Day 4 but add fish.

Day 6
As for Day 5 but add offal, poultry or game.

Day 7
Return to your diet as discussed with a nutritionist.

FATS

Fats are good for you, in fact fats are essential to our well-being. That is not the impression we would get from the media although explanation of the concept of good and bad fats is becoming clearer.

Fat is only a problem if it exceeds more than 15 to 20 per cent of our diet. Having said that, it is important that the fat that we eat is 'good' fat, containing the sort that we can utilize, and has associated with it the vitamins known as the fat-soluble vitamins that cannot be found in water-based foods.

Firstly let us understand the different terms that we so frequently read about.

- *Essential fatty acids (EFA)* – are those that humans cannot synthesize and must therefore be obtained through the diet. Fats are made up of fatty acids, which are principally carbon, hydrogen and oxygen molecules joined together in a variety of combinations.
- *Triglycerides (TG)* – are three fatty acids joined together, which vary in their length and carbon:hydrogen ratio. Dietary fat is mostly composed of triglycerides. These are found in both animals and vegetables.
- *Phospholipids and glycolipids* – these are triglycerides that contain phosphorus and other molecules. These are important constituents of biological membranes, blood plasma and most cell walls. Nervous tissue is made up of a type of phospholipid known as sphingomyelins and it cannot function without them.
- *Cholesterol and its derivatives* – cholesterol is in fact a steroid. Are we not generally led to believe that steroids are bad? Absolutely so if they are artificially manufactured (although

certain conditions require steroid treatment), but in fact life depends upon them. Cholesterol is the starting point for hormones of the adrenal glands and sex glands, vitamin D and the bile acids, all of which are essential to life. Cholesterol is discussed elsewhere (*see* **Cholesterol**).

- *Vitamins A, D, E and K* – are all fat-related vitamins that do not dissolve in water and can only be found in fats.
- *Saturated and unsaturated fats* – if a fatty acid chain has all of the carbon atoms linked together with a single electromagnetic link, it is said to be saturated. If the chain is joined by more than one bond, it is unsaturated. The fewer the links, the harder it is to break down the chains, making saturated fats more difficult to utilize as energy (because it is the breaking of the bonds that releases energy) and increasing the tendency for the body to store these poorly utilizable fats. The more saturated the fat, the easier it binds together and a simple way to understand whether a compound is heavily saturated or not is by its solidity at room temperature. Beef, pork or lamb fat is hard, butter less so and olive oil is a fluid. There are more saturated fats in animal proteins than in vegetables.

Fats – strong and weak bonds

SATURATED	$(CHO)_x$—$(CHO)_y$
UNSATURATED	—$(CHO)_x$=$(CHO)_z$
POLYUNSATURATED	$(CHO)_a$=$(CHO)_b$=$(CHO)_c$—$(CHO)_d$—

- It is important to remember that many fats are necessary and good for us, particularly those known as the omega 3 and omega 6 oils found in fish oils, eicosapentaenoic acid (EPA) and linseed. Getting the gist? Saturated fats are 'bad', unsaturated fats are not.
- If a fatty acid chain has many bonds it is said to be polyunsaturated and having more bonds is weaker as a chain and thus more readily broken down. As a general rule, these are therefore healthier and are recognized by remaining a liquid at room temperature, as mentioned

above. Polyunsaturated fats also have the additional benefit of being cholesterol-free and although this is not necessarily a good thing (see **Cholesterol**), as a general rule low-cholesterol foods are liable to do us less harm.

- *Hydrogenated fats* – unfortunately there is another twist in the tale and this is the term *hydrogenated fats*. A hydrogenated fat is one that has had additional hydrogen ions added to it, usually by being exposed to heat and altering its natural structure. An otherwise 'good for you' polyunsaturated fat may become harmful by being heated. Much to our misfortune, the food processing industry takes healthy polyunsaturated vegetable oils and processes them in such a way that they are exposed to high temperatures, oxygen and light (the latter two also hydrogenate fats) and sell them to us proclaiming great health benefits.

- *Trans-fatty acids.* Lastly, we are hearing about products that are free of *trans*-fatty acids. These are altered forms of the EFAs, altered by the heat and oxygen exposure of processing. *Trans*-fatty acids cannot be used by the body and actively interfere with the biochemistry of one of the body's protective compounds, known as prostaglandin E_1.

So where are we? We should not eat animal fats, including butter, because of its saturated status and cholesterol, but we cannot eat the vegetable oils that are provided to us because the processing of these otherwise healthy polyunsaturated oils is generally hydrogenated. Unfortunately, these are the facts.

We need to reduce the amount of fat in our diet to an absolute minimum until the 'powers that be' can produce an easily available *non-treated* polyunsaturated fat. At the moment these are called 'cold-pressed' and are available in health-food stores and some supermarkets.

If polyunsaturated, cold-pressed, non-hydrogenated and low or no *trans*-fatty acid fats and oils are not available (and, heavens above, you really have to have your thinking cap on when you buy your

spread for your morning toast), you may choose to give up. Do not do this. Persevere. The 'good stuff' is available and at the end of the day if you have small amounts even of the most refined and dangerous compounds your healthy body will deal with it efficiently and extract the necessary EFAs and vitamins. Purified supplements can be used on a daily basis and eating the occasional oily fish (such as salmon, mackerel, herring) will provide the necessary requirements. Remember that the body must have fats to survive, and bad is better than none!

Synthetic fats

Recently there has been research into production of a fat that carries the taste and flavour associated with the food group but does not have the capability of being stored in fat stores. The food industry is looking forward to the fortune that such a food product may confer since it would allow everyone to enjoy their cream teas and fried foods without worrying about weight.

Be very wary. There have been no long-term studies and we have little idea of how the body will react to this extremely artificial substance. Like genetically engineered food (*see* **genetically altered food**), this is a compound that should be avoided for at least the next 20 years. Then, if no adverse affects have been reported, we may be able to use it. Be very sceptical about 'scientific studies' because those that show negative aspects are not likely to be published. Millions of dollars have gone into the production and assessment of this food and the food industry is not going to give up their profits easily.

FOOD ADDITIVES

The body has developed an enzyme and biochemical system over millions of years of evolution. We are the most complex of organisms and, some would say, the most successful on the planet. We did this because we learned and developed abilities over a long period of time, allowing us to deal with most things that nature threw at us. Now our bodies are compromised by an array of unnatural chemicals that are changing at an alarming rate.

Our evolutionary capabilities to deal with these compounds cannot keep up and in an attempt to defend ourselves we are storing these additives, preservatives, insecticides, pesticides, household chemicals and airborne pollutants, which are known, in many cases, to alter our genetic material and trigger diseases as serious as cancer. Wherever possible, just do not eat them.

FOOD ALLERGY AND INTOLERANCE
– *see* **Allergies**

It is important to differentiate between food allergy and food intolerance. An *allergy* is a blood response to a foreign body. A substance that is in the bloodstream that does not belong to the body will have immunoglobulins produced against it. These immunoglobulins, more commonly known as antibodies, attach to foreign matter and make that particle more recognizable by the white cells that ingest such invaders. An *intolerance* is less well defined by the orthodox world but holistically would be considered to be a substance to which the body responds badly in any number of ways, such as nausea and vomiting, skin rash, diarrhoea, frequent urination and any other eliminative process. I believe an intolerance to be an energetic confrontation. All cells in the body resonate at a particular frequency and any foreign molecule whose electrons resonate in such a way as to inhibit or block the body's natural resonance is going to create an intolerance. The orthodox attitude to intolerance is discussed below.

In my opinion, food allergy and intolerance is far more prevalent than even holistic practitioners, as a general rule, consider. Symptoms of food allergy/intolerance may be mild or may even trigger serious disorders such as diabetes and cancer.

The orthodox world divides allergy into four major components, type one being anaphylaxis and type four being delayed-allergy response.

The development of allergies/intolerance

The bloodstream should have in its flow only compounds that are made and derived by the body or those that are absorbed through the lungs and bowel (and to some extent the skin). The latter organs filter out unwanted particles and, in the case of the digestive system, break down foods into the smallest of components, such as amino acids and peptides (small chains of amino acids), basic nutrients, small chains of carbohydrates and fatty acids. When these reach the bloodstream they are not considered to be viruses or bacteria and the immune system leaves them alone. If any of these break down or selective mechanisms are inhibited or fail, the larger molecules are absorbed, the body cannot differentiate between them and invading organisms and sets up an allergic response. In the case of intolerance, even some small peptides may carry a resonance or vibration that is harmful to the body, but these do not set up an allergic response.

Any action or reaction that inhibits the protective or digestive mechanism can lead to a prolonged, possibly lifelong allergy or intolerance. Most commonly, bowel infections or the use of antibiotics that inhibit the body's natural flora and damage the delicate bowel membranes can lead to larger molecules being absorbed through the intestinal wall in a process that is now termed the 'leaky gut syndrome' (*see* **Leaky gut syndrome**). Literally, the bowel inflames and loses its selectivity, causing larger molecules to be absorbed. Pollutants and inhalants such as cigarette smoke cause inflammation in the lungs and allow larger molecules to enter the bloodstream and commonly inhaled components such as pollen and pet hair will follow and potentially set up an allergic response. The skin is subjected to more cosmetics and chemicals than it used to be, creating more inflammatory responses such as eczema, which in turn allows compounds into the bloodstream to trigger allergic or intolerance responses.

It is, therefore, important to understand that allergies and intolerances are not about the causative agent but are reflections of our lifestyle, habits and environmental pollutants. We should establish an idea of those foods that may be creating problems. To do this requires some form of investigation or testing, and the choices are listed in the section on allergy testing.

The terms allergy and intolerance have become somewhat synonymous in the holistic world. This is a sad reflection of the lack of education in science that many complementary medical practitioners receive, through no fault of their own. The independent colleges should pay more attention to the basics of psychology, but that is another discussion.

An intolerance is simple: a lack of capacity to endure or an oversensitivity to a compound. This is generally created by a direct chemical reaction between a foodstuff and chemicals or cells in the body, this is mediated by a chemical release from the tissues that are intolerant. This is quite a separate concept from an allergy, which is an acquired condition initiated by exposure to a compound (known as an allergen) that creates a blood cell response to produce histamine-like chemicals or immunoglobulins (antibodies).

It is quite possible to be intolerant without being allergic, and have allergies without intolerance. An example is somebody who drinks coffee and eats wheat and creates an acidic indigestion or an irritated skin. There may be no changes in the bloodstream or white blood cells of the tissue and the person is therefore intolerant but not allergic. Alternatively, the immune system may produce antibodies against a compound with no symptoms being exhibited whatsoever.

The differentiation between intolerance and allergy is only relevant if allergy testing is undertaken because many people are surprised when allergy tests come back as negative despite frank reactions occurring.

Applied kinesiology (muscle testing) and all bioresonance computers and techniques are testing for intolerance. Hair samples, often tested in the alternative world by the unproven techniques of the pendulum or radionics, only show levels of compounds that have been eliminated and therefore suggest an intolerance within the system. Blood tests are the only method of registering allergy.

FRUIT JUICE

Fruit juice is without doubt one of the best and healthiest products available to human beings. Fruits are nature's vitamin suppliers, eaten by most herbivores in preference to any other foods. Each fruit contains a variety of vitamins, nutrients, minerals and even proteins, which make it a vital part of the food chain. In juiced form they are easily available, not hard to digest and easy to transfer across the bowel membrane.

The above statement applies to fresh fruit or fresh fruit juices. Read on . . .

Juices that are prepared, processed, packaged and provided to us through the shops are at best, from a nutritional point of view, worthless and at worst harmful. Without many exceptions they have added sugar. Even those that state 'no added sugar' may have up to six teaspoonsful of refined glucose added. I am not sure of the political mechanics but it is something like this. The food manufacturers (a most powerful industry) claim that the manufacturing process removes sugar that would otherwise be present. Adding sugar back in (albeit not exactly the same sort that is taken out) is merely replacing the fruit's own store. There is, therefore, no added sugar. The governments believe this and we and our children are subjected to refined, artificial sugar additives in these 'natural' fruit juices.

To conform to most hygiene standards, fruits from which juices are made are generally put into contact with some form of preservative. The fruits themselves are mass produced and most often artificially chemically encouraged to grow larger (often at the expense of flavour). Many chemicals are added to remove the unpleasant flavour of the skin and pips (seeds) that are all pulverized in the juice-making process. One of these chemicals is formaldehyde, a chemical used for preserving bodies!

Many vitamins are denatured or altered through the process, especially vitamin C, which alters when exposed to air. The addition of artificial vitamin C at a later stage is the food industry's answer but this is not absorbed as well as orange's original vitamin

C because it imbalances the proportion of bioflavonoids that are needed to help absorption.

In conclusion, freshy extracted and immediately drunk fruit juice is one of the best forms of nutrition, as opposed to the easily available artificial fruit juices that are sold to us in the belief that they are of benefit. At best, our body will deal with the chemical poisoning and high sugar content that we take in, and at worst it will not. There is a dramatic increase in the UK of diabetes, especially in the age group under five years, and I suspect that the increase in white sugar through fruit juices is a primary factor in this finding.

GENETICALLY ALTERED FOOD

Over the last decade the enormously powerful food industry and its political lobbyists have been researching, producing and promoting genetically altered food. Scientists have methods of altering the genes in the nucleus of the cells of the foods that we eat. This provides the foods with abilities such as faster growth, yeast and fungus resistance and even insect-repellence. Lauded as the first step towards eliminating worldwide food shortage (a farce as there is plenty of food; it is just not distributed as it should be, because of the poor profits involved), the technique is, in principle, a good idea. The problem lies in the inability of the scientific world to assure us that the techniques (chemical and radiation) used to alter the food genes will not carry on their effect within the human body. There is also the fear that the genetically altered genes may, in some way, incorporate themselves into our own cells and alter the function. A man-made (super-bionic) tomato or soya gene may instruct a liver cell to produce chemicals that the plant cell would make.

RECOMMENDATION

General Advice
- *Until we have had 10 or possibly 15 years of well-controlled studies on animals and volunteer human populations, avoid genetically altered foods.*

GLUTEN AND GLIADIN (GRAIN PROTEINS)

These two proteins are found predominantly in wheat but also in varying amounts in other grains. They are accepted as the main cause of allergic, intolerant or inflammatory responses in the human being, often caused by introducing wheat too early in an infant's life, the large quantity of grain that is eaten, or to the diminished ability in the human gut to break down these complex protein molecules.

Gluten sensitivity manifests in a condition known as Coeliac disease (*see* **Coeliac disease**) and it is probable that other proteins such as gliadin may cause similar problems, although a specific disease process has yet to be attributed to them.

MILK

Opinion is divided as to whether milk is of great benefit – only to calves or a wonderful multi-faceted food?

The proteins casein, lactalbumin and lactoglobulin (the milk proteins) are known to be the cause of allergies and are not easily broken down by the human gut. If a protein is not well broken down it can be absorbed in its entirety and the body will recognize it as a potential virus or bacteria and produce an antibody response. If the partially broken down protein resembles the proteins within our body, then this immune system response may well attack our cells.

Milk sugar, lactose, is not well tolerated by many races. Ninety per cent of Filipinos, 50 per cent of Indians and approximately 8 per cent of the USA and the UK populations do not have the necessary enzyme to break down lactose. To these people this makes the sugar useless as an energy source and encourages fluids to stay in the bowel, leading to dehydration.

Homogenization, a process to 'sterilize' milk to ensure safe consumption, leads to the production of a chemical called xanthine oxidase, which destroys a compound in the blood called plasmogen, which in turn leads to the loss of a protective factor in the arterial walls. This, in turn, encourages atheroma.

Milk is often considered to be a major source of calcium and indeed the calcium content of milk is very high. Several studies, however, show that the calcium in milk is not easily absorbed into the bloodsteam and does not increase calcium levels as profoundly as we would assume (*see* **Calcium**).

Milk has been related to a myriad of symptoms and conditions, including problems associated with mucus, such as respiratory infections, ear, nose and throat problems, sinus congestion, asthma, colitis, acne and eczema, arthritis, heartburn and ulcers, to name but a few.

Milk has a complex chemical make-up and some authorities consider that some of these chemicals have a strong biochemical effect on tissue growth. Insulin growth factor IGF-1 increases the rate at which cells divide and reproduce. Milk also contains oestrogen-like hormones and prolactin, any of which can effect cellular growth in the breast. There are grounds to believe that milk may promote breast cancer.

Milk has found its way into our diet and a majority of us enjoy a breakfast cereal (despite its acid-forming tendencies, especially when we liberally add refined sugar). It is an integral part of breakfast and alternatives are hard to find: goat's and sheep's milk have a distinctive taste that may not be acceptable; soya has a grainy texture; and fruit juices on cereals simply do not hit the spot for those of us who are accustomed to cow's milk. It is worth, however, trying to prepare a 'milk' from a variety of nuts and seeds by following the instructions below:

- Try almonds, cashews, hazelnuts, sesame, pumpkin or sunflower seeds.
- Soak overnight in enough water to cover the seeds by at least half an inch.
- The next morning, pour the soaked seeds and water into a blender and pulverize. (Discard the overnight water that the almonds have been in,

as the taste is not pleasant.) If the solution is too thick, add more water.
- If the flavour is not to your taste, add a spoonful of honey or blend in raisins earlier on in the preparation.

I do not think that milk is a good food. If it does not cause obvious symptoms then there is probably no harm in drinking it, but organic milk, to avoid homogenization, is a prerequisite for anybody whose family has any cardiovascular disease. I do not recommend it as a food for young children, preferring, despite recent scares, formula preparations and weaning on to a wholesome diet.

NITRATES

Of all additives and preservatives, one of the most prominent found in our food are the nitrates. They are used to colour and preserve foods, especially meats. It has been found that these destabilize the body's oxygen supply, with potentially fatal results if eaten in sufficient quantities.

Blackouts are uncommon but can occur because of a drop in blood pressure due to nitrate ingestion. As usual, the orthodox world has set a safety level of 200ppm in any food and thereby suggest that taking in 190ppm is safe but 201ppm is not. There is, as always, a grey area and some people are more sensitive than others. Beware and avoid any foods containing nitrates.

SALT

Salt is made up of two elements: sodium and chlorine. It is the sodium component that is particularly relevant because this small molecule controls a multitude of biochemical processes but principally maintains the bloodstream and tissue-fluid integrity.

Dehydration of the body, blood pressure and permeability of nearly every cell in the body is dependent on sodium and fortunately sodium is found in nearly everything we eat. The problems arise with *excess* salt. Salt is essential and must never be considered toxic unless taken over and above the necessary requirement.

The vital essence of sodium has encouraged our evolutionary development to make the taste of salt a great pleasure and even a comfort. Our mind–body connection knows that salt is essential and therefore likes to take it in and encourages this by making it taste nice.

Unfortunately not only does our mind–body connection know this but so does the food industry. The outcome is an abundance of salt in everything that is manufactured for mass production and sale. Go for a browse through a supermarket alley and find me a product that does not have salt added and you will bring me a natural food or one that sells poorly.

RECOMMENDATIONS

General Advice

- *Avoid adding extra salt to meals and limit any addition to cooking. It may take up to two weeks but a diet with no salt added will become tasteful after the excess has been removed.*
- *Look closely at any bought product and reduce the intake of naturally salty foods, such as sea fish.*

SOYA

There is a lot written and discussed concerning soya, the bean originally grown in the East. Commonly found in its natural form, soya sauce, tofu and soya milk, it contains protease inhibitors and isoflavins and other chemicals, all or any of which may act as an anticancer and anti-atheroma compound.

Soya has been the main vegetable crop to be experimented with using gene altering or genetic tampering techniques. Ensure that any products containing soya come from a natural, organic source and do not contain genetically altered substance (*see* **Genetically altered foods**).

Soya products contain chemicals called phyto-oestrogens. These chemicals are known to inhibit an enzyme that converts not so active oestrogen-like compounds into the more potent oestradiol.

These chemicals also occupy receptor sites on cells. Both of these reactions stop oestrogen from acting and exhibiting its effects.

The Japanese and Chinese have used soya in large quantities as part of their normal diet and show no detrimental oestrogen effects. In fact, soya may be responsible for the lowered levels of breast cancer in the Japanese race. It is suggested that some property of soya combines with oestrogen receptors and prevents oestrogen from affecting the growth rate of particular oestrogen-sensitive cancer cells. The paradox occurs because we use soya for its oestrogen-like effect in menopause but use it as an oestrogen blocker in cancer.

Until clearer evidence is available as to whether or not soya works as a weak oestrogen or as an oestrogen blocker (or both), enjoy it as a food but do not consume it in excessive quantities. If you are an oestrogen-sensitive cancer risk you need to be aware that safe doses and the efficacy of using soya products have not been established and there is a slight possibility that current theory is wrong and that the isoflavones may be harmful. Keep an eye on the popular press that will, no doubt, advise us as research develops.

It may be wise not to use high quantities of soya products in infants and children following studies in animals in New Zealand around 1994. There have been no studies performed on human beings and therefore there are no known risks, only assumptions. It is worth noting that the levels of oestrogens that a foetus is subjected to *in utero* are probably much higher than any level caused by soya food products.

Soya is a valuable protein source and essential in vegan diets. It is always worthwhile spending time with a nutritionist if any particular diet format is to be used where a balance may be compromised.

SUGAR

Sugar is a carbohydrate (*see* **Carbohydrates**). In its natural form it is enjoyable to taste and a swift and excellent source of energy. Sugar, whether in the form of glucose or fructose (fruit sugar), or a variety of combinations, is usually found in nature in association with a variety of other nutrients and is bound up with larger molecules. This means that the body, at the same time as absorbing sugar, is also absorbing useful building blocks and does not absorb the sugars too quickly because a considerable amount of digestion is necessary to break down the complexes to get at the sugar molecules.

All of this is lost with refined sugar. The complexes are already broken down so the glucose is absorbed rapidly. This creates a fast insulin response, which causes sugar levels to be stored as fat more swiftly and blood sugar levels to drop, thereby providing short bursts of energy only. All the nutrients are stripped so the body gets a sudden surge in energy but no building blocks are necessarily there to do the building. Refined sugar is much sweeter than natural sugar and the taste buds accommodate rapidly, taking away the pleasure of the sweetness of, say, a carrot or an apple. Very swiftly do we 'hook' ourselves and especially our children, onto un-nutritious sweetness, much against the preferences of nature. Sugar is not bad for you. In fact it is extremely good, but not if refined.

The mechanism of insulin production leads to states of hypoglycaemia with a myriad of symptoms: fatigue, depression, irritability, muscle weakness, shakiness, headaches and even asthma. Diabetes is encouraged, arteriosclerosis is propagated and blood pressure is elevated. Sugar requires vitamins and minerals to be utilized and high doses of white sugar keep the metabolism going but, without a nutrient supply, deficiencies will arise. Worst of all, perhaps, refined sugar makes us fat, along with all of the social and health implications that this brings. Believe me, I have only scratched on the surface of metabolic and health dangers of refined sugars. (*See* **Hypoglycaemia**, **Diabetes** *and* **Weight loss**.)

SPICY FOODS

Like all food groups, spicy foods have their place. They are generally eaten in hot climates where they raise the body temperature, making the external heat comparatively less intense.

Those in cooler climates who enjoy spicy foods should eat them only in moderation and preferably with a cooling (raw or lightly steamed) food to compensate. Excess heat in the system, according to Eastern philosophies, will arise from excessively spiced foods and there are problems associated with inflammation. (*See* **Yin and Yang foods**.)

VITAMINS

Vitamins are a group of organic compounds that are present in variable, minute quantities in natural foodstuffs and are required for normal growth and maintenance of life. As a rule the human is unable to synthesize these compounds, thus encouraging the term 'vital' to be part of the name. Vitamins are generally needed only in small amounts and have no calorific value, therefore they do not furnish energy but are essential for transformation of nutrition into energy and the regulation of most, if not all, biochemical processes in the body.

It is not necessary for the individual to have much of an understanding of vitamins despite what the popular press and complementary medical journals might suggest. A balanced diet containing five portions of fruit or vegetables, not overcooked, in association with non-refined carbohydrates, protein and a small amount of the right sort of fats will probably not lead people into deficiencies. The body is remarkably good at absorbing what it needs from the most unlikely sources and if food is eaten by instinct, most vitamins will be taken in as required.

I use the word 'probably' in the paragraph above since there is now evidence suggesting that our fruit and vegetables are not absorbing all the nutrients they should. Over-farming and the leaching of minerals from the soil, combined with picking our fruit and vegetables before they are ripe may mean our food is deficient. Economic pressures demand that our soil is overused and this means that fewer fields are left to lie fallow,

VITAMINS – Dosage and Toxicity

Vitamin	Maximum permissible dosage	Toxic signs and symptoms
Vitamin A	Infants 10,000iu Adults 50,000iu	Appetite loss, headache, blurred vision, unusual bleeding, dry cracked skin, loss of hair, muscular stiffness and pain
Vitamin B group	*See* individual compounds below	
Niacin (vitamin B_3)	100mg	Flushing, headaches, cramps, nausea, vomiting and burning or itching skin
Niacinamide	100mg	As above
Pantothenic acid (vitamin B_5)	Not tested	Occasional diarrhoea
Pyridoxine (vitamin B_6)	200mg*	Numbness, tingling and other sensory nerve effects
Riboflavin (vitamin B_2)	No toxic effects	
Thiamine (vitamin B_1)	No toxic effects	
Vitamin B_{12}	No toxic effects	
Beta-carotene	No toxicity recorded up to 250mg per day	
Biotin	No toxic effects reported	
Vitamin C	10g per day, except under supervision	Nausea, diarrhoea, flatulence
Vitamin D	1,000iu/kg of body weight	Nausea, vomiting, appetite loss, diarrhoea, headache, excessive urination, constipation, pallor
Vitamin E	800iu	Severe weakness and fatigue, may worsen hypertension
Folic acid	15mg	Abdominal distension, appetite loss, nausea and vivid dreams
Vitamin K		No side effects if given orally

There is controversy about this dosage and legal guidelines may state that 10mg or more is toxic. This continues to be a contentious issue.

and consumer demand to have fruit looking perfect on the shelves means that a tomato picked when ripe will be rotten by the time it gets to the shelf. Picking it green and ripening it in artificial light, after it has been transported in a freezer, may interfere with its nutritional content. I suspect that it may be necessary to supplement diets in the near future with vitamin and mineral supplements, but evidence on this matter is currently equivocal.

For that reason, no more is mentioned in this section on this vast and fascinating subject. Every condition that would benefit from vitamin supplementation will have recommended dosages or guidelines within the text of this book. The recommendations are based on 'natural' products that, sadly, tend to separate individual supplements from their coenzymes and other compounds that help their absorption. I therefore strongly recommend the use of natural food-state vitamins. These are available and are made by extracting all the nutrients from a natural source and not separating them. Vitamin E is a prime example of this. D-alphatocopherol is twice as absorbable as the synthetic vitamin E – DL-alphatocopherol.

Loss of nutrients between 1940 and 1991

Mineral	Vegetables	Fruits
Copper	76% content loss	19% content loss
Sodium	49%	29%
Calcium	46%	16%
Iron	27%	24%
Magnesium	24%	15%
Potassium	16%	22%

Vitamin toxicity

As more knowledge filters through to practitioners of complementary medicine concerning the beneficial effects of high-dose vitamin therapy, it is necessary for practitioners and individuals to be aware of possible side effects or toxicity.

Principally, it is difficult to overdose on a vitamin, especially if it is a natural food state vitamin as mentioned above. I have listed here the maximum permissible amounts that can be taken on a daily basis and some of the signs and symptoms to watch out for if taking vitamin supplements.

WATER

The importance of water is discussed in the section on dehydration (*see* **Dehydration** because it is the most important part of this book).

The quality of the water that we take in is of extreme importance to our health. It is very rare that natural sources of water are available and most Western societies are now drinking water that may have been recycled up to seven times. Water should arrive from the skies to fill our lakes and reservoirs in a pure state but of course air pollution is altering that factor. Atomic fall-out is creating radioactive clouds and earth through which the rain must pass. Pesticides, insecticides and other agrochemicals are filling our soil and rivers and finding their way into the food chain. The water companies (under governmental regulations) in many parts of the Western world are treating our water with chemicals, traces of which find their way into our nervous systems. The less-developed countries have water contaminated by faeces because of a lack of recycling plants, and overpopulation is making matters worse.

Sounds gloomy, does it not? We have to rely upon the strength of our body's constitution and on our immune system to deal with the toxins that we inevitably take in. Bottled water has its critics but is, probably, safer than most tap water. Human cells are found in occasional samples but I dare say that these would be found in tap water too. One arguable criticism of bottled water is its mineral content. Whilst the body does need minerals, the absorption of these is energy-consuming and a water that actually tastes salty is probably best avoided. All bottles are now labelled and anything with a sodium content over 5mg/l should be replaced with one with less.

Filtration systems that can be fitted under the kitchen sink certainly remove a lot of the contaminants, and none more so than the reverse-osmosis filters that are beginning to come into circulation. These are, at the time of writing, expensive but worth it for those who can afford it. The more we buy, the more will be produced and the more the price will come down and be affordable by the masses.

Water has extremely special properties that are not fully explained by physics and is one of the prominent features and categories in Eastern philosophies of medicine. Homeopathy will probably be found to have its 'unscientific' effects and success based on the unique properties of the electrons within the water molecules.

Drink plenty and drink it pure.

YOGHURT BACTERIA – *see* **Acidophilus.**

DIAGNOSTIC TECHNIQUES

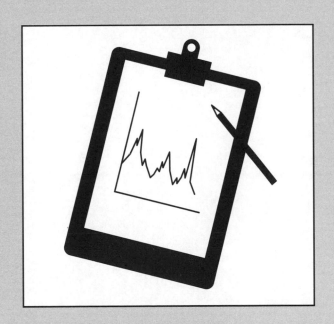

CHAPTER 8

DIAGNOSTIC TECHNIQUES

If there is one area of modern medicine that has to be lauded it is the advance in diagnostic investigation and technique. Whether it is through indirect means such as a blood test or direct visualization through ultrasound or endoscopy, the ability of today's doctors to diagnose a problem is incomparable with the options available even only 50 years ago. Computers are creating an ever more rapid advance on our diagnostic capabilities.

Unfortunately, in this technological rush much bedside manner and clinical diagnostic abilities seem to be diminishing. It is quite feasible for a doctor to make accurate diagnoses without touching the patient, and with the advent of television screen consultations, the doctors need not even be in the same country.

From an orthodox point of view this may not be a problem because diagnosis is generally superficial, with most concern being paid to the immediate cause of a symptom rather than any long-term, underlying cause of an illness. The holistic view has to be that modern diagnostic techniques need to be integrated with clinical examination, experience, intuition and 'sixth sense'. This abstract concept is probably closely linked with an individual's healing ability. There is no lack of evidence that healing exists and even the most interventional surgeons may have part of their success manifested by their innate, but not consciously accepted, healing ability.

A holistic physician will take a patient through four stages of examination.

- Observation
- Listening
- Touching
- Investigating

There should be no difference whether you are visiting an acupuncturist or a yoga teacher. These four stages should be considered to the best of the practitioner's ability.

Some aspects of a diagnostic consultation may be awkward for both the practitioner and the patient. Complementary medical practitioners integrate observation far more into the diagnosis than orthodox physicians and it is not unusual to find the consulting room of an osteopath or chiropractor without a screen behind which a patient may undress. The practitioner may sit and watch, which can be quite embarrassing and unnerving for a patient. A sensitive therapist will explain the reasons for doing so but as many do not, I have done so in the sections below.

Questions will be asked, the answers to which may not even be known to your spouse or best friend and the concept of even discussing these matters may be at least embarrassing and at most shocking. The relevance of some questions will defeat immediate logic but a practitioner with a knowledge of mind–body energy and medicine will need to know your state of mind even if you only have a fungal infection of your toe nail. Questions about gynaecological matters may be asked when the complaint is about depression. There is generally a reason for these connections even if they are not apparent.

An examination should be complete. Every part of the body is linked directly or indirectly with every other part and any practitioner using meridian or Hara diagnoses (*see* **Hara diagnoses**) will examine the abdomen, back and limbs even if the problem is associated with the nostril. Intimate examination is generally not required unless the problem is associated with that area. Traditional Chinese practitioners, especially those of a particular school, may not allow any conversation from the patient. The little ivory statuettes often found as ornaments here in the West were originally designed for the patient to point to the part that hurts or is afflicted. The practitioner would, from tongue and pulse diagnosis only, make a full diagnosis and offer treatment. This too may be done in silence, simply writing out the script and handing it to the patient who takes it to an assistant. This attitude is not accepted by the Western patient and with so much media coverage of alternative medicine, individuals are, quite rightly, asking questions and demanding to know the basis of the suggested treatment.

RECOMMENDATIONS

General Advice

- *Do not hesitate to ask a practitioner why they are watching, asking or examining any part of your mind–body space. No practitioner should object, although some may prefer silence.*
- *If you do not 'click' with your practitioner, discuss your difficulties or change your practitioner. Healing is far more likely to take place in the hands of someone you like and trust.*
- *Do not be put off by the thought of examination and investigation. Burying your head in the sand (the ostrich syndrome!) may delay the diagnosis of an underlying condition and hinder the choice of a correct treatment programme.*
- *Leave your inhibitions at home. Discuss your condition fully and frankly and answer any questions, however odd or irrelevant they may seem.*

OBSERVATION

All practitioners of healthcare will start their examination as soon as you enter the consulting room or they meet you in the waiting room. They will be watching the way you walk or how you sit, establishing any obvious structural irregularity. Attention will be paid to the quality of the hair, skin and eyes and even to the choice of the colour of clothes. Sallow or pale complexion, jaundiced

eyes and the way that an individual may walk into a consultation, perhaps with a limp, are examples of how an initial observation will guide the practitioner to diagnoses. A psychological case of depression or anxiety may be reflected in somebody choosing to wear black and even the type of clothes may be covering up anorexia or obesity.

Aura reading

The aura is a fuzz around the body. Anybody can be taught to read an aura. There is nothing mystical or magical about this. There is a skill in associating what is seen with underlying illness, but this too is taught and learned through experience.

Most of us are subconsciously aware of an aura and this manifests in several ways. We have all walked into a room and instantly 'clicked' with someone as our auras match. Auras have a sense of a colour (and some aura readers can see this), which is why some people suit certain colours. We all have an awareness, especially of those close to us, if something is not right with an individual. It is not just about their lack of a smile or a glint in the eye, it is a feeling or sensation that we cannot explain. Instinct would be a suitable label. Whilst the aura is generally seen within a few inches of the body, its ability to transmit may have no boundaries. An instant attraction across a room is liable to be the joining or meeting of two sympathetic wavelengths and the term 'telepathy' may also be part of the aura. Have we not all experienced an absolute certainty of the telephone being about to ring only to find that your best friend calls that instant.

The aura is yet to be measured to the satisfaction of the orthodox scientific world. As it is part of the vital force I doubt if we will be able to measure this field of energy in the near future. Kirlian photography is the process of taking pictures of energy radiating in spikes from the surface of the body. Unlike highly sophisticated orthodox medical technology, which can measure heat, the Kirlian photograph can sense not only temperature but also other electromagnetic fields.

This is the closest, I believe, that we may get to converting the energy of the aura into a two- or three- dimensional picture.

Those who read auras are capable of seeing colours and use this to establish general health or they compare the aura to the superficial points known as meridians or energy channels that travel through the body.

A 'black' area is often seen above the head in depression because energy (often discussed as 'white light') fails to pass through the chakra and reach the top of the body. If an aura is diminished along a meridian, a dip will be noticed.

Aura reading is a useful tool when considered with other diagnostic techniques but should not be an acceptable form of diagnosis on its own.

Learning to read the aura

The first step is to be able to visualize it. Take a cardboard box and line it with a black material. Place the box on a table with a candle behind it and close the room off from external light as much as possible. Training should start at night.

Place your hand in the box and your hand should appear to have a small fuzz around it. This may only be one to two centimetres in width and may in fact blend in between the digits. If nothing can be seen, light another candle and continue to brighten the room from behind the box until this fuzz is noticed. Try to focus on the energy layer and appreciate the amount of defocusing that is necessary. When you feel confident, start examining other parts of the body using the same principle of keeping the candle light shielded from the area examined.

Next, ask a friend or relative if you can examine their hand and after a short while you will be able to focus the eyes immediately on an aura by meeting somebody in a darkened room. Eventually, with practice, auras can be seen in any light, although in a darkened room will always be easier.

You may see or sense a colour in an aura and this colour will generally reflect the individual's health. If they are well then this is probably the colour of their aura. If they are not then the colour may change as they improve (or get worse). There is no colour that is healthier or unhealthier but as a general rule brightness reflects well-being. There is some correlation with the colours green and yellow producing a soothing effect on the brain (as established through electrical brain tests), but whether this means that a yellow/green aura is a healthy one I cannot comment.

To use this technique in a diagnostic manner requires an individual practitioner to correlate the aura with energy meridians or channels and also to have a sound anatomical knowledge.

The eyes

The colour of the sclera (the whites of the eyes) and the general sparkle can give both orthodox and instinctive clues. Do not be put off or embarrassed by a practitioner who seems to be staring intently at your eyes. *See* **Iridology** for a discussion of the iris.

Medical practitioners will examine the back of the eye, known as the fundus, with an ophthalmoscope. Blood vessels are clearly visible at the back of the eye and give the observer information on the patency (openness) of vessels in general. High blood pressure causes the arterial wall to thicken and this shows up under an ophthalmoscope as a 'railway track' appearance.

The tongue

'Show me your tongue' is a popular phrase amongst TV doctors and is occasionally muttered by the orthodox practitioners. Its colour, moisture and the amount of fur may convey a little knowledge to a Western-trained physician, who will simply use this to confirm a previously considered diagnosis.

Ayurvedic, Chinese and Tibetan practitioners will all pay marked attention to the tongue and the table (p 597) gives some examples of the use of tongue observation for many different conditions. In Ayurveda the main organs of the body are actually mapped out on the tongue and patches may represent an energy lack or excess within an organ or system.

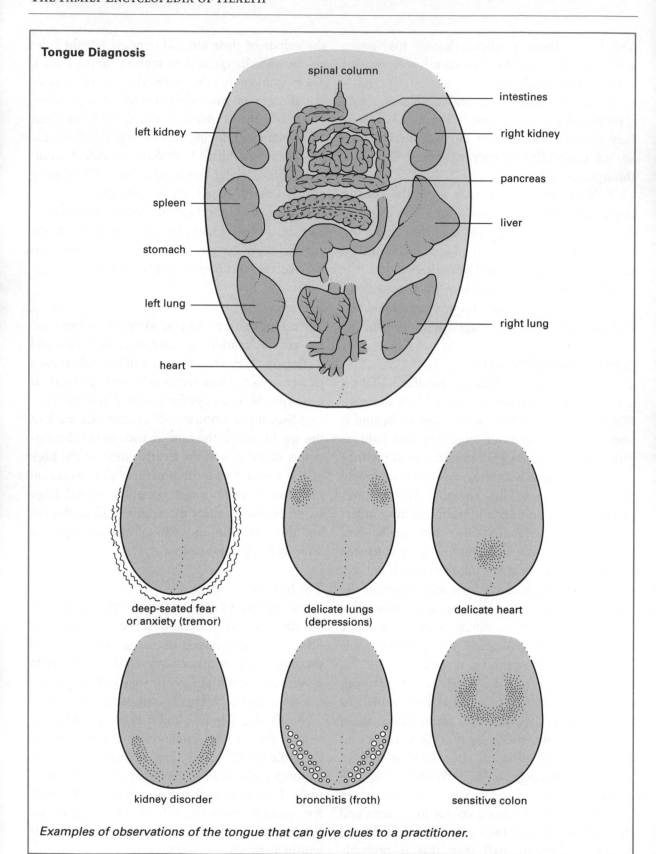

Tongue Diagnosis

spinal column

intestines

left kidney

right kidney

pancreas

spleen

liver

stomach

left lung

right lung

heart

deep-seated fear
or anxiety (tremor)

delicate lungs
(depressions)

delicate heart

kidney disorder

bronchitis (froth)

sensitive colon

Examples of observations of the tongue that can give clues to a practitioner.

Clinical Examination of the Tongue

Colour

Very red	Imminent or present fever
Red and dry	Inflammation of the brain and/or of its membranes, inflammation of stomach, intestines or organs within the chest
Red, glossy	Excess heat
Pale	General exhaustion and anaemia (loss of vital fluids)
Bluish	Poor circulation, anaemia, scurvy, heavy metal poisoning (especially mercury)
Yellow	Gallbladder and liver afflictions
Dark Brown	Oral bleeding
Black	Liver/spleen weakness, dysentery and serious viral infections, abscesses

Humidity

Moist or excessively damp	Exhaustion
Dry	Excessive heat and psychological disturbances, especially anxiety, but also depression

Temperature

Hot	Excess heat
Cold	Lacking heat, cancer
Cold + fever	Impending death

Coating

Often normal	After sleep, tobacco and tea/coffee
On the tip	Phthisis
One-sided	Unilateral disease, liver, spleen
Patchy or map	Stomach affliction
Thick, white	Upper respiratory tract, stomach
Leathery	Enteritis, hepatitis, tonsillitis

Form and size

Small	Cachectic diseases
Sudden shrinkage	Inflammatory disease of lungs or liver, formation of abscesses, general exhaustion
Gradual diminution	Obstinate disease, cranial problems
Broad	Calcium/vitamin D deficiency, lymphatic or abdominal afflictions
Narrow, pointed	Internal inflammations
Thick, swollen	Calcium/vitamin D deficiency, lung complaints, gastritis, catarrhal problems, mercury poisoning

Consistency

Hard	Congestion, inflammation in upper torso
Soft	Catarrhal or chronic mucus afflictions, gastric problems, mercury poisoning

Cracks and fissures

(Usually normal but may indicate swelling)

Dry and bleeding	Severe illness
Down the middle	Back or spinal problems

Movement

Lack of, or trembling	Central nervous system problem, high fever, septicaemia, Motor Neurone Disease (MND)
Uncontrolled	Normal
On extension	Points to side of central nervous system lesions

Other areas of examination

The Eastern philosophies will pay attention to most parts of the body in their observation of a patient. Ayurvedic and Tibetan physicians can glean a lot of information from the face. Examples are: dark circles under the eyes – deficient kidney Qi; puffiness – kidney/spleen; uneven features – long-term Yin/Yang imbalance.

The hands tell many stories. The colour of the nail beds, ridging or discolouration of the nails themselves, the dryness or moisture and the muscularity of the hands give many clues. The feet are equally informative.

The structure of the back, the balance of the shoulders and the pelvis are all important clues to the possible underlying cause of disease.

RECOMMENDATIONS

General Advice

- *When visiting a practitioner, avoid wearing make-up or nail varnish and select clothes that you would normally wear. Do not try to appear to be what you think a physician would expect, but when you enter the consulting room be your normal self.*

- *Whilst basic cleanliness and hygiene must not be shirked, do not apply deodorants or strong-smelling cologne or aftershave. The smell of an individual can be demonstrative of any underlying illness and part of observation is body odour.*

LISTENING

Orthodox doctors are taught that 90 per cent of diagnoses are concluded from the history of the condition and the story the patient tells. Eastern philosophies, as I mentioned with regard to experienced Chinese physicians who only take the pulses, often pay little heed to the patient's complaint and concentrate on the signs and diagnostic techniques through observation and palpation (touching).

It will come as no surprise to find that I think a mix and balance of the two is the answer. There is no doubt that listening to a story will lead to an understanding of the condition, especially of its origins, provided that the right questions are asked. It is important not to assume that an illness originated from when the patient first started to feel symptoms. The onset of a headache may be because of drinking the night before. The symptoms of cancer or diabetes may only become apparent at the last stage of the disease.

I feel that it is also important for a patient to express his/her concerns and the way that this is expressed should give the practitioner clues as to how to respond and answer a patient's concerns. A tearful report should not be answered by a brusque response. A patient who is clearly a matter-of-fact type who gives clear and concise symptoms probably does not want to hear about the ethereal imbalances within his/her Qi. A symptom report is not just about the symptoms but also about assessing the needs of the individual.

From the patient's point of view, therefore, it is important to present the problem in his/her own way and not as the patient would expect the practitioner to want it. Try not to be a 'Oh and another thing . . .' patient. A holistic physician is interested in the 'whole' and it is important for all the symptoms to be made available, however irrelevant they may seem to the individual. A good practitioner should elicit all the information needed but sometimes serious symptoms are not owned up to by the patient and may be so removed from the reason for the consultation that a practitioner may not ask. An example is a patient of mine who sat with me for 40 minutes whilst we discussed all the possible underlying causes for her insomnia. As we were parting company I heard the physician's dreaded comment 'Oh, another thing doctor, I have been passing blood whenever I have gone to the toilet for the last three weeks'. Needless to say, I worked late that day.

Use of instruments

The stethoscope is a prerequisite for the archetypal physician to wear around the shoulders. In fact most doctors will tell you that the stethoscope is of limited use in diagnosis except for a cardiologist. Very few treatment protocols change because of the findings from a stethoscope examination. A physician can tell whether a lung is well-congested or a bowel is blocked by listening directly with the ear. The stethoscope makes things easier or confirms diagnosis. Modern machines can allow us to hear and monitor heart beats within a foetus and can certainly be beneficial in obstetrics.

RECOMMENDATIONS

General Advice

- *If you do not think that your practitioner is listening to or hearing your complaints or symptoms, then make mention of this and be satisfied with the explanation or change your practitioner.*
- *Make a list of complaints because even the smallest factor may make an enormous difference in the ability to diagnose or prescribe. This is particularly the case in homeopathy.*
- *A copy of your list handed to the practitioner on entering the consulting room may make things easier for you both.*

TOUCHING

A lot can be gleaned from physical examination. The orthodox world uses the term 'palpation' for the pushing and poking that goes on over the abdomen and a doctor will tap around the chest and abdomen to test for the amount of air contained. This is called percussion. Congestion in the lungs will sound like a dull thud, whereas excess air in the bowel will sound much like a drum. Stretching joints and pushing on painful areas in the musculature and skeleton of the body will tell a physician a lot about injury and inflammation. All this is a necessity and, whilst mildly invasive, should be allowed regardless of how remote the examination may be from the area of

discomfort. Examination of the lower back and upper thigh is essential for a pain in the foot, for example, and is very important in making a firm diagnosis. The neck may be the reason for cramping in the calves. This is known as referred pain.

Eastern-trained physicians will utilize all these Western approaches but then have a few tricks of their own. Observation by physicians over thousands of years has suggested that different parts of the body reflect energy flow through the system as a whole. Acupuncturists plant their needles in the points through these meridians or energy channels and Shiatsu practitioners and reflexologists apply pressure to alter the flow of energy. Shiatsu practitioners study the hara, reflexologists study the reflex points in the feet and hands, and applied kinesiologists will test muscle groups to monitor their strength or weakness, which varies depending on the compound that the body is in contact with.

Hara diagnosis

The Japanese have developed their art of healing from a clear and distinct belief in energy flow through the system. Their practitioners have noted and taught for thousands of years the ability to diagnose by the excess (Jitsu) or deficiency (Kyo) of various systems or organs in the body. Each organ or system is represented by a position on the abdomen or back and is described in the diagrams on page 600. Gentle application of pressure will either be resisted (Jitsu) or allow the practitioner to push in with very little resistance (Kyo) and this represents the energy within the organ. Specific abdominal pains may or may not be related to the energy area, and muscles on the back that are pulled may have nothing to do with the system or organ either. A practitioner who uses this together with pulse technique, tongue diagnosis and such like can pick up the subtle differences that will tell whether the deficiency has been long-standing or is acute. As a general rule the pulses may change rapidly but Hara changes are slower. This may account for why a Shiatsu

Hara diagnosis

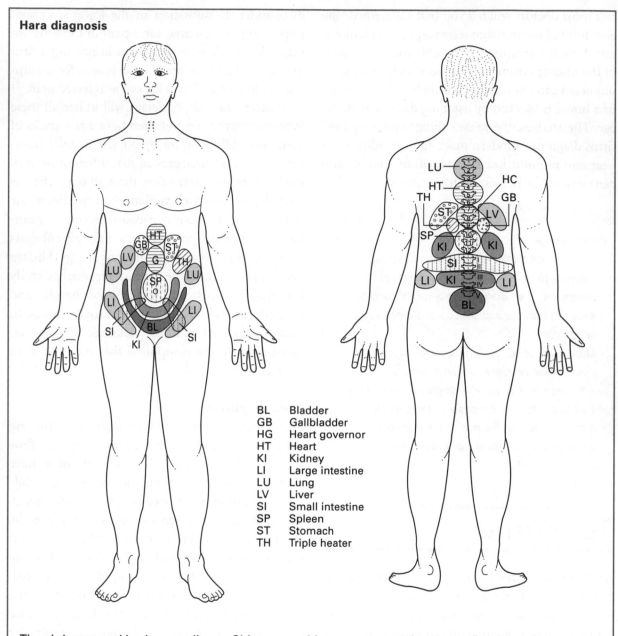

BL	Bladder
GB	Gallbladder
HG	Heart governor
HT	Heart
KI	Kidney
LI	Large intestine
LU	Lung
LV	Liver
SI	Small intestine
SP	Spleen
ST	Stomach
TH	Triple heater

The abdomen and back, according to Shiatsu practitioners, map out the energy flow to various organs.

practitioner may pick up one set of strengths or weaknesses, whereas a pulse-taker will pick up another within an hour or so of examination or even at the same time.

It is also relevant to note that pressure on a Shiatsu point or on a weakened or excessive pulse point may actually be a treatment or therapy and therefore alters the energy flow quite markedly.

Pulse taking

The orthodox world considers the pulse in the wrist an accessible point to test for a variety of cardiac functions. We are able to tell the rate of the heart, the rhythm and, with experience, glean some idea of the arterial pressure. The feel of the artery may give clues as to the development of arteriosclerosis but beyond this the orthodox world goes no further.

Ayurvedic, Tibetan and Chinese philosophy believes that different systems and organs reflect their intrinsic vital force in different parts of the body. The wrist is an extremely accessible pulse point and is the most documented of areas for practitioners to learn how to measure the energy in the system. In principle, all these disciplines share the same fundamental beliefs but have different names and ways of describing the energies.

The Eastern philosophies believe that the body is made up of humours, organs, systems and elements. The practitioner will be checking for pulse rate, missed beats and 'quality'. An orthodox training will teach about a 'full' pulse or a pulse with a double beat, for example, and correlate this with the function or structure of the heart. An Eastern-trained practitioner might describe the pulse as full or empty, having excess fire or damp, or as being thready.

The practitioner, using whichever technique he or she has been taught and possibly by correlating different philosophies in one pulse-taking technique, can perform the examination with the patient sitting or lying. It is important that no part of the body is crossed (legs or ankles) and that nothing that affects the pulse rate has been ingested. This includes caffeine, alcohol and refined sugars in particular, but also excessively spicy foods or those that may cool the body, such as an iced drink or ice-cream.

Whilst the orthodox pulse-taker is interested only in the function of the heart or the influence of chemicals on the heart rate, the Eastern practitioner will take this into account but also consider the effects on a much broader diagnostic scale.

The Chinese philosophies believe that the pulses not only reflect the physical but also the emotional and psychological states. You may hear a practitioner describing a weak spleen or a full liver, which will not necessarily correspond to the normal orthodox function of that organ.

Another Eastern philosophy suggests the following psychological and spiritual correlations with the organ pulses.

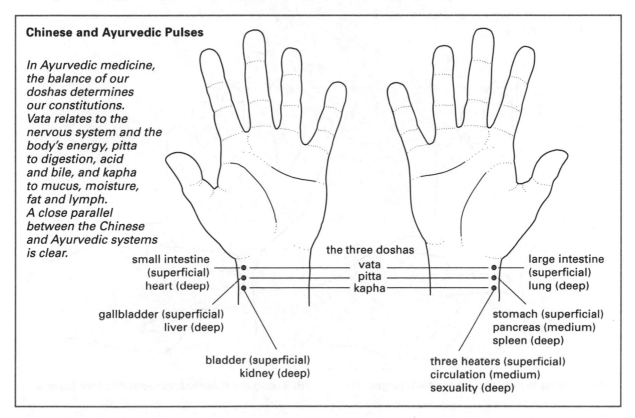

Chinese and Ayurvedic Pulses

In Ayurvedic medicine, the balance of our doshas determines our constitutions. Vata relates to the nervous system and the body's energy, pitta to digestion, acid and bile, and kapha to mucus, moisture, fat and lymph.
A close parallel between the Chinese and Ayurvedic systems is clear.

small intestine (superficial)
heart (deep)

gallbladder (superficial)
liver (deep)

bladder (superficial)
kidney (deep)

the three doshas
vata
pitta
kapha

large intestine (superficial)
lung (deep)

stomach (superficial)
pancreas (medium)
spleen (deep)

three heaters (superficial)
circulation (medium)
sexuality (deep)

ORGAN PULSES	POSITIVE ATTITUDE	NEGATIVE ATTITUDE
Lung	tolerance	disdain, prejudice, contempt
Heart	happiness, joy	unhappiness, sorrow, sadness
Gallbladder	love	rage, fury
Spleen	faith in future	anxiety about the future
Kidney	sexual security	promiscuity
Large intestine	self worth	guilt
Circulation/Sexual function/ Heart protector	renunciation of past, generosity, relaxation	jealousy, regret
Liver	love, forgiveness	anger
Stomach	contentment	disappointment
Triple heater	happy	depressed, lonely, grieving
Bladder	peace, harmony	restlessness, impatience

Taking your own pulse

In each wrist there is a bony prominence about two finger widths up from the wrist crease on the side of the thumb (*see* diagram below). (A) Place the third finger of the opposite hand on this lump and move inwards slightly. A pulse should be felt.

(B) Place the second and fourth fingers either side and press as lightly as is necessary to establish a pulse in all fingers. Push down deeply with each finger in turn and then altogether and you will be feeling the superficial and deep pulses characteristic of Chinese pulse-taking.

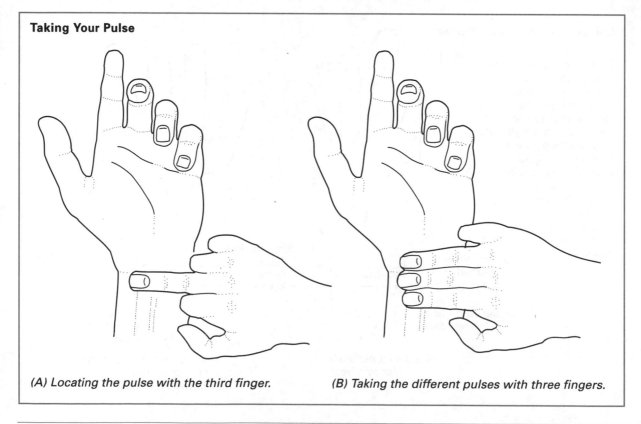

Taking Your Pulse

(A) Locating the pulse with the third finger.

(B) Taking the different pulses with three fingers.

Ayurvedic physicians state that the right-hand side of the body is the masculine side and gives out energy and the left-hand side of the body is feminine and receives energy. Imbalances in specific organs or humours can be detected by comparing each point with all of the others and a generalized weakness in one set of pulses as opposed to those of the other wrist may represent a general lack or excess of masculine or feminine energy. Masculine energy represents aggression, achievement, drive and ambition, whereas feminine energy represents nurturing, love, homemaking, tolerance and acceptance. All of us have a balance and we should all strive for an equality of energy. Pulses change through the day, depending upon the amount of energy that is used. Kidney energy is said to be an energy store and should be diminished towards the end of the day. Each point represents a spiritual, psychological and physical aspect and therefore when you hear a practitioner talking about kidney energy he does not necessarily mean the possibility of kidney problems. Lung energy may represent sadness and grief, stomach energy the ability to absorb a concept, and gallbladder energy about digesting facts.

The subject is both fascinating and immense and can take a lifetime to even attempt to understand and practise accurately.

Reflexology – The Foot

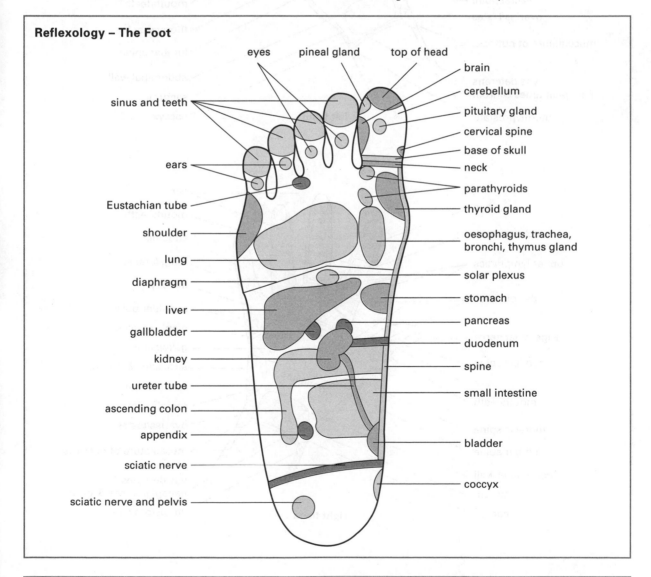

Reflexology – The Hands

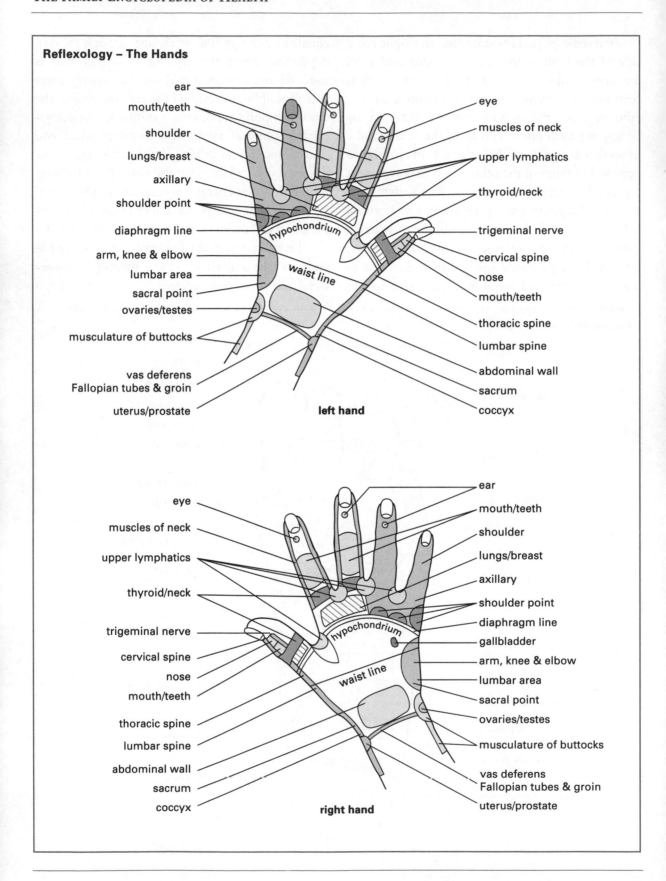

ear
mouth/teeth
shoulder
lungs/breast
axillary
shoulder point
diaphragm line
arm, knee & elbow
lumbar area
sacral point
ovaries/testes
musculature of buttocks
vas deferens
Fallopian tubes & groin
uterus/prostate

eye
muscles of neck
upper lymphatics
thyroid/neck
trigeminal nerve
cervical spine
nose
mouth/teeth
thoracic spine
lumbar spine
abdominal wall
sacrum
coccyx

hypochondrium
waist line
left hand

eye
muscles of neck
upper lymphatics
thyroid/neck
trigeminal nerve
cervical spine
nose
mouth/teeth
thoracic spine
lumbar spine
abdominal wall
sacrum
coccyx

ear
mouth/teeth
shoulder
lungs/breast
axillary
shoulder point
diaphragm line
gallbladder
arm, knee & elbow
lumbar area
sacral point
ovaries/testes
musculature of buttocks
vas deferens
Fallopian tubes & groin
uterus/prostate

hypochondrium
waist line
right hand

Reflexology

Gentle pressure applied to the feet and hands may give vital information about the underlying areas of weakness from an energetic point of view. Training is academically quite simple but experience is what counts. There may be very subtle differences in the texture of the tissue where the energy point lies and a lump or pain is not necessarily reflective of weakness in the system or organ. The diagrams on pages 603 and 604 gives a basic representation and gentle self-manipulation may be useful in self-treating.

RECOMMENDATIONS

General Advice

- *Overcome any concept of shyness before you enter a complementary medical practitioner's rooms. Physical examination will include pulse-taking and pushing on acupuncture points throughout the body.*
- *A complementary medical examination, whilst it may be informal, should never be invasive. Any internal examination or examination of the breasts, anus or genitals should only be performed with a member of the same sex chaperoning the practitioner and present throughout the entire examination.*
- *If a practitioner uses the pulse technique ask for their findings and discuss them on the basis of their spiritual, psychological and physical meaning.*

INVESTIGATING

What does that young doctor mean on the TV series *ER* when he blurts out 'We need a CBC, Chem 7 and lytes, LFT, drug screen, AP and Lat, swab and call the OR tell'em we'll need a room STAT'? Answer: He is asking for blood and urine samples to be taken and sent to the laboratory for testing, ordering various X-rays, asking for an operating room to be prepared and raising next year's health insurance premiums by 15 per cent.

He is, however, also gleaning the information that he will potentially need to save a life.

Most investigations are warranted and are, without argument, modern medicine's gift to health. Understanding the balance of certain minerals in the bloodstream tells us the state of the kidneys and liver, sugar levels tell us the state of the pancreas, the level of white blood cells tell us how the immune system is functioning – the list goes on. There are many sophisticated tests that an individual may only come across should they become unwell but a certain array of investigations may be used as a screening process and might even be encouraged to enable a healthcare practitioner to monitor the well-being of the patient. I list below some of the basic tests that may be of benefit or be mentioned to give the lay-person a guideline to what information is being sought. The main problem with investigations is the concept of a 'normal' range of results. Normality is measured by testing a large number of people and drawing up a standard deviation curve.

What this means is that the top or bottom three per cent of any group are automatically considered too high or too low. This may not be the

Standard Deviation Curve

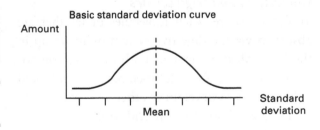

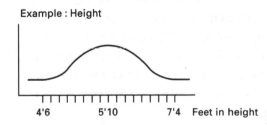

While 'normality' might be a reasonable reflection of a population as a whole, it can be very misleading when applied to an individual.

case and a result that suggests an abnormality may in fact be perfectly normal for the individual. Also, someone with a result within the 'normal' range may in fact be quite abnormal. For example, if a haemoglobin level of 11.5 is found, the orthodox world would say 'normal'. But if that person *should* have a level of 15, then it is considerably lower than it should be and yet may not be treated.

There is no black or white in health. The orthodox medical world tends to lose sight of that grey area and may rely too heavily on results. Investigations should be integrated into a full clinical setting, story-taking and examination and not viewed on their own merits.

Blood tests

Medics have been studying blood since the advent of the microscope and possibly before. High-power magnification and computers have now made the observing and measuring of the components of the bloodstream extremely easy and swift. Almost anything can be measured, ranging from the number and type of red blood cells to the presence of pesticides or other toxins. The following gives an insight into some of the more common tests.

Cholesterol and triglycerides

Triglycerides are small molecules of fat that are absorbed via the digestive system or made up in the liver. Measurement of both of these components can tell us about fat metabolism, intake and risks such as of developing atheroma, which may lead to high blood pressure and strokes.

Cholesterol is subdivided into several groups – high-density lipoproteins (HDL), low-density lipoproteins (LDL), and very-low-density lipoproteins (VLDL) are the most common. All forms are needed for survival but as a general rule too much LDL is dangerous (*see* **Cholesterol**).

Electrolytes (also known as urea and electrolytes or Us and Es)

Atoms with positive or negative charges are known as electrolytes. These include sodium, potassium and calcium, which are positive, and chloride and bicarbonate ions that are negatively charged. The balance of these electrolytes controls the amount of fluid in our system and the levels are maintained by the functioning of the kidneys and the amount of water and nutrients that we take in. Measurement of these electrolytes, which should be within narrow bands, enables a practitioner to assess water balance and kidney function.

Urea is the byproduct of protein metabolism and is a compound that gives the name to urine. Measurement of urea enables a practitioner to assess kidney function and is usually assessed with a specific protein known as creatinine, which is maintained as a normal level only if the kidney is functioning properly.

The ESR

The erythrocyte sedimentation rate (ESR) is a non-specific test for a variety of conditions. The investigation is performed by placing a blood sample in a tube and measuring the speed with which the red blood cells settle. This sedimentation should run at a rate of about 1cm/hour but alters under various conditions. Pregnancy may cause the ESR to 'rise' (the speed may rise from 10mm to anywhere up to 20 or 25mm). Destructive conditions such as arthritis or cancer may cause the ESR to rise higher and certain inflammatory conditions may actually cause the ESR to reach over the 100 mark. An ESR rises due to a decrease in the viscosity of the serum in which the blood cells survive. A healthy bloodstream reacts similarly to placing a coin on the top of a pot of honey, as opposed to on a glass of water.

Full or complete blood count (FBC, CBC)

This test measures red and white cell numbers and also microscopy is used to examine the shape, size and colour of the cells. This can give information about the presence of anaemia, how the red blood cells are taking up iron, B_{12} or folic acid, the number and type of white blood cells (the body's

BLOOD VALUES REPORT

Haematology	Sample Values			Male Range
Haemoglobin	14.9		g/dL	13.0 – 17.5
HCT	44.3			38 – 52
Red Cell Count	5.14		$\times 10^{12}/l$	4.5 – 6.3
MCV	86.3		fL	76 – 97
MCH	29.0		pg	27 – 33
MCHC	33.6		g/dL	32 – 36
RDW	15.3			11.0 – 17.5
Platelet Count	194		$\times 10^{9}/l$	140 – 440
White Cell Count	6.0		$\times 10^{9}/l$	3.6 – 11.5
Neutrophils	52%	3.12	$\times 10^{9}/l$	2.0 – 7.5
Lymphocytes	36%	2.16	$\times 10^{9}/l$	1.0 – 4.0
Monocytes	8%	0.48	$\times 10^{9}/l$	0.0 – 1.5
Eosinophils	3%	0.18	$\times 10^{9}/l$	0.0 – 0.4
Basophils	1%	0.06	$\times 10^{9}/l$	0.0 – 0.2
(Comment: *All cell populations appear normal.*)				
ESR	2		mm/hr	0 – 11

Biochemistry

Sodium	138	mmol/l	135 – 145
Potassium	4.0	mmol/l	3.6 – 5.0
Chloride	109	mmol/l	98 – 111
Bicarbonate	25	mmol/l	18 – 31
Urea	4.6	mmol/l	2.9 – 7.0
Creatinine	78	umol/l	60 – 125
Bilirubin	8	umol/l	2 – 22
Alkaline Phosphatase	43	iu/l	30 – 95
Aspartate Transferase	17	iu/l	10 – 35
Alanine Transferase	26	iu/l	8 – 45
HBD	88	iu/l	70 – 135
CK	73	iu/l	33 – 186
Gamma GT	23	iu/l	5 – 50
Total Protein	66	g/l	60 – 80
Albumin	38	g/l	32 – 50
Globulin	28	g/l	23 – 39
Calcium	2.25	mmol/l	2.20 – 2.60
Phosphate	1.12	mmol/l	0.65 – 1.55
Uric Acid	327	umol/l	159 – 475
Random Blood Glucose	6.1	mmol/l	3.5 – 7.9
Triglycerides	1.68	mmol/l	0.50 – 2.10
Cholesterol	4.42	mmol/l	Optimum<5.20
HDL Cholesterol	1.14	mmol/l	0.8 – 1.9
HDL % of total	26	%	20 and over
LDL Cholesterol	2.52	mmol/l	Up to 4.0
Iron	22	umol/l	11.0 – 32.0

Endocrinology

Total Thyroxine (T4)	83	nmol/l	58 – 154
Thyroid Stimulating Hormone (TSH)	1.32	miu/l	0.35 – 5.00

bloodborne immune system). A differential count refers to the types of white blood cells and can tell a practitioner whether an infection is bacterial, viral, fungal or absent. Excessive white blood cells are usually present in infection or more serious conditions such as leukaemia. In the latter case the cells look different as well as being in abundance.

Liver function tests (LFT)

If liver cells are damaged their contents spill into the bloodstream and can be measured. The liver also produces proteins known as albumins which indicate the state of function rather than level of damage. Tests for these albumins are all grouped together and known as LFTs. Conditions such as hepatitis, alcoholism and cancer affecting the liver will all alter the LFTs by damaging the cells. Different intracellular chemicals come from different parts of the cell and the extent of the damage can be measured by defining which liver enzymes are actually present in the bloodstream. Some chemicals exist in the substance of the cell, whereas others live within the nucleus or brain of the cell. These latter chemicals are not released unless severe cell damage has taken place, so measuring the amounts in the bloodstream is as important as measuring their presence.

Thyroid function tests (TFT)

Thyroid function tests measure thyroxine, which is the main hormone produced in the thyroid gland, and another form of thyroxine called triiodothyromine (TH3). TH3 is produced in smaller amounts but is far more important in its effect. The levels of these two hormones indicate the function of the thyroid gland.

Also measured is the controlling hormone, known as thyroid-stimulating hormone (TSH), which comes from the pituitary gland (*see* **Thyroid**).

Toxicity tests

A few laboratories are sophisticated and forward-thinking enough to be checking blood samples for toxins. Most chemicals can be detected but may require special requests. These few laboratories actually have panels to test for heavy metals, pesticides, insecticides and other environmental toxins. Any neurological condition or chronic problem, such as postviral fatigue syndrome or even cancer, needs to be assessed from the toxicity point of view.

Other tests

Most known compounds can now be assayed (assessed) through blood testing. Levels of glucose, iron, toxins and prescribed drugs and special chemicals produced by particular inflamed tissues can all be isolated and used in the process of assessing organ function and body deficiencies and toxicity.

SPECIMENS AND SAMPLES
Urine samples

Urine is the filtration product of the blood, which, in turn, picks up toxins from around the system. Measurement of the toxicity and contents of urine gives a clear indication of the state of the body. In days gone by, simple examination by visual assessment, microscopy, measurement of density and even taste were of great advantage to the physician. Nowadays, computers have given practitioners insights into the very functioning of the body's cells.

A basic urine analysis measures the acidity, water level, the presence of sugar or glucose and certain biochemical products manufactured by the liver. Measurement of these latter compounds – bilinogen and urobilinogen – is a simple non-invasive method of assessing the health of the liver. Basic analysis also includes checking for red and white blood cells and protein, none of which should be found in the urine because it is indicative of ill-health.

Ketones are breakdown products of fat metabolism. They show up in the urine if there is any suggestion of starvation or poor fat/sugar metabolism control.

URINALYSIS

Urine Chemistry

pH	7.0
Protein	+ (0.30g/l)
Glucose	Negative
Ketone	Negative
Blood	+

Microscopy

WBCs	>100/hpf
RBCs	Not seen
Casts	Not seen
Epithelial cells	+
Crystals	Not seen
Organisms	++
Culture	No bacterial growth

First morning urine samples are generally preferred for assessment of the body's metabolism but for any suggestion of infection a mid-stream urine (MSU) is preferred. This reduces the chances of contamination of a sample by bacteria that may have bred at the opening of the urethra and, in the male, elements of seminal fluid that may pass into a sample with the final contractions of the urethra. Such samples undergo what is known as culture, microscopy and sensitivity (CMS). The sample is looked at under a microscope and then a portion is placed in a laboratory dish containing a special medium that allows bacteria to grow. If any bacterial growth occurs it is known as a culture, and then different antibiotics are placed on the dish to see which ones kill the bugs. This technique allows physicians to assess which antibiotics a particular breed or strain of bacteria are resistant to and select out those that are effective in killing the bugs. A bacterium is said to be 'sensitive' to these agents.

Other samples

A sample of any excretion or discharge may be collected either directly into a sample pot or using a swab. These are then provided to a laboratory or technician who will prepare them (known as 'fixing'). Certain stains may be applied to colour particular bacterial agents or the presence of other compounds and a variety of technical assessments may be used.

Anything that is coughed up or spat out is collectively known as a sputum sample and certain skin samples may be taken by gently scraping the skin – known as skin scrapings. Other areas may be swabbed by a medical 'ear bud' and, as one bible for the junior doctor describes, 'there is no body cavity that a sample cannot be taken from by using a long needle and a brave attitude'.

Biopsy

Biopsy is the sampling of a tissue for examination under a microscope or for some other test. Theoretically any part of the body can be biopsied, but the risk/benefit ratio has to be examined. Tissue biopsy from the skin, or needle-aspiration from a cyst can be done in the doctor's surgery but other tissues need to be biopsied under anaesthetic. Local anaesthetic is used for muscle biopsy of organs that are more easily accessible with a long biopsy needle and an acceptable level of experience. General anaesthetic is required if brain tissue samples are required or if a suspicion of cancer is high, in which case a further procedure may be required wherein the tissue sample is sent to the pathologist immediately and a report produced swiftly to enable the surgeon to proceed with the operation if necessary. This is common in suspicious breast lumps during lumpectomy.

Biopsies are generally to be considered necessary because they can create a firm diagnosis and allow a treatment protocol to be accurately prescribed.

ORTHODOX MEDICAL TECHNOLOGY
Blood pressure measurement

Blood pressure is measured using a sphygmomanometer. An inflatable 'cuff' is placed around the upper arm and air pumped into it until a level of 250mm/Hg is reached, as seen on the dial. This pressure occludes the underlying arteries. The practitioner places the end of the stethoscope over the front of the elbow and listens. Nothing should be heard.

The air is slowly released from the cuff and as the pressure drops there comes a point when the strength of the heartbeat overrides the pressure in the cuff and blood is squirted down the arteries.

This blood hits the wall of the artery with a thump, which can be heard through the stethoscope. As the cuff pressure continues to drop and less impedance ensues, the blood flow becomes smooth and the thumping stops. Cardiologists

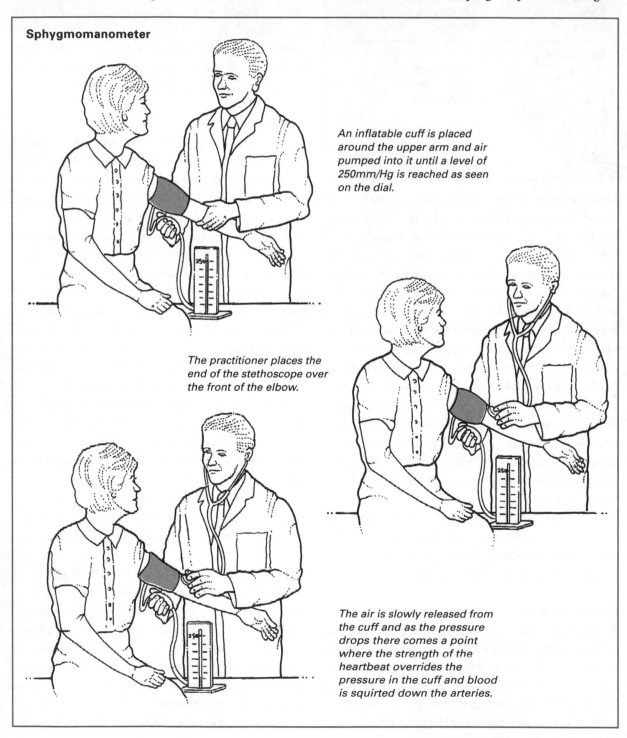

Sphygmomanometer

An inflatable cuff is placed around the upper arm and air pumped into it until a level of 250mm/Hg is reached as seen on the dial.

The practitioner places the end of the stethoscope over the front of the elbow.

The air is slowly released from the cuff and as the pressure drops there comes a point where the strength of the heartbeat overrides the pressure in the cuff and blood is squirted down the arteries.

teach us that there are five sound stages, ranging from stage I – the initial thump – to stage V – a return to silence.

Simple and 24-hour blood pressure machines

Sensitive computers are now being used to take blood pressure and can be bought at any medical outlet. These generally comprise a finger-sized cuff that slips over a digit and measures the underlying pressure in the arteries. These are fairly accurate and can be used to check an individual's blood pressure at different times throughout the day.

Twenty-four-hour blood pressure measurements are of benefit in diagnosis if sporadic symptoms such as dizziness or blackouts are associated with blood pressure. A small computer is carried for 24 hours with leads attached to the body to measure blood pressure. A patient records the time of any symptoms and this is compared, by computer, with the blood pressure measurements. It is worth noting that many individuals who may have high blood pressure when visiting the doctor's surgery (white-coat hypertension) or at times of stress may spend much of their time with normal blood pressure and incorrectly be prescribed treatment. Many hypertensives have normal blood pressure during the night, which suggests to a holistic physician that the stress of consciousness is the underlying cause and that a relaxation or meditation programme may be of benefit rather than drugs.

Doppler test

C J Doppler was an Austrian physicist who noticed that sound waves (and light waves) change if bounced off something that is moving. This is a very simplified description of what is known as the Doppler principle. A Doppler machine passes out a sound wave that bounces off moving blood within a vessel and can show the speed of flow. As this is very dependent upon the patency of the vessel, this technique can be used as a non-invasive investigation to check for arteriosclerosis or occlusion within arteries.

Electrocardiogram (ECG, EKG)

An ECG is the measurement of electrical conductivity in the heart muscle. For an explanation of the origin, initiation and travel of these electric impulses, *see* **Heart, irregular beats.**

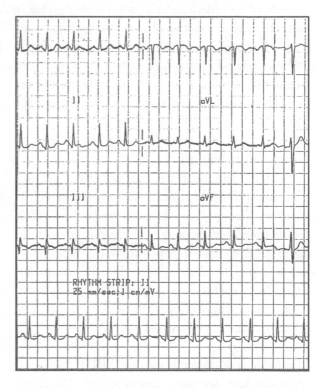

An ECG is a non-invasive technique that can be of great benefit in diagnosing heart diseases. There is no reason to avoid such an examination although results need to be correlated with symptoms, as with all investigations.

An ECG produced while somebody is on a treadmill is known as a stress ECG and shows the electrical conductivity when the heart has an increased need for oxygen. This test can be very useful in demonstrating cardiac muscle disease because any injury from, say, a heart attack will damage some of the heart muscle and prevent conduction through that part.

Electrodes are placed around the heart and on both wrists and ankles because the electrical impulse will be picked up even at distances. The computer within an ECG will correlate all the information from all the leads and print out a pattern that requires a certain amount of expertise to interpret.

Holter monitor

The Holter monitor is a small box that attaches to the side of an individual and is connected to leads that are placed on the chest. The monitor will record the heart rate and electrical pattern over a 24-hour period. The individual notes down any periods of cardiac symptoms, such as chest pain or tachycardia, and any associated heart irregularity can be ascertained.

Electroencephalogram (EEG)

The brain conducts its function through the transmission of chemicals from one nerve to another. This process releases electricity, which can be measured by placing electrodes around the scalp. An EEG can demonstrate not only function but also structural changes or damage within the brain. Very useful in conditions such as epilepsy or in diagnosing tumours, the EEG is a safe and effective method of diagnosis.

Magnetic resonance imaging (MRI)

Over the last decade a technique of visualizing internal organs and structures has been developed using magnets rather than sound or X-ray. The technique is complex, and computer imaging from the information sent by powerful magnets, which surround the body part to be investigated, is required.

The MRI has its critics, suggesting that the imaging is not all that accurate in certain areas of the body (the prostate or the coronary arteries) and it is often necessary to use 'dyes' which are magnetic substances that may cause problems that we have yet to understand. These dyes are, however, far safer than the known damage created by the CT scan dyes containing iodine (*see* **Radiography**).

Magnetic resonance imaging usually involves the patient being passed into a body-sized tube and being asked to keep absolutely still. Whilst

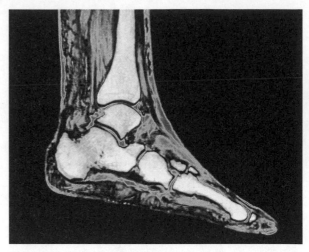

MRI scan of a woman's ankle (age 58).

claustrophobic, the technique is not in any way invasive or painful but may take up to an hour to complete a full body scan. These MRI scans are extremely sensitive and can be used in place of CT scans (*see* **Radiography**) in many if not most investigations.

Magnetic resonance imaging may impart certain dangers as we now begin to see that magnetic energy may disrupt electromagnetic function in the body but at the moment it is safer than X-rays. If confronted with a need for hi-tech investigation, always ask whether MRI would be available and as accurate.

Radiography (X-rays)

Radiography (colloquially and commonly now known as X-rays) is the most common, and potentially most damaging, of modern medicine's investigations.

X-rays are very high frequency waves that pass through most compounds. A radiogram is basically a photograph created by X-rays hitting a wave-sensitive plate. As X-rays are passed through the body, the denser the tissue the more X-rays are absorbed. The less dense tissue allows more X-rays to pass through, which hit the plate and show up as a white/grey area. Bones, being dense, are seen as white on an X-ray because no X-rays hit the plate, whereas air space in the lungs is seen as black because all the X-rays hit the plate. X-rays are harmful, there is no debate over that whatsoever. The argument concerns whether the amount we receive through an investigation is harmful or not (*see* **Radiation**).

Angiography

Angiography is a frequently used X-ray technique. A radio-opaque dye is injected into the bloodstream and X-rays are taken of the arteries that are suspected of being diseased or narrowed. This technique is popular but has its critics. Some rarely-repeated studies have shown that angiography is open to misinterpretation or actually imparts false information. Unnecessary operations are therefore conducted. This, combined with the potential risk of an X-ray, should make angiography a last-choice investigation rather than a first choice, but overall is likely to be of benefit in the right case.

Myelography

Myelography is an X-ray technique used on the spinal column that also uses radio-opaque dyes. When injected into the spinal column to show disc lesions, a percentage may cause inflammation leading to persistent pain and problems with movement. The dyes themselves may be toxic to the kidneys and may have a direct effect on the nervous system, leading to paralysis. Dyes used for CT scans contain iodine, which is known to be toxic to the thyroid gland if taken in excess. The trouble is, everyone is different and nobody is certain how much is too much for any individual patient. Try other techniques of imaging before allowing dyes to be used.

Densitometry

Bone density scanning (Densitometry) is becoming popular and whilst it carries a low risk of X-ray exposure the scan itself is not a particularly reliable investigation. A variety of studies have suggested that the accuracy is questionable and that bone density can change, depending upon

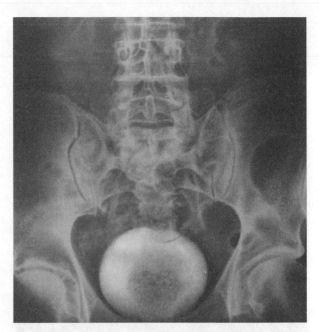

Cystogram – a specialized X-ray to show up bladder deformities.

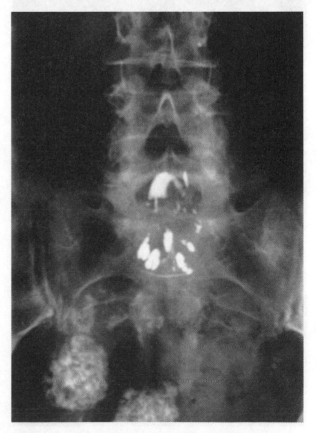

X-ray of the spine two years after undergoing myelography showing oily contrast material (as white patches) still present in the spinal cord.

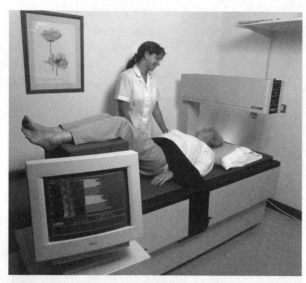

Bone density scanning for osteoporosis.

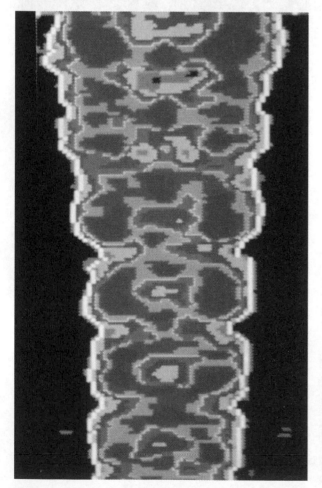

Densitometry scan of the spine, used to measure mineral density of bone in the assessment of osteoporosis.

such factors as movement and recent diet, so that general or yearly screening is not reliable. One study followed up a group of 1,000 women who were considered to be at high risk of osteoporosis via a scan, only to find that they had fewer hip fractures than the control group. Neither group were given any orthodox treatment.

There are other alternatives (*see* **Osteoporosis**) for measuring bone density and, in principle, these other ultrasound techniques can be done with safety.

Computed axial tomography (CAT or CT)

Computed axial tomography (CAT or CT) scans are formed by passing an X-ray image through a computer that is highly sensitive and therefore produces much more detailed pictures. These scans use a three-dimensional picture, thereby giving the physician an idea of the depth and size of a tumour with far more accuracy than a two-dimensional X-ray film.

A CT scan provides an enormous amount of radiation, especially if the procedure is repeated because of movement of the patient, error within the computer system or because the technique is being used to monitor a changing situation.

Whilst extremely accurate, many of the results can be obtained through magnetic resonance imaging but with lower risks. Also, CT scans are

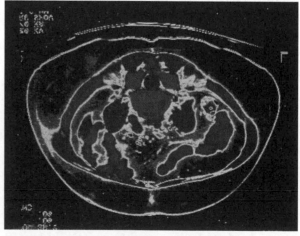

Computed axial tomography (CAT) scan of the spine, kidneys and intestines (female).

often used despite the fact that whatever the results, no change in treatment is likely. It simply gives a prognosis.

Ultrasound

Ultrasound or sonography has been developed over the last 30 years within the medical fraternity. The principle has been around a lot longer and was used by geographers to chart the depth of oceans. The principle is simple. A sound wave is emitted from a transmitter into tissues and rebounds back to a receptor lying next to the transmitter. A less dense tissue will reflect less sound waves, whereas a solid object will bounce back all of the waves. This information is transformed into a visual picture by a computer, much like a radio will pick up inaudible radio waves and transform them into sound through mechanical means.

One trial has shown that using ultrasound eleven times in a pregnancy may produce babies that are small for their age, but otherwise no other detrimental effect has been demonstrated. I suspect that because the foetus is a highly sensitive state of being, the ultrasound is disturbing and creates a stress response rather than having any direct detrimental effect upon tissue growth.

Ultrasound can be used for most diagnoses except for organs such as the brain, which is encased in a solid shell, or organs that are too deep in the body to be imaged without other organs being in the way. Basically, problems may be imaged and a diagnosis made on any part from the neck down with the use of ultrasound. Bone density can be measured without X-rays using this method.

Ultrasound machines vary in size but the actual transmitter/receptor is rarely larger than a mobile telephone and is placed over the area to be investigated. A sound-transmitting gel is applied to allow a freer movement and less interference from the skin surface. Ultra-sound diagnosis rarely takes more than a few minutes in the hands of a skilled technician and reports can be read immediately.

ALTERNATIVE DIAGNOSTIC INVESTIGATIONS

If Madame Curie had listened to the derision piled upon her we would not have X-rays. Her experimentation carried the price of her life because she died from the effects of radiation. She is the most well-known example of scientists who have come up with ideas in medicine that have been doubted, ridiculed and ostracized. However, because of their determination we have an astounding array of investigative procedures.

Today, there are investigations that have been born out of sound scientific and medical hypotheses but are finding it difficult to attract funding *because* the techniques may be very accurate and inexpensive. This would suggest that they would be popular, but indeed the financial state of play in medicine inhibits study and research into new techniques. I list below some of those that I believe have a future. This is partly because the study and research carried out so far is positive or because I have used them in my practice for anywhere up to 12 years. In one or two cases the investigation has been around for many decades but has been either suppressed or vilified to such an extent that it is only recently that they have been able to gain some credibility.

I stress that the techniques below are not well established from a scientific or double-blind viewpoint and therefore should not be considered suitable diagnostic techniques if used by themselves. But, in conjunction with other orthodox techniques or when current investigative procedures are inadequate, they may be of benefit.

ALLERGY TESTING

Orthodox medicine uses the skin to reflect the possibility of allergies more so than it does the use of blood tests. These prick or scratch tests seem to be sensitive to allergens found in the air (airborne) but are generally less sensitive than blood tests for food allergy.

It is important to distinguish between an intolerance and an allergy (*see* **Food Allergies and Intolerance** *and* **Allergies**).

I also recommend that, before food allergy testing is undergone, a physician with knowledge of the leaky gut syndrome is consulted because allergies may alter rapidly due to this condition, making some of these expensive tests irrelevant within a month of eliminating the foods (*see* **Leaky gut syndrome**).

Self-testing

Select the five foods you most enjoy, the five foods you most crave, the five foods you eat most and the five foods that you eat through convenience rather than through enjoyment. These foods may overlap and you may have a list of 10 or so that are the most likely to be culprits if you suspect food allergy or have persisting ailments.

I am often confronted with quizzical looks when I bring forward this paradox that the foods you most desire are those that are liable to cause problems. It is important to remember that a body, when it is not well, will encourage reactions because reactions are usually curative. The body, not being a perfect machine, when it realizes it is unwell will ingest foods that create either a bodily reaction or a psychological sense of well-being in order to encourage a reaction or suppress psychological angst. This is why we eat foods that are not good for us and we tend to move towards alcohol and drugs to escape our awareness of illnesses.

Eliminate these foods for one month and note the changes. If improvement is forthcoming then reintroduce each food one at a time over a week and see which foods are more aggressive towards your well-being. Over a period of time you may be able to assess that you can eat certain foods if you take them only on a weekly basis, whereas others will create a reaction immediately and persistently.

Self-testing through exclusion diet regime

There are certain hypoallergenic diets based on foods that are rarely the cause of allergies/intolerances. In my experience of having tested hundreds of individuals, I do not agree with this principle. One popular hypoallergenic diet enforces patients to eat only lamb, rice, watery vegetables, apples, virgin olive oil, goat's products and honey. I have come across many patients who have had allergies to these foods and, as you can see, the diet is extremely restrictive.

I prefer people to experiment and find regimes such as the Hay diet (food non-combining diet), stone age diet or any specific diet picked off the shelf. Find one that suits you and makes you feel better, stay on it for 4–6 weeks and then reintroduce suspected culprits one by one each week; the reactions will occur much more quickly and be noticed within a few days.

Food allergy tests
Applied kinesiology or pulse testing

These techniques are reliant upon the sensitivity of a practitioner. In principle, a food compound is placed in the patient's mouth or on the body and a muscle group such as the shoulder muscles are tested for strength. A food that disagrees with the patient will momentarily create a weakness, which can be assessed by the practitioner. A similar response is noted in the pulse, which will either speed up or slow down in response to the compound.

These tests have been well substantiated in trials but one has to bear in mind the skill and sensitivity of the individual practitioner. At its extreme, practitioners have suggested that if a patient simply reads the name of a compound the muscles or pulse may alter. This has not been proven through any trials that I have come across, but I know practitioners and popular healers who are very successful with these techniques.

Hair analysis

A sample of hair is taken and tested against preprepared antibodies. In principle, the body will eliminate foods that it does not like and the hair has been established as containing (within its keratin fibres) unwanted molecules of foods. The antibodies will react with these foods and can be measured.

I am not particularly convinced by the accuracy of this test because certain molecules may not find their way into the hair particles as the skin is only a secondary mechanism for toxin removal and the hair is merely an adjunct to that. Chemicals in shampoos may also alter the structure of the food molecules or even remove them, thereby leading to false results.

Be wary of hair analysis being performed by some energetic or dowsing technique. Whilst the use of energetic measurement and the pendulum (the more popular technique for dowsing tests) is well established, the patient is once again dependent upon the skill of a practitioner and not any scientific reasoning.

Blood analysis

Food allergy cellular test (FACT). This is the development of a simple hypothesis. Most tests for food allergy are done on immunoglobulins, specifically IgG4 and IgE. These are made by specific types of white cell and can alter in the bloodstream depending upon the hydration of the person and when they last ate the food. However, the bloodstream carries memory cells, which are white cells specifically geared to remembering past infections. These do not vary to the same degree and may recognize a food allergen years after it has been eaten. Therefore, FACT is more sensitive than other food allergy tests.

Radioallergosorbent test/procedure (RAST/RASP). This is a specific blood test to check for IgG4 or IgE antibodies in the bloodstream and has been surpassed by the enzyme-linked immunosorbent assay (ELISA) (*see below*).

The test for IgG4 or IgE must, in my opinion, be combined: IgE is a fairly short-lived response but IgG4 tends to last in the bloodstream for a few weeks. A small study done by myself compared very accurate IgE testing with IgG4 and the results were quite different. I do not wish to get bogged down in the science but it is important to have both immunoglobulins tested and as these tests are quite expensive do not waste your funds on an assay that only covers one.

There is no doubt that this test will pick up an allergic response in the bloodstream but there is no guarantee that the allergy is relevant to an individual's illness. Being strongly allergic to eggs may simply make the patient sneeze once a day and may not be the underlying cause of their chronic fatigue syndrome. Conversely, a mild allergic response may be the cause of a cancer. It is important, therefore, to have these tests reviewed by a complementary practitioner who has a strong understanding and overview of the patient's case.

Enzyme-linked immunosorbent assay (ELISA). This is a common enough term in medical circles. It is a method by which blood is mixed with specific chemicals that bind in a particular way with certain blood components, especially immunoglobulins (antibodies), which can then be detected by a sensitive, computerized machine. The RAST (*see* above) is still available in some laboratories but has been surpassed by the more sensitive ELISA test. This is the best technique for assessing food allergy.

RECOMMENDATIONS

General Advice

- *Having selected your choice of food allergy testing, do not hesitate to sit with a complementary practitioner for an overview.*
- *Do not place total emphasis on a food allergy result because a healthy body may well be able to deal with any food allergy given an underlying level of good health.*

Electromagnetic testing

The Voll and Vega machines have been surpassed in recent years by American/German computers that pass electromagnetic frequencies through the body, and in many cases through the acupuncture meridians, and measure frequency fluctuations when the body is confronted by food and other compounds. These machines do not test for allergy (as explained before) but are, in my opinion, profoundly efficient in testing for intolerance, which may also cover allergy.

A patient sits with the practitioner who will connect him/her to the computer and a painless electromagnetic impulse is passed through the system. Different compounds are applied to the patient or the computer and the energy flow will diminish or enhance depending on the beneficial or adverse effect of the food. This is a simple and relatively inexpensive technique which I think is highly accurate in the right hands.

Bioresonance

A scientist in the 1930s by the unusual name of Royal Rife created a device that was capable of passing energy waves through a body. He noted that this created changes that were beneficial to health. Over the last six decades scientists and technological research companies with an interest in his original work have developed more and more sophisticated transmitters associated with complex computers. Research and studies have been done into the concept of disease having a particular energy wavelength or resonance, and this fact has been well established for many bacteria, viruses and conditions such as cancer.

It has been shown that passing a wavelength that antagonizes or blocks the natural wavelength of a condition can kill the organism or diseased cell. Much of Royal Rife's work was destroyed by a fearful medical fraternity and since then there have been several stories of practitioners having their records confiscated and doors are closed with regard to the availability of finance for research purposes. Other techniques such as Vega and Voll tests have supported the theory.

Machines, nowadays, are capable of diagnosis by comparing wavelengths picked up from a body being compared to wavelengths stored in the memory of the computer. If an individual resonance matches, say, tuberculosis then a diagnosis of a tubercular-like condition can be made. At this juncture, firm diagnosis is difficult but the process can be used to support an orthodox finding or help to steer a practitioner in the right direction.

The computer has a set treatment programme for particular diseases that have individual resonances and this is correlated with the body's own natural wavelengths, computed and passed back into the patient.

The two systems that appear most advanced and which work both diagnostically and as a treatment technique are the BiCom and the Quantum CI computers. Their availability is becoming much more widespread and, in the right hands, are of great benefit to diagnoses and healing.

Vega and Voll tests

Two machines named after their inventors, the Vega and Voll, were the basic forerunners to more sophisticated bioresonance computers. The same principle is used, whereby a small electric current is passed through a patient and an electricity-sensitive machine. A sensitive gauge measures the flow and different compounds are put into the machine to see if the electricity is hampered or enhanced. Many practitioners still use these machines with great accuracy but the process is much slower than the computers available nowadays.

GASTROGRAMS AND PANCREATICOGRAMS

A gastrogram is a measurement of the amount of hydrochloric acid produced by the stomach and a pancreaticogram measures pancreatic enzyme release. At the moment the assessment of this is an invasive procedure requiring samplings from the stomach. However, a non-invasive method is being developed that involves nothing more than drinking a particular solution which is measured

BIORESONANCE REPORT

Primary Diagnosis: *Leukemia*
Secondary Diagnosis: *None*

Additional Complications: *Does not appear to be energetically reacting to her Leukemia*
Possible Causes of Disease/Nosodal Suggestions: *Multiple psychological stress and also a lot of house renovations, good possibility of Geopathic stress also*
Alersodal: *Molds and Dust . . . aromatic hydrocarbons*
Isodal or Toxic Possibilities: *See summary*
Nutritional Problems: *Fatty acid deficiency possibly enzymes also*
Behavioural Problems: *None noted*
Trauma: *None noted*
Stress: *Psychological*
Perverse Energy Exposures: *Reacts to radiation exposure*
Inherited Tendencies or Disorders: *See report*
Mental Problems or Emotional Clinging: *None noted*
Sarcoidal Suggestions: *None noted*

Patient report

High items on Main screen
C:19 Fatty acid deficiency
Soponaria . . . sore throat
Catalase ID'S free radical Ca risk
Belladonna
Nux vom
Coxsackie . . . virus
Hepato liq
Tinea . . . Fungus

Auricle . . . ear
Gelsemium
Dulcamara
Lecithinase

Kidney liq
Algin Radiation
Aesculus Hlpp
Lyco
WBC Weakness and defiency
Diethylstilbesterol
Grass
Miasm Cholera
Miasm Allergy

C:14 Fatty acid
Carbonic anhydrase
Zingiber . . . for digestion
Aconite . . . Mental anguish
Sycosi
Chromosome 16 Q Cataract, MPS
Dysentery
Passiflora
Lymph, Spleen, Mammary

Nutrition
Vit F
Internal enzymes 80
Minerals 86

Allergy screening
Food allergy 109
Inhalant 98
Animal hair 88
Dairy sens 124
Grains 105
Pollen 104
Sulfites 123
Molds 96
Sugar 110

Specific allergens
Tomato
Pollens
Grass
Dog

Energy screening shows possible reaction to Geopathic stress

Other remedies
Alkaplex G
Bone C Dent
B 12 and Liver
Adreno neucleo

MNX anterior pituitary and E
Enzastatin

Homoeopathy
113 Nux Vom
Uranium 106
Dulcamara 109
Gels 109
Lyco 105
Lobelia 91
Myristica 97
Uva Ursi 101
Iris Vers 89
Machine recommends Nux vom as most similar at this time

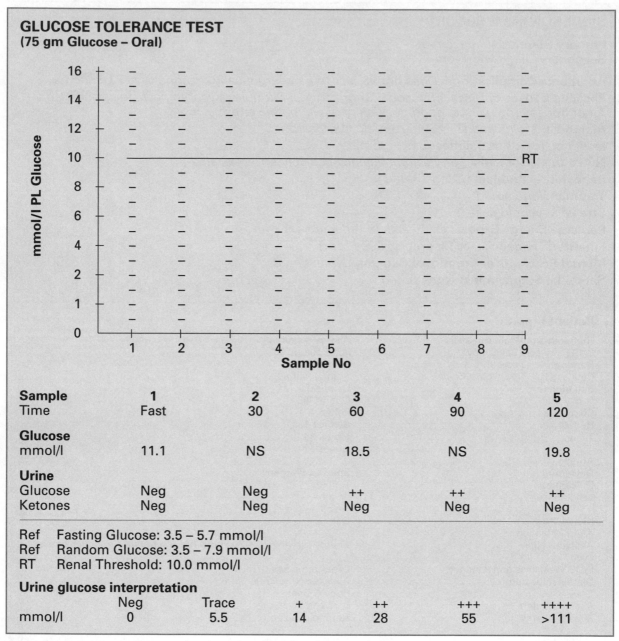

GLUCOSE TOLERANCE TEST
(75 gm Glucose – Oral)

Sample	1	2	3	4	5
Time	Fast	30	60	90	120
Glucose					
mmol/l	11.1	NS	18.5	NS	19.8
Urine					
Glucose	Neg	Neg	++	++	++
Ketones	Neg	Neg	Neg	Neg	Neg

Ref	Fasting Glucose: 3.5 – 5.7 mmol/l
Ref	Random Glucose: 3.5 – 7.9 mmol/l
RT	Renal Threshold: 10.0 mmol/l

Urine glucose interpretation

	Neg	Trace	+	++	+++	++++
mmol/l	0	5.5	14	28	55	>111

by an external monitoring machine. Many bowel problems and dyspeptic symptoms may be associated with a lack of hydrochloric acid rather than an excess and this simple test can illustrate this.

GLUCOSE TOLERANCE TEST (GTT)

This test is generally used to show a tendency towards diabetes. The holistic practitioner can also use the GTT to confirm a hypoglycaemic state (*see* **Hypoglycaemia**). An individual is given a 75-ml loading dose of a glucose solution after having fasted for at least 6 hours. Blood samples are taken every 30 minutes for 2.5–5 hours to establish whether or not the body's sugar control is being maintained. The blood sugar level should rise initially and drop as insulin levels rise to combat this change. The sugar level should drop below the normal threshold at which blood glucose is maintained and then rise again as the insulin levels drop.

GUT PERMEABILITY TEST

Fraction	Molecular weight	Dose (Mg)	Recovery in urine (6 hour collection)		
			Mg	%	Reference range
1	198	4.0	1.3	31.5	26.6–33.4
2	242	9.0	2.7	30.2	26.5–31.6
3	286	39.0	11.2	28.7	25.2–29.4
4	330	96.0	25.7	26.8	21.1–25.0
5	374	157.0	35.6	22.7	17.9–22.0
6	418	171.0	30.4	17.8	12.5–16.2
7	462	176.0	18.0	10.2	6.4–10.8
8	506	145.0	7.8	5.4	3.6–6.0
9	550	105.0	1.9	1.8	1.0–2.4
10	594	67.0	0.5	0.7	Up to 1.4
11	638	31.0	0.1	0.2	Up to 0.7
	TOTAL	**1000.0**	**135.2**	**13.5**	**10.0–13.3%**

Comment
Some increase in permeability up to molecular weight 450.

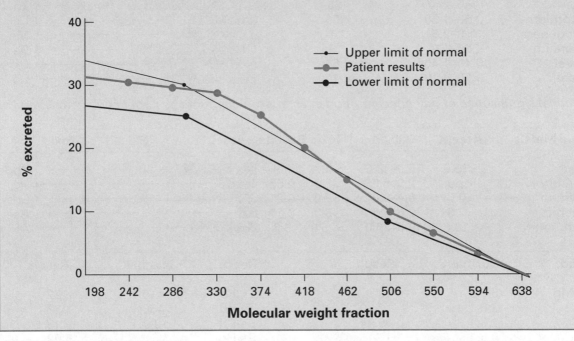

GUT PERMEABILITY TEST

This investigation is being pioneered at a laboratory in London. Brilliant in its simplicity, it is a test to assess the permeability of the intestine and is particularly important in establishing leaky gut syndrome (LGS), which may be responsible for food allergy that can lead to so many disorders.

A patient passes the first morning urine and follows this by drinking a solution that contains a range of molecules of different sizes. Depending upon the gut permeability, these molecules are absorbed into the bloodstream. The kidney will filter these and a collection of urine can be assayed to measure the size of the molecules that were absorbed. If larger molecules are found then a leaky gut can be diagnosed and curative treatment obtained.

At this time the availability of this test is limited, but access to it is being increased and I believe this will be one of the most important tests available.

HAIR MINERAL ANALYSIS REPORT

Reference: SHB/ASJD/N91   **Sample Date:** 10-02-1998

Age: 30
Sex: Male

Height: 5'2"   **Shampoo:** Baby   **Conditioner:** None
Weight: 14st 8lbs   **Bleach:** None   **Highlight:** None
Hair colour: Black   **Perm:** None   **Tint:** None

	Reference range:	Results: (Parts per million)	Low	Reference Range:	High
Calcium	200–600	442			Ca
Magnesium	30–95	38			Mg
Phosphorus*	100–210	187			P
Sodium*	90–340	202			Na
Potassium*	50–120	34			K
Iron*	20–60	27			Fe
Copper	10–40	18			Cu
Zinc	150–240	196			Zn
Chromium	0.60–1.50	0.56			Cr
Manganese	1.0–2.6	1.1			Mn
Selenium	1.5–4.0	2.8			Se
Nickel	0.40–1.40	0.66			Ni
Cobalt*	0.10–0.70	0.19			Co

Clinical significance of hair concentration of asterisked elements has not been established.

Toxic Metals	Accept	Raised	Toxic	Results	Acceptable	Raised	Toxic
Lead	<15.0	15.0–40.0	>40.0	8.9			Pb
Mercury	<2.0	2.0–5.0	>5.0	0.55			Hg
Cadmium	<0.5	0.5–2.0	>2.0	0.21			Cd
Arsenic	<2.0	2.0–5.0	>5.0	0.11			As
Aluminium	<10.0	10.0–25.0	>25.0	5.2			Al

Ratio:	Normal:	Result:	Ratio:	Normal:	Result:
Ca/Mg	6.1:1	12	Zn/Pb	>10:1	22
Ca/P	2.6:1	2.36	Zn/Cd	>400:1	933
Na/K	2.3:1	5.94	Se/Cd	>3.4:1	13
Zn/Cu	8.5:1	11	Se/Hg		5.09

HAIR ANALYSIS

A tablespoon amount of hair may be used for two investigations.

Mineral and toxic metal analysis

Hair analysis for mineral deficiency or excess has an established scientific background but it is poorly used by orthodox medicine. Hair is known to be an excretion and therefore its composition can be a useful indicator. Many minerals can be measured although the clinical significance of some of them has not been established. Analysis of hair can be inaccurate due to environmental or occupational exposure. Many shampoos have compounds, such as selenium, which can alter the results. Hair mineral analysis is particularly useful as it reflects long-term metabolism, unlike blood and urine that can change within a matter of hours. Measurement of metal levels is therefore of particular use.

Food intolerance

I am highly sceptical of the use of hair analysis in food intolerance/allergy testing (*see* **Allergy testing**).

HUMORAL PATHOLOGICAL LABORATORY TEST (HUMORAL LABORATORY BLOOD TEST)

The HLB test, I am sure, will be one of the most beneficial investigations in the future of holistic medicine. It, like so many great ideas, was based on a simple observational fact, which is that blood, its cells, plasma and serum, change and react in relation to chemical factors released from diseased tissue.

A pinprick of blood is placed as four drops on a microscope slide. This is placed underneath a high-power microscope that magnifies the blood up to 1,500 times. The pictures produced are passed into a computer which compares the samples to thousands of other samples taken from known conditions. Deficiencies, poor oxygenation

---

HUMORAL PATHOLOGICAL LAB TEST (HLB Method)

NAME: **DATE:**

Interpretation:
Notice: These interpretations are based on Newtonian Laws and have been developed by Heitan, Legard and Bradford (1930). It is widely used in the biggest Cancer Research Institute of USA the Bradford Institute, and in various Institutes in Europe.

Results could be altered by the influence of antioxidants, chemotherapy or radiation therapy. To have an exact reading, it is advisable to refrain from the above mentioned for two weeks, otherwise, slight alterations in the results are possible.

SYMPTOMS	RESULT	SYMPTOMS	RESULT
oxidation leading to allergies	✓	vitamin C deficiency	✓
anaemia of qualitative origin	✓	oxidation MS origin	✓
oxidation leading to arthritis	✓	Heinz bodies	✓
lack of ability to assimilate food	✓	hypo-Calcemia	✓
asthma cellular origin	✓	physical stress	✓
degenerative state I, II, III, IV	✓	increased acidity in stomach	✓
dehydration of kidney	✓	congested lymph system	✓
Free radicals activity	✓	psychological stress (catecholamine)	✓
oxidation patterns indicating fungus	✓	indications for hormone imbalance	✓

Next proposed Humoral pathological control in six weeks

Humoral Pathological Laboratory Blood Test

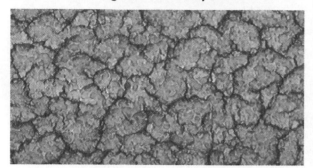

Normal blood cluster

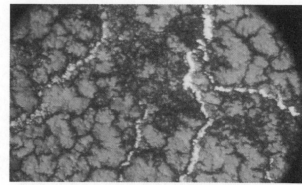

Lymph and bowel toxicity

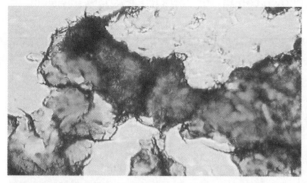

Strong oxidation

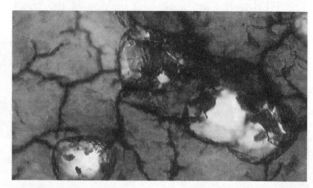

Fungi in blood

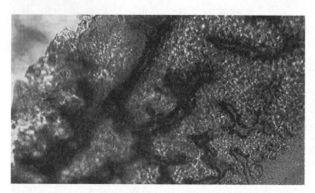

Fungi infested blood

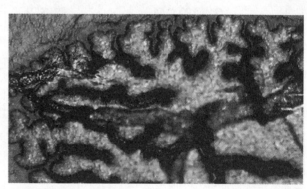

Fungi in blood

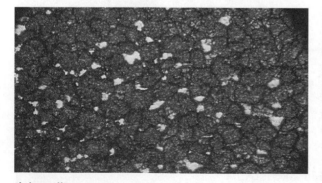

Adrenalin stress

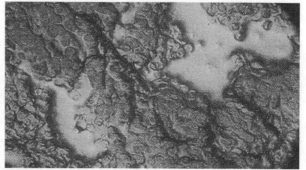

Blood from cancer case

Iris Topograph

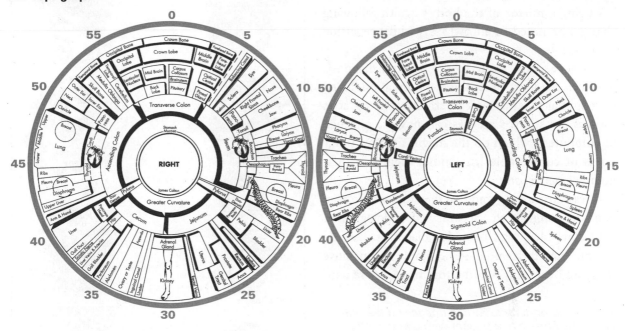

and the presence of chemicals from cancer cells are just examples of the huge bank of conditions that any sample is compared to. The computer prints out the possible diagnoses and, if programmed correctly, may offer advice on treatments that have been successful and have returned abnormal blood back to a normal status.

The availability of this test is increasing but at present it is available in only a few centres. Please contact the 101 Group (*see* **Useful addresses**).

IRIDOLOGY

Iridology is the study of the colour and patterns on the iris of the eyes. This technique has been in use for thousands of years and probably has its origins in the East. However, a Hungarian doctor,

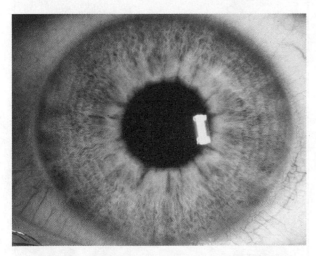

Tendency to rheumatism and arthritis. Stress rings. Pseudoparathyroidism – excess calcium in the stomach.

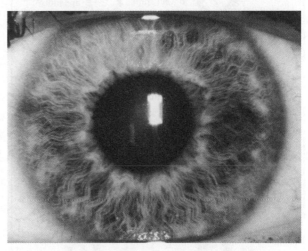

Tendency to toxicity of the lymph glands. Spots showing difficulty with metabolism – overweight. Left hand side (15°) – weakness of the lungs – asthma.

Ignacz von Peczely, studied the possibility of the iris being a mirror of the body's health following changes he noted in an owl's iris whilst repairing its broken leg.

Until recently, study of the iris and diagnosis has been made by practitioner observation, aided by a special magnifying camera that photographs the iris for study. Cameras can now be attached to computers, which do the diagnosis from thousands of comparable iris studies logged in their memory banks.

I was surprised to find that few studies have been done to compare the accuracy of iridologists or their computers with orthodox diagnosis. I would assume that this would be a simple comparative study and can only assume that finances are hard

The computer-derived Kirlian images on the right are of the fingers of a patient with chronic fatigue syndrome. The second print-out is significantly worse as the patient has had flu. Below is a table used in diagnosis.

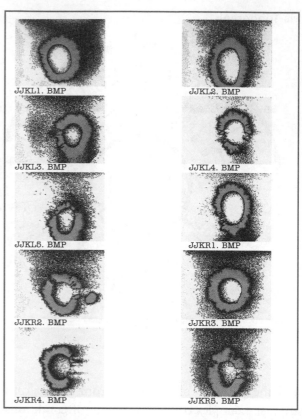

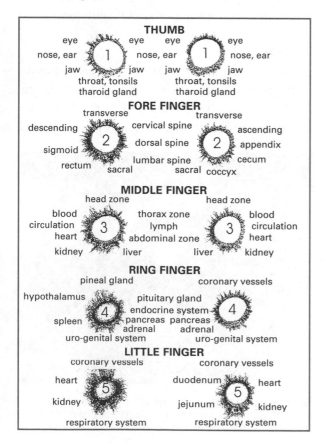

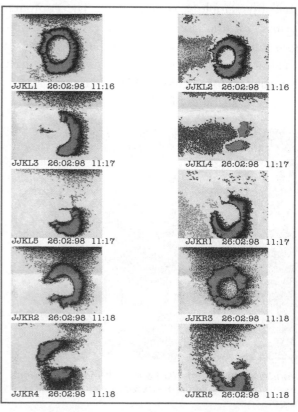

to find. I am sure that research will be done in the future to show firmly where iridology may be of benefit. As a diagnostic technique in conjunction with other tests and clinical observation, iridology can be a great eye-opener!

KIRLIAN PHOTOGRAPHY

The Kirlian photograph technique takes 'pictures' of the aura (*see* **Aura reading**). Initially created as a diagnostic technique by a Russian engineer, Semyon Kirlian, the original equipment consisted of an electric coil, an aluminium plate and photo-sensitive film covered by glass. Modern-day cameras, based on the same principles, send a high-voltage charge that measures energy release when part of the body is placed in contact with it. Whole-body auras are now taken without actual contact.

An individual's aura will change depending upon their health and certain patterns are correlated with certain diseases. As with iridology, I wonder why a clear correlation has not been made between certain patterns and particular diseases but I do know that trials are underway in Europe and the UK. I suspect that auras will not correlate to specific diseases but will alter depending upon an individual's response to a particular disease process. Until proven otherwise, Kirlian photography should only be used in conjunction with clinical assessment and other investigations. *See also* **Aura Reading**.

PANCREATIC EXOCRINE TESTS
See **Gastrograms and pancreaticograms**

It is of immense benefit for a complementary medical practitioner to know the individual patient's ability to digest foods. Many conditions may be associated with deficiencies that may be due to a lack of digestive capability rather than insufficient ingestion of a particular compound that is deficient. The orthodox world pays little attention to this factor and, until recently, practitioners of complementary medicine had to use their clinical judgement and experience to assess the possibility that a patient is not digesting properly. A non-invasive test that involves the patient doing no more than swallowing a particular fluid to assess digestive capabilities and enzyme production is available at this stage, but patients need to visit the laboratory in London and there is currently limited availability and a long waiting list. Availability will, hopefully, become greater. Practitioners rather than patients should contact The 101 Group for information if they feel a patient would benefit.

ALTERNATIVE THERAPIES

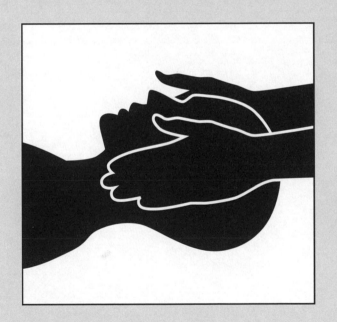

CHAPTER 9

ALTERNATIVE THERAPIES

This chapter provides a synopsis of the different alternative therapies that bind together with orthodox medicine to give us the choices that make up holistic medicine.

CHOOSING YOUR HEALER

Most main branches of complementary or alternative medicine have a regulatory body or a college to which a practitioner may be affiliated. Some are more officious than others but all demand a basic standard of technique and stipulate a certain amount of time spent in training to be able to join.

Unfortunately, many healing arts do not have any form of association and there is currently no legal requirement to have studied the subject that a practitioner may claim to practise. I believe that this will change in the near future. For now, however, the best method of choosing a practitioner is through word of mouth. Qualifications do not necessarily ensure that a practitioner has healing qualities but if they have helped someone they are likely to be able to help others.

If you cannot find somebody in this manner, then select a practitioner from a reputable clinic. It is unlikely that a practitioner who is not safe or effective will flourish within a group. Other practitioners will hear any detrimental information and either correct the failing or recommend to the clinic owners that the practitioner is not suitable.

A waiting list is usually a good sign. You need to ask how many days a week that an individual may work with patients. I know of a practitioner who has a remarkable reputation based on a six-month waiting list. He only works one day a week! Most practitioners should expect a six-day waiting list!

Good practitioners are busy practitioners who, as a rule, do not need to advertise. Accepting that everybody has to start somewhere and that advertising is a method getting one's presence known, an advert may represent an unexperienced or failing practitioner. An advertisement may be drawing your attention to a new field of practice or a unique technique but selecting a practitioner by this method may not be the best. It is better to go on articles that you may read, because journalists are generally quite scrupulous and have experience. Always, however, look for the political motive in anything that is being written about complementary medicine. I may be overzealous in my belief that the orthodox world would not like to see complementary medicine flourish but I do feel that many articles on the subject are overcritical and do not compare the down side of orthodox medicine when criticizing an alternative technique.

At the end of the day you need to be comfortable with your chosen practitioner. If the area in which they work, the room in which they practise or their character feels uncomfortable then look again. Trust your instincts.

ACUPUNCTURE

Acupuncture is one aspect of Chinese and Tibetan medicine. (*See* **Chinese and Oriental medicine**.) Using acupuncture outside of the full discipline of these medical philosophies can be likened to using physiotherapy and no other treatment when dealing with orthodox medicine.

Acupuncture is thought to have originated from the observations by Chinese physicians of their warriors who had been stabbed, speared or injured in battle. Specific wounds seemed to create changes, depending on their placement superficially in the body.

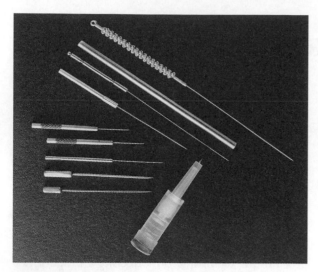

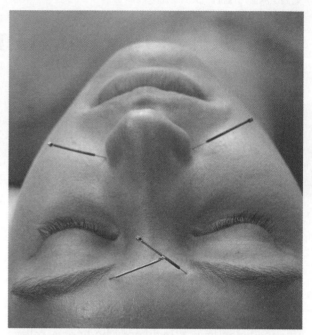

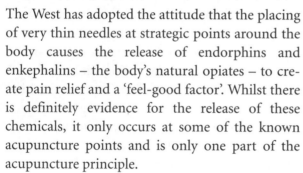

(above) There is a large variety of acupuncture needle designs. (right) A patient receives treatment for hay fever. (below) An acupuncturist inserts needles to 'tonify' the kidneys.

The West has adopted the attitude that the placing of very thin needles at strategic points around the body causes the release of endorphins and enkephalins – the body's natural opiates – to create pain relief and a 'feel-good factor'. Whilst there is definitely evidence for the release of these chemicals, it only occurs at some of the known acupuncture points and is only one part of the acupuncture principle.

In truth, and perfectly scientifically provable on the basis of observation, the acupuncture points are stimulatory areas along energy lines known by the Chinese as meridians and the Tibetans as channels. The Tibetans have many points along known nerve routes, whereas the Chinese have little correlation with these. Stimulation of these points increases, decreases or varies the energy in these lines. These channels or meridians represent organs or systems within the body, mind and soul of a human being.

Acupuncture treatment consists of inserting fine needles into the skin to correct the imbalances or disharmony discovered in your meridians or channels. The acupuncturist will first ask you questions and examine you in ways that other medical systems may not find

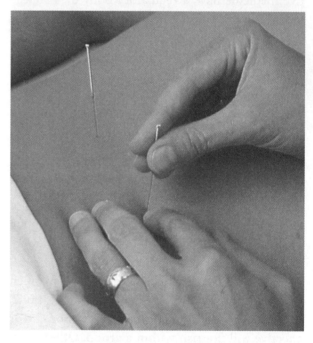

important. For example, he may feel the palms of your hands and look at your tongue. He will also feel your pulses at both wrists. On the basis of his understanding of the 'symptom picture', he will will decide where to place the needles, the depth to which they need to be placed, the application of heat and the need to apply movement to the needles (see **Pulse taking**).

ACUPRESSURE

Acupressure is an ancient healing art based on the same principles as acupuncture except that, instead of needles, finger or thumb pressure only is used to harmonize the flow of energy through the body. There is evidence that acupressure was used even earlier than acupuncture, when the Indians first documented some basic principles of massage over 5,000 years ago. The Japanese have advanced this therapeutic application of massage

Acupuncture/Acupressure Meridians

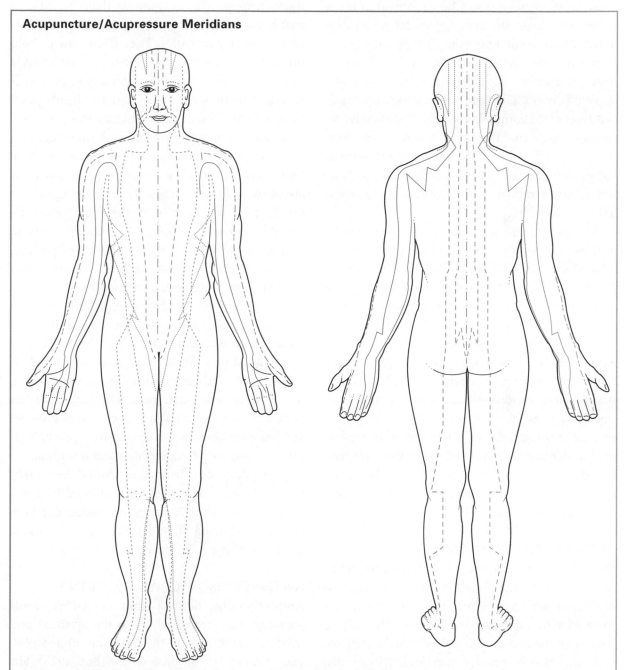

There are twelve principal meridians, each corresponding to an organ or function of the body. In addition there are two special meridians, the Conception vessel, and the Governor vessel. In the Chinese tradition, each meridian is associated either with Yin or Yang, and with one of the five elements.

and from it developed the technique now known as Shiatsu.

Application of pressure, either gentle or deep, to specific pressure points can stimulate the meridians or channels in the same way as acupuncture. Unlike acupuncture, it can be performed at home either as a self-treatment or to treat other members of the family. If you know the right pressure points to use it makes an effective first-aid measure for pain or cramps. Acupressure massage will also boost the immune system, relieve stress and fatigue and treat many common ailments. It is effective for chronic conditions including insomnia and joint pain and stiffness, and for acute ailments such as indigestion and headaches. In addition acupressure will release lymphatic blockages and help relieve 'knots' in muscles.

The points and meridians, which correspond to those in acupuncture charts, are pressed for at least 20 seconds with the thumb, middle or index finger, whichever feels most comfortable. This pressure may be varied in intensity according to the condition being treated. For example, for fatigue or lack of energy the point needs to be stimulated and this is achieved by applying deep clockwise pressure; to sedate a point for pain or stress-related conditions, somewhat lighter, anti-clockwise pressure is applied. When the person you are treating feels slight discomfort or tenderness under pressure you will know that you have found the exact point. Points on the body will usually need firmer, more prolonged pressure than those on the face.

ALEXANDER TECHNIQUE

The Alexander Technique was developed in the 1890s by an Australian actor named Frederick M Alexander who found that he could correct his voice loss by adjusting his posture. He realized how his poor habits of movement had interfered with the body's healthy functioning, and that learning to move well and with the head and neck correctly aligned he derived many beneficial effects, not just on his voice but on his general health. From his observations he was able to formulate the Alexander Technique, which he taught to other actors and singers and then to a wider public.

Today, specially trained teachers all over the world help people to improve their health and well-being by changing the way they use their bodies in everyday activities. They teach how to hold the body and breathe more efficiently, which oxygenates the body better. Re-alignment of posture is necessary in all of us. Unless you are already practising a physical technique, the chances are that I could ask you at this moment to sit up straight. In doing so you would probably find that you have been slumped, and can increase your height by about two to three inches. This 'slumping' closes up the chest and may block the energy channels that flow through the body. The technique aims to change permanently these poor habits of posture, movement and thought, replacing unconscious tensions with thoughtful movement.

Practising the Alexander Technique offers a wide range of health benefits. In addition to reducing stress, and improving the voice and breathing, it may improve lung conditions such as asthma and persistent postural problems causing, for instance, low back pain. The technique has been shown through trials to lower blood pressure and has even been shown to deal with psychological problems such as depression and insomnia.

The Alexander Technique should be taught within a course of ten lessons, followed by occasional extra lessons. Visiting the teacher regularly is a bit like having piano lessons – you practise if you know that you are going to be assessed!

ANTHROPOSOPHICAL MEDICINE

Anthroposophy, derived from the Greek words meaning man and wisdom, is the spiritual and mystical teachings of the Austrian philosopher and scientist Dr Rudolf Steiner (1861–1925). His ideas have been particularly influential in education, but they also inspired a new approach to healing. Anthroposophical medicine is practised mainly in continental Europe, although there are doctors and clinics in other parts of the world.

Steiner realized that the human being was not just a physical or biochemical organism but contained 'etheric' and 'astral' bodies. These were non-measurable energies that made up our emotions and 'vital force'. Steiner used the term 'ego' to define our spiritual core. Steiner's concepts harmonize with Eastern philosophy: he believed that the body is made up of earth, water, fire and air which are connected through the digestive and movement structures, the sensory system and the rhythmic system. The physical and etheric energies control digestion and movement; the ego and the astral body control senses; and the rhythmic system controls the circulation and breathing.

Steiner believed that health was governed by a balance of all of these. He had a holistic view of healing, and warned of the limitations of scientific medicine. He saw healing primarily as an art, and the patient as a human spirit finding its way amid its relationships with the body, with other people and with nature, and not simply as an object separated from everything else in the universe. Steiner simplified illness into inflammatory and degenerative conditions, but wished to stress the meaningfulness of each illness by putting it into the context of the individual's biography and surroundings.

Treatment is by altering spiritual and emotional consciousness, through diet, exercise and remedies. Healing possibilities are enriched by artistic and other therapies such as painting, eurythmy, sculpture and music. Anthroposophical medicine uses a mixture of herbal, mineral and homeopathic remedies.

APPLIED KINESIOLOGY – *see* Kinesiology

AROMATHERAPY

Aromatherapy is the use of plant extracts, known as essences or essential oils, to treat a range of common ailments and for their effect on the emotions and mental well-being. There are about 30 commonly used oils, ranging from basil and

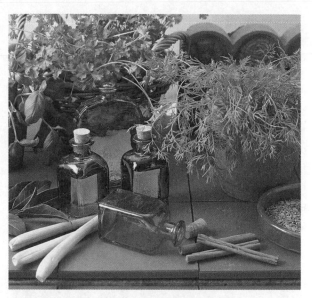
Aromatherapy oils with herbs and other ingredients.

bergamot to lavender, rose, sage and tea tree. These highly aromatic oils can penetrate the skin when used in the bath or in conjunction with massage (when dispersed in a carrier oil), but more probably have a greater therapeutic effect through inhalation, when they are absorbed into the body through the nose and lungs.

Aromatherapy is one of the most ancient of the healing arts, and has been documented from the East for thousands of years. The ancient Egyptians used aromatic substances in medicine (and for the mummification process) as far back as 4500 BC. It was not until the twentieth century, however, that the healing powers of essential oils were studied and fully appreciated.

Some of the oils are expensive to buy (a huge number of plants is needed to make just a small amount of oil), but only a few drops are needed to provide an effective treatment, so a little goes a long way. Provided the right oils are used in the correct quantities and are not ingested (unless on the advice of a qualified therapist), the techniques are safe. Many of the oils may be used in combination, which will increase the beneficial effect. For relaxation and to enhance your mood, choose the oil whose fragrance you prefer.

The most successful results have been seen in wound healing, treating skin problems such as acne, PMT, poor circulation, respiratory disorders, and headaches and other stress-related disorders. Some of the most useful oils include: eucalyptus (for colds, flu and rheumatism), tea tree, pine or lemon (for sore throats, colds, flu and bronchitis), lavender (for eczema, acne, minor wounds, insomnia and tiredness) and geranium (for skin problems, neuralgia, sore throats and tonsillitis). There are many good books available, listing the main essential oils and their uses.

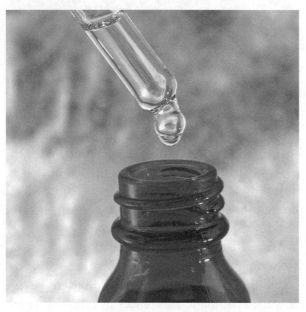

One of the most effective ways of using aromatherapy oils is to place a few drops into the water of an oil burner. As the water heats up the aromatic vapours are released.

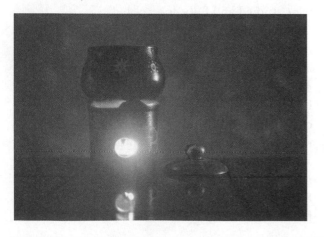

ART THERAPY

A branch of psychotherapy (*see* **Psychotherapy**), art therapy is used as a means of understanding emotional and psychological problems and gaining release from them. People know intuitively that creative self-expression is a way of healing oneself, and artistic expression is one such way of doing so. No artistic skill is needed, but through the creative process itself many problems can be addressed, including depression, low self-esteem and relationship difficulties. Art therapy is especially effective with severely disturbed people who find it difficult to express their feelings verbally.

An art therapist, through interpreting the meaning of the art produced by the client or patient, can uncover problems that may be deeply buried and that might otherwise take years of regular counselling to uncover. The therapist hopes to come to an understanding of the client and thereby help him or her towards making fresh discoveries about the self and about life. The process of creating something through visual means can help people to detach themselves from feelings or problems that might be difficult or impossible to express verbally or that are otherwise too overwhelming to deal with.

Art therapy utilizes colour and patterns using pencils, crayons, paint and any other colourful medium to try to bring whatever is lying in the subconscious to the visual consciousness. Collages, sculpture, paintings and drawings can all express unexpected angst in the artist in a very immediate way, and this method often bypasses the self-censoring process with which we may block out disturbing feelings and thoughts.

The British Association of Art Therapists is an expanding group and registered therapists can be found throughout the UK, USA and many other countries. Art therapists will differ in their interpretive approach depending on their school of thought, which could be Freudian or Jungian, or might put more emphasis on interpretation of the artwork by the clients themselves.

AURICULAR THERAPY

Like many parts of the body, the ear reflects and maps out the rest of the body. The diagram below shows the many acupuncture points found on the external ear (*see* **Acupuncture**). Auricular therapy generally involves the insertion of acupuncture needles into these points, but can deal with most health matters (usually in conjunction with more mainstream treatments) by acupressure. Points are located in the ear by pressing with a fine, blunt

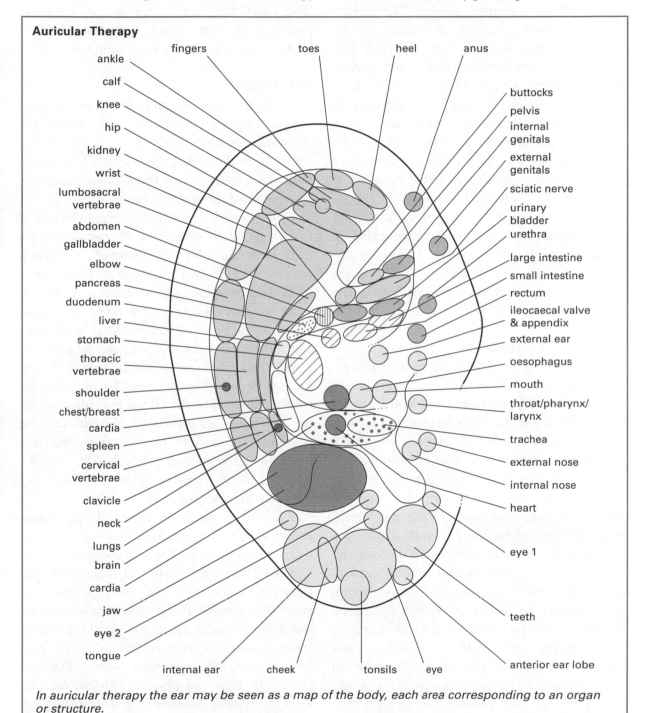

Auricular Therapy

fingers · toes · heel · anus

ankle · calf · knee · hip · kidney · wrist · lumbosacral vertebrae · abdomen · gallbladder · elbow · pancreas · duodenum · liver · stomach · thoracic vertebrae · shoulder · chest/breast · cardia · spleen · cervical vertebrae · clavicle · neck · lungs · brain · cardia · jaw · eye 2 · tongue

buttocks · pelvis · internal genitals · external genitals · sciatic nerve · urinary bladder · urethra · large intestine · small intestine · rectum · ileocaecal valve & appendix · external ear · oesophagus · mouth · throat/pharynx/larynx · trachea · external nose · internal nose · heart · eye 1 · teeth · anterior ear lobe

internal ear · cheek · tonsils · eye

In auricular therapy the ear may be seen as a map of the body, each area corresponding to an organ or structure.

instrument to locate sensitive spots or by using an electrical sensor. There are more than 120 points on each ear and for treatment to be effective it is important that they are located exactly.

The point is then stimulated by acupressure or with small acupuncture needles. The needles remain in place for about 15 minutes and are manipulated now and then. Some therapists may use electrical stimulation, which is not painful, and experiments are now being tried using laser. Continuous treatment lasting several days may be obtained if the therapist, using acupressure, attaches a small press needle or seed with adhesive tape to the point in the ear. During treatment a dull or tingling sensation may be felt in the ear or on the same side of the body.

Auricular therapy is particularly useful for treating addictions (such as help with giving up smoking) and for pain control. Respiratory disorders, musculo-skeletal disorders and chronic conditions such as arthritis and skin problems have all been shown to benefit from this treatment.

AUTOGENIC TRAINING

The word 'autogenic' is derived from the Greek for 'coming from within' and is principally a self-relaxation/hypnosis technique. Devised in Berlin by Dr J Schultz in the 1920s, the training consists of learning a set of six simple exercises designed to induce deep relaxation and thereby promote self-healing. The exercises include the repetition of certain phrases to bring on feelings of general warmth, an abdominal glow, a feeling of heaviness, and heartbeat and breathing control. Schultz also recommended a technique for cooling the forehead.

Autogenic training involves learning how to control the body's involuntary nervous system, and needs to be taught by a specially trained therapist. It can be used to treat many disorders, from anxiety and tension to asthma and tendonitis. Autogenics is an effective alternative to using tranquillizers or sleeping pills. It is not only an excellent self-help addition to the treatment of any chronic condition, but also one of the most

positive antidotes to everyday stress. By practising the exercises for only a few minutes you can release yourself from the stresses in your life, and allow the body to restore itself and become more resistant to illness. Its long-term effects are to lower heart-attack risk factors such as high blood pressure and high blood cholesterol, and to improve emotional balance and willpower.

AYURVEDA

Ayurveda is a word derived from one of the oldest known languages, Sanskrit, and means the 'knowledge of daily living'. There is mention of Ayurveda in the Vedas, the world's oldest literature, which suggests that this healing system has been practised for over 5,000 years.

Ayurveda considers human beings to be part of the 'whole', indivisible from all else. There are many authorities who define Ayurveda in different ways but in principle it is a way of life rather than a medical doctrine and includes spiritual, emotional, social and physical concerns. As much importance is given to sleep as to activity, to diet as to ablutions and hygiene, and to exercise as to meditation.

Ayurvedic medicine cannot be separated from a consciousness of one's entire lifestyle. Ayurveda is only properly practised if the individual is willing to change all aspects of ill-health-creating activities. The current fad of using Ayurvedic remedies is like taking painkillers for a badly injured limb. It is only one part of the necessary treatment to regain function.

Ayurveda is based on three principal forces known as the *tri-dosha*. *Vatta* represents air and space, *pitta* represents fire and water, and *kapha* represents water and earth. All these overlap to some extent and none can survive without the other. For example, fire cannot burn without air and without some substance (earth) to burn. Water becomes stagnant without air and fire cannot be controlled without water. Different emotional states and physical activities fall into these categories. Movement and breathing are vatta, temperature and digestion are pitta, and energy and stability are kapha. Emotionally, dreams and intentions are represented by vatta (head in the clouds), ambition and drive by pitta ('he is all fired up') and nurturing and forgiveness are covered by kapha (nesting and nurturing).

All people are made up of all doshas but usually one or two predominate. Most books on Ayurveda help individuals to understand their constitutional type, and knowing this can help balance the tri-dosha. People who are predominantly vatta/pitta may benefit from having more kapha, for example. All foods have their own elements. Chillies and hot soups are generally pitta, whereas red meat is predominantly pitta and kapha. Knowing one's constitutional dosha allows a diet to be set for that particular body type.

Ayurveda is a complex philosophy, made more so by the use of Indian terminology, but once the basics have been grasped, the common sense attitude and approach are simple and can have a profound effect on well-being. Unfortunately, in the West the necessary dedication to an all-around lifestyle is not easily formed or followed and, I think, Ayurveda is probably only of benefit to those with time to dedicate to their health and not to those looking for a 'quick fix'.

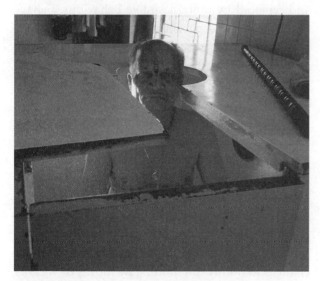

Steam baths are one of the five Ayurvedic purification therapies. The three doshas – vatta, pitta and kapha – are brought to a balanced state, thus promoting well-being.

BACH FLOWER REMEDIES

These are herbal remedies derived from flowers. They promote healing by reducing negative states of mind, seen as the cause of disease, and increasing positive emotions. Physical problems are thought to derive from a mind/body energy imbalance that nature can correct through its effects on plants when they are taken in the right combination. The remedies are extracted from the flowers and buds of common plants by the action of sunlight or heat, and preserved in brandy.

The system was devised by Dr Edward Bach (1886–1936), a pathologist and bacteriologist who, following an illness of his own in the early 1900s, discovered that plants contain compounds or energy that affect the psyche. He found that different diseases seemed to be linked to different temperamental types, and classified these types into seven main groups, each with a habitual negative emotional state. These states are indicated by a key word or phrase, and are: loneliness, fear, uncertainty, lack of interest in the present, over-sensitivity, despondency, and over-concern for others.

Working intuitively, Dr Bach set out to find plants that made these negative states positive, and eventually found 38 in all, ranging from agrimony to willow. For the purposes of prescribing he further subdivided each state of mind so that, for example, under the heading uncertainty, aspen acts on fear of the unknown, cherry plum on fear of losing control and rock rose on terror or self-abandonment. Under the category of over-sensitivity, agrimony acts on worry and anxiety hidden under a brave face, centaury is for weak will and a 'doormat tendency', and holly works for jealousy and anger.

The remedies should therefore be selected to correspond to the state of mind and the personality. The experience of a practitioner may be helpful if you find it difficult to decide on the appropriate remedy. Since they are completely safe for any age, the remedies are commonly used for self-help at home, particularly the 'Rescue Remedy' which is a mixture of five of the flower remedies and can be used after a shock or in an emotional crisis.

BATES METHOD FOR EYES

The Bates method of eyesight training, named after Dr W H Bates, an eye specialist of New York, is a natural way of improving and maintaining eyesight using particular exercises to relearn proper habits of vision. Dr Bates published his bestseller, *Better Eyesight without Glasses*, detailing these exercises, in 1919. He argued that perfect vision was the product of completely relaxed eyes, and that it was misuse of the eyes that led to defects of vision.

Bates's methods found many advocates, including the writer Aldous Huxley who as a young man could hardly see to read. Huxley's book, *The Art of Seeing*, explains how he was helped by this method. Followers of the method, found throughout the world, argue that the exercises benefit people of all ages, however poor their eyesight. Many practitioners of other complementary therapies use the Bates method during treatments.

There are seven main exercises which should be practised daily. They can be learned easily by obtaining a book or, more simply, by consulting a Bates practitioner, who will usually recommend a course of weekly training sessions. The exercises aim to relax tension in the eye muscles, and include 'palming', covering the eyes with the palms of the hands for ten minutes two or three times a day; 'splashing', splashing the closed eyes repeatedly with warm and then cold water, morning and evening; and 'shifting and swinging', consciously imitating the minute shifting movements of the eyes around objects. Bates also believed in blinking frequently, once or twice every ten seconds. In addition he considered the importance of diet, supplements and homeopathy in maintaining the health of the eyes.

BEHAVIOURAL THERAPY

This is one of the four main branches of psychotherapy (the others are the psychoanalytic, the humanistic and the cognitive). Sometimes known as stimulus/response psychology, the behavioural approach is based on 'learning theory' which grew out of research with animals. Basing his work on Pavlov's earlier studies of conditioned reflexes in dogs, the American psychologist B F Skinner (b. 1904) made further studies of animal behaviour from which he developed his 'laws of learning', the theory of reinforcement on top of conditioning.

Behaviourists emphasize how the environment 'conditions' us to behave in certain ways, and that we modify our behaviour to suit our surroundings. In principle, anything that we do is reinforced by a reward or punishment. We tell a joke and people laugh, so we tell it again. We chatter in the theatre, everybody stares at us with a scowl, so we do not do it again. Behavioural therapy uses this simple fact to encourage correct behaviour and discourage bad behaviour. A good example is a disruptive child who manages to attract the attention of his parents by misbehaving. If the parent ignores the child the behaviour goes unattended (the equivalent to not being rewarded) and the child's attitude will change.

Since all behaviour is learned, behaviourists argue that undesirable behaviour can be unlearned and replaced by more desirable behaviour. Behavioural therapy is particularly useful for phobias, breaking habits, obsessive–compulsive behaviour and even bed-wetting. The most successful and widely used form of the therapy is desensitization or flooding for specific phobias: in the first method the patient is lightly hypnotized, relaxes deeply and imagines a progressively more frightening series of fearful stimuli; in the second the patient confronts the most frightening stimulus, either in reality or imagination, for 20 minutes or so.

BIOFEEDBACK

Biofeedback is a method of monitoring minute changes in bodily functioning by means of various small electronic machines. The machines are attached to an individual via electrodes and may be used to measure heart rate, brain-wave patterns, body temperature or respiratory rate. This information – about the autonomic nervous system – shows the level of relaxation or arousal in the body, and can be used consciously to influence bodily processes that were once thought to be beyond voluntary control. Biofeedback is not itself a therapy, but is used in conjuction with the teaching of relaxation or meditation techniques, often including breathing and visualization therapy. By being able to monitor your level of relaxation, it is possible to learn how to change your physiological responses and vice versa.

The machine will register certain bodily activities by a high-pitched sound or a dial. In response to a reduction in the stress response in the body, the dial will register a lower level or the high-pitched sound will become low-pitched. The technique reinforces an individual's success with their relaxation method. Biofeedback training may be given in groups or on a one-to-one basis. It aims to accelerate the process of learning how to relax or meditate, so that one can quickly become independent of the machines while using the knowledge gained from them.

Biofeedback can be used to treat stress-related conditions such as insomnia, anxiety, fears, raised blood pressure and asthma. It is also useful, in conjunction with cardiovascular drugs, for controlling an irregular heartbeat. Migraines and muscular tension can be soothed with meditation techniques and biofeedback can reinforce this. It has also been found to be effective in relieving chronic pain, and for retraining muscles if their function has been lost after an illness or accident.

BUTEYKO THERAPY

A scientist in Russia by the name of K P Buteyko has spent his life showing that breathing can alter the acid/alkaline levels in the bloodstream by adjusting the oxygen and carbon dioxide levels. In principle, hyperventilation (overbreathing) causes a depletion of carbon dioxide (CO_2). Low levels of CO_2 cause blood vessels to spasm and tissues to be deprived of oxygen. This can, in theory, create any

disease process ranging from arthritis to ulcerative colitis. The body's metabolism will often slow down in response to this decreased CO_2 level. By counteracting this, the Buteyko breathing technique can be very beneficial in increasing energy and reducing weight.

Buteyko therapy aims to retrain breathing patterns to increase the oxygenation of the blood and tissues. Asthma is particularly susceptible to Buteyko breathing methods. Research carried out in Australia, showing a remarkable response in asthmatics using drugs to control their problem, is soon due to be published. There has been some delay and I wonder if this is a block by the orthodox medical world, who would lose millions of dollars if a breathing technique were found to be more effective.

The Buteyko method needs to be taught over a number of sessions, generally given on a daily basis over a few days. Buteyko teachers have been fed information suggesting that this method of breathing may affect many different maladies and those that I know have been, in my opinion, overzealous in suggesting that patients 'throw away their crutches' (including stopping prescribed medication) sooner rather than later. It is best to follow a Buteyko method under the guidance of an independent physician or complementary medical practitioner.

The Buteyko method is based on training an individual to breathe less deeply than most Eastern breathing philosophies, and this creates a direct confrontation. I think that the answer lies in following the advice of yoga, Qi Gong, or meditation teachers whilst relaxing, exercising or meditating, but perhaps incorporating the Buteyko concepts into regular life.

CHELATION THERAPY

Chelation is the bonding together of a toxin, usually a metal, into another molecule. Nature has many compounds that chelate, but chelation therapy uses a chemical called ethylene-diamine-tetra-acetic acid (EDTA). This is used to remove heavy metals and toxins from the bloodstream.

This compound, given by intravenous drip, is used in the orthodox world to bind with metals such as mercury and lead that may be ingested or inhaled unintentionally. Chelation therapy was first used in the 1940s to treat lead poisoning. Physicians also noted several decades ago that EDTA treatment was useful in opening up blood vessels, possibly by reducing the calcium deposits or plaques of arteriosclerosis (atheroma).

Chelation therapy may be of benefit in removing industrial toxins that we take in through our food and from pollution. A session of the therapy takes about three hours, and is usually administered a few times a week over two or three months. Chelation therapy is now being used in combination with oxygen and high-dose vitamin therapy in fighting cancer. Treatment is only licensed to fully qualified medical practitioners because EDTA may be toxic, and specific amounts must be given depending upon certain kidney functions.

DMSA (meso-2, 3-dimercaptosuccinic acid) is a sulphur-containing amino acid that binds to metals. This larger molecule tends to be flushed out through the kidneys and the bowel and it can be taken as an alternative to the more interventional EDTA therapy.

CHINESE AND ORIENTAL MEDICINE

The ancient traditions of Eastern medicine have developed over many centuries. While there are differences between them in terms of methods of diagnosis and treatment, they all have the same basic philosophy. This has its foundation in a belief that the body is controlled by energy, and not by anatomy or physiology as it is in the Western tradition. The human body is seen as a microcosm of the universe, governed by the same energy and the same five elements. This energy or life force flows through the body in channels or meridians and ill-health is a disruption of this energy flow. The body, like the universe, is made up of five elements through which cosmic energy is manifested: ether, earth, water, fire and air in Ayurvedic medicine, and earth, wood, metal, fire and water in Chinese medicine.

In Chinese medicine there is an emphasis on balancing the life force, known as *Qi* or *chi*. Good health is maintained when the opposing principles of the chi, called Yin (negative) and Yang (positive) are in balance. Ill-health is seen as a disturbance of this balance, or disharmony, so that the life force cannot flow freely through the body. Treatment is aimed at strengthening Yin or Yang or eliminating excess Yin or Yang. This is done by various methods, from making lifestyle changes via nutrition, diet, exercise and meditation, to herbal remedies and bodywork which includes manipulation and acupuncture/acupressure.

Medicinal herbs are a small part of Oriental medicine and vary depending on the plants grown in the area. Thai and Vietnamese medicine, for example, differ from Cambodian or Tibetan in the plants used, although the underlying belief system is similar. The Chinese use a different meridian chart from the Tibetan one, which follows much more closely the routes travelled by nerves.

Like Ayurvedic medicine, Chinese, Tibetan and Oriental medicine should be considered only

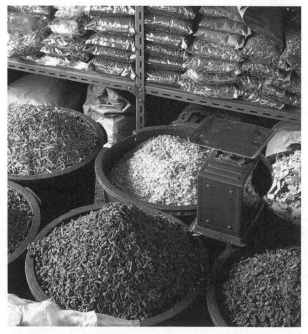

Chinese medicinal herbs and sliced horns ready for weighing and packing.

if a total lifestyle change is possible and acceptable because these disciplines do not have a 'quick-fix' answer.

CHIROPRACTIC

Chiropractic, derived from the Greek words 'kheir' (meaning hand) and 'praktikos' (meaning practical), is a manipulative technique which corrects the alignment of the bones of the spine in order to treat a wide range of health problems. By adjusting the position of the spinal bones and joints, and thereby the muscles and nerves attached to them, mobility is restored and pain relieved.

The system was devised in the United States at the turn of the century by Dr David Daniel Palmer (1845–1913). Palmer was a gifted healer who discovered the power of spinal manipulation. By adjusting spinal vertebrae he cured one patient of deafness and treated heart disease in another. He became convinced that the displacement of vertebrae caused disease, and developed a theory that displaced or 'subluxed' vertebrae restricted the spinal nerves, blocking the flow of nervous energy through the body. Although some of Palmer's ideas are no longer seen as correct today, many research studies in recent times have confirmed the therapy's effectiveness. In particular, an eight-year clinical trial, published by the Medical Research Council in 1990, clearly established the superiority of chiropractic over hospital treatment for lower back pain.

Chiropractors generally work on musculoskeletal problems such as back and neck pain or complaints created by structural misalignment such as headaches, migraines, sciatica and sports injuries. It is not only very effective for mechanical problems causing pain in the joints, muscles, ligaments, discs and nerves in the back, but it has also been used to improve asthma and other breathing problems, to lessen allergies and alleviate digestive disorders. One chiropractor has recently published a short study of nine patients with tinnitus (ringing in the ears) and claims some success. It may be that manipulation of the neck can benefit many different internal problems.

Chiropractic has much in common with osteopathy (*see* **Osteopathy**). Osteopaths use similar manipulative techniques but have a much broader training in physiology and they manipulate soft tissues as well as the skeleton. Chiropractic, in well-trained hands, is a safe and extremely effective treatment.

CLINICAL ECOLOGY

Clinical ecology, also called environmental medicine, developed from research into allergies in the early 20th century. I believe that it was Hippocrates in the 5th century BC who suggested 'let food be your medicine and medicine be your food'. Most practitioners of holistic medicine would agree that the bulk of our ill-health stems from that which we put into our bodies. This includes not only food itself, but with it the persistent and almost unavoidable ingestion of agrochemicals (such as pesticides, fungicides and weedkillers), as well as airborne pollution from petrol and diesel fumes and household cleaning compounds. All these environmental factors are very likely to be detrimental to our well-being, weakening our immune system and making us susceptible to allergies and intolerances.

Clinical ecology takes this into account, and pays special attention to the probability of the development of intolerances and allergies to toxic substances in foods that we commonly eat. Symptoms may well be associated with leaky gut syndrome in most cases, and irritants and allergens may create any number of illnesses, including respiratory problems, digestive disorders, infertility, headaches and migraines, and even cancer.

Using techniques ranging from applied kinesiology, iridology, bioresonance techniques and blood tests, a clinical ecologist will try to isolate problem foods or toxins. The practitioner uses elimination diets, desensitization techniques and any other preferred naturopathic treatments, such as herbal medicine or homeopathy, to remove these. Practitioners will also suggest changes in lifestyle to avoid exposure to environmental irritants such as dust, pollen and chemicals. Mild forms of sensitivity or intolerance may respond well to antioxidant supplements, as well as to drinking filtered tap water.

COLONIC IRRIGATION AND ENEMAS

Colonic irrigation, also known as colonic hydrotherapy, is becoming an increasingly popular technique for clearing out the bowel. Water is passed through a tube into the bowel via the rectum, and used to flush out the bowel contents. Most people report feeling distinctly refreshed and more energetic after having the procedure. The principle is that many toxins build up in the colon where they may fester or even be absorbed into the bloodstream, and the individual invariably feels better for having these removed. The physical benefits commonly reported include relief from constipation, diarrhoea, bloating and wind, intestinal pain, skin problems, stress and general sluggishness. Many practitioners also offer advice on nutrition as well as other therapies such as massage.

I remain somewhat doubtful about colonic irrigation. I have often seen pictures of the remarkable amount of debris that is removed following the procedure but I wonder what it was doing there if the individual was having regular bowel motions. What is more, during my time in hospital, I have seen many colons that have been prepared for colonoscopy or bowel surgery that look immaculately clean once the scope has been passed. The bowels are generally cleansed by taking large amounts of water and a potent laxative 12 hours before the procedure. It appears to me that a fast with some fibre and a natural laxative may be just as effective as the artificial technique of flushing a fluid the wrong way around the colon.

Colonic irrigation and enemas have their place, especially if the bowel is stagnant for any medical reason and, provided that the technique is performed under the watchful eye of an experienced practitioner, is not particularly dangerous. A series of four to eight irrigations is usually recommended, and each procedure takes about half an hour. There are tales of bowel rupture if colonics are performed on individuals with a friable colon but I dare say that the incidence is far less than for those undergoing colonoscopy in an orthodox hospital.

COLOUR THERAPY

Colours affect the mood and emotions, and can therefore influence health. Many studies have shown that colour can have a profound effect on the function of brain waves and on the levels of circulating stress hormones such as adrenaline and cortisol. Colour therapists use colour or coloured light to treat illness. At a simple level, green has been shown to be calming and is actually used as the main wall colour in most hospitals. Blue light is also calming and lowers blood pressure, while red light is stimulating and increases blood pressure.

The use of colour to aid healing involves the whole spectrum of colours. The therapist may diagnose the colour a person needs by noting which colours they like and dislike, by looking at their 'aura' to see what colour it is, and by taking a medical history. When the colours most suited to an individual have been identified and isolated, the therapist will administer the treatment in various ways. For example, you may be bathed in coloured light, or asked to eat food of a certain colour. Some therapists will advise you to change the colour of your home environment or to wear clothes of a particular colour.

It is difficult to use colour therapy as a self-help treatment without detailed advice, and a practising colour therapist or a simple book on the subject is recommended. It is certainly worth exploring as an adjunct therapy to other treatments.

COUNSELLING – see Psychotherapy

CRANIOSACRAL THERAPY

Craniosacral therapy, effectively a branch of osteopathy (and similar to the technique of cranial osteopathy), supports the view that the skull bones (cranium) are not completely fused and immobile. Whereas the orthodox world considers the only mobile joints involving the skull to be at the point where the cranium attaches to the spinal column and at the jaw, this is in fact not the case: minute movements are measurable all over the skull. The craniosacral therapist considers this movement to be relevant because the covering of the brain – the dura – will move with the skull bones. Movement will therefore apply pressures to the brain and thereby affect the entire nervous system.

By exerting very light pressure on the cranium the therapist treats the whole craniosacral system, which also includes the membranes and cerebrospinal fluid that surround the brain and spinal cord. Firstly the cranial pulse is palpated, to give information about the condition of the craniosacral system, and then the skull bones are gently manipulated in order to release any distortions. These can be the result of the cranial bones becoming misaligned or jammed after birth, injury, or even dental work. Pain anywhere from the head all the way down the spinal column can arise, and gentle traction of these bones, by releasing the internal tensions, will relieve it.

Any problem involving neurological supply may be created by cranial misalignment and successfully treated by this form of therapy. In principle most, if not all, health problems will have some neurological involvement and therefore craniosacral therapy may benefit most conditions. It has been found to be particularly useful in treating chronic pain, migraines, sinusitis, certain eye problems, twisted spine and joint stiffness. Craniosacral therapy works with the body's own healing ability, improves the functioning of the nervous system and brain, and so enhances general health and well-being.

CRYSTAL AND GEM THERAPY

The ancient belief that certain stones and crystals have healing properties has been held by many cultures. For example, the American Indians were given special stones at birth which were thought to have particular powers. We now know that all objects have a vibrational action: the electrons in the most 'dead' of substances are vibrating and maintaining an equilibrium within the molecules. It is theorized that gems and crystals give off a frequency that can affect the human body's resonance and may, indeed, be curative. This theory may combine with colour therapy (*see* **Colour Therapy**) and be of benefit as an adjunct to more mainline treatments.

Many practitioners today use the energies emitted by precious and semi-precious stones to enhance the body's ability to heal itself. Different stones are considered to have different therapeutic powers. For instance, a green stone (such as an emerald) will have a stress-reducing effect, while jade has long been used in traditional Chinese medicine to treat disorders of the kidneys and bladder. Quartz and amethyst crystals are thought to be particularly powerful. The healer will either place the stones around the patient, or give them to be worn or carried. Crystals placed in a room are also felt to have a positive effect on the atmosphere.

Crystals can also be used in colour therapy, using a special light box. Light shone through different crystals will intensify their healing energy and give an array of colours that stimulate different parts of the brain. Electro-crystal therapy involves transmitting pulses of high-frequency electromagnetic energy through crystals and on to the part of the body to be treated. Gem essences or elixirs may also be taken, so that the healing energy of the stones is absorbed directly into the body.

DANCE THERAPY

We are all aware of how body movements can relate concepts and express feelings. When trying to communicate with a speaker of another language, for example, sign language and gestures are invaluable. Eastern cultures, especially the Indian and Balinese cultures, integrate movement and dance very much more than the West into their lifestyle. Most tribal cultures have long included dance as part of their way of life, not only to express feelings but also as a means of reaching a higher level of consciousness. Both performing and watching such movements is known to be relaxing and transforming.

Dance therapy aims to release the natural flow of bodily self-expression in each individual, concentrating on natural, spontaneous and unrestricted movements rather than on formal dance patterns. Dance therapists support and motivate their clients to use this healing art form to connect to their unconscious mind, and many are integrating the possibility of an association with the stretching of meridians or energy channels that allow the vital force to move more freely.

A wide variety of situations are appropriate for this therapy. Music may or may not be used. Sometimes the creative aspects of dance are emphasized, sometimes the therapeutic aspects. It can be useful for people who would otherwise find it difficult to talk about their feelings, and is effective for most forms of psychological illness, mild or serious. Theoretically, physical illness affecting mobility such as Parkinsonism may benefit from the movement of Qi. Physical symptoms related to stress can also be helped by dance therapy.

Dance therapy takes many different forms and approaches. Eurythmy, an art of movement to music and speech developed in the Rudolph Steiner schools to foster the children's sense of rhythm, and Gabrielle Roth's Five Rhythms freestyle dance are both forms of therapy designed to encourage self-expression and creativity.

DOWSING

Dowsing is the use of an instrument, be it pendulum, rods or a fork-shaped stick, that picks up some presently immeasurable energy. At the end of the nineteenth century it was realized that, if dowsers can locate the sites of water, metal and other substances under the ground, then they ought to be able to locate the sites of disease in the body in the same way. Tests were carried out, mainly in France, and it was discovered that they could. The orthodox world continues to be sceptical, but as we delve more into quantum physics I

would not be surprised if, in the near future, we find some justifiable explanation of why a pendulum should swing or a divining rod rise or fall in a different pattern depending upon the substance over which it is held. The process does not seem to work if the instrument is attached to a non-organic (non-living) object, raising even more doubts in the scientist.

In the medical use of dowsing there seems to be an interplay between the energy of the practitioner and of the patient, or sample of the patient's hair or blood. The pendulum or divining instrument merely reflects this. It is a bit like attaching a voltmeter to two ends of a battery: there need to be two opposing or different energies to create a movement.

Dowsing may also be used to determine the most effective treatment against the disease. The success of the technique relies largely on the skill and sensitivity of the practitioner rather than on the instrument used. Some dowsers do not need to use a pendulum at all, but simply by holding their hands over the patient's body will be able to sense a change in vibration or heat and thereby detect the site of an illness. Healers, in this way, are in fact dowsers.

This is a diagnostic technique that may be useful in conjunction with more orthodox techniques but should not be relied upon by itself. This is not because I doubt the efficacy of the technique but because the assessment is very subjective, depending upon the practitioner.

ENZYME-POTENTIATED DESENSITIZATION (EPD)

Those doctors who practise enzyme-potentiated desensitization would probably be surprised at my putting this treatment into a section on alternative therapies. I do so simply because at the time of writing this is not a well-established therapy, even though the first treatments were carried out at St Mary's Hospital Allergy Clinic in Oxford, UK, in 1966.

The principle of desensitization is based on a

release of a chemical called beta-glucuronidase by specific white blood cells involved in the immune response. This beta-glucuronidase is attached to a known allergen and kept next to the skin for several days or injected into the system. The body becomes tolerant of the allergen and any allergic response is reduced.

Enzyme-potentiated desensitization is currently licensed only for use in asthma by the NHS, and the boffins in Oxford are adamant that the technique should not be used for anything else. This is because they do not want 'cowboys' to use the technique incorrectly and discredit the work. If this treatment is successful billions of dollars will be wiped off the pharmaceutical companies' profits because of the decreased necessity of asthma drugs and any other compounds used in allergic-responsive conditions. We await the future with interest.

FELDENKRAIS METHOD

Moshe Feldenkrais (1904–84) was a Russian physicist and engineer who came to England in 1940. He theorized that from infancy our brain develops patterns of movement. Bad posture or gait in a parent could therefore be passed on to a child, and this incorrect structure can have an effect on the neurological and muscular systems. His exploration of the dynamics of movement in the human body led to the development of his movement method.

The Feldenkrais method teaches gentle sequences of movement which aim to reorganize previous patterns of action so that the body may be used more effectively. Feldenkrais believed that the body and mind were connected and profoundly affected one another, and that changing negative habits of movement and posture would not only enhance physical well-being but also have positive influence on the mind and emotions. As with the Alexander Technique, pupils learn how to change their restrictive patterns and habits of movement using an awareness technique, and this leads to an increased sense of

relaxation and a reduction in stress which benefit the mind as well as the body.

The method is taught in two ways: in a group class called 'awareness through movement', the teacher guides students verbally through a series of slow exercises, carried out at first while lying down so that the strain on the body is minimized. Then, in an individual lesson called 'functional integration', the teacher guides the student by means of touch, in conjunction with gentle manipulation and massage. Individual lessons are particularly beneficial for those with disabilities or painful injuries.

Anyone can gain from the Feldenkrais method. It is helpful in cases of chronic pain and helps recovery from physical trauma. Because it is such a gentle therapy, it is suitable for stroke patients and children with cerebral palsy. The method is very popular among athletes and those in the performing arts.

FENG SHUI

The Eastern philosophies, but particularly the Chinese and Japanese, believe strongly that the universe is connected through immeasurable energy. This *Qi* emanates from all living organisms and permeates all matter. The forces of the universe, the movement of water, light, wind and everything else in the natural world – all these things have an energy which has an influence on everything else. The scientist who recently suggested that the flapping of a butterfly's wings in the Amazon may cause a storm in Central America was merely validating an age-old concept.

Feng Shui, meaning 'wind and water', evolved from these ancient principles, and is concerned with the movement of energy in one's immediate surroundings. It is the art of establishing the correct position for the body to be in at particular times of the day, so that negative energy can be curbed and positive healing energy increased. (This is a gross oversimplification but nevertheless describes the technique practically.) The position of the desk at work, the bed at night and the height of trees around the house all come into play, with a need to understand and vary colours and the shapes of household objects. Nearby water, visible or underground, is also significant. Water is associated with difficulty, and the flow of water can create ionic (charged particles) changes that strongly influence an individual's Qi.

More books are becoming available on Feng Shui but practical advice from an expert is always the best. He or she can look at your personal space and give advice on all aspects of placement for optimum harmony, seeing the good, and bad spaces for different areas of life within your home or office so that relationships, health, wealth, children, career and creativity may all be enhanced.

FLOTATION

The body and mind are constantly under 'sensory attack'. In the West, especially, it is very difficult to obtain a state of sensory deprivation. We are constantly surrounded by noise, sights and smells, and we are generally touching something all the time, even if it is merely the ground through our feet or our clothes which are in contact with our bodies.

A good meditation technique can remove us

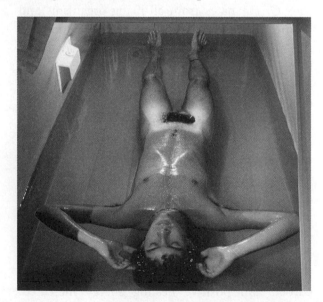

The water in this flotation chamber contains Epsom salts heated to body temperature. Silence is usual although soothing sounds may be channelled through underwater speakers.

from our senses, but an easier method is the Flotation Tank. This is a bath or pool containing a concentrated saline solution deep enough to allow the body to float, and enclosed in a capsule or cubicle. Floating in a high concentration of salt gives an individual greater buoyancy, allowing the body to be completely and effortlessly suspended and thereby relaxing all the muscles. The uniform surroundings thus created for the body by the water markedly reduce the sensation of touch. The tank is usually completely dark (although those who fear claustrophobia can benefit from a gentle light), is soundproof and should have no strong odour. The whole effect is of a warm, cosy environment which feels inviting and safe. By minimizing stimulation of all the senses, any tensions and anxieties can easily be let go. The feeling of deep relaxation that occurs usually endures for some time – up to several days – after the float.

This is a safe therapy which has been shown by research studies to lower high blood pressure and the level of stress-related chemicals in the body. It can also help reduce pain, because it stimulates the production of endorphins, the body's own pain-reducing hormones. Those who find other relaxation methods such as meditation difficult often find that floating is the answer, since it is passive and requires no effort. It can be used either as a substitute for meditation or as a way of stimulating the ability to meditate.

GEM THERAPY – *see* Crystal and gem therapy

GERSON THERAPY

Gerson therapy was developed by Max Gerson, a German who emigrated to the United States. He initially treated tuberculosis through a low-salt diet and then modified his recommendations for treatment of more chronic conditions, especially cancer. He believed that his regimes reversed the conditions that were necessary to support the growth of malignant cells. He promoted the elimination of toxins, protected and supported the liver and paid special attention to the balance of sodium and potassium in the body. Gerson therapy also encourages the use of thyroid supplements containing iodine and potassium but is principally a set dietary regime.

The diet proposes fresh, raw juices of vegetables and fruits taken regularly, in conjunction with a restricted fat and salt intake, a high intake of complex carbohydrates and a low proportion of protein foods. Coffee enemas are part of the treatment and, if organic liver is available, raw liver juice is prescribed. The diet is a strict one, and the regime, which also involves counselling, demands commitment on the part of the client.

The guidelines on diet now officially recommended by governments for optimum health follow the Gerson principles, and the therapy has been shown to enhance mood and well-being, promote faster healing of wounds and relieve pain. Research supports the Gerson concept as an anti-cancer therapy, but because there is no element within it that would create profits for a pharmaceutical company, little money goes into further studies (*see* chapter 7).

GESTALT THERAPY

This is a form of psychological therapy that creates a strong self-awareness. It is based upon the idea that an event not experienced by both logic and emotion is not completely experienced and causes an imbalance which leads to behavioural problems. A simple example is that of a child brought up in an abusive household. The conscious mind may make excuses for why he/she is being beaten, but to do so feelings of hurt and despair must be pushed aside. If this is done successfully then this trait carries over into other emotional experiences and the child will grow up suppressing and unable to express feelings.

The founder of Gestalt therapy was Fritz Perls, a Freudian-trained psychoanalyst who became disenchanted with psychoanalysis. His aim was to enable people to learn from their own experience to acknowledge previously denied or suppressed feelings. Rather than paying attention to *why*

clients behaved in a certain way he was more interested in *how* they behaved and what that behaviour meant to them. He was more attentive to non-verbal than verbal cues, and insisted that clients take responsibility for their behaviour and feelings. He also wished to help people see the effects of their behaviour on others, and this is why Gestalt therapy takes place in groups, sometimes called encounter groups.

A hallmark of Gestalt therapy is 'talking to the empty chair'. The client is asked to imagine that a person to whom they wished they had expressed certain feelings is sitting in the chair. They then have an opportunity to express those feelings. They may also be asked to place a part of themselves, for example an emotion or characteristic that they find uncomfortable, in the chair, and have a dialogue with that side of themselves. Other techniques include the highlighting of negative internal 'messages', also making clients speak always in the present tense and in the first person, in order to increase self-awareness. Interaction between the members of the group is encouraged, as is the discarding of inhibitions, although the leader of the group also aims to keep the environment safe and unpressured.

HEALING

All forms of treatment are healing, whether they are surgical, chemical or holistic therapies such as acupuncture or chiropractic. The term itself, however, describes one of the oldest forms of medicine, and means the technique of 'the laying on of hands' by healers who see themselves as the medium for a healing energy. Healing is thus a form of energy therapy based around some immeasurable force. Healers see the source of this force in various ways: some feel that it is a universal psychic energy that passes directly from them into the patient, while others believe that the force is divine in origin and that they are the conduit through which it flows. Faith healers believe that it is the power of God working through them, and this kind of healing has a long Christian tradition.

Healing can be effective regardless of personal beliefs; much more important are the quality of communication between healer and patient and the patient's receptivity and desire to get well.

The healing technique used may involve physically placing the hands on the body or by holding the hands over but somewhat away from the body. Practitioners can sense or feel a lack of energy and may focus their attention upon the energy centres or chakras. Some practitioners will actively vibrate their hands and others may go into a form of trance while they communicate with the 'spirit' or energy source that is transmitting the energy. Healing may also be performed or transmitted without any form of contact, as the practice of radionics shows.

Subjects react differently to healing sessions, which usually last for about half an hour. Some people feel a tingling, or a sensation of heat or cold under the healer's hand. They may feel better immediately, or need a series of sessions before noticing an improvement.

Healers report a sense of changes in their own energy field while healing, and research has shown that the effect of a healer's hand is similar to that of a strong electro-magnetic field. Other measurable physical changes in healers include a common pattern of brain waves that occurs during the healing process.

Every medical philosophy or therapy is utilizing healing energy and none can be considered any better than any other. There may be, however, a cumulative effect should a healer also prescribe homeopathy or practise osteopathy.

HELLERWORK

This is a form of bodywork founded in the late 1970s by Joseph Heller, an engineer. Based on the ideas of Ida Rolf with whom Heller had worked closely (*see* **Rolfing**), its purpose is to provide the individual with a sound foundation for good health by structurally realigning the body through movement and massage. It offers an education in the principles of movement that will help maintain and improve this balance once achieved. The goal, however, is not only to produce physical results as with Rolfing, but by emphasizing psycho-emotional aspects of the therapy, to empower clients to grow, change and improve their total well-being.

The therapy usually consists of eleven 90-minute sessions of deep-tissue bodywork and movement 're-education'. Specific to Hellerwork is dialogue between client and practitioner to explore the mind–body connection and uncover where unconscious thoughts and feelings may have created restrictive patterns in the body. The bodywork is a deep form of massage that concentrates on the interstitial or connective body tissues rather than the muscles or the skeleton itself. The aim is to release toxic and tension build-up, releasing stored stress and restoring balance. The client is also taught how to move in ways that increase body awareness and improve posture, so that everyday movements become easier, freer and smoother. Each session concentrates on a different part of the body and the emotions related to it, starting with the outer parts of the body such as the arms and legs, and going on to the 'core' areas deep within the body. Final sessions deal with the whole body, integrating all the work done previously.

By balancing the mind and body, Hellerwork aims primarily to prevent rather than treat health problems. Practitioners claim that the method relieves aches and pains, increases relaxation and improves general mobility and flexibility. Many medical conditions also respond well to this therapy, including headaches and migraine, chronic fatigue, disorders of the musculoskeletal system, respiratory problems such as asthma and stress-related conditions.

HERBAL MEDICINE

There are two sides to herbal medicine. The first is the pharmaceutical aspect and the second is the innate energy within the plant itself. In the West the therapeutic use of herbs is very much based on their chemical effects, and there is much

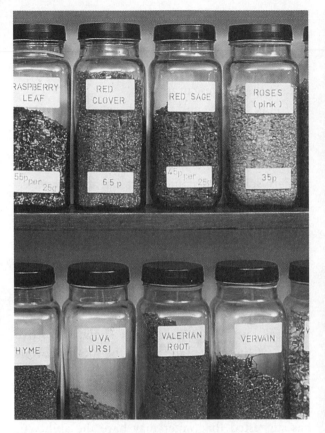

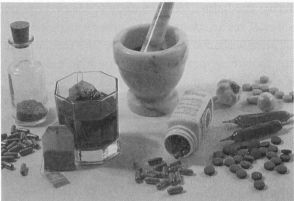

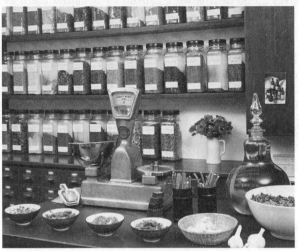

The shelves of a well-stocked herbalist and (above right) a selection of pills, capsules, preparations and teas made from the herbs.

research to suggest that the pharmaceutical benefits of herbal medicines are greater than those of orthodox drugs. Being naturally occurring chemicals, they seem to be broken down by the body more efficiently and with fewer side effects than seems to be the case with many artificially made drugs. Because they create fewer toxic metabolic byproducts, these chemicals can be broken down by the the liver and kidneys more easily.

A herbalist may follow the Western tradition and use plants native to Western Europe, or follow the Eastern philosophies and use traditional herbs from China or India. Eastern traditions seem to take into account both the chemical aspects of plants and also the energy within the plant cells and its structure. More emphasis is placed upon the plants' masculine/feminine, Yin/Yang and the earth/water/fire/air aspects.

Plant extracts contain steroids and other drugs such as salicylic acid (aspirin), and thereby work in exactly the same way as the proprietary drugs. Injudicious use or overuse can be just as harmful as regular drug-taking and may act by suppressing symptoms rather than dealing with the underlying cause, which is the principle of holistic medicine. The notorious success of Chinese herbs in eczema is an example of this. Most herbalists are scrupulous about sticking to the concept of natural medicine but many are not. The Eastern philosophies will rarely prescribe a herb without looking at the lifestyle as a whole but I have noticed that many practitioners of Eastern medicine are simply providing remedies with little or no insight into the person as a whole. Such herbalists should be avoided.

There is occasional 'bad press' concerning

herbal medicine. Very recently a major London hospital reported six deaths among people using Chinese herbs for skin problems. The media made out that these deaths were caused by unlicensed practitioners and that the whole of alternative/complementary medicine was a risk. In fact, all six cases were related to people overdosing on the compounds and should have created no more of a stir other than to press for the correct labelling of prescriptions. It is worth putting this piece of information into context by understanding that over 2,000 deaths were caused by over-the-counter (non-prescribed) medicines in 1994. There are no statistics to show the number of deaths caused by prescribed drugs that are taken incorrectly. Basically, herbal medicine is safe when prescribed in the right dosages by the right practitioner.

HOMEOPATHY

The term homeopathy is derived from the Greek words 'homo' meaning like and 'pathy' meaning illness. It is based on the idea that an illness which produces certain symptoms can be cured using a substance that produces the same symptoms in a healthy person. The term 'like cures like' explains this treatment in a simple manner.

The founder of this system was Christian Samuel Hahnemann, a respected German physician practising in the latter part of the 18th century. He noticed that individuals with aggressive symptoms of illness seemed to recover better than those who only had a mild response. He initially experimented by using the bark of the chinchona tree on individuals who had what we now know to be malaria. This bark caused the same symptoms as malaria, and when given in minute quantities seemed to stimulate the body's symptoms, which in turn defeated the affliction. Hahnemann was unaware of the existence of microbes but he stuck to this basic observation and experimented on himself, friends and patients and built up what is now known as a *Materia Medica* of plant, mineral and animal extracts that exhibit symptoms similar to diseases.

He found that using large amounts of a compound actually poisoned a system, but that using very small amounts would stimulate the body's own defences and enhance reactions that were in themselves curative.

To his surprise and to the disbelief of scientists today he found that by shaking the original substance vigorously in water he could dilute down the compound much more. With the advent of modern scientific techniques we can actually measure the amount of a substance within a solvent and in most homeopathic remedies over 'potency 20' there are no molecules of the original substance left. This defies the Law of Mass Action and therefore science discredits homeopathy as being a placebo effect. There are, however, over 160 papers on homeopathy published in reputable medical journals, all of which show a positive effect. Of these, 22 stand up to the most vigorous scientific standards, but the orthodox world still disbelieves the effects.

The work of a Professor Benveniste from Paris has suggested that water may have the ability to imprint upon its electron structure the electron energy from another substance. Professor Benveniste is a scientist and not a homeopath and has been ostracized from the scientific world because of his findings. He goes to great lengths to point out that he has no homeopathic bias and that he is only reporting his own scientific experiments. He is currently considered a maverick but his work is probably the most important alternative study taking place at the moment. I, personally, wish him the very best and hope that he can find the funding necessary to continue his experiments.

Homeopathic remedies prepared by vigorous shaking, known as succussion, are diluted 10 or 100 times before being succussed again. Each time this happens the potency increases a number. Most remedies come in potencies of 6, 7, 10, 12, 30, 200, 1,000 (better known as 1M), 50,000 (LM) or 100,000 (CM). Remedies and their potency often have the letters X or D after the potency number and these denote a dilution of 1 in 10, whereas the letter C denotes a dilution of 1 in 100. These letters should not be confused with LM and CM which represent the number of times a remedy is diluted, as described above. There is, generally, little difference in an X or a C dilution. The lower the potency the more physical the effect; and the higher potencies are generally reserved for psychological aspects of a patient.

A homeopath chooses a remedy based on a symptom picture of the person as a whole. There are, for example, over 400 remedies that have a fever, of which 200 will include sweating, 50 include flushing, 25 include trembling or shaking, 10 will be thirstless, 7 associated with diarrhoea, etc. The more symptoms presented, the more likely a remedy will be accurately prescribed.

A homeopath will also look at the constitution of an individual, which describes the temperament and personality of the person when well. A homeopath needs to have an understanding of where a patient needs to be returned to when choosing medication accurately. If one person is naturally a sweaty type, then remedies that are particularly dry may move the individual away from their constitution and slow down the healing process.

Homeopathy is a complicated matter and modern pharmacies try to simplify it by advising that, for example, Arnica is good for bruising, Belladonna for fevers, and Pulsatilla for earache. Homeopathy cannot be prescribed in this way because it must take into account the whole person and not just the symptom. When it is so used it often fails. This gives the practice a higher level of failure than it deserves.

Homeopathy can be safely used in any condition where the vital force of the individual is strong or intact, because a remedy will create reactions of healing from within. Homeopathy should not be used where the body is particularly weak because the underlying energy may not be strong enough, which at best will render homeopathy useless or may worsen an individual's health by using up the remaining energy more quickly.

HYDROTHERAPY

Water has many properties that are poorly understood by science. It is the only natural compound that is lighter when it is solid than as a liquid (ice floats). Water is also considered a universal solvent, which means that it will eventually break down any compound immersed within it. (Homeopathy is beginning to have some scientific justification based on the intrinsic electronic movement within water molecules.)

Hydrotherapy is the use of water to promote healing. It may be used as a liquid or steam, taken internally or externally either by immersion or by inhalation, and taken hot or cold. The water may have a high level of salts or be extremely pure, depending upon the reason for its use.

The healing benefits of water have been known for thousands of years and are well documented in ancient literature, Roman baths being most famous. These were built at the sites of natural springs, often where the water was hot or minerally rich. The popularity of the spa was at its height in Europe during the 18th and 19th centuries, and hundreds of towns became famous for their waters. Water is now a popular therapy in health farms and hospitals throughout Europe, and the increasing number of whirlpools, hot tubs

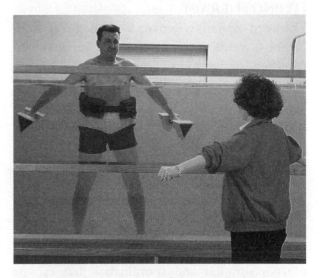

A patient exercises with weights in a hydrotherapy pool in order to build up strength and improve joint mobility.

and jacuzzis in hotels and sports clubs is testimony to the immediate beneficial effects of immersion in water.

Therapies include wrapping, baths, douches or showers, sitz baths (where only the lower part of the body is immersed) and steam or Turkish baths. Herb and mineral baths and sea-water baths (thalassotherapy) are also used. Sprays and steam may be used externally and inhalations with or without essential oils may be of benefit (*see* **Aromatherapy**). Hot water is used to stimulate and then relax, while cold water invigorates. Alternate use of hot and cold water stimulates blood and lymph circulation, tones tissues and relieves congestion. Sitz baths are used in this way to treat pelvic and abdominal disorders, liver and kidney problems, constipation and piles. Hydrotherapy is also beneficial for people with physical disabilities since the buoyancy of the water allows an increased range of movement.

Hydrotherapy is one of the safest and cheapest ways of relieving common ailments, and is therefore ideal for self-help treatment. Exercising in water brings relief from aches and pains, increased relaxation and greater flexibility, and also promotes fitness and a sense of well-being.

HYPNOTHERAPY

The word *hypnosis* is derived from the Greek word 'hypnos', meaning 'to sleep'. It was brought into common parlance by Scottish surgeon James Braid in the 1840s. Hypnotherapy techniques were used with operative procedures before the use of anaesthetic and had developed from the theories of a Dr Mesmer from 60 years before.

Hypnotherapy is the production of a trance-like state that is not dissimilar to daydreaming. In effect, the consciousness leaves the body, which continues to be controlled and protected by the subconscious. An example is thinking of a beach in Rio while driving a car. Driving demands a lot of concentration and coordination but can be done without thinking about it. If a child were to run in front of a car the subconscious would not

have the ability to avoid it. The consciousness is called back into the body, which deals with the situation, and Rio is forgotten!

I divide hypnotherapy into two techniques. The first is suggestive and the second is 'part'. In both techniques the individual is taken into a deep relaxed state through imagining a comfortable and enjoyable place. The suggestive hypnotherapist will then plant an idea into the subconscious, such as that an onion is an apple or a cigarette is nauseating. When the consciousness returns the subconscious holds this concept and the individual will bite into the onion with relish (as often seen in shows) or may wish to stop smoking (as is seen in therapeutic hypnosis). 'Part' hypnotherapy is geared towards discussing matters with the subconscious and finding out which part of the individual's past has triggered the unnecessary or unwanted psychological problem. Part hypnotherapy should not be undertaken by those who cannot afford or intend to follow through with the psychological support that is often necessary when something deeply buried comes forward and which can markedly affect their life. Suggestive hypnotherapy is safer but may not be quite so effective. I would like to stress that these definitions are my own and would need to be explained to a hypnotherapist to find out which form of treatment they intend to use.

KINESIOLOGY

Kinesiology is a manipulative therapy, based on diagnosing imbalances or deficiencies in nutrition or energy flow by testing the strength of muscles. Applied kinesiology was developed during the 1960s by Dr George Goodheart, an American chiropractor. He discovered that massaging the neuro-lymphatic reflexes strengthened muscles. He linked his discoveries with oriental medical ideas of the Qi, or vital force, which flows through the body and can be stimulated by using pressure points. To this extent kinesiology is not very different from acupressure.

Goodheart was more convinced that the

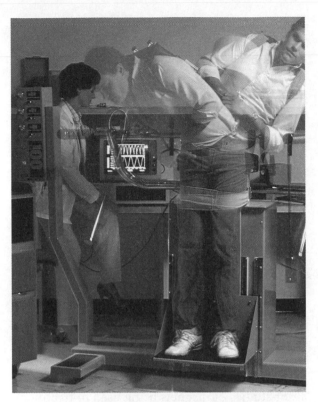

A volunteer undergoing kinesiology tests. A computer displays the flexion of the spine from left to right as the subject performs bending movements.

technique's effectiveness was based on spinal reflexes but, whatever the underlying cause, he found that one stimulated muscle can affect others in a different part of the body. This idea has since been expanded, and it has been noted that the strength of a muscle will vary momentarily in response to the body coming into contact with a product to which it is intolerant or allergic, as well as responding in a positive way to compounds in which it may be deficient.

A practitioner will test a muscle group (either trying to force apart opposed index finger and thumb or testing shoulder muscles by having the patient hold out the arm as it is pushed down) while the patient has a variety of different foods placed on the tongue, one at a time. Some kinesiologists have taken the step of simply placing a compound on the abdomen or even only using the homeopathic form. Theoretically the resonance of a substance is passed into the watery solution when it is prepared as a homeopathic remedy. Even further removed is the belief that the thought of a compound will affect the muscular energy. Some practitioners simply ask an individual to read a list of compounds one word at a time and test the muscle group. Even the word 'yes' as opposed to 'no' can strengthen or weaken a muscle group. Used in conjunction with more orthodox diagnostic techniques kinesiology can be a most supportive diagnostic investigation. Its therapeutic effects are based on acupuncture and acupressure.

KIRLIAN PHOTOGRAPHY

This is high-frequency photography used to produce a photograph of the 'aura' of energy that surrounds a person. Semyon and Valentina Kirlian, who discovered and developed the method for diagnostic purposes, found that photographs made using this technique showed differences in the energy field of healthy and diseased subjects. It is said that a healthy person emits a strong aura, while a person with disease, whether manifest or latent, emits a weak aura. Any imbalances requiring treatment will be identified after interpretation of the aura by the practitioner.

Under strictly controlled conditions a Kirlian photograph of the two hands of the patient is usually taken. The resulting print will show a furry effect surrounding the outline of the hands, with flares of energy and areas of blockage that can be used to diagnose certain illnesses (*see* **Kirlian photography** *in chapter 8*).

LIGHT THERAPY

Light has a direct effect on the workings of the body and on our moods. When the sun comes out our spirits rise and we feel more energetic, while insufficient light can lead to depression and lethargy. Light is known to stimulate the pineal and pituitary glands, which correspond to the highest two chakras (energy centres) in yogic medicine. There is much scientific evidence to show that certain chemicals such as melatonin are produced or suppressed by sunlight. Melatonin controls our sleep patterns but an excess can lead to depression and tiredness. Seasonal Affective Disorder (SAD), a depression that occurs through the winter, can easily be improved by subjecting an individual to bursts of full-spectrum light. This mimics natural sunlight, exposure to which increases the amount of serotonin (the 'feel-good' hormone) produced by the body.

Light therapy is used to treat a range of other problems associated with hormone imbalance. Menopausal and premenstrual problems, infertility and loss of libido have all responded well to light therapy which works directly on the eyes stimulating the pineal gland in the brain. The body needs sunlight in order to manufacture vitamin D, essential for maintaining the health of the bones and skin. Skin disorders such as acne, eczema and psoriasis, as well as the debilitating bone disease osteoporosis, may all benefit from light therapy. In these cases the light is shone on to the skin as well as the eyes. Light therapy is also used to boost the immune system and improve blood circulation.

Each session of therapy involves lying on a couch under an overhanging light, and lasts for about 45 minutes. For acute cases a weekly session is usually recommended at first. People usually respond very quickly to the therapy and after a few sessions find that they only need 'top-up' sessions occasionally.

Light therapy is also part of crystal therapy (*see* **Crystal and gem therapy**).

MAGNETIC THERAPY

The earth has its own electromagnetic field, aligned to the poles, and the cells of the human body also have subtle magnetic forces. Conventional medicine uses electromagnetic energy in imaging equipment, harnessing this force (MRI scans) for diagnosis, and also in order to influence the body's own electrical currents to promote healing, particularly of fractures. Complementary therapists claim that ordinary magnets can also

do this, and many are beginning to use magnets as part of a healing programme.

The body has many electromagnetic energies travelling through it which are measurable or assumed, as in Eastern meridian channels, and magnetic therapy is particularly well known in Japan. The use of powerful magnets placed close to the body for a short or long period of time can influence blood flow, improving the oxygen supply to the area being treated, and stimulating the metabolism and speeding the elimination of waste products. Magnetic therapy may be used as a self-help treatment, and many magnetic products, such as shoe insoles, mattresses, pillows and car-seat covers are available. A practitioner will suggest the most suitable items for your needs, and show you how to use them. Special supermagnets may be used for specific points on the body, often over lymph nodes or acupuncture points.

At this time we still await some reasonable trials or studies of magnets being used in treatment. If a practitioner has had some experience or training then I can see no risk, except that I would avoid magnetic therapy in conditions that might have been triggered by electromagnetic energy, such as cancer.

MARMA THERAPY

A Marma point is defined in Ayurvedic medicine as a site on the body where flesh, veins, arteries, tendons, joints and bones meet. There are 107 of these 'vital points' throughout the body, and it is believed that an injury to any one of them – such as a puncture wound, burn or impact injury – will lead to permanent damage or even death. Marma therapy is an ancient form of massage which uses the fingers to stimulate the Marma points, thereby promoting physical and mental healing and well-being.

The Ayurvedic system emphasizes the preventive aspects of healthcare, and part of this is Marma massage, which increases blood flow to the neuromuscular junction of each point and tones the surrounding muscles. Results of a Marma massage include increased levels of energy, reduced stress and freedom from tension and anxiety.

There are also many medical applications for Marma massage. It has been shown to be of particular benefit to stroke victims, because it can clear away obstructions which delay information being communicated between muscles, nerves and brain, and thus help the brain relearn the use of the parts of the body paralysed or debilitated by the stroke. Other symptoms that are alleviated through Marma massage include muscular aches and pains, light-headedness, numbness and tingling in the extremities, and a metallic taste in the mouth, as well as stress-related conditions.

The Marma therapist also checks the acidic levels of the tongue with a litmus paper (a healthy result is 60 per cent alkaline to 40 per cent acid) as well as the muscle and nerve reflexes. A course of between two and six weekly sessions is usually recommended in order to restore full physical and mental health. Stroke victims usually need more treatments, often to be carried out over several months.

MASSAGE

Massage is the manipulation of the soft tissues in the body, particularly muscles, in order to promote relaxation and healing. There are many different massage techniques, and some practitioners may use or base their technique on different body therapies such as Shiatsu, Rolfing or physiotherapy, while others use a more intuitive approach. All branches of massage are effective, either in removing cramps, pain and tension from the muscles or in stimulating the lymph glands (part of the body's immune system) to eliminate toxins.

The massage session usually takes place at a health centre or at the home of the therapist, but in some circumstances the masseur will come to your home. Some practitioners work with the client lying on the floor but most will use a massage table. The therapist will work with oil on their hands, to facilitate the smooth, flowing movements of their hands over your skin. A variety of strokes are used, including kneading, rubbing, pummelling, circling and stroking, using fingertips, thumb or the whole hand.

Choosing a massage technique or practitioner is very much a subjective decision. It is worth experimenting with different types of bodywork until a preferred technique or practitioner is found. Some therapists employ more vigorous techniques than others. There is some concern that massage should not be employed in cancer because this may spread the tumour, although there is no evidence to back this up. I think it wise to avoid lymphatic drainage techniques in a cancer that is known to have spread through the lymphatic system, but massage that employs acupressure such as Shiatsu should be fine.

The use of aromatic essential oils in conjunction with massage brings together two forms of healing therapy, combining the benefits of massage with those of the oil, which acts directly on the bloodstream (*see* **Aromatherapy**). Whichever type of massage you choose, the experience is pleasant because it feels nurturing, soothing and relaxing, and at the same time is often invigorating. Its benefits are often felt for hours or even days afterwards, especially when used as part of a programme for combating stress.

MEDITATION

Meditation is a way of transcending the everyday level of consciouness by emptying the mind of conscious thoughts and concerns. It involves training your awareness so that your mental processes come under conscious control. There are many forms of meditation but their goal is always to enhance physical and mental well-being.

Meditation has been practised for at least 3,000 years. Most of the forms we know today are of Eastern origin and associated with spiritual practice, but for most people in the West meditation is seen as a simple self-help technique for which no religious beliefs are necessary. The practical advantages of meditation are that it can be performed in any comfortable place where you

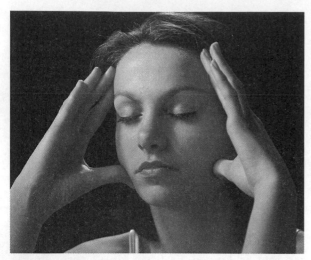

Any comfortable position that aids relaxation is suitable for practising meditation.

will be undisturbed for 20 minutes or so, and that any sitting or lying position that suits the individual may be adopted.

There are two stages in the meditative process: the first is physical relaxation and the second is focusing and emptying the mind. Concentrating on your breathing is an ideal way of doing this, as it makes you focus on something calming which also blocks out other thoughts and quietens the mind. Some people find it more helpful to repeat a single word or mantra, or focus on a single object such as a flower or a candle. Whatever the method used, breathing should be unforced and slow, with the stomach gently rising and falling and the shoulders staying still. When you are relaxed, close your eyes and continue to concentrate on each in and out breath, excluding all other thoughts, until you gradually become more and more relaxed, eventually reaching a trance-like state. At this point the mind is calm yet alert; the brain is producing an even pattern of alpha and theta brainwaves which is the 'relaxation response'. You have reached a state of the utmost balance and harmony and let go of all tensions.

Research has shown that regular meditation, for about 20 minutes once or twice a day, lowers blood pressure and relieves depression and anxiety. Other benefits include improved concentration, creativity and memory and increased energy levels. Meditation has also helped people overcome addictions to drugs such as tranquillizers and alcohol.

Meditation is discussed more fully elsewhere in this book (*see* **Meditation**).

MUD THERAPY

Immersing oneself in mud for its medical benefits is a form of hydrotherapy (*see* **Hydrotherapy**). Mud contains high levels of vitamins and minerals, small amounts of which will be absorbed through otherwise impregnable skin. There is certainly external benefit and mud therapy may be useful for treating skin conditions such as acne, eczema and psoriasis. The internal benefits are suggested but not well documented, and it is probable that the small amounts that are absorbed are dealt with by the efficient liver and kidney before any therapeutic benefit can be experienced. The nerves in the skin may well set up reflex responses through the spinal column.

Mud therapy is an excellent form of treatment, particularly for dermatological conditions, but is not easily available since very few mud spas exist. The Moor in Austria is one highly regarded spa, based beside a boggy lake and marshland which is home to hundreds of unique medicinal herbs whose lipids, enzymes, minerals and vitamins are dissolved in the water and mud of the lake. These have been shown to have many healing properties when applied to the skin, and their anti-inflammatory quality makes Moor treatment particularly useful for rheumatism and arthritis. Research into the benefits of mud therapy is currently going on and the results look promising.

Products from the Moor and from other spas are now becoming available for use at home, either in the form of powders or in tubs and tubes. Ideally the mud should be applied to the skin as a soft paste, but since this is an extremely messy procedure it is probably better to use a liquid mud extract in the bath. Follow the instructions on the container and soak in the hot bath for about 20 minutes. Afterwards, take a shower and get into a warm bed. You will sweat as the impurities and toxins in the body are drawn out.

MUSIC THERAPY

The ability to appreciate and respond to music is an inborn quality in human beings. Rarely is this ability affected by handicap, injury or illness, and it is not dependent on music training. For people who find verbal communication difficult, particularly those with mental illness or physical, learning or sensory disabilities, music therapy offers a safe, secure way of releasing feelings.

Fundamental to music therapy is the development of a relationship between the therapist and client, in which music becomes the basis for communication and a way of promoting change and growth. There are different approaches to the use of music in therapy, depending on the needs of the client as well as the preferred style of the therapist but they all involve playing, singing and listening, either in group or individual sessions. The therapist does not teach the client to sing or play an instrument, but encourages improvization with percussion and other accessible instruments as well as the voice in order to explore the world of sound and create a personal musical language. By responding musically, the therapist supports this process and encourages positive changes in behaviour and well-being.

Music therapists work with adults and children of all ages, in hospitals, special schools, day and community centres and in private practice. Involvement in creative music-making is particularly useful in psychological treatments for children with behavioural problems, language impairment and birth defects, since it promotes physical awareness and develops attention, concentration and memory. For people with emotional difficulties, music therapy allows the safe expression of otherwise repressed or 'difficult' feelings. By offering support and acceptance, the therapist can help the client work towards emotional release and self-acceptance. Increasingly, music therapy is being sought by people who do not have any specific difficulties but who would like to enhance their creativity and gain insight into themselves and their ways of relating to others (*see* **Sound therapy**).

NATUROPATHY

Naturopathy is a broad term used to describe a multi-disciplinary approach to illness and health. Its practitioners have expertise in a variety of medical therapies, and follow many of the same principles as the Eastern approach to medicine. Ayurvedic, Chinese, Tibetan and other Eastern philosophies of medicine all share a view of life and health that looks at the whole person rather than at just the symptoms. Naturopathy is the Western equivalent, in which a fundamental idea is that the body has the power to heal itself through its 'vital force', and that illness is a reaction to disharmony and imbalance in the body.

The aim of naturopathy is to help the body to regain health by restoring its natural balance rather than by addressing specific symptoms. Indeed, modern research confirms the naturopath's belief that many symptoms such as fever and inflammation do have a healing function. The naturopath teaches the patient how to help to boost the body's own defences, mainly through giving advice on lifestyle adjustments and diet. A healthy wholefood diet, fresh air, an unpolluted environment, exercise, adequate rest and sleep, a reduction in stress and a positive mental attitude will all strengthen the body's immune system and enhance its self-healing abilities.

Naturopaths see themselves as teachers as much as healers, believing that everyone should take personal responsibility for their own health. The body will heal itself and fight off invading organisms when its homeostatic balance is reinstated. The methods used to do this emphasize good nutrition with vitamin supplements, exercise, bodywork, relaxation and breathing techniques, all of which work with nature rather than against it. Natural medicines (herbal or homeopathic) are also used in naturopathy. Theoretically, a homeopath who spends time on adjusting the lifestyle of an individual is practising naturopathy. Naturopaths have training in some form of body-work, usually osteopathy in this country. Fasting, massage and hydrotherapy are also important features of naturopathic therapy.

Most health problems, acute or chronic, may be treated by naturopathy and many research studies have shown that naturopathic methods are an effective alternative to conventional medical treatment. The therapeutic value of a healthy lifestyle, a vital part of the naturopathic philosophy, is now being confirmed by modern research and is widely accepted.

NEURO-LINGUISTIC PROGRAMMING (NLP)

Neuro-linguistic programming is a form of psychotherapy that was developed from the work of several well-known therapists in the 1970s. It accurately describes its principle within its own name: the nerves (neuro) are affected by language (linguistic) and, like a computer, can reprogram the thought process. Basically, NLP reorganizes how people think and allows emotions to flow in a way that they perhaps have never previously done.

The technique depends for its success on the patterns of communication in the relationship between therapist and client, rather than on the particular theories about therapeutic change held by the therapist. The practitioner approaches each client as a unique individual, noting the minutiae of the client's behaviour and body language, in order to understand that person's mechanisms of perception. For example, by observing changes in pupil size, direction of gaze, head movements and breathing, the therapist can identify whether a person is using visual or auditory recall. The therapist can then communicate with the client in the appropriate way, encouraging rapport.

NLP can be used to change deeply-buried emotional states and is therefore generally practised by experienced psychotherapists who can deal with what changes are necessary. Practitioners

are often trained in hypnotherapy, allowing access to the deepest areas of the subconscious. The client learns some of the skills used by the therapist, such as mirroring, reframing, disassociation and anchoring.

Anchoring is the recalling of good or positive experiences and using them as resources for the future, so that they can be superimposed on a situation that has unpleasant feelings and make those bad feelings less potent. In this way clients increase awareness of how their thoughts, beliefs and values influence how they perceive the world and that they can learn new thought patterns in order to make changes to unhelpful ways of functioning and thereby increase personal happiness. NLP is a method of thinking and acting more effectively, in order to succeed in any area of life, whether it is work, relationships, self-esteem or creativity.

NEUROTHERAPY

This form of treatment is new to the West. It is a branch of Ayurvedic medicine, utilizing all aspects of prayer/meditation, dietetics and nutrition, exercise and lifestyle changes in conjunction with a specific form of therapy involving the meridians of the body.

A neurotherapeutic practitioner will lay the patient on the floor and, while bearing most of their body weight on two chairs beside the patient, will apply pressure on the back through the feet. Particular trigger or acupressure points will be pushed by specific parts of the practitioner's feet, thereby stimulating reflex responses and passing energy from the practitioner's reflexology meridian points directly into meridians in the patient's back. This treatment is yet to become well established but can be useful for an array of conditions, either on its own or in conjunction with more mainline treatments.

ONANI

Onani is a form of medicine practised in Northern India and Pakistan. It is principally derived from Ayurvedic medicine but also includes ideas based on Greek and Arab sources. Onani differs from Ayurvedic practice in some of the medicinal herbs prescribed, and it also incorporates the therapeutic use of minerals.

OSTEOPATHY

Osteopathy is a manipulative technique in which the bones, muscles, ligaments and nerves are restored to their proper alignment and functioning. It is probably the most widely used of the complementary therapies, and certain States in the USA consider an osteopath to have equal training to a doctor.

Osteopathy was devised by an American doctor, Andrew Taylor Still, at the end of the 1800s. In principle, Still felt that the disease process occurred because of structural misalignments. He postulated that when vertebrae slip out of position the nerves around them become oversensitive and affect surrounding tissue. This in turn affects blood circulation, and since the blood carries substances to protect against disease, the blocked circulation leads to illness. His theories can be well supported because poor structure may obstruct blood flow, nerve conduction and, from an Eastern perspective, Qi or energy flow.

A treatment session, which lasts about half an hour, involves using various manipulative techniques depending on the condition being addressed. You may be asked to take up a variety of positions while the practitioner pushes, pulls and applies pressure to your back, head, arms or legs in a number of ways. It is not usually painful but may sometimes feel a little uncomfortable. The number of treatment sessions needed will depend on the severity of the problem.

Many people consider osteopaths to be 'bone crackers' but this is simply not the case. Osteopathy is geared towards work on soft tissues and blood flow through manipulation. This rarely includes 'cracking' the spine. Many people only think of an osteopath when dealing with a structural problem such as an ache or a strain, particularly of the back and neck. There is no doubt that osteopathy is probably the best form of manipulative medicine for such structural problems but that is not where it ends. Osteopaths, often in conjunction with other forms of complementary medicine, can deal with all health problems, including headaches and migraine, digestive complaints, respiratory difficulties such as asthma, glue ear and sinusitis, and gynaecological conditions. Osteopathy may even be able to prevent surgery in some cases of injury.

OXYGEN THERAPY (INCLUDING HYDROGEN PEROXIDE AND OZONE THERAPY)

There is much scientific evidence to support the belief that disease may stem from poor oxygenation of cells. Oxygen therapy is about increasing the availability of oxygen to the body tissues. Pedantically, one may argue that breathing techniques and oral supplementation with antioxidants are actually oxygen treatments and one would be right. However, oxygen therapy is generally the term used for intravenous therapies. Ozone (which is three molecules of oxygen attached together) and hydrogen peroxide (two molecules of oxygen with two molecules of hydrogen) can be introduced directly into the bloodstream and increase the availability directly.

Oxygen has been shown to be of some benefit in cardiac disease, vascular disease, including strokes, and cancer. Work is being done at the moment on HIV and AIDS. Theoretically, enhancing oxygen intake may be of benefit to any condition.

There are risks, however, and intravenous work should only be carried out by qualified medical practitioners or those with experience in emergency resuscitation. It is not so much the oxygen itself that could cause a problem but the fact that the introduction of any chemical directly into the bloodstream can alter the biochemistry rapidly.

Low-oxygen treatments

Athletes are known to travel to high places to train before major events. This is because of the rarefied atmosphere. Training at that level encourages the body to make more red blood cells to carry more oxygen because there is less available in the air. When the athlete returns to sea level normal atmospheric oxygen appears, to the increased number of red blood cells, to be in abundance. The athlete will potentially benefit by having the oxygen availability increased. There is some evidence coming from the former Soviet Union suggesting that short bursts of low-level oxygen each day (delivered through a machine) may trigger a similar response.

Low blood-oxygen levels at the time of radiation treatment may enhance its effects. It appears that cancer cells are much more susceptible to radiation in the presence of low oxygen, whereas the normal body cells seem to be more prepared to fight its effects. This theory has been put forward following several studies in both Eastern Europe and France but the treatment is not yet widely available. I hope to put the theory into practice through a trial in the very near future.

POLARITY THERAPY

Polarity therapy is a holistic system of healing that draws on elements of both Eastern and Western medicine to promote well-being. The body is seen as made up of universal energy or *Qi*, which forms both the material and spiritual universe. The body is a system of energy fields which keep the life energy in constant motion, and it is believed to be the disruption or stagnation of this energy that leads to illness. Developed in the late 19th century by Dr Randolph Stone, an osteopath, chiropractor and naturopath working in the USA, polarity therapy combines different healing techniques to bring about the state of balance and health in the body, mind and emotions.

There are four aspects of polarity therapy: body awareness, posture and balance which are all retrained; cleansing diets and nutritional advice; awareness and counselling skills; and stretching exercises with specific bodywork based both on superficial and deep massage. Touch and manipulation are used to relieve stagnation and encourage energy to flow round the body. Since poor nutrition and digestion may often be a factor in physical problems, detoxifying diets are prescribed, followed by a health-building dietary regime. The patient's state of mind has a direct impact on physical health, and so counselling is used when the practitioner feels that negative thoughts are impeding energy flow. Stretching exercises, or 'polarity yoga', are prescribed to release and harmonize energy.

Polarity therapy is not designed to treat specific symptoms, but to encourge healing through rebalancing the flow of energy. It requires some effort on the part of patients, who are asked to take responsibility for their own health by changing harmful habits. Polarity can be used to benefit many conditions, including allergies, ME, respiratory disorders, cardiovascular problems and aches and pains caused by stress. It may be used either by itself or in conjunction with other forms of more medicinally orientated therapies such as herbal medicine or homeopathy.

PSYCHONEUROIMMUNOLOGY

Scientific evaluation of the components of the immune system in the bloodstream have been shown to alter in response to psychological or emotional changes. Most emotions are associated with chemicals that are released within the structure of the brain. These chemicals trigger impulses along the central nervous system that then travel out to the peripheral nerves and exert an influence on the tissues of the body. The immune system is no different; the thymus (which produces the T cells) and the bone marrow (producing other white blood cells) are particularly influenced.

The fact that the personality and emotions affect the nervous system which in turn affects the immune system is the basis of psychoneuroimmunology. Poor stress-management skills and negative emotions are immune-suppressing and predispose the subject to infection and ill-health. Studies show that people who remain healthy in spite of stressful life experiences have a more positive attitude to life in general than those who succumb to frequent illness.

Psychoneuroimmunology is a diagnostic therapy, combining modern scientific knowledge with psychotherapy. It aims to help prevent illness or aid recovery from existing ill-health by positive emotional counselling and methods of mind control, including visualization and guided imagery techniques. A sense of control and happiness, relaxation and a positive outlook are among the desired outcomes. The therapy has proved helpful for people with cancer and AIDS, and is often highly effective for those with less serious health problems.

Psychoneuroimmunologists may also use any other healing technique or medicinal therapy but always work on the principle that a 'distress-free' state of mind is essential for strong immune function, since the psyche, through the neurological system, affects the body's defence mechanisms.

PSYCHOTHERAPY

The use of conversation and discussion to illustrate, understand and sort out underlying psychological problems is a vast subject. The broad term psychotherapy is used to denote a wide variety of methods to deal with emotional problems. It covers everything and anything from counselling (listening and giving basic advice) to psychoanalysis (deep-seated therapy to establish underlying causes of psychological imbalances stemming from childhood). There are four main branches of psychotherapy: psychoanalytic, humanistic, cognitive and behavioural. Within these branches are many more types or 'schools' of psychotherapy, but all of them (some of which are discussed in more detail in this chapter) use talking to stimulate and support the process of achieving mental health.

Psychotherapy is not only suitable for people in crisis or conflict, but can also be used as a method of achieving personal growth and realizing full potential. Undergoing therapy requires that you make the choice to do it yourself (rather than being pressured by someone else), and that you are open to change and to new feelings and experiences. A basic rule of thumb is to trust your psychotherapist or counsellor and to let him or her use whichever therapy is felt to be the most suitable. A few practitioners have training in more than one type of psychotherapy and these are probably the practitioners with whom to work. Whatever theories or techniques they may espouse, all the psychotherapies have one aim in common – that is, to enable their clients to understand themselves and their relationships with others, and to explore new ways of behaving and dealing with conflicts and difficulties.

QI GONG

The Chinese word for vital force or energy is *Qi*, pronounced chi. *Gong* means 'working with'. Any energy therapy is therefore Qi Gong. The phrase is, however, used mostly to define a vast number of sets of movement that allow energy to flow freely through the body. The Eastern philosophies believe in meridians or channels containing energy that supply the life force to organs and systems. Qi Gong is about moving this energy by following particular patterns of movement and exercise.

Qi Gong's system of exercises, positions and breathing techniques is even more ancient than yoga, originating in China more than 5,000 years ago. Like yoga, Qi Gong is aimed at integrating the mind and body so that a state of harmony is achieved, but unlike yoga it concentrates on moving energy within the body rather than externally. The exercises relate to the acupuncture or pressure points found on the meridians of the body through which the vital energy flows. There are seven basic exercises with hundreds of variations, and all are suitable for health and relaxation. Different sets of movements concentrate on different body organs and systems, and they may be used to alleviate specific health problems such as arthritis and digestive or circulatory disorders.

Ba Duan Jin – a form of Qi Gong

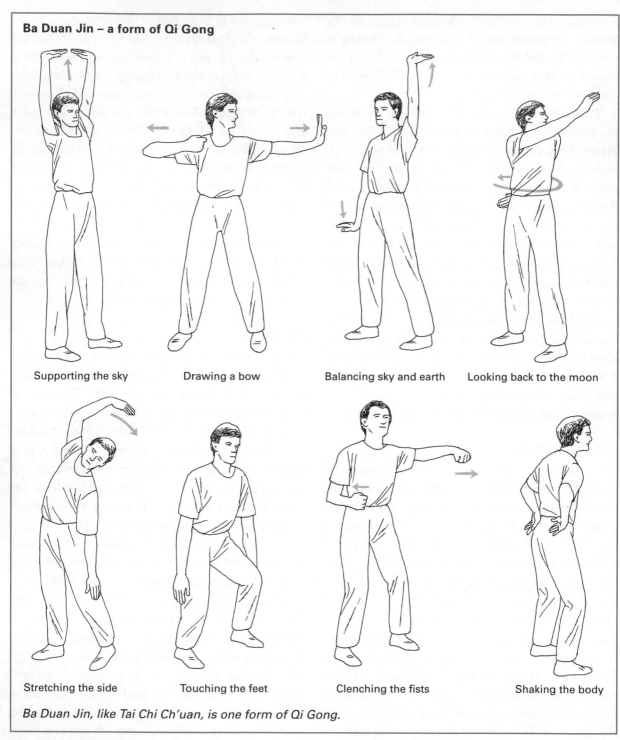

Supporting the sky | Drawing a bow | Balancing sky and earth | Looking back to the moon

Stretching the side | Touching the feet | Clenching the fists | Shaking the body

Ba Duan Jin, like Tai Chi Ch'uan, is one form of Qi Gong.

The breathing exercises may be used to relieve asthma and other breathing difficulties. Both sports injuries and low back pain can be healed without strain by the exercises, which strengthen the muscles and improve general mobility and flexibility.

Remedial Qi Gong is taught on a one-to-one basis in one-and-a-half-hour sessions, and exercises are chosen on the basis of the problem or problems to be addressed. Ten sessions are usually recommended and these will involve general bodywork, breathing exercises and relaxation. You will be expected to practise at home between sessions. People who practise Qi Gong regularly make rapid progress, and invariably find that their health, stamina, energy level and alertness improve, along with their sense of inner power, well-being and joy in life.

RADIESTHESIA

Radiesthesia, meaning 'the perception of radiations', was developed by a Swiss priest, Abbé Alexis Mermet, at the turn of the 20th century. It is a form of dowsing at a distance for medical purposes, whereby the practitioner responds to changes in the energy field produced by patients using a pendulum and charts. The success of the technique, however, depends more on the skill of the therapist than on the instruments used. The practitioner works by detecting and correcting the disharmonies or distortions in energy patterns, often from a great distance. One of the great advantages of the technique is that the hidden causes of disease, which may be undetectable by other methods, can be discovered and treated.

If you decide on radiesthesia treatment, you need never meet the practitioner. You simply send a medical questionnaire giving your symptoms and case history, along with a sample (called 'a witness'), which might be a spot of blood or a lock of hair, to the therapist. He or she will place the sample on a diagnostic instrument, mentally tune into you and pose mental questions about your health, and then hold a pendulum over the instrument in order to receive the answers. Healing energies are then focused on you from a distance (*see* **Dowsing**).

RADIONICS

Radionics is, like radiesthesia, a technique of healing from a distance, and the two therapies are often used in conjunction with each other. As with radiesthesia, the principle is based on a universal energy flow connecting all living things. Radionics was developed early in this century in California, but banned in the USA during the 1960s. Since the 1950s the UK has been the world centre of radionics, but there is poor scientific research on the subject. The therapy does seem to be particularly effective for certain conditions such as asthma and allergies, however, and many practitioners are extremely popular, which suggests some success. Toxins in the body that are not detectable by conventional means can be identified and dispersed by radionics as well as radiesthesia.

There is certainly no danger in the therapy other than the convictions of the practitioner, who may try to persuade a patient to stop or avoid other treatments that may in fact be successful. Be wary, but by all means use this treatment of distant healing in conjunction with other forms of therapy.

REFLEXOLOGY

The body has many energy lines running through it known as meridians or channels. Different parts of the body reflect these channels, which supply energy to the organs and systems. The entire body can be mapped out on pressure points on the feet as is shown in the diagram on page 603. In reflexology the area of the foot (the 'reflex point') that corresponds to the body organ is palpated for diagnostic purposes and then, if treatment is needed, massaged in order to stimulate the healing energies.

The origins of reflexology go back to the time of the ancient Egyptians, and the art was also practised by healers in ancient Greece and China. Use of the therapy in the West was developed in the early 20th century by two Americans, Dr William Fitzgerald and Eunice Ingham. Fitzgerald proposed the theory that 10 zones of communication run the length of the body from head to toe, and that stimulating an area of the foot in one zone affects other parts of the body along the same zone. Eunice Ingham developed his ideas and her research on thousands of pairs of feet confirmed his findings.

Treatment is carried out with the patient lying or sitting barefoot, either on a couch or a reclining chair. A session typically lasts 30–40 minutes. The reflexologist uses the thumbs, fingers and hands to isolate any points that are particularly empty (the finger falls into them easily) or full (generally a tender lump). By this means diagnosis of internal energy weakness can be made. It is important not to confuse a reflexologist's comment that the kidney is weak with any suggestion that the kidney has a disease process. As in pulse-taking, the comment reflects the energy of the system and not the physiology. The therapist will then seek out and treat any painful areas with a compression technique, which clears congestion in the corresponding organ by improving lymphatic, blood and nerve circulation. It is thought that the sensitive lumps felt beneath the skin are crystalline deposits, and it is not uncommon to feel some pain during massage, as these deposits are dispersed.

Reflexology can help almost any condition, especially if used in conjunction with other more mainstream procedures. It is a highly effective way to detoxify the body and treat a wide variety of health problems, including skin disorders, digestive and menstrual problems, glue ear and colic in children, urinary and kidney disorders, migraine and chronic aches and pains. A recent study showed that reflexology helped knee operations to heal more quickly. Further trials need to be done but, in principle, reflexology is safe, pleasurable and, undoubtedly, of benefit.

ROLFING

Rolfing is a body therapy named after its founder Dr Ida Rolf, an American biochemist who suggested that many health problems are caused by poor posture. The principle of improving the body's alignment in order to enhance well-being is not dissimilar to that of the Alexander Technique, but Dr Rolf devised a complex manipulative technique in order to realign the body's structure so that it can work with, rather than against, gravity. This she termed structural re-integration. Deep massage of the body's connective tissues and muscles realigns the system, encouraging energy flow, circulation and better nervous conduction.

Rolfing is a deep massage, sometimes using the elbows or knuckles, that can be uncomfortable or even painful, but undoubtedly has great benefits. Rolfing stretches the pliable connective tissue, or *fascia*, of the body. If it has contracted, it will have adhered to neighbouring structures, impeding freedom of movement and the proper functioning of the organs and other structures of the body.

Treatment usually consists of a course of 10 hour-long sessions spread out over a period of time that is dependent upon the response of the patient. Each session builds on the last one and works on a different part of the body, starting with areas where the muscles are close to the surface and moving on to deep-tissue work in later sessions. The Rolfer may take photographs at the beginning and end of the course to document the changes that happen. The effects of a course of Rolfing include increased vitality, a better range of movement and visibly improved balance and ease of posture. Relief of chronic structural aches and pains also results. It is not, however, a treatment for a particular ailment but a system of preventive therapy.

SHIATSU

Shiatsu is a combination of massage and acupressure that has derived from the Japanese use of Chinese medical philosophy. The word Shiatsu means 'finger pressure' in Japanese. Stretching meridians and manipulating acupuncture points can feed vital energy, or *Qi*, into organs and systems within the body to create health. The therapy is becoming increasingly popular in the West, as people come to realize the importance of maintaining their own health and reducing stress.

This is my favourite form of bodywork because it incorporates the concept of Qi, acupressure and massage. A session with a Shiatsu practitioner consists of first learning the case history of your complaint and taking the pulses. A diagnosis is then made by palpating the abdomen, the so-called 'Hara' diagnosis. The abdomen is seen as a map of the body which is a guide to the energetic state of the person and the relative strength or weakness of its major systems. The process, which

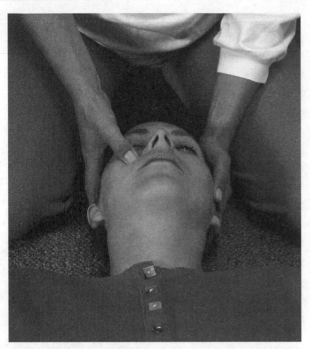

Shiatsu facial massage.

takes about five minutes, can tell the therapist which meridians to work on to rebalance the energy flow through the body. Treatment takes place with the client lying fully clothed on a mat or futon on the floor. The practitioner applies sustained pressure, which varies in intensity, to the appropriate points using the hands, elbows, knees and feet. Gentle manipulation may also be used to loosen joints and stretch the meridians, the energy pathways. Shiatsu treatment takes about an hour or so and is deeply relaxing.

Used in conjunction with other forms of alternative or orthodox treatment, Shiatsu will make people feel better and speed up the healing process. Shiatsu also helps to maintain health by toning up the body's energy and promoting relaxation. Shiatsu can be used safely in all conditions and with all ailments including cancer, because lymphatic drainage is only a part of the treatment programme and can be put aside.

If you know the right pressure points to use, Shiatsu can be used as self-help first aid treatment to use on yourself or your family to relieve pain or cramps.

SOUND THERAPY

Sound is an energy. The human body is made up of energies and therefore sound affects the body. This principle has been known for thousands of years and its health-promoting aspects have been harnessed through the use of singing, chanting and making music from instruments. Sound is our principal method of communicating and expressing, and works directly upon the nervous system which branches into every part of the body.

Sound is used through chanting to create vibration within the main chakras or energy centres in the body, but can also be used in conjunction with movement, as in dance therapy. The theory is that everything in the universe is in a state of vibration, including human beings. There is a natural resonance or frequency of vibration for each part of the body, and certain sound waves directed towards specific areas can affect the frequency of these vibrations and thereby restore the energy balance.

Many different practitioners will use music and chanting as part of their therapy, and even doctors' waiting rooms may play music as part of the holistic approach (*see* **Music therapy**). Sound therapy may involve the voice, music or a variety of tonal sounds, and sometimes all three combined. Sound therapy may utilize special machines that transmit 'healing vibrations'. A special chair known as the acoustic chair has been developed and is undergoing trials for a variety of conditions. Sound can be used in any condition as an adjunct to other therapies or in the form of chanting, as part of daily life and for maintaining health. It is an effective therapy for use with the mentally and physically disabled of all ages.

TAI CHI CH'UAN

Abbreviated frequently to Tai Chi, this is one group or set of movements among a vast number of exercise protocols that make up Qi Gong. Tai Chi can be practised at any age and allows the free flow of Qi through the meridians and channels, many of which are utilized by acupuncture.

Tai Chi works on the body and mind at the same time, relaxing the muscles and calming the nerves. The exercises consist of flowing movements that are performed slowly and gently, and each exercise begins and ends with standing still for a few seconds. It has been described as 'moving meditation'. The emphasis is not on strength or exertion but on balance, grace, concentration and becoming centred. The knees are kept bent and the body's weight slowly shifted from one foot to the other, while the hands make careful circling and pushing gestures. Attention is also paid to the breathing.

As well as helping to promote and maintain good health and well-being, Tai Chi is often recommended as a therapy for those suffering from high blood pressure, tension and anxiety and heart complaints, because of its relaxing effect on the body and mind (*see* **Qi Gong**).

VISUALIZATION

The mind has a powerful influence on the body. Whether this is through psychoneuroimmunology (*see* **Psychoneuroimmunology**) or through a direct mind/body connection as the Eastern philosophies suggest, the mind can be used to cure problems. Visualization, or forming meaningful images in the mind, is a visual approach to meditation that can have a therapeutic effect in several ways, especially in conjunction with hypnotherapy.

Most of us will note that a pain is far less severe if we are happy or doing something we enjoy rather than sitting around focusing on a discomfort. We can harness this positive mental attitude to overcome stress and other problems by using visualization techniques. Imagining yourself in beautiful surroundings (a sunlit forest or a wide sandy beach, for example) while using relaxation and breathing techniques has the power to counteract negative thinking, anxiety, fear and low self-esteem. It can also be used to defuse a stressful situation, such as going to the dentist; the use of positive imagery can help us to overcome apprehension and help us face challenges.

Just as the mind can override psychological problems, the same energy can be used to heal physical complaints. Visualization is a taught technique that trains the body to visualize the destruction of a problem. Forming a clear image of the part of the body in need of healing can cause actual improvement to take place. An example would be to imagine a small man with an axe chopping away at a tumourous lump. A hose can be imagined to be flushing out the sinuses and a tailor to be stitching up a hernia. See the part of your body that needs healing or strengthening becoming strong and whole again. In cases of infection, you could see the white blood cells in your bloodstream as attacking warriors destroying disease organisms and new healthy cells multiplying in their place.

As a therapy on its own, it may have limited value, but in combination with other more orthodox or mainstream alternative therapies it can speed up healing. It is now increasingly used in this way in many hospitals and clinics alongside conventional treatment.

WATER THERAPY– *see* **Hydrotherapy**

YOGA

Yoga is a system of movement which has been practised in India for 5,000 years. Yoga is derived from the Sanskrit word for union and is principally geared towards uniting the spiritual, mental and physical aspects of the being. Yoga works on the body, mind and soul, and is part of an entire philosophical system, the ultimate aim of which is enlightenment and union with the divine. Different branches of yoga have different names depending on the part of the 'being' that they affect.

- Hatha yoga – works on the physical aspects by using postures and exercises in conjunction with breathing techniques. This is the most popular branch and is what the West considers to be yoga.

- Raja yoga – is a series of techniques that focus on understanding the mind and how it exerts its control over the body.
- Jnana yoga – focuses on intellect, academia and the understanding of the whole through meditative techniques.
- Karma yoga – concerns itself with the 'reason for being' and moral concepts.
- Bhakti yoga – is that part of the being that focuses on a devotional or religious aspect.
- Tantric yoga – is a branch of Hatha yoga that incorporates sexual union between two consenting individuals. Certain sexual positions are formed and held in conjunction with spiritual meditation.

Yoga can be used as a way of relaxing and keeping fit, as well as a meditation technique. All the different types involve learning breathing techniques, and adopting and holding different poses such as

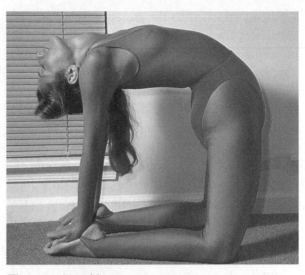

The camel position.

'cobra', 'tree' and 'corpse'. The poses stretch and strengthen the muscles and ligaments, increasing suppleness, and also stimulate the internal organs. Yoga has been found to benefit certain diseases, particularly arthritis, asthma, backache, high blood pressure and digestive disorders such as irritable bowel syndrome. It is also a very effective way of dealing with stress.

Yoga is not just about standing on your head but is an integrated mind/body activity that connects the material with the ethereal. Books and tapes can introduce people to the basics of Hatha yoga but a teacher with experience is required to access the true benefit of other forms of yoga.

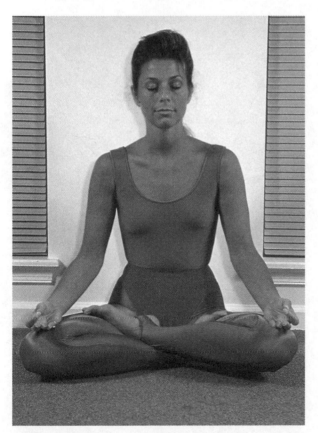

Lotus position.

ZEN

Zen is a Japanese school of Buddhism, of 12th-century Chinese origin, teaching that contemplation of one's essential nature to the exclusion of all else is the only path to pure enlightenment. It is a philosophy of life, promoting self-discipline through insight, self-awareness and mindfulness, both of the self and others. Buddhism, simply put, sees the body and personal identity as a 'block' to spiritual enlightenment.

Zen meditation helps an individual to understand that the soul or spirit is a separate entity from the body, and that illness or disease is merely a process attached to the material world and not to the self. It encourages a joyful acceptance of the impermanent nature of existence, leading to contemplation of the 'reality of emptiness', and complete freedom and transcendence of suffering. Concern for others and the development of compassion are also crucial aspects of the Buddhist philosophy. Of the many approaches to Buddhism, Zen is anti-rational, teaching an acceptance of ordinary life and encouraging direct experience. Zen influences daily life through *zazen* (meditation), and encourages correct nutrition, hygiene and exercise.

Zen is perhaps the most well-known form of Buddhism in the West. More information can be obtained from Buddhist Centres which show how Zen practice can be suited to modern living. They offer meditation and study programmes through classes, workshops and retreats.

ZONE THERAPY

Dr W H Fitzgerald, the founder of reflexology, divided the body vertically into ten zones and isolated the acupressure points within them (*see* **Reflexology**). Pressure applied creates changes throughout the entire body. Whereas reflexology uses points on the feet, a zone therapist works throughout the whole system, using reflex areas all over the body. Pressure is applied to a point corresponding to an organ elsewhere. For example, there is an acupoint on the inner forearm just below the wrist, used for nausea and motion sickness (and utilized commercially in 'Sea Bands' worn on the wrist as a preventive measure). Both the fingers and the toes have several points that help the head area, and pressure on the medial edge of the little finger will relieve headaches and a stiff neck. The hand reflexes mirror the position of those on the feet, and are very convenient for self-help treatment.

DRUGS

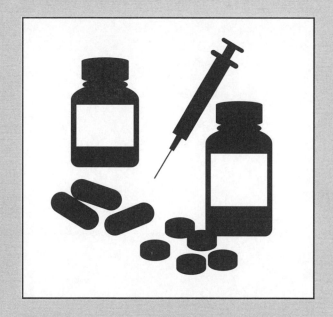

Chapter 10

Drugs

'If you have to take drugs, here are some facts you should know . . .'

A trial reported in the *British Medical Journal* in November 1996 showed that research sponsored by pharmaceutical companies performed in general practice does not appear to generate a high level of scientifically valid or clinically relevant findings. A report by WHAT DOCTORS DON'T TELL YOU in their journal *Proof* states that 80 per cent of drugs are not proven to be safe. The BMA paper also stated that 27 per cent of the trials paid for by the pharmaceutical companies were never published, which raises the probability that unsuccessful trials are not put forward in the hope that the next trial on the drug will show the treatment in a better light.

Despite the use of the terms complementary and holistic, many people and doctors consider non-orthodox treatments to be alternatives to the use of regular drugs. This is not the case. The best treatments can come in many guises, both orthodox and naturopathic, and good medicine is all about knowing which to use and when. There are many situations throughout this book that illustrate the need to use orthodox medicines. The biggest difficulty is answering two questions:

- If drugs are dangerous why are they prescribed?
- Why does my doctor not know this?

The answers are simple. The pharmaceutical industry accepts that there are dangers, which is why they print side effects and contra-indications on the packaging of drugs. The pharmaceutical industry is a business, not a caring profession, so they do not draw attention to the dangers, only to the positive aspects. Doctors are aware of the dangers but are limited as to what else they could prescribe. Only 1,000 out of the 120,000 doctors in this country have any complementary knowledge and most of those are trained only in one technique, such as acupuncture or homeopathy. General practitioners cannot be blamed for prescribing antibiotics if they think that an infection is present, because there is little else they can give. In this chapter I shall discuss some of the major drug groups and point out their negative aspects. This does not mean that they should not be used in specific cases but illustrates how alternatives should be looked at before rushing into using them.

It is important to remember that many drugs are withdrawn after passing safety tests. I tried to obtain the number of such withdrawals but, surprise, no-one had that statistic. I tried to contact various pharmaceutical companies to request this information with regard to their own products – my calls were never returned. I say this to ensure that the reader accepts that my comments are accurate to the best of my knowledge at the time I write this, but they are only my opinion.

I have added at the end of several of the individual drugs and drug groups mentioned in the next few pages, the vitamins and minerals that should be taken alongside the drugs to counteract the deficiencies created by them. The amount to take should be on the product label or prescribed by a complementary medical practitioner or doctor.

ADRENALINE

Adrenaline is a naturally occurring hormone made in the adrenal glands. It is used as a drug to treat allergic reactions in such events as insect stings, medical drug reactions and hypersensitivity to certain foods, most commonly eggs and peanuts. The most serious form of allergy reaction is called anaphylaxis, where the bronchial tree tightens up, the blood pressure rises and the heart beats excessively fast.

Adrenaline needs to be given by injection and strengths of 1 part adrenaline to 1,000 or 10,000 parts of water are available through a doctor and should be kept in the house if anyone has had a strong reaction to anything at all in the past. Adrenaline is given by subcutaneous injection into any muscular part of the body and is very easy to administer.

AIDS DRUGS

Zidovudine, also known as azidothymidine, and therefore referred to as AZT, was manufactured many years ago as an anticancer, chemotherapeutic agent. It was too toxic for use and therefore never marketed. Wellcome, the pharmaceutical giant, discovered that AZT was detrimental to the human immunodeficiency virus (HIV).

In fact the initial trials suggested very little about its curative aspects and shortly after its release onto the market, it was suggested that if taken early (after HIV infection and before AIDS had started) patients would live longer and delay the onset of AIDS. There was evidence to support this but a more recent and conclusive study – the Concorde Trial – has shown this not to be the case and in fact early use of AZT may be detrimental in the long term.

The pharmaceutical industry are now suggesting that AZT in combination with other drugs such as didanosine (DDI) and zalcitabine (DDC) is everything they thought AZT was ten years ago. This time, they say, the combination is definitely delaying the onset of AIDS.

New groups known as protease inhibitors and nucleosides are coming forward and seem at this time to be as effective, if not more so, as AZT.

It is very difficult to elicit accurate figures concerning the effectiveness of AIDS drugs. Official reports vary from hospital to hospital but my personal experience and those of the holistic physicians with whom I work is that the majority of patients using AIDS drugs do not use them for long because of side effects and, on a more sinister note, the majority of AZT users do not do very well and have problems eventually.

Azidothymidine is highly toxic and may well be damaging to the immune system, which goes against the holistic view of AIDS and its treatment.

AMPHETAMINES

Amphetamines are rarely prescribed except by hospital physicians in a few specific types of disease. Amphetamines are, however, commonplace as a drug of abuse. Uppers, speed and reds are examples of the varying forms of amphetamines. Derivatives of amphetamines were popularly prescribed as diet pills. Unwise physicians may continue to do this but they lead their patients into risky territory.

Amphetamines act by stimulating adrenaline receptors, thereby exciting and keeping the user awake. These are exceptionally dangerous drugs. Their direct effect on the adrenal system can lead to heart attacks, strokes and burst blood vessels due to increased blood pressure. The body does not remove these artificial stimulants easily and dependency can occur quite quickly.

ANAESTHETICS

The development of anaesthetics has come a long way since biting the bullet and strong slugs of brandy. Ether was a godsend in comparison to the pain relief offered by the barber surgeons. No physician would encourage the use of anaesthetics if surgery can be avoided but on the whole they are safe and necessary. The orthodox world accepts that they are dangerous drugs but rarely has anything to say about protecting patients from the effects.

Anaesthetics have strong effects on both the nervous system (causing it to lose consciousness) and the liver, as does any toxic compound. Anybody who is going under anaesthesia should consider this and use naturopathic compounds to support both the liver and nervous system (*see* **Operations and Surgery**).

ANALGESICS

Analgesics can be divided into non-opioid analgesics which include aspirin, paracetemol and acetaminophen, and other non-steroidal anti-inflammatory drugs (NSAIDs), which are discussed in their own section.

If modern medicine has come up with anything particularly worthwhile, it is the ability to numb most pain. All the drugs have side effects but principally these are clearly labelled and short-lived. The second group of analgesics are known as opioids and are discussed in their own section.

ANTACIDS

The stomach produces acid to initiate the breakdown of ingested food. The stomach has a lining that produces a thick protective mucus, which prevents the very high acid content from breaking down the stomach wall. A variety of illnesses and poor life-style can lead to the breakdown of this mucous membrane which in turn leads to discomfort and pain. Many people also have hiatus hernia (*see* **Hiatus Hernia**), which allows acid to reflux up into the oesophagus and cause a burning sensation.

Antacids fall into two categories:

- Compounds that neutralize the acid (alkalis) – calcium, magnesium and aluminium salts.
- Drugs that stop acid production – such as cimetidine, ranitidine and omeprazole.

These treatments are very much geared towards blocking the symptoms by reducing the acid rather than looking at the cause of the damaged mucosa, the reflux or the excess production of acid. They are not harmful to any great extent if taken for a short period of time but continual use suggests that the cause of the problem is not being dealt with and this can lead to difficult and dangerous illnesses.

Supplements required drugs that suppress acid production, i.e. proton pump inhibitors – vitamin B_{12}; medication that neutralizes acids, such as magnesium/aluminium – calcium.

ANTIBIOTICS

Antibiotics are produced to fight bacterial infection.

The drugs may be bactericidal – where bacteria are killed – or bacteriostatic – where the treatment prevents the germs from multiplying. There are many antibacterial compounds in nature, garlic, ginger and honey being three very common ones. Manufactured antibiotics come about through the fabled tale of Sir Alexander Fleming and his accidental discovery of penicillin at St Mary's Hospital, London. This simple drug collected from mould has undoubtedly been the forerunner of a group of medicines that have saved lives and relieved discomfort beyond all imagination. Sadly, their misuse has now led to far greater dangers.

The problem lies in the fact that bacteria, like any organism on the planet, will fight tenaciously to hold on to life. Bacteria multiply at an astounding speed and through this process create slight changes as their genes copy themselves. As one bacteria splits into two, minor changes occur in the genetic make-up and because of the billions of these divisions occurring every minute there eventually comes along a bacteria whose genetic make-up is resistant to the antibiotic that kills the rest of its colony.

In the presence of an antibiotic this resistant strain finds that it has more food to eat because of the loss of its brothers and sisters. It is unaffected by the antibiotic, multiplies more quickly and within a short space of time the colony is made up predominantly of this resistant strain. As new antibiotics are developed to kill this new strain it too mutates and once again develops resistance. We are now faced with strains of bacteria that are resistant to most antibiotics, and in the case of some strains of tuberculosis and the so-called 'flesh-eating' staphylococcal infections we have no antibiotic to kill them.

This state of affairs has come about because of the injudicious choice of antibiotics made by doctors who 'best guess' without taking a sample of the infection for analysis, and because of the distribution of antibiotics to Third World, and some First World, countries that allow them to be bought over the counter without a doctor's prescription. All doctors are beseeched at medical school by their professors of microbiology never to prescribe an antibiotic unless a sample of the bacteria has been sent to a laboratory, grown or cultured and tested against a range of antibiotics. On an individual basis the use of an antibiotic in a patient who has a strain of bacteria that is even partially resistant will lead to a resistant strain developing and possibly a more difficult infection to treat.

Despite my comments above, do not hesitate to use an antibiotic in a condition that your doctor considers serious. Ensure that your physician is as certain as he can be, clinically, that the infection is bacterial. You can request a culture and antibiotic sensitivity test before using an antibiotic and then, having established with your doctor whether or not delaying the start of the antibiotics is dangerous, consult a complementary practitioner for the use of an alternative. Bromelain has been shown to increase the absorption of antibiotics but should be prescribed by a complementary practitioner.

A second misunderstanding about antibiotics is the assumption that even if they are ineffective they are not harmful. This is simply not true. An antibiotic is indiscriminate. It does not focus its attention on the 'bad' bugs. It will have a go at all bacteria. Our bodies are entirely dependent upon our own bacteria for survival. Skin bacteria are essential to defend against unwanted invaders, as well as being essential for the maintenance and integrity of the skin. Our ears, eyes, mouth, nasal passages, bronchial tree and lungs are all coated and protected by our own 'commensal' bacteria. Our alimentary tract, from our lips to our anus, is covered with bacteria (even in the high acid content of the stomach), which collectively have a vital role to play in our well-being.

These bacteria compete with unwanted bugs for food and prevent their multiplication, they kill many other bacteria and also viruses, they break down food to allow proper absorption and produce chemicals that are both protective and nutritious to our systems.

Without them we die. Most people who use antibiotics will feel some side effects, ranging from tiredness and lethargy to diarrhoea and thrush. These symptoms are all due to the unwanted destruction of our own body flora.

A course of antibiotics can have a profound effect on the bowel bacteria. The effect on large numbers of bacteria can lead to the loss of the protective effect and can prevent nutrients being absorbed (through lack of breakdown of food or production by the bacteria themselves). This can lead to a mild malnutrition which in turn enhances the depressed immune system that allowed the infection into the body for which the antibiotic was being used. A vicious circle is started up with recurrent infections occurring, leading to more antibiotics *ad infinitum*.

Remember to focus on the fact that an infection represents a breakdown in the body's immune system and is not the fault of the germ. If an antibiotic is taken, protect the bowel flora by using high doses of *Lactobacillus acidophilus*. Loss of bowel bacteria allows fungal growth such as *Candida* and an anti-*Candida* treatment should be followed whilst taking the antibiotics. Assume that your bowel flora have been affected and that you are not absorbing as well as you should. Take a high dose of a multivitamin/mineral supplement.

Supplements required – B_{12}, essential fatty acids.

ANTICANCER DRUGS

There is no doubt that these drugs can be life-saving and have their place in holistic medicine. Their mode of action varies but in principle they tend to stop fast-replicating cells from doing so. This is usually done by interfering with the chemistry or the chromosomes of the cancer cells. Unfortunately, no cancer drug is that specific and they will have effects on other cells. The stronger ones will stop the cells in the bowel, hair follicles and bone marrow from behaving normally because all of these are fast-replicating cells as well.

If there is any big disappointment concerning

cancer drugs it is that they are used in various combinations and quantities by different cancer specialists. Very few protocols are clearly defined and set up. We are still in a very early stage of anticancer drug development and many patients today are unwitting guinea pigs.

As in most pharmacological developments, anticancer drugs are geared towards killing the cancer and not dealing with the cause. It is imperative that anybody using an anticancer drug sees a specialist in complementary medicine for the best advice on how to avoid the side effects, help build up the body's immunity, speed up the removal of the toxic drugs once they have performed their action and, most importantly, isolate the possible causes of the cancer and treat them (*see* **Cancer**).

ANTICOAGULANTS
The blood system has a complex and fascinating cascade – one reaction triggers another in a course of approximately 15 different stages – that allows the blood to clot. This process is essential to prevent blood loss if any vessels are damaged externally or internally but it can become a problem if clotting occurs within a blood vessel. If this does occur, anticoagulants can be life-saving.

Anticoagulation therapy can only be initiated by a physician and should never be stopped without specialist approval. The most common anticoagulants are heparin, which works swiftly but is generally used only in the short term, and warfarin and coumarin, which are used for longer-term prescribing.

ANTIDEPRESSANTS
Volumes have been written about the pros and cons of antidepressants. *See* **Depression** to understand the continual abuse of these drugs by individuals and the doctors who prescribe them. Discussion on each group and type of antidepressant would require a book this size again, so those using antidepressants should discuss the matter with a medically qualified practitioner of alternative medicine to learn the full pros and cons.

There is no antidepressant of any variety that does not have a myriad of side effects. When diazepam (most commonly taken as Valium) was first produced in the 1950s and considered to be the 'housewife's miracle', the public and doctors were told that side effects were few and minor. It now takes over 2 minutes to read out the list of the side effects that have been registered on this one drug alone in the last 40 years.

As I have explained in the section on depression, the use of antidepressants has its place in truly endogenous depression. When an individual is incapable of producing his/her own 'happy juice' and alternative measures have failed, then these drugs can alter a life very much for the better – perhaps more so than any other medical invention.

Supplements required – Vitamin B complex and CoQ 10.

ANTIEMETICS (ANTI-SICKNESS DRUGS)
If the body is feeling sick it is generally an indication that the individual has taken something in that it needs to throw out, or it is busily processing a toxin and does not need anything else going in to detract from that biochemical process. Once the cause has been established, it is better to use homeopathic medication to encourage a cure rather than a drug that stops the sensation of nausea.

In cases where nausea is part of a treatment course, such as anticancer drugs or radiation, antiemetics are essential to allow the appetite to be maintained. Not eating during serious illness will not allow the body to repair as well as it should. The use of antiemetics is also permissible if it is for short-term use such as travel sickness.

ANTIFUNGAL AGENTS – *see* Antibiotics
The body is coated internally and externally with fungi. It sounds awful but, like the bacteria in the body, they are essential to our well-being. They prevent foreign fungi, which may be very toxic to our system, from gaining a foothold by what is called competitive inhibition. Fungi thrive on

sugars and other nutrients and our own fungi are not harmful to us. If we kill them off by the use of antifungal agents or poor diet, unhealthy fungi will find themselves with more food to eat because of the absence of the good guys and will multiply quicker, producing their toxic effects.

Yeasts are fungi. The most infamous is monilia, more commonly known as *Candida*, which produces the symptoms of thrush. Thrush is controlled due to the phenomenon of cross-species competitive inhibition. To put it more simply, antibiotics and unhealthy lifestyle kill off our own fungi and bacteria leaving more food for the tougher varieties. *Candida* lives in a high percentage of our bodies (up to 50 per cent of women will carry *Candida* vaginally) and will not cause us a problem unless we destroy its competitors. This is why people in immuno-compromised states and those who have taken antibiotics can end up with thrush.

As in the case of antibacterial agents, resistant strains occur and we are seeing more virulent, aggressive and faster-replicating yeast and fungi species developing due to the over-prescribing of antifungal and anti-*Candida* preparations.

ANTIHISTAMINES

When the body is irritated or invaded by a foreign substance, special cells release histamine. This chemical causes the arteries in the area to open up allowing more blood to travel to the damaged part and thereby allowing the white blood cells, vitamins, minerals and other necessary factors for healing to reach the area quickly. Unfortunately, this increase in blood flow is experienced as inflammation, which is irritating to the nerves and causes redness, rashes, itching and pain.

The complementary medical view is that if this is encouraged the problem will be dealt with swiftly in a healthy body. The orthodox view is to take away the irritation by blocking the healing effect of the histamine release. Antihistamines, whilst effective and if taken in the right doses not particularly harmful, are in fact preventing the body's natural healing mechanism. Antihistamines have several side effects but predominantly cause drowsiness and should not be taken whilst driving or using machinery.

ANTI-PARKINSON'S DRUGS

Parkinson's disease is created by a lack of a neurotransmitter called dopamine in the central nervous system. Treatment is by replacing this with a compound called levodopa, which when given in the right quantities is a safe drug to take. Another drug called dopa-decarboxylase inhibitor prevents natural dopamine from being broken down. The two in combination help people with Parkinson's disease and can be a very effective treatment.

The problem lies in the fact that the body gets used to these compounds and after a few years may no longer respond. New drugs are constantly being brought in, such as selegiline, lysuride, amantadine and pergolide. All are beneficial but avoid the use of these drugs until alternative avenues have not succeeded. Use these drugs as late in the condition as possible because resistance to their efficacy will develop and lead to a decrease in usefulness after five to ten years.

ANTIPYRETICS

As a general rule fever is considered by holistic practitioners to be a friend. Most bacteria and viruses do not fare well at higher temperatures whilst the body, although it may not feel too comfortable, can generally survive fevers up to around 103°F (40°C). The best-known antipyretics are aspirin and paracetamol (or Tylenol® in the USA). Their mode of action is varied between direct action on blood vessels, the effects on mediators called prostaglandins and effects on white blood cells that release chemicals that increase the body's temperature in the presence of infection.

The holistic consensus would be to avoid any drug that goes against the body's natural reaction unless the body is losing control. The pain- and discomfort-relieving aspects of antipyretics must be balanced against the potential for these drugs to prevent or slow down the healing response. Occasional use is not likely to be harmful but a need to use these drugs beyond 48 hours or their apparent ineffectiveness in allowing the body to heal strongly suggests a visit to your health practitioner.

ANTIVIRAL DRUGS

There are very few effective antiviral agents that can be taken by humans. Killing a virus is not difficult, but the problem is the drugs will kill humans equally efficiently. Acyclovir is the most commonly used antiviral agent against herpes and shingles. This is, without doubt, an effective drug but probably kills many other viruses that may be of use to the body. It is also unable to penetrate the nervous system well, so it is only superficially effective and is in no way curative against herpes and shingles, which live in the nerve centres. The body's best defence against antiviral agents is its own immunity, and promotion of this through complementary techniques is a safer and possibly more effective method of antiviral treatment (*see* Vaccinations).

Antiviral drugs are predominantly ineffective unless given in very toxic doses. The concept of an antiviral agent sustains the myth that ill-health is created by germs. In reality, the human immune system has the most efficient antiviral techniques, and correct maintenance and stimulation of this part of our bodies continues to be more effective than drugs.

ANTIWORM (ANTIHELMINTHIC) AND ANTIPARASITE DRUGS

Threadworms and pinworms are very common amongst schoolchildren and spread through families very easily. They are generally not harmful although an excessive number can cause poor absorption and affect growth and development in children. These parasites lay their eggs at the anus and travel through the gut, usually overnight, to do so. This gives the characteristic itching. Other worms and parasites, such as tropical worms and amoeba, can be very devastating and cause serious illnesses.

Most of these live in the gut, at least initially. Early treatment is advisable and the drugs which are prescribed by doctors stay in the gut and are poorly absorbed. This makes them very effective and non-toxic, although some people can struggle with stomach upsets, nausea and diarrhoea. These drugs should be used if a diagnosis of infestation has been made or if infestation is likely, as in family groups or schools.

ASPIRIN – *see* Analgesics

Aspirin is being tested as an effective treatment against bowel cancer because a reduction in the incidence of these tumours has been noted in a group who had been taking aspirin for its anticoagulant and therefore antistroke aspects. We watch and wait for the outcome.

Supplements required – CoQ 10, Vitamin C, folic acid, iron, potassium and sodium.

ASTHMA DRUGS – *see* Asthma

Do not forget that asthma is a potentially lethal condition. Adjusting of asthma drugs is not recommended without medical supervision.

There are no orthodox asthma medications that are curative. The pharmaceutical industry has preferred to research into medications that keep asthma at bay but are not curative. This is a perfectly acceptable situation for an industry that is geared towards profit and not healthcare. Feel no anger towards the pharmaceutical industry on this count; they are very clear in their attitude.

The drugs used in asthma treatment are all geared towards decreasing mucus production and opening the narrowed bronchial tubes. Most are effective, relieving and in many cases life-saving. Do not underestimate their importance in medicine but do not consider their use in health maintenance. Nearly every branch of complementary medicine will have a treatment for asthma. If one is already being taken or you are being threatened with the use of asthma drugs, always consult a complementary practitioner before continuing or starting to use these drugs. *Do not stop your use of antiasthma drugs unless monitored by a medical practitioner.*

BARBITURATES

These are rarely prescribed these days except for specific paediatric conditions. However, they are found in several European-manufactured painkillers and should be avoided at all costs. Barbiturates are highly effective as tranquillizers and as toxins to the system. There is no need to use them because far better and less dangerous drugs are available for all their potential uses.

BETA-BLOCKERS

Beta-blockers are so called because they block adrenaline beta-type receptors in certain cells around the body. These beta-receptors respond to adrenaline produced by the adrenal glands and nervous system in response to anxiety, shock and fear.

Beta-blockers are commonly used in heart patients (*see* **Cardiac drugs**) but are also used by people who have palpitations through anxiety or metabolic diseases such as hyperthyroidism. In themselves they are not particularly dangerous drugs unless taken in overdose or taken by asthmatics. It is contraindicated to use these drugs if you have any suggestion of asthma.

Once again, these drugs deal with the symptoms and not the underlying cause and alternative treatments are available but withdrawal should be done only under medical supervision.

CALCIUM-ABSORBING DRUGS (BISPHOSPHONATES)

There has recently been a surge of interest in drugs that maintain calcium levels in bones. These drugs are not always effective and need to be taken continuously if any effect is to be maintained. They are often prescribed together with hormone replacement therapy (HRT). Complementary measures should be tried before resorting to either of these drugs.

There are currently three oral bisphosphonates – etidronate, alendronate and risedronate. These are comparatively new drugs and long-term effects are poorly studied. They are generally well tolerated but they do have adverse effects.

CARDIAC (HEART) DRUGS

Cardiac drugs can only be prescribed by medical practitioners. In principle, if you are prescribed them, take them. They may have many side effects and may be unnecessary, but most often they are life-saving. Further discussion on the use of cardiac drugs should be undertaken with a medically qualified practitioner of complementary medicine or a complementary practitioner in conjunction with the medical doctor who prescribed them.

There are many naturopathic and holistic medicines and treatments that can be used for most heart conditions so one may not need to stay on the drugs once a safe and comprehensive holistic view has been taken.

CHOLESTEROL LOWERING DRUGS (INCLUDING STATINS)

There is strong evidence that, for patients with heart disease who have symptoms resulting from the blockage of arteries, lowering LDL cholesterol improves the outcome. By extrapolating these results, the orthodox medical world assumes that further studies will show that lowering raised cholesterol levels will reduce the chances of heart attacks and angina even in those without symptoms. Fair enough.

Fibrates, ispaghula husks and the drug colestyramine reduce fats in general and thereby reduce cholesterol levels. However, a group of drugs known as statins are more effective at reducing LDL cholesterol. They have few side effects, the most frequent being muscular aches, headache, stomachache, flatulence, diarrhoea, nausea and vomiting. Rash and skin sensitivity are occasionally reported as is a correlation between their use and an increased desire to commit suicide. This latter report has not been substantiated.

For those patients who have found that diet, exercise and either naturopathic or other medication has not helped bring down cholesterol levels *and* there *is* a need to lower cholesterol levels, then statins should be considered.

CONTRACEPTIVES – *see* **Oral contraceptive pill**

CORTISONE – *see* **Steroids**

COUGH MEDICINES

A cough is the body's natural response to removing an object, excess mucus or infection from the lung. Cough medicines inhibit this process by desensitizing the nerves that recognize an irritant and, whilst soothing, will allow the cause of the problem to stay in the lungs.

The general use of these suppressants should be curtailed unless the patient is losing sleep or coughing so much that bruising and further damage to the lungs seems inevitable. Even then, the cough suppressants should be used sparingly and the natural fluid-extract preparations available from healthfood stores and complementary practitioners are supposedly easier for the body to break down than the more pharmaceutically manufactured chemicals.

CYSTITIS PREPARATIONS

The orthodox practitioner will swiftly prescribe antibiotics for cystitis, very often without taking a urine sample to see if the bacteria are sensitive. This is leading to the production of resistant strains of bacteria, which is detrimental to the individual and society as a whole.

Cystitis can be dealt with by altering the acidity of the urine and making it more alkaline. Over-the-counter preparations of alkaline compounds are effective, useful but expensive. An alternative is the use of sodium bicarbonate, as described in the section on cystitis (*see* **Cystitis**). Excessive use of the alkalizing compounds can cause other problems and therefore should not be overused, but I recommend the use of them in preference to antibiotics.

DECONGESTANTS

Congestion of the nasal passages and sinuses is generally a natural body response to the presence of irritants or infection. The swelling and mucus production is there to protect the body from invasion. Decongestants suppress this body healing response and should therefore only be used in extreme cases. If a patient, particularly a child, is unable to sleep or if the congestion is such that it is preventing breathing to a dangerous extent, then decongestants should be used.

Decongestants come as oral formulations, nasal sprays or drops and all should be avoided with equal effort. Natural decongestants carry the same suppressant activity but are easier for the body to break down because of their plant origins.

DEHYDROEPIANDROSTERONE (DHEA)

This hormone, found in most cells in the body, is thought to be responsible for maintaining a cell's ability to repair and maintaining its integrity. Its action is possibly by mediating the permeability of the cell wall to glucose.

This hormone is now extracted and manufactured and is being touted as a potential elixir of youth. Doctors who have researched it and those who stand to benefit from its sales are adamant about its safety and efficacy. So were the doctors who invented thalidomide! My view is that, until further studies are done, this drug should only be taken under the care of a physician who genuinely believes in the curative properties of DHEA, not so much because it will make the drug safer but they are liable to know of the most recent reports. I am sure that DHEA has its place but at the moment not as broadly as certain sources would have us believe.

DIABETIC DRUGS – *see* **Insulin**

Diabetic drugs should only be taken under the guidance of a qualified doctor, and even then only after an original prescription by a hospital specialist. The two forms of diabetic drug either stimulate the cells in the pancreas, called the islets of Langerhans, to produce insulin or affect cells generally and encourage the membranes to let more glucose in.

It is advisable to establish whether diabetes can be controlled through diet and other naturopathic methods, but if not the use of these drugs is definitely preferable to uncontrolled or high levels of glucose in the bloodstream.

Supplements required (biguanides) – Vitamin B_{12}.

DIURETICS

The kidney has several parts in its miraculously complex make-up. Different diuretics work in different ways but principally encourage the excretion of potassium, which causes water to leave the bloodstream and also causes the dehydrating effect of diuretics. There is no doubt that diuretics, along with antibiotics and steroids, have made a profound impact on the survival and well-being of many different types of patient with a variety of conditions. Prescribed by the right people and used in the right way, diuretics are life-saving. When abused, such as in weight loss, they can be surprisingly rapid in creating very dangerous states of health. The abuse of diuretics is a leading cause of death and disease in the list of dangers from prescribed drugs.

Most often used in cases of hypertension (high blood pressure) and cardiac conditions, alternative measures should be reviewed but prescriptions should not be stopped without the support of a GP or specialist.

Supplements required – Magnesium and zinc (potassium is generally lowered but many of these types of diuretics have potassium added so ask your doctor).

DYSPEPTIC DRUGS – *see* Indigestion drugs

EAR DROPS

Antiwax compounds melt the wax build-up in the ear and are perfectly safe to use. Anti-bacterial, antifungal and steroid drops can all be used with some confidence in their safety provided that the prescription has been given by your physician. Please review the relevant sections depending on the type of drug being used and always look for a naturopathic alternative before using them.

EMOLLIENTS

Emollients are principally soothers, smoothers and hydrators of the skin and can be used in all conditions that cause scaling or dryness. Those that are unmedicated, such as aqueous cream, and those that are extracted from natural sources are beneficial and safe. They do not claim to be curative but are generally very soothing, especially in eczema, and can be applied directly or through bathing.

EPILEPSY DRUGS

Antiepileptics work by altering the sensitivity of the cells in the brain. This reduces their firing off an electrical impulse when instructed to do so, incorrectly, by the area in the brain that is triggering the fits. Antiepileptic drugs have side effects, including drowsiness and reduced concentration, but need to be used for at least two years of fit-free life. Being put on and coming off these drugs must be governed by a medical specialist because removal from the drug suddenly can actually trigger fits.

EYE DROPS AND CREAMS

Optical applications are antibiotic, antifungal, steroidal or for reducing the pressure in the eye as in glaucoma. The first three groups can be referred to in the relevant sections and, in principle, avoided if such advice is supported by a medically qualified alternative practitioner. Eye drops to combat glaucoma must be taken, although they do not confront the cause of the condition. Untreated, this condition may cause blindness.

FEVER DRUGS – *see* Antipyretics

FINASTERIDE

This drug interferes with testosterone metabolism and is an alternative to the more commonly used

Alpha-blockers in the treatment of Benign Prostatic Hyperplasia. Recent studies have shown that it has reduced the risk of needing surgery by 55 per cent, reduced urinary flow obstruction and reduced one of the main problems which is urinary retention. The study suggests that it produced no serious adverse effects but impotence and decreased libido are more serious to some than others.

GAMMAGLOBULINS – *see* Immunoglobulins

GLYCERINE SUPPOSITORIES
Glycerine is a stool softener and is used by gently inserting a suppository into the rectum. There are no contraindications for this use provided that they are not needed too often. Persisting hard stool is generally a matter of hydration or poor diet and referral to a nutritionist would be recommended.

GLYCERYL TRINITRATE (GTN)
This is used as a sublingual tablet, spray, oral tablet or transdermal patch. It is a cardiac drug (*see* Cardiac drugs) that opens up the blood vessels which can instantly reduce the pain of angina. Like any cardiac drug it should only be used once advised by a medically qualified specialist and should only be stopped with that expert's approval. It is not curative of heart disease and a complementary medical view should be obtained in an attempt to remove the necessity of any of these drugs.

GOLD
Gold is used as an antiarthritic drug prescribed by hospital specialists and usually after other treatments have failed. It is a toxic drug that should only be considered by those whose quest for relief has failed through basic drugs and extensive alternative treatments.

GOUT DRUGS
The drugs used to combat gout are divided into those for acute and those for chronic situations. Alternative treatments are often very effective in both, whilst the orthodox drugs are geared towards relieving the pain or cutting down the causative uric acid crystals by artificial means, paying little attention to the underlying metabolic defect or dietary imbalance. Treatment for acute gout often includes anti-inflammatories (*see* Nonsteroidal anti-inflammatory drugs).

Supplements required (colchicine) – beta-carotene, vitamin B_{12}, potassium and sodium.

HAY FEVER DRUGS – *see* Antihistamines *and* Decongestants

HEAD LICE PREPARATIONS
Head lice are a common and irritating infestation that are often amenable to complementary medical treatments. The topical drug preparations have been cited as causing illnesses, possibly cancer, although these compounds have been withdrawn from the market in the UK. If an alternative treatment schedule does not solve the problem swiftly then I think the use of these compounds is perfectly acceptable and safe on occasions.

HEARTBURN DRUGS – *see* Indigestion drugs

HEPARIN – *see* Anticoagulants

HIGH BLOOD PRESSURE DRUGS (ANTIHYPERTENSIVES) – *see* Diuretics *and* Beta-blockers
Treating high blood pressure is discussed fully in the main text. Diuretics and beta-blockers are discussed elsewhere in this chapter and should be the first-line treatments from GPs and specialists. If complementary methods and these basic drugs do not work, people with high blood pressure will be introduced to calcium antagonists or ACE inhibitors.

Calcium antagonists block the movement of calcium in the muscles surrounding the blood vessels. Calcium is responsible for the tension in these muscles and thereby the width of the arteries. The narrower the tubes, the higher the pressure.

Angiotension-converting enzyme (ACE)

inhibitors block the production of a chemical produced by the kidneys that works directly on blood vessels again to narrow the lumen. By blocking this enzyme the blood vessels remain wider, thereby artificially reducing blood pressure.

Both of these drugs have their place in modern medicine for uncontrolled high blood pressure but both should be considered only when other treatments have failed and only under the care of a specialist initially. Other antihypertensive drugs are being discovered, analysed and introduced regularly and my comments on last-resort and specialist care apply to these as well.

Except in acute and sudden cases of raised blood pressure, alternative treatments should be tried initially because all these drugs are geared towards suppressing the high blood pressure without any interest in dealing with the underlying cause.

HORMONE REPLACEMENT THERAPY (HRT) DRUGS

These drugs are principally oral contraceptives and the pros and cons can be read about in the relevant sections (*see* **Oral contraceptive pill** *and* **Hormone replacement therapy**).

In principle, 50 per cent of ladies who embark upon HRT will not be using the medication within the first year. The side effects are pronounced and efficacy against the symptoms of menopause is limited. The protective benefits against osteoporosis and cardiovascular disease are still poorly evaluated and need to be balanced against the carcinogenic (cancer-causing) risks of breast and uterine cancer.

The pharmaceutical industry has gone to great pains to promote the lack of oestrogen as being the main factor in menopausal symptoms although there is strong evidence that progesterone is strongly associated and special reference should be made to the section on the menopause (*see* **Menopause**) where HRT is discussed at great length. Much research continues into HRT and a new form is being examined known as a Selection Oestrogen Receptor Modulation (SERM). This type of HRT acts on tissues such as bone but, apparently, does not affect other oestrogen receptors such as those found in the womb thereby reducing the incidence and risks of cancer. The same, apparently, may be the case for Breast Oestrogen Receptors. Unfortunately, these SERMs do not have such a strong effect on the hot flushes and night sweats that encourage people to take such drugs.

HYDROCORTISONE – *see* **Steroids**

HYDROGEN PEROXIDE

Used most commonly in a dilute topical solution against acne, this molecule containing two oxygen atoms is also found in intravenous techniques for increasing oxygen levels in the blood.

The topical applications are safe provided that the solution is dilute enough, although they will only treat the symptoms and not any underlying cause of skin conditions; the intravenous solution can only be administered by doctors trained in the subject and is, therefore, of potential use.

HYPNOTICS – *see* **Sleeping pills**

IMIGRAN – *see* **Sumatriptan**

IMMUNOGLOBULINS

The body has a remarkable defence system. Part of its immunity is the production of specialized molecules called immunoglobulins that attach to invading or foreign matter within the bloodstream to form a larger molecule that is removed from the system by entrapment in lymph glands or envelopment by white blood cells specialized in recognizing immunoglobulin–antigen complexes. Immunoglobulins are often referred to as antibodies.

Science has been able to replicate very few immunoglobulins, which can be injected into an individual and generally offer protection against specific diseases such as hepatitis A for up to six months. Some complementary AIDS protocols include the use of immunoglobulins such as gamma globulin which can also be used in other immunosuppressive conditions.

Immunoglobulins have their place in modern medicine. If the body is failing to defend itself then these compounds can be life-saving. There is some anecdotal evidence that immunoglobulins, being foreign proteins themselves, may stimulate an immune response from the body and problems may be associated with the other compounds that are injected during the manufacturing process. I feel that if an individual is liable to be in a situation where the disease is present, from which the immunoglobulin is due to protect them, there are grounds to use these short-lived treatments.

IMPOTENCE DRUGS

There are no oral drugs that are legally prescribable to help the formation of erections. Certain combinations of drugs of abuse can be erection-enhancing but carry potential dangerous side effects. The drugs most commonly used are injected and work by constricting the venous blood vessels. This allows blood into the penis but not out, thereby creating an erection. These will last for a few hours and are not reversible, a little painful to give and the erections may ache. These drugs can only be offered after review by specialists and are worth a try if alternative measures have not worked.

INCONTINENCE DRUGS

These are specifically prescribed by specialists and work by blocking the contraction of the detrusor (bladder) muscles. These drugs should only be used in patients with intractable incontinence. Use only as a last resort.

INDIGESTION DRUGS

Indigestion is a very broad term covering anything from a sensation of bloating and mild discomfort to severe acidic, burning pains felt in the epigastrium, the area just below the breast bone. The discomfort can travel up into the chest and throat and can be associated with diseases such as stomach ulcers, duodenal ulcers, hiatus hernia and gallbladder problems. Persistent indigestion should be thoroughly examined by a GP or specialist and once a diagnosis is made please review the relevant section in this book. Indigestion medicines fall into two categories:

- Antacids (already discussed; see **Antacids**).
- Drugs that prevent acid production.

This latter group, containing common drugs such as cimetidine, ranitidine and omeprazole, works by stopping the production of hydrochloric acid (the acid normally found in the stomach) by the special cells lining the stomach wall. These drugs are dealing with the symptom of pain created by an acid burn and in no way are they working on the cause of the loss of protection that the gut normally produces against acid.

In many cases a six-week course is 'curative', although if the underlying reason for the diminished gut protection is not dealt with, the problem will return and very often people are kept on a daily or nightly dose of the antacid preparation.

This is not good medicine and antacids of this nature should only be used if alternative or complementary medical treatments are not working or if the necessary lifestyle changes, such as stopping smoking and reducing alcohol and spicy foods, are not taken into consideration. I suspect that over the next 20 years we will see an increase in stomach cancer because the cause of indigestion is rarely dealt with and other, hopefully less sinister, problems arising because we are not producing enough acid to break down our foods.

Some of these drugs are used in the popular triple and double therapies to fight *Helicobacter pylorus* in conjunction with antibiotics. This once again returns to the principle of the germ theory where everything that goes wrong with us is caused by a bug rather than our depressed immune system and is, in my opinion, missing the point. Use triple therapy only after alternative treatments have failed.

INFERTILITY DRUGS

Infertility drugs for both men and women are principally hormonal in character and stimulate the production of sperm in men and eggs in women. These drugs have considerable side effects and are only prescribed by specialists.

Try alternative treatments before using these progressive drugs and if you do use them use complementary therapy alongside to help negate the side effects.

INSULIN – *see* **Diabetic drugs**

Insulin is prescribed when investigations suggest that the pancreas is unlikely to be able to produce enough insulin and/or diet and antidiabetic drugs are not working.

Most types of insulin are extracted from pigs, although newer types are obtained from humans. The latter are proving to be more effective but also have more side effects. Specialists will prefer certain types and diabetics requiring insulin should follow their advice. I have never seen a case of insulin-dependent diabetes improved to the point that insulin is not required. Alternative therapies may reduce the daily injectable requirement but under no circumstances should insulin injections be stopped without your doctor's approval.

LABOUR AND DELIVERY

One of the few things that doctors can do is remove pain. I am a great supporter of natural childbirth but, for the very small risk that drugs may carry, removing the pain of delivery is, in my opinion, a perfectly safe option to consider.

Pain relief in the first part of labour needs to be minimal so that mother can be aware of the progression. As the contractions become more severe and frequent, the use of nitrous oxide ('gas') is safe and effective.

If this ceases to be effective then the mother may be offered an epidural (an anaesthetic injected into the lower spinal column) or, more rarely these days, pethidine – a painkiller on the same level as morphine. Pethidine can cause respiratory depression in the child and is therefore not commonly offered. Epidurals when administered properly are safe and carry few risks of side effects.

The biggest problem is if the anaesthetic travels up the spinal column (the chances of this are reduced to negligible by keeping the mother sitting up) because if the anaesthetic hits the lower part of the brainstem it may stop respiration. This effect, should it happen, is temporary and a medically equipped delivery centre will deal with the problem very efficiently.

The use of local anaesthetic when repairing any tears or for an episiotomy, if required, should also be taken with no fear of risk.

Use alternative methods primarily but if in pain you can feel happy and safe in using orthodox drugs. Ask your complementary medical practitioner for a 'washout' treatment for both you and baby if drugs are used.

LAXATIVES

Laxatives are principally of four kinds:

- Compounds that increase bulk
- Compounds that pull or keep water in the bowel
- Drugs that stimulate peristalsis (contractions) of the large bowel
- Stool softeners

As discussed in the section on constipation (*see* **Constipation**) these drugs should be avoided if possible. If dietetics and a complementary medical practitioner cannot solve a problem of constipation then laxatives should be used from as natural a source as possible and as infrequently as possible. Laxatives that cause gut contraction should be avoided in particular, because the bowel-training habit will alter very swiftly with these.

LEVODOPA – *see* **Anti-Parkinson's drugs**

LIGNOCAINE

This cocaine-like drug is used as a local anaesthetic either with or without adrenaline. Some people have sensitivity to lignocaine but most have no problems. It is broken down in the liver which allows the small amount that may be absorbed through its use as a local anaesthetic to be tolerable and acceptable. Provided that you have no specific problems with lignocaine, its occasional use is not a problem.

LITHIUM

Lithium carbonate is a drug used specifically in psychiatry for people with psychotic or schizophrenic disorders. It is generally prescribed by psychiatrists initially and these specialists and GPs will monitor levels very accurately because too little will be ineffective and too much can be toxic, causing liver and bone marrow problems.

It is a remarkably effective drug although it carries dangers and should be used only if other drugs and alternative measures have not proven effective. This is not the safest of drugs and should be used only under specialist guidance.

MALARIA DRUGS

More accurately termed antimalaria drugs, this group of chemicals is beneficial for travellers, although their use for longer than three months is generally not recommended. The drugs kill the malaria parasites at varying stages of their lifecycle, which includes time spent in the red blood cells as well as in the bloodstream.

Treatment is by quinine, intravenously if the condition is serious or by tablet if not. Other drugs such as mefloquine or Fansidar may also be necessary and these drugs should be used if so advised.

Prophylaxis is with mefloquine, chloroquine, Paludrine or proguanil hydrochloride. Mefloquine has recently had some bad press and ideally should be avoided, but many strains of malaria parasite are now resistant to other drugs and it is better to try mefloquine and keep a close eye on your general health through your GP or healthcare professional.

Prophylaxis against malaria is generally safe.

The pills are taken once a day or once a week because the body clears out the drugs within that time frame. If you do not react badly to them then it is safer to run the risk of the drug causing a problem than to run the risk of malaria.

Homeopathic remedies, specifically Natrum muriaticum, are often mentioned as an alternative. There is no strong evidence to support this although the use of Natrum muriaticum and vitamin B_6 (100mg per day for an adult) may help the body to fight any malarial infestation.

MAXOLON – *see* Antiemetics

MEBENDAZOLE – *see* Antiworm drugs

MORPHINE

Morphine is the most potent pain reliever. It is similar to the body's own painkillers known as endorphins and enkephalins, and also similar in structure and efficacy to heroin.

Morphine is profoundly addictive, not so much psychologically but certainly physiologically. This means that when its use is stopped the body will be much more sensitive to pain for a short while. The body does readjust. Morphine is usually introduced when terminal conditions are creating pain that is unrelenting with other painkillers.

I, amongst other holistic physicians, suspect that the use of morphine is suppressive not only of pain but also of the body's natural vital forces. Morphine should only be used when other painkillers are failing to succeed.

MOUTHWASHES

Mouthwashes are principally antiseptic solutions. They kill bacteria but do not differentiate between the good guys and the bad guys. Our mouths are protected by a variety of useful bacteria that mouthwashes may kill off, leaving us open to unwanted bacterial effects. The loss of bacteria also encourages the growth of fungi and yeasts. Avoid the use of mouthwashes except for short periods under dental or medical advice.

NALOXONE

This drug is given to block the effects of opiates, principally in those who have overdosed on heroin, opium or morphine. An excess of these compounds can cause respiratory depression and they are therefore potentially fatal; naloxone plays its part in emergency medicine.

NALTREXONE

This drug is currently prescribed in specialist clinics and is given at around 50mg daily to help prevent relapse in opioid (heroin) dependent patients. Currently, complementary medically-qualified practitioners are using doses around 3mg a day in the treatment of a variety of conditions. These include lymphoma and pancreatic cancer, HIV positive patients, psoriasis, chronic fatigue syndrome, other cancers and neurological conditions such as multiple sclerosis as well as inflammatory conditions such as rheumatoid arthritis. It is postulated that low-dose naltrexone may increase endorphin production and encourage nutrition and oxygenation of the nervous systems.

NANDROLONE

At the time of writing, an illegal performance-enhancing drug nandrolone is being found in athletes. In many cases, the sportsperson is astounded by the accusations of cheating. As research is ongoing I cannot comment conclusively, but there is evidence to suggest that certain plant extracts may contain anabolic (build-up) steroids that can be changed into this drug. An athlete cannot assume that a manufacturing company will not tamper with their product in an attempt to enhance its reputation. To that end all athletes who wish to remain healthy should avoid anabolic steroids of any sort and ensure that any supplements they are taking are guaranteed free from contamination and that they contain only natural ingredients.

NEBULIZERS

These are instruments that enable patients with lung problems who do not have the necessary skills to use an inhaler to receive inhalations (*see* **Antiasthma drugs**).

NICOTINE PRODUCTS

Nicotine is a highly addictive compound found in all tobacco. It is conceivable that some cigarette companies might put extra nicotine into their brands to 'hook' users.

The pharmaceutical industry has produced nicotine products in the form of patches and chewing gum in an attempt to remove the need for people to obtain nicotine from smoking.

This is simply transferring the addiction from one method of administration to another. However, it is probably better to use a nicotine patch or chewing gum rather than smoking because you will be protecting the lungs, but dependence on these products maintains the addictive aspect and is less likely, therefore, to reduce the smoking craving in the long term. Many people are allergic to the patches and struggle with nausea when nicotine is chewed. *See* **Smoking**.

NIFEDIPINE

Nifedipine is a cardiac drug and if prescribed should be used, unless an alternative therapy proves successful and even then withdrawal should only be under a doctor's supervision.

Nifedipine had some bad press because it was causing suicide and a worsening of symptoms and cardiac failure in a larger than acceptable number of users. Other drugs may be preferable but this decision must be made with the expertise of specialists.

NITRATES

The most commonly used nitrate is glycerine trinitrate (GTN). This is a potent arterial dilator that has its most beneficial effect on the arteries supplying the heart muscle. It is commonly used in angina and, like any cardiac drug, should be used as instructed unless alternatives can be found.

Like any drug that affects the cardiovascular

system it has side effects, including dizziness, headaches and nausea, and any such symptoms should be discussed with your GP.

NITRAZEPAM

This hypnotic drug is more commonly used as Mogadon (*see* **Sleeping pills**).

NITROUS OXIDE

Nitrous oxide, commonly known as laughing gas, is used as an inhaled painkiller most commonly through delivery. It is absolutely safe to use.

NON-STEROIDAL ANTI-INFLAMMATORY DRUGS (NSAID)

These drugs, as the name suggests, are anti-inflammatory drugs. They are a step up from aspirin, paracetamol and acetaminophen, and a step down from steroids.

Inflammation is the body's natural healing process and should only be suppressed as a last resort. Alternative and complementary medical treatment should be tried first before an anti-pain drug is used.

What is more, the British Medical Research Centre recently stated: '. . . (the) high level of prescribing is still not justified' and '. . . the therapeutic role of topical NSAIDs is unclear'. This is based on the poor trial evidence there is and the fact that they showed a 'marked placebo response'.

Paracetamol and aspirin are often as effective as NSAIDs and seem to have fewer side effects.

Supplements required (indomethacin) – Folic acid and iron.

NYSTATIN – *see* **Candida**, **Thrush** *and* **Fungal infections**

Nystatin is a very popular prescription for candidal or thrush infections because it kills yeasts but, like any such drug, has a capability of creating resistant strains. Avoid the use of nystatin whenever possible.

OESTROGENS

Oestrogens are a group of hormones manufactured in both males and females but more so in women. Produced predominantly in the ovaries (testes in males) and the adrenal glands, they affect many different cells in the body. Until the age of puberty, oestrogen levels are low in girls, they rise and fall through the normal menstrual cycle and their production tails off at menopause.

Artificial oestrogens are used in the oral contraceptive pill and in hormone replacement therapy (*see* **Oral contraceptive pill** and **Hormone replacement therapy**). Artificial oestrogens are much more potent than natural oestrogens and carry side effect risks in those who are susceptible. These include minor symptoms such as headaches, water retention and mood swings but may also have an influence on more serious problems such as blood clotting, raising blood pressure and cancer.

The use of any oestrogen should be considered with a complementary practitioner who is knowledgeable in this area. Alternative options do exist in the form of oral and topical oestrogen compounds derived from certain plants that contain phyto-oestrols, such as hops, fennel, rhubarb and soya products.

OPIOID ANALGESICS (INCLUDING MORPHINE, DIAMORPHINE)

The body produces natural painkillers, the most effective of which is a group called endorphins and enkephalins. These powerful analgesics are produced when the body is in severe pain or has undergone trauma, but can also be produced through heavy muscular exercise. These hormones also carry a sense of euphoria.

'Man-made' opiates have a very strong resemblance to the body's natural opiates and therefore tend to be handled well by the body. Unfortunately, opiates are addictive and are usually prescribed only in very severe pain for short periods or for pain created by terminal disease where addiction does not matter.

The euphoric affect of opiates is well established

but less well documented is morphine's effect on willpower. Very often opiates are used in terminal diseases and I have found that the conscious willpower to fight the battle diminishes, as well as a subconscious willpower that I think is very necessary in the fight against disease. It is almost as if the subconscious or the soul shrugs its shoulders and says 'well this is not too bad, why bother fighting'.

Opiates should only be considered when all other orthodox and complementary medical options have been exhausted.

ORAL CONTRACEPTIVE PILL

When the 'Pill' was first produced in the late 1950s its claims were: socially enormous and medically safe. Nearly 40 years later the social implications have been supported and indeed the number of unwanted pregnancies and the serious complications that go with this, such as terminations (abortions), will also support its beneficial claims.

It takes over 2 minutes, however, to read the list of the variety of side effects and dangers that the Pill can create. Although the problems associated with the Pill are less numerous and less risky than the immediate dangers of a termination, and incomparable on a social basis to unwanted pregnancies, the side effects are nonetheless potentially lethal.

There is an increased risk of a variety of cancers with the use of the Pill although supporters would point out that the Pill also has protective effects. No conclusive trials are advertised against the use of the Pill because of the enormous financial gains made by the pharmaceutical industry from its sale.

The consensus of holistic opinion is against the use of artificially created hormones taking the place of the body's natural cycle. The nature of the Pill's effect is, broadly speaking, to convince the body that it is already pregnant and therefore does not need to produce the natural fertility hormones. There is little doubt that if other contraceptive methods are usable then the Pill should be avoided.

If a holistically-minded GP or a knowledgeable complementary medical practitioner has fully pointed out the risks and side effects and can see no reason why your past history, family history, lifestyle or general health would make you more prone to the side effects, then I feel that the use of the Pill over a nine-month period (the body's normal pregnancy time) with a 3–6-month break afterwards offers a happy medium.

Please ensure that you read the list of side effects before going on the Pill.

Oral contraceptive pill – Supplement with vitamin B complex, vitamin C, folic acid, magnesium and zinc.

PALUDRINE – *see* **Malaria drugs**

PARACETAMOL

Paracetamol is a mild but potent analgesic similar in its effect and strength to aspirin but with far less anti-inflammatory effect. Because, holistically speaking, inflammation is part of the body's repair mechanism, paracetamol is preferred to aspirin as a first-line pain relief.

Paracetemol is, however, far more toxic to the liver than aspirin (although aspirin has far greater chances of causing gastritis or ulcerous conditions in the stomach) and should not be taken too frequently or in excess (*see* **Analgesics**).

PENICILLIN – *see* **Antibiotics**

PEPPERMINT OIL

Used as an aromatherapy oil, peppermint can be most beneficial. From an orthodox point of view peppermint has been found to be helpful in relieving bowel spasm, especially in irritable bowel syndrome. It has its place in holistic treatments and if effective can be used without anxiety, although one must remember that peppermint will negate the effect of homeopathic remedies.

Topically, peppermint oil can be very relieving for haemorrhoids and phlebitis but remember to dilute the peppermint oil considerably before applying it to the sensitive anal area.

PETHIDINE

Pethidine is a commonly employed opioid analgesic. It used to be quite commonplace in childbirth, although like any opiate derivative it may have a suppressive effect on respiration and is therefore no longer encouraged because of the risk to the foetus or baby.

Commonly found in the emergency medical bags of doctors, pethidine can be used in emergency and for pain with great relief and safety.

PHENERGAN (PROMETHAZINE HYDROCHLORIDE) – *see* Antihistamines

Phenergan is the trade name of the most common antihistamine used in Britain: promethazine. Promethazine is used all over the world as a first choice for hayfever and other allergic symptoms. It deserves special mention because it is used as a sedative preoperatively and also for children who are exhibiting sleep pattern difficulties. This latter use as a sedative is based on one of Phenergan's side effects, which is drowsiness.

Basically Phenergan will suppress symptoms of allergy and is in no way a treatment or cure. It is best to try to treat the cause of an allergy rather than suppress the symptoms. If necessary, however, it can be used safely if taken short term. The same can be said for its sedative effects, and for children I would recommend that no more than three nights should be affected by promethazine without at least a one-week gap.

PHENOBARBITONE – *see* Barbiturates

Phenobarbitone is one of the few barbiturates still utilized for certain conditions. It is generally only prescribed by specialists and only if other more effective drugs with less addictive properties are not available. If you are using a barbiturate you probably need to and you should continue to do so unless an alternative treatment is effective.

PHENYTOIN

This is an anticonvulsant or antiepileptic drug. It acts by reducing the sensitivity of neurological cells, thereby preventing the electrical impulses that flash through the brain causing epilepsy. It is an extremely effective and successful drug, although some side effects are associated.

Phenytoin is usually only prescribed by specialists when no other options are available. Treatment, once started, should be continued until your specialist or GP removes you from the drug. It is worthwhile discussing the underlying problem with a complementary medical practitioner but stopping any anticonvulsant is a risky business.

PIPERAZINE

Piperazine along with mebendazole are the two most frequently used antihelminthic (worms) drugs. Although there is a myriad of herbal treatments that have been used for centuries in dealing with infestation by worms such as roundworms and threadworms, these two drugs are safe and effective.

I recommend the use of these drugs because they are poorly, if at all, absorbed into the system and stay in the bowel, killing the parasites. Very few people have any side effects or problems.

PIRITON (CHLORPHENIRAMINE MALEATE) – *see* Antihistamines

This drug receives a specific mention because it is one of the more popular antihistamines used for hayfever and urticarial symptoms. Like any drug aimed principally at symptomatic relief, Piriton should be used as a last and not first choice.

PODOPHYLLUM

This is an antigenital wart lotion that is painted on topically. A very effective treatment but the warts may return. Podophyllum is also toxic if used too much because it damages normal skin. It is important to avoid the area around a wart.

PONSTAN – *see* Non-steroidal anti-inflammatory drugs

PREDNISOLONE – *see* Steroids

PREMARIN – *see* **Hormone replacement therapy**

PROGESTERONE – *see* **Hormone replacement therapy** *and* **Osteoporosis**

Progesterone is infrequently used because of the artificial forms being 40 times stronger than naturally made progesterone. Certain conditions require its use but plenty of alternatives exist for all but the most serious of problems.

Natural progesterone is available in a cream and may be far more effective than oestrogen in many hormone-related conditions, including premenstrual syndrome, breast cancer, osteoporosis and cardiovascular disease.

PROPRANOLOL – *see* **Beta-blockers**

PROSTAGLANDINS AND OXYTOCICS

Prostaglandins are commonly found in many biochemical pathways within the body but artificial prostaglandins are principally reserved to induce abortion or induce labour. These drugs are prescribed by a specialist and generally have no alternative.

PROVERA

This is a modified progesterone drug that is used by specialists in the treatment of endometriosis and other gynaecological problems. It is sometimes used to try to induce periods if they have stopped. Provera has many unpleasant side effects and should be used only when alternative treatments have failed.

PROZAC – *see* **Selective serotonin re-uptake inhibitors**

QUININE

Quinine is used in severe cases of malaria and differs from antimalarial drugs (*see* **Malaria drugs**) simply because it is used as a treatment and not as a prophylactic.

Quinine is the most effective of antimalarial drugs and that is not speaking too highly. Used in conjunction with complementary therapies its effects may well be enhanced but this is a drug that may save lives and should not be resisted.

RANITIDINE – *see* **Antacids**

Ranitidine is an antacid drug that blocks receptors in the stomach lining that trigger acid production. It is of benefit in relieving symptoms and supposedly gives the stomach time to repair any damaged membrane.

REGAINE (MINOXIDIL)

This topically applied drug, minoxidil, has gained fame by acting as a hair follicle stimulant in male-pattern baldness.

The drug was initially discarded from its original intended use as an antihypertensive drug because of severe side effects. One of these was hair growth. Some clever boffin applied it directly to the skin and a whole new pharmaceutical angle is born.

Minoxidil works by producing a fine, downy hair growth in over 70 per cent of individuals but less than 15 per cent have an acceptable type of hair and to maintain it they need to continue to use the drug, at approximately £1 a day. The drug is absorbed and therefore side effects are possible as well as the compound causing local irritations.

REGULAN (ISPAGULA HUSKS) – *see* **Laxatives** *and* **Constipation**

RENNIES – *see* **Antacids**

RETIN-A

This compound, tretinoin, is the acid form of vitamin A. It is a topical application used in acne that causes a drying effect and temporarily reduces the problem of acne. It is frequently used in association with Roaccutane (isotretinoin), again in acne. It is an extremely aggressive topical treatment and is in no way curative. Avoid if possible.

RIFAMPICIN – *see* **Antibiotics**

Rifampicin is a first-line antituberculosis drug. More and more strains of tuberculosis are becoming resistant to this compound but it should still be used in the initial fight.

RITALIN

This drug is sold as part of a treatment programme for attention deficit disorder (ADD) and hyperactivity disorders. The manufacturers suggest that it should only be used as a last resort, although, especially in America, its use is becoming much greater.

The drug must be prescribed by a specialist and even then the safety is questionable. It is known to retard growth and no trials have been done on long-term therapy. The principle of the drug (methylphenidate hydrochloride, which is derived from amphetamines) is to stimulate the central nervous system, thereby increasing attention. The paradox of the success of a stimulating drug in overstimulated children is unclear, but it clearly stimulates some part of the brain that counteracts the cause of hyperactivity. The belief is that hyperactivity is a compensatory mechanism for a poor concentration ability (*see* **Hyperactivity**).

ROACCUTANE (ISOTRETINOIN)

This is a powerful and toxic anti-acne drug based on a derivative of vitamin A. The side effects take approximately 2 minutes to read out and this drug is generally only prescribed by a hospital consultant. Try every avenue to treat acne other than with this drug.

ROHYPNOL – *see* **Sleeping pills**

This potent hypnotic receives a mention separate from sleeping pills in general because of its use as a drug of abuse. When taken with alcohol and the initial soporific effect is fought off, an exciting buzz is said to occur and with a prolongation of time before orgasm during sexual intercourse. This may be so but the amount of chemical neurotransmitters that need to be produced to override both the soporific effects of the alcohol and this immensely powerful drug are enormous. The drain on the nervous system is intense and the long-term effects of such abuse are unknown but certainly not liable to be healthy.

SALAZOPYRIN

A salicylic acid or aspirin-based derivative, this drug works as a potent anti-inflammatory agent used predominantly in bowel inflammation and particularly ulcerative colitis. Salazopyrin definitely has a beneficial effect in inflammatory bowel disease and may reduce inflammation and prevent operations if taken either alone or in conjunction with steroids.

If prescribed, withdrawal should be under very careful control and the return of any bowel condition should be assessed immediately.

Supplements required – Folic acid, sodium bicarbonate and potassium.

SALBUTAMOL – *see* **Asthma drugs**

SALICYLATES AND SALICYLIC ACID

These are aspirin by another name (*see* **Aspirin**).

SEDATION – *see* Anaesthetics *and* Tranquillizers

SELECTIVE OESTROGEN RECEPTOR MODULATORS (SERMs)

These drugs are a specific type of HRT that, in trials to date, have been shown to increase bone density in postmenopausal women. The drugs also appear to lower LDL-cholesterol and do not increase the risk of endometrial cancer. These are marked benefits over and above regular HRT. SERMs drugs may be beneficial in avoiding the side effects of other conventional HRT therapies – in particular, breast pain – but they do have the increased risk of developing clots, as do all the HRTs.

SELECTIVE SEROTONIN RE-UPTAKE INHIBITERS (SSRI)

The SSRI drugs are relatively new and work by blocking the breakdown of the body's main 'happy juice' neurotransmitter, known as serotonin. If ever a drug was to have a holistic approach, this must be it.

This group is less sedative than its better-known rivals, the tricyclic antidepressants, and have fewer side effects. Fewer side effects does not mean side effect free and the group can cause quite severe symptoms and has been cited as the cause of marked and severe anorexia. If an antidepressant has to be used, this group is a good starting point but work as hard as you can to find alternative treatments.

SELSUN

Selsun is an antidandruff shampoo that contains a high quantity of selenium. This is toxic to certain skin fungi and is used topically. This is an extremely effective and safe treatment.

SENNA – *see* Laxatives

SEPTRIN – *see* Antibiotics

This is a common antibiotic that is used less because of its toxic side effects. It is popular for urinary tract infections and is now used as a prophylactic antibiotic against *Pneumocystis carinii*, a common infection in AIDS. Only use this drug on the recommendation of a specialist because others are less toxic and just as effective.

SLEEPING PILLS – *see* Insomnia

There is a variety of different chemical compounds that can be used to put people to sleep. There is no 'safe' sleeping pill because any of them in excess can cause brain damage or death. From a more holistic point of view sleeping pills are a quick solution for a deep biological imbalance.

Sleeping pills generally work by telling the brain and nervous system that it should be asleep. This overrides the body's natural chemicals that are being produced to keep you awake for some underlying reason or taking the place of the body's natural 'sleepy' chemicals. In both cases sleeping pills work against the body's natural processes and are, therefore, generally contra-indicated.

If you use sleeping pills for any length of time the underlying cause of the sleeplessness will become more deeply buried and harder to deal with and the body will quickly become quite dependent and take more time to reproduce its own sleeping chemical. As these pills do not stop the production of the compounds that keep us awake, the brain is subjected to both stimulus and suppression at the same time, making the sleep shallow and unrefreshing at a deeper level.

Sleeping pills should only be used under the supervision of a medically qualified and holistic-thinking practitioner. They can be used for up to three nights to break sleep patterns on rare occasions without too much risk of longer term problems.

SOLPADEINE

A common painkiller containing paracetamol and codeine (*see* Analgesics, Paracetamol and Opioid analgesia).

STELAZINE – *see* Antiemetics

STEMETIL (PROCHLORPERAZINE)

A most popular antiemetic (*see* Antiemetics).

STEROIDS

The human body makes its own steroids. These may be anabolic (body stimulating) or catabolic (inhibiting). The body maintains an intricate balance of these chemicals and different types are produced for different functions, accurately and rhythmically. Steroids that encourage repair are produced through the night when we are sleeping and those that stimulate activity are produced in abundance in the early hours of the morning. Conversely, those involved in the breakdown of unwanted products and elimination have their set times to be produced at high or low levels. This delicate balance is maintained by command hormones produced in the pituitary gland and adrenal glands and, provided that we maintain good health, this balance is undisturbed. Steroids have an immunosuppressive action. In the same way that they balance the body's blood flow, they also prevent overstimulation of the body's immune system.

As one can see, steroids have many effects but one of their main methods of action is by constricting blood vessels, thereby decreasing blood flow. If a body part is injured the nervous control and histamine release cause arteries to open up to carry the blood into the area, thus bringing in vitamins and other nutrients – white blood cells to kill invaders and scar tissue-forming cells to heal damage. The action of steroids is to keep this in balance.

The use of steroids, whether topical or systemic (taken into the body), is damaging from five points of view:

- The delicate balance of healing is disturbed.
- The control mechanisms are blocked.
- The natural healing process is inhibited.
- The steroids themselves are shrouded with side effects, some of them lethal.
- The immunosuppressive action of steroids can lead to recurrent or persistent infections.

The most common steroids in use in Western medicine are hydrocortisone (a molecule similar to but more potent than the body's naturally produced cortisone) and prednisolone. In the East many plant extracts contain steroids that are equally potent, equally suppressive and make a mockery of the concept that natural medicine is safe if injudiciously used or over-prescribed. Self-medication with herbs is often dangerous because of this steroid effect.

The orthodox world concerns itself with removing discomfort, often at any price, and with little concern for the underlying cause. For instance, the use of steroids in asthma removes the inflammation in the bronchial tree thereby opening the passages. In life-threatening conditions this is invaluable but it does not profess to be a cure. The use of steroids in less severe cases of asthma is, undoubtedly, relieving and often necessary. However, without a complementary medical view steroids may have to be used in perpetuity or until the body repairs itself regardless of the medication.

When a steroid is prescribed by a physician *it must not be stopped* except under medical supervision. The inhibition created by steroids on the control mechanisms in the body may stop natural steroid production. Ceasing medication may leave the body without steroids and this can be fatal. Anyone taking or who has been recommended to take steroids should review the situation with a complementary medical practitioner and under medically qualified supervision either withdraw or assess the efficacy of not taking them. The pharmaceutical industry would have us believe that topical steroids are poorly absorbed through the skin and therefore have little if any effect. They do thin the skin if used persistently, they reduce the immunity in the area and, without any doubt, are absorbed in quantities that can affect the system as a whole. One must be particularly wary if using a steroid cream on an area of skin that is weeping or bleeding.

Supplements required – Vitamin C and D, folic acid, calcium, magnesium, potassium, selenium and zinc.

STILBOESTROL
This drug is prescribed by specialist units in rare cases now to treat prostate cancer. It has many side effects and is less used than other oestrogens such as fosfestrol. Its use should be continued if started unless side effects are noted, in which case the specialist involved should be advised.

STREPTOKINASE
This is an injected drug carried by most GPs and emergency doctors for use within a few hours of a myocardial infarction (heart attack). Streptokinase is also used for deep vein thrombosis

and other clot problems such as embolism. It is considered to increase the chances of survival following heart attack. Further studies are required but at this juncture it is worth taking.

SUDAFED

Sudafed is an adrenaline-like drug called pseudoephedrine. It is used as a topical nasal decongestant and should only be considered after alternative treatments have failed for situations such as rhinitis and hay fever.

SUDOCREM

God's gift to nappy rash. This zinc-based synthetic beeswax cream acts as a marvellous barrier to prevent infection for nappy rash and open sores. Used in conjunction with an *Arnica* or *Calendula* cream, it will protect whilst the other heals.

SULPHASALAZINE

This is the generic name for Salazopirine (*see* **Salazopyrin**).

SUMATRIPTAN

Initially an injectable drug used in acute attacks of migraine, it is now available orally but has many side effects and little long-term experience. It should be used only after all other alternatives and orthodox antimigraine treatments have been tried.

SUN SCREEN

An ever-increasing market is being found for these creams, which contain agents that block ultraviolet light. Their effect is only as a barrier cream and most people do not apply the lotion thickly enough. This means that the effects are much shorter lived than described on the bottle. Limited exposure to sun and reference to the section on sunburn (*see* **Sunburn**) should be used in conjunction with sun screens.

TAGAMET (CIMETIDINE)

This is a drug that blocks acid production (*see* **Antacids**).

TAMOXIFEN

Tamoxifen blocks oestrogen receptors and is the first-line hormonal treatment in breast cancer that is sensitive to oestrogen. It is also used in postmenopausal women because of an effect other than oestrogen blocking (postmenopausal women have low levels of oestrogen and therefore the oestrogen-blocking action is not the method of defence). Side effects are rare but include menopausal symptoms and will, of course, stop the normal cycle.

Tamoxifen appears to lose its defensive capabilities after five years. It is thought that tamoxifen alters the oestrogen receptor on a cancer cell, but after a few years the cancer cell adjusts and makes the tamoxifen appear like an oestrogen stimulant. The pharmaceutical industry is working on adjusting the tamoxifen molecule to make it last longer.

TEMAZEPAM

This is a most popular sleeping pill (*see* **Sleeping pills**).

TEMGESIC

This is a sublingual opioid-like painkiller (*see* **Analgesics**).

TERFENADINE

Until recently this was the most popular antihistamine because it had a weak sedative effect. It is now known to create marked arrhythmias (irregular heart beats) and should be avoided.

TESTOSTERONE

Testosterone is only provided by specialists and for particular conditions. The use of this drug is very limited and should only be used if other treatments fail.

TETANUS TOXOID

Tetanus toxoid is given if a wound is liable to be infected. Tetanus toxoid is likely to be administered to anyone with a wound or cut that is likely to have been infected by the tetanus causing bacteria (*see* **Tetanus**).

Its use in serious wounds is sensible but minor abrasions seem to receive the same dosage, although it is probably safe.

TETRACYCLINES

These are powerful antibiotics with many side effects and should only be used after a firm diagnosis, culture and sensitivity have been established on any infection. This is sadly not done and many strains of bacteria are proving to be resistant to this antibiotic (*see* **Antibiotics**).

Supplements required – Calcium, iron and magnesium.

THEOPHYLLINE

This is a second-line antiasthma drug, traces of which are found in black tea. Use it if prescribed, but consider complementary medical therapies to aim at a cure for asthma rather than this drug, which simply relieves symptoms.

THIAZIDES – *see* **Diuretics**

THYROXINE

This is not strictly a drug although it is manufactured. It is a combination of an amino acid and iodine and is used as a replacement therapy in thyroid deficiency. Commonly needed and safe to use in the right dosage.

TIBOLONE

This drug is due to be pushed strongly as an anti-osteoporosis drug because of its oestrogen and progesterone activity. Initially used to block flushing after surgically induced menopause, the pharmaceutical industry have recently had it licensed for this other use.

Avoid this drug until it has been on the market a little bit longer, in case it comes up with serious side effects and review the section on osteoporosis in this book (*see* **Osteoporosis**).

TRANQUILLIZERS

This term has now been superseded by hypnotics (*see* **Sleeping pills**) and anxiolytics. A tranquillizer is principally a drug that takes away anxiety and is now synonymous with anxiolytics.

These drugs can be divided into the benzodiazepines and barbiturates. The latter are very rarely used nowadays because of their side effects and rapid addictive qualities. The former are less addictive – but only just. Diazepam (Valium) is the most common drug indicated for the short-term relief of severe anxiety. The benzodiazepines can be long- or short-acting drugs but are being replaced by sustained serotonin re-uptake inhibiters (SSRIs), principally Prozac.

TRICYCLIC ANTIDEPRESSANTS

Until recently, tricyclics were a preferred form of antidepressant drug. More recently the serotonin re-uptake inhibitors have surpassed them.

Tricyclics may still be prescribed by psychiatrists who stick with their known, tried and tested drugs and if they work and no alternatives are successful their use should be maintained.

TRILUDAN

This is the most popular tradename for the drug terfenadine, which is an antihistamine (*see* **Antihistamines**).

TRYPTOPHAN

Tryptophan is an essential amino acid and is used by the brain to produce serotonin, one of the body's major calmants and sleep chemicals. L-Tryptophan was a most popular and successful antidepressant and is found in cottage cheese, milk products, meat, fish, fowl, bananas, dried dates, peanuts and most other protein-rich foods.

It is now only prescribable by hospital specialists and registered doctors because it was linked to a potentially fatal blood disease. This was following a contaminated batch supplied by one single Japanese manufacturer. Despite many other trials showing tryptophan to be safe (after all, we are eating it constantly), the pharmaceutical industry took advantage to take this easily available and extremely inexpensive supplement off the market, thereby requiring the increased sales of more artificial and expensive drugs. Sometimes I despair.

UNGUENTUM MERCK

A popular ointment made up of paraffin, neutral oils and alcohols and brilliantly marketed by the pharmaceutical company Merck, who attached their name to the Latin 'Unguentum' for ointment. It is safe to use as a barrier cream, preferably in conjunction with a naturopathic ointment such as *Arnica* or *Calendula,* which can be used instead of Unguentum.

VACCINES – *see* Vaccinations

VALIUM

The most popular tradename for diazepam, the tranquillizer (*see* **Tranquillizers**).

VANCOMYCIN

Vancomycin is an antibiotic that deserves special mention. It can only be given intravenously and is used as a last resort against multiresistant bacteria. Its use is becoming more needed because of hospital-induced resistant strains, especially of staphylococcal infections. Special mention is given because it is our last-resort antibiotic. We now have resistant strains to this as well. Beware the coming plague!

VASELINE

Vaseline is a safe barrier cream and lubricant.

VASOCONSTRICTORS

These drugs are used as local anaesthetics when given by injection and in the treatment of migraine if vasodilation is considered. Use if needed.

VASODILATORS

Principally anything that opens up blood vessels is a vasodilator, which includes alcohol. Peripheral vasodilators are used in an attempt to treat Raynaud's disease and others affect the blood vessels in the brain and are being unsuccessfully tried in Alzheimer's disease and other dementias. Use only if alternative therapies do not work because these drugs may be too powerful causing an overdilation leading to weakness and fainting.

VENTOLIN – *see* **Antiasthma drugs**

VIAGRA

This drug, released in America in the early part of 1998, encourages the production of a firm erection by influencing a chemical (cGMP) that, in turn, constricts the contraction of the veins in the penis as opposed to relaxing the muscles in the arteries. Highlighting the large number of men with erectile problems this drug sold more in its first six weeks of being available than any other drug yet produced.

Like all drugs that make it to the market, strict and stringent tests have been performed to monitor its safety. Initial reports quoted some deaths but longer-term studies suggest that this is a safe enough drug.

VICKS

Vicks is a collection of painkillers and decongestants under a tradename. The use of naturopathic treatments is preferred.

VOLTAROL

This is a popular non-steroidal anti-inflammatory drug (*see* **Non-steroidal anti-inflammatory drugs**).

WARFARIN

Warfarin is a drug that interferes with the body's clotting mechanism. It takes some time to kick in, unlike heparin, and is given to prevent clotting in deep vein thrombosis or emboli.

Careful monitoring of blood clotting time s required but it may be a life-saving compound. Naturopathic treatments are available but should only be prescribed by a competent and experienced complementary medical practitioner with experience in herbal medicine.

XANAX
Xanax, a short-term anxiolytic (*see* **Tranquillizers**).

ZANTAC
Zantac is the tradename for ranitidine (*see* **Ranitidine**).

ZIDOVUDINE
Also known as azidothymidine and best known as AZT (*see* **AIDS drugs**).

Supplements required (AZT) – Carnitine, vitamin B_{12}, copper and zinc.

PART THREE

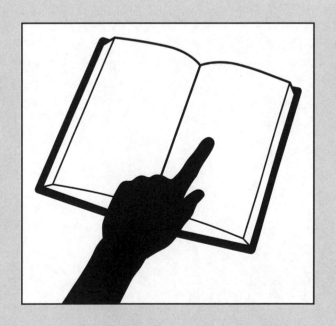

GLOSSARY

Acute – a term used to describe a disease that is sudden, short-lived and relatively severe.

Aetiology – the cause or origin of a disease or disorder.

Allergen – a substance capable of inducing an immune response and producing an immediate hypersensitivity (allergy).

Analgesia – the relief of pain without loss of consciousness.

Anaphylaxis – a manifestation of immediate hypersensitivity in which exposure of a sensitized individual to a specific antigen results in life-threatening respiratory distress.

Antihelminthic – an agent that is destructive to worms.

Antioxidant – a vitamin-based molecule that neutralizes negatively charged particles (free radicals) in the bloodstream, thus delaying or preventing degradation by oxidation.

Antipyretic – an agent that relieves or reduces fever.

Arteriosclerosis – a group of diseases characterized by thickening and loss of elasticity of the arterial walls.

Asymptomatic – showing or causing no symptoms.

Atopic – allergic response occurring in a site other than the area of contact with allergen.

Aura – an energy 'fuzz' around the body that changes colour and density according to general health.

Autoimmunity – a condition characterized by a specific humoral or cell-mediated immune response against constituents of the body's own tissues.

Autonomic – self-controlling or functionally independent.

Beta-blockers – drugs that combat hypertension by slowing the heart rate or preventing arterial contraction.

Bioflavonoids – compounds present in plants that maintain the walls of small blood vessels in a normal state.

Bioresonance – the use of electromagnetic energy, in conjunction with a computer, in the diagnosis and treatment of disease.

Calcium channel blockers – drugs that interfere with intracellular calcium flux and reduce the contraction of arterial muscle, thus acting as vasodilators.

Calculus – an abnormal concretion occurring within the body that is usually composed of mineral salts.

Calisthenics – a system of physical exercises for promoting strength and cardiopulmonary fitness.

CT scan – computed tomography scan: reconstruction of cross-sectional images of the body made by a rotating X-ray source and detector that move around the body and record X-ray transmissions throughout the 360° rotation.

Catecholamines – compounds that function as neurotransmitters.

Chalazion – a small nodule on the eyelid due to chronic inflammation of a sebaceous gland.

Chancre – a hard swelling that constitutes the primary lesion in syphilis.

Chemotherapy – the treatment of disease by chemical compounds selectively directed against invading organisms or abnormal cells.

Chronic – a term used to describe a disease that persists over a long period of time.

Circadian rhythm – a cyclical variation of about 24 hours in the intensity of a metabolic, physiological processes and other facets of behaviour.

Clinical – founded on actual observation and treatment of a patient rather than theory or basic science.

Commensals – organisms that feed off or within a host organism but do not harm the host.

Complementary medicine – systems of treatment that 'complement' orthodox methods but are not fully accepted by orthodox medical science.

Constitutional remedy – a remedy that affects the whole body.

Contraindicated – a term applied to any condition that makes a particular line of treatment undesirable.

Desensitization – a method of abolishing the sensitivity of a person to an allergen by injecting graded amounts of the same allergen.

Diuretic – an agent that promotes the excretion of urine.

Douching – use of a jet of water to wash a body cavity or opening.

Embolus – a clot or mass formed in one part of the circulation that is moved in the bloodstream to become impacted in another part of the circulation.

Endemic – a disease permanently established in moderate or severe form in a defined area.

Endocrine gland – an internally secreting gland whose function is to secrete into the blood or lymph a substance (hormone) that has a specific effect on another organ.

Endorphins – peptides synthesized in the pituitary gland that have analgesic (painkilling) properties associated with their affinity for the opiate receptors in the brain.

Epidemic – an outbreak of an infectious disease spreading widely among people at the same time in any region.

Exocrine gland – a gland that secretes into some cavity in the body or onto the external surface of the body by ducts.

Expectoration – the coughing up of mucus or sputum from the air passages.

Free radicals – negatively charged particles capable of free existence in special conditions, usually only for short periods.

Goitrogens – foods that inhibit thyroxine production, thus causing a swelling of the thyroid gland known as a goitre.

Gynaecology – the branch of medicine that deals with functions and diseases of the genital tract in women.

Haematology – the branch of medicine that deals with the study of the blood and blood-forming tissues.

Heimlich manoeuvre – a procedure used to force an obstruction out of the airway of someone who is choking.

Holistic – the concept of a person being considered as a functioning whole in terms of body, mind and spirit.

HRT – hormone replacement therapy whereby the hormones, oestrogen and progesterone, are taken as a supplement to alleviate the symptoms associated with the menopause.

Iatrogenic disease – a doctor-induced disease, usually occurring as a side effect of prescribed drugs.

Immune – protected against an infectious disease.

Immunocompromised – having the immune response reduced by immunosuppressive drugs, irradiation, malnutrition or a disease.

Immunoglobulins – proteins that function as antibodies and combine with antigens.

Immunosuppressant – an agent that suppresses immune responses.

Intussusception – the pushing down, or telescoping, of one part of the intestine into the part below it.

Jala Lota – an Eastern technique of nasal washing.

Karma – the force generated by a person's actions that is held in Hinduism and Buddhism to be the motive power for all the rebirths and deaths endured until that person has achieved spiritual liberation and is free from the effects of such force.

Laparoscopy – the insertion of a rigid or flexible device to inspect the abdominal cavity.

Learned response – a biological response that has been learned by association with a stimulus, ie a conditioned response.

Lipoproteins – lipid–protein complexes that serve to transport lipids in the blood.

Magnetic resonance imaging (MRI) – the use of nuclear magnetic resonance of protons to produce proton density maps or images of the human body for diagnostic use.

Miasm – a supposed noxious emanation from the soil or earth, at one time alleged to be the cause of diseases endemic in certain areas, such as malaria.

Neti pot – a small watering can used for nasal washing (Jala Lota).

Nirvana – the state of freedom from karma.

Obstetrics – the branch of medicine that deals with the problems and management of pregnancy and labour.

Orthodox techniques – the tried-and-tested Western medical techniques for treating the symptoms of a disease or condition.

Palliative – affording temporary relief from pain or discomfort, but not a cure.

Palpation – physical examination by touch.

Palpitation – a subjective awareness of a rapid or irregular heartbeat in the chest.

Parasites – organisms that live on or within a host organism to the detriment of the host organism.

Pathogen – a disease-producing microorganism or substance.

Pathognomonic – indicative of a particular disease.

Percussion – the act of striking with one finger, lightly and sharply, against another finger placed on the surface of the body so as to determine, by the sound produced, the physical state of the part beneath.

Phthisis – a wasting away of the body or part of the body.

Physiology – a study of the functions of the living organism and its parts, and of the physical and chemical factors and processes involved.

Phyto-oestrogens – natural oestrogens from plants.

Placebo – a pharmacologically inactive substance administered as a drug either in the treatment of psychological illness or in drug trials.

Prophylactic – tending to prevent or protect against disease, especially infectious disease.

Proprietary – any chemical, drug or similar preparation used in the treatment of disease that is protected against free competition by trademark, copyright or other such means.

Protozoa – an organism that exhibits both bacterial and viral activity.

Psyche – the human faculty for thought, judgement and emotion.

Qi – according to Eastern philosophy, Qi (or the Vital Force) is an immeasurable energy emanating from all living organisms and through all matter, connecting the whole universe.

Radiography – the making of film records (radiographs) of internal body structures by the passage of X-rays or gamma rays through the body to act on specially sensitized film.

Radiotherapy – theory and practice of medical treatment of disease, particularly cancer, with large doses of X-rays or other ionizing radiations.

Reverse osmosis – purification of water by forcing it under pressure through a membrane that is not permeable to the impurities to be removed.

Sequela – any condition or affliction following or caused by an attack of disease.

Silent – a term used to describe a disease that produces no detectable signs or symptoms.

Subclinical – without clinical manifestation; used to describe an infection or other disease or abnormality before symptoms or signs become apparent or detectable by clinical examination or laboratory test.

Subluxation – an incomplete or partial dislocation.

Symbionts – organisms that live together or in close association for mutual benefit.

Systemic – pertaining to or affecting the body as a whole.

Tens – transcutaneous electrical nerve stimulation: the passing of an electrical impulse through nerves to stimulate the body's pain-relieving chemicals.

Tetracyclines – a group of biosynthetic antibiotics with wide spectrum activity isolated from certain species of *Streptomyces* or produced semisynthetically by catalytic hydrogenation of chlortetracycline or oxytetracycline.

Tofu – a Japanese food preparation from the soya bean.

Transcendental – beyond human knowledge or independent of experience.

Trichology – the study of hair.

Triple heater – in Eastern medicine an energy line that controls the head of the body via its influence on the adrenal and thyroid glands.

Ultrasound scan – the visualization of deep structures in the body by recording the reflections (echoes) of pulses of ultrasonic (high-frequency) waves directed into the tissues. This technique is widely used in the diagnosis of disease of the abdomen and heart and in the management of pregnancy.

Urogenital – pertaining to the urinary and genital systems.

Urology – the branch of medicine that deals with the urinary tract in both male and female and with the genital organs in the male.

Vessel of Conception – the Chinese meridian or energy line that flows from the top of the head down the mid-line of the body, connecting the pituitary gland, thyroid, pancreas and uterus.

Vital Force – according to Eastern philosophy, the Vital Force is the immeasurable 'energy for life' or Qi.

Yang – the masculine and positive principle (as of activity, height, light, heat or dryness) in nature that, according to Chinese cosmology, combines and interacts with its opposite 'Yin' to produce all that comes to be.

Yin – the feminine and negative principle (as of passivity, depth, darkness, cold or wetness) in nature that, according to Chinese cosmology, combines with its opposite 'Yang' to produce all that comes to be.

Yoga – a discipline by which the individual prepares for liberation of the self (mind and body) and union with the universal spirit (soul). This is achieved by a system of exercises for attaining bodily or mental control and well being so that the self may be liberated from all pain and suffering and unite with the universal spirit.

Further Reading

GENERAL

A–Z of Natural Healthcare
Belinda Grant
Optima, 1993

The Alternative Dictionary of Symptoms and Cures
Dr Caroline Shreeve
Century, 1987

The Alternative Health Guide
Brian Inglis and Ruth West
Michael Joseph, 1983

ACUPUNCTURE/ACUPRESSURE

Acupressure Techniques
Dr Julian Kenyon
Thorsons, 1987

Acupuncture
Peter Mole
Element Books, Shaftesbury, 1991

Acupuncture: A Comprehensive Text
J O'Connor and D Bensky
Eastland Press, Seattle, 1981

Acupuncture: Energy Balancing for Body, Mind and Spirit
Peter Mole
Element Books, 1992

Acupuncture for Everyone
Dr Ruth Lever
Penguin, 1987

Acupuncture Medicine
Dr Y Omara
Japan: Japan Publications, 1982

Traditional Acupuncture, The Law of Five Elements
Dianne Connelly
Center for Traditional Acupuncture, Columbia, 1979

ALEXANDER TECHNIQUE

Alexander Technique
C Stevens
Optima, 1987

The Alexander Technique: Natural Poise for Health
Richard Brennan
Element Books, 1991

The Alexander Technique Workbook
R Brennan
Element, 1992

Better Health through Natural Healing
Ross Tratler
McGraw-Hill, USA, 1987

Body Learning
M Gelb
Aurem Press, 1981

Choices in Healing
Michael Lerner
MIT Press, USA/UK, 1994

The Encyclopaedia of Alternative Health Care
Kristen Olsen
Piatkus, 1989

Encyclopaedia of Natural Medicine
Brian Inglis and Ruth West
Michael Joseph, 1983

Encyclopaedia of Natural Medicine
Michael Murray and Joseph Pizzorno
Macdonald Optima, 1990

Gentle Medicine
Angela Smyth
Thorsons, 1994

The Greening of Medicine
Patrick Pietroni
Gollancz, 1990

Guide to Complementary Medicine and Therapies
Anne Woodham
Health Education Authority, 1994

The Handbook of Complementary Medicine
Stephen Fulder
Oxford Medical Publications, 1988

How to Live Longer and Feel Better
Linus Pauling
W H Freeman, USA, 1986

Maximum Immunity
Michael Wiener
Gateway Books, 1986

Reader's Digest Family Guide to Alternative Medicine
Dr Patrick Pietroni (ed)
The Reader's Digest Association, 1991

Will to be Well
Neville Hodgkinson
Hutchinson, 1984

ANTHROPOSOPHICAL MEDICINE

Anthroposophical Medicine
M Evans and I Rodger
Thorsons, 1992

AROMATHERAPY

Aromatherapy
Christine Wildwood
Element Books, 1991

Aromatherapy: An A–Z
Patricia Davis
C W Daniel, 1988

Aromatherapy Blends and Remedies,
Franzesca Watson
Thorsons, 1996

The Aromatherapy Book
Jeanne Rose
North Atlantic Books, 1994

Aromatherapy for Healing the Spirit
Gabrielle Mojay
Gaia, 1996

Aromatherapy for Pregnancy and Childbirth
Margaret Fawcett
Element Books, 1993

Aromatherapy from Provence
Nelly Grosjean
C W Daniel, 1994

Aromatherapy: Massage with Essential Oils
Christine Wildwood
Element Books, 1991

The Complete Aromatherapy Handbook
Susanne Fischer-Rizzi
Stirling, 1990, USA

The Complete Illustrated Guide to Aromatherapy
Julia Lawless
Element Books, 1997

The Fragrant Mind
Valerie Anne Worwood
Doubleday, 1996

The Fragrant Pharmacy
Valerie Anne Worwood
Bantam Books, 1995

The Illustrated Encyclopedia of Essential Oils
Julia Lawless
Element Books, 1992

Massage and Aromatherapy
Andrew Vickers
Chapman and Hall, 1996

ART THERAPY

Art as Therapy
S McNiff
Piatkus, 1994

AYURVEDA

A Handbook of Ayurveda
Vaidya Bhagwan Dash and Acarya Manfred M Junius
New Delhi, India: Concept Publishing Co, 1983

Ancient Indian Massage
Harish Johari
Munshiram Manoharial, 1984

Ayurveda
Scott Gerson
Element Books, 1993

Ayurvedic Medicine, Past and Present
Pandit Shiv Sharma
Calcutta, India: Dabur Publications, 1975

Basic Principles of Ayurveda
Bhagwan Dash
New Delhi, India: Concept Publishing Co, 1980

The Complete Illustrated Guide to Ayurveda
Gopi Warrier and Dr Deepika Gunawant
Element Books, 1997

The Handbook of Ayurveda
Dr Shantha Godagama
Kyle Cathie, 1997

Health Essentials: Ayurveda – The Ancient Indian Healing Art
Scott Gerson MD
Element, 1993

Indian Materia Medica: Volumes One and Two
Dr K M Madkarni

Prakrti: Your Ayurvedic Constitution
Robert E Svoboda
Albuquerque: Geocom Press, 1988

Quantum Healing
Dr Deepak Chopra
Bantam Books, 1989

Return of the Rishi
Dr Deepak Chopra
Houghton Mifflin Co, 1988

The Seven Pillars of Ancient Wisdom
Dr Douglas Baker
Douglas Baker Publishing, 1982

The Yoga of Herbs: An Ayurvedic Guide to Herbal Medicine
Dr David Frawley and Dr Vasant Lad
Lotus Press, 1988

BATES METHOD FOR EYES

Bates Method
P Mansfield
Vermilion, 1995

BODY WORK

Bodywise
Joseph Heller and William A Henkin
Tarcher, 1986

Job's Body: A Handbook For Bodywork
Deane Juhan
Station Hill, 1987

CHINESE MEDICINE

Arisal of the Clear – a simple guide to eating according to Traditional Chinese Medicine
B Flaws
Blue Poppy Press, Boulder, 1991

Between Heaven and Earth
H Beinfield and E Korngold
Ballantine, New York, 1991

Chinese Herbal Medicine
Richard Craze and Stephen Tang
Piatkus, 1995

Chinese Herbal Medicine, Ancient Art and Modern Science
Richard Hyatt
Wildwood House Limited, 1978

Chinese Herbal Medicine, Formulas and Strategies
D Bensky and R Barolet
Eastland Press, Seattle, 1993

Chinese Herbal Medicine, Materia Medica
D Bensky and A Gamble
Eastland Press, Seattle, 1993

Chinese Herbal Patent Remedies:
A Practical Guide
Jake Fratkin
Institute for Traditional Medicine, 1986

Chinese Medicine
Tom Williams
Element Books, Shaftesbury, 1995

Chinese Medicine, The Web That Has
No Weaver
Ted Kaptchuk
Rider, London, 1983

The Chinese Way to Health
Dr Stephen Gascoigne
Hodder Headline, 1997

The Complete Family Guide to
Chinese Medicine
Tom Williams
Element Books, 1997

The Foundations of Chinese Medicine
Churchill Livingstone
Giovanni Maciocia
London, 1989

The Fountain of Health: An A–Z of
Traditional Chinese Medicine
Dr Charles Windrige and
Dr Wu Xiaochun
Mainstream Publishing, 1994

The Fundamentals of Chinese
Medicine
Ellis Wiseman and Zmiewski
Paradigm, Brookline, 1985

The Practice of Chinese Medicine
Churchill Livingstone,
Giovanni Maciocia
London, 1994

The Web That Has No Weaver
Ted J Kaptchuk
Congdon and Weed, 1983

CHIROPRACTIC

Dynamic Chiropractic Today
M Copland Griffiths
Thorsons, 1991

CLINICAL ECOLOGY

Clinical Ecology
Dr George Lewith and Dr Julian
Kenyon
Thorsons, 1985

COLONIC IRRIGATION

Principles of Colonic Irrigation
J Collings
Thorsons, 1996

COLOUR THERAPY

Colour Me Healing
Jack Allanach
Element, 1997

Colour Therapy
Pauline Wills
Element, 1993

The Colour Therapy Workbook
Theo Gimbel
Element, 1993

FELDENKRAIS

Awareness Through Movement
Moshe Feldenkrais
Penguin, 1990

FENG SHUI

The Complete Illustrated Guide to
Feng Shui
Lillian Too
Element, 1996

The Elements of Feng Shui
Man-Ho Kwok and Joanne O'Brien
Element, 1991

Feng Shui
S Rosbach
Rider, London, 1984

The Feng Shui Handbook
Lam Kam Chuen
Gaia, London, 1995

Feng Shui Made Easy
W Spear
Harper Collins, London, 1995

Interior Design with Feng Shui
S Rosbach
Rider, London, 1987

FLOWER REMEDIES

A Guide to Bach Flower Remedies
Julian Barnard
C W Daniel, 1987

The Bach Flower Remedies:
Illustrations and Preparations
Victor Bullen and Nora Weeks
C W Daniel, 1964

The Collected Writings of Edward
Bach
edited by Julian Barnard
Flower Remedy Program, 1987

Flower Remedies: Natural Healing
with Flower Essences
Christine Wildwood
Element Books, 1991

Heal Thyself
Dr Edward Bach
C W Daniel, 1931

The Original Writings of Edward Bach
Judy Howard and John Ramsell (eds)
C W Daniel, 1990

The Twelve Healers and Other
Remedies
Dr Edward Bach
C W Daniel, 1936

HEALING

The Complete Healer
D Furlong
Piatkus, 1995

The Healer's Hand Book
Georgina Regan and Debbie Shapiro
Element, 1988

Healing Words
Larry Dossey
HarperCollins, 1993

Spiritual Healing
Jack Angelo
Element, 1991

HERBALISM

A Modern Herbal Vols I and II
Mrs M Grieve
Dover Publications, 1971

British Herbal Pharmacopoeia
British Herbal Medicine Association,
1990

The Complete Family Guide to Natural Home Remedies
Karen Sullivan
Element Books, 1996

The Complete Illustrated Holistic Herbal
David Hoffman
Element Books, 1996

The Complete New Herbal
Richard Mabey (ed)
Penguin Books, 1991

The Complete Woman's Herbal
Anne McIntyre
Gaia Books, 1994

The Dictionary of Modern Herbalism
Simon Mills
Inner Traditions, 1985

The Encyclopedia of Herbs and Herbalism
Malcolm Stuart
Orbis Publishing, 1979

Family Medical Herbal
Kitty Campion
Dorling Kindersley, 1988

The Golden Age of Herbs and Herbalists
Rosetta E Clarkson
Dover Publications, 1972

Green Pharmacy
Barbara Griggs
Inner Traditions
International Ltd, 1991

Healing Power of Herbs
Michael Murray
Prima Publications, 1992

The Herbal for Mother and Child
Anne McIntyre
Element Books, 1992

Herbal Healing for Women
Rosemary Gladstar
Fireside, 1993

Herbal Medications
Priest and Priest
L N Fowler and Co Ltd, 1982

Herbal Medicine
Rudolf Wess
Medicina Biologica, 1988

The Herb Society's Complete Medicinal Herbal
Penelope Ody
Dorling Kindersley, 1993

Herbal Medicine: The Use of Herbs for Health and Healing
Vicki Pitman
Element Books, 1994

Herbal Remedies: A Practical Beginner's Guide to Making Effective Remedies in the Kitchen
Christopher Hedley and Non Shaw
Paragon, 1996

Herbs for Common Ailments
Anne McIntyre
Gaia Books, 1992

The Home Herbal
Barbara Griggs
Pan Books, 1995

Male Herbal
James Green
Crossings Press, 1991

Natural Medicine for Women
Julian and Susan Scott
Gaia Books, 1991

Neal's Yard Natural Remedies
Susan Curtis, Romy Frasher, and Irene Kohler
Arkana, 1988

The New Holistic Herbal
David Hoffman
Element Books, 1983

Out of the Earth: The Science and Practice of Herbal Medicine
Simon Mills
Viking Penguin, 1992

Potter's New Cyclopaedia of Botanical Drugs and Preparations
R C Wren
C W Daniel, 1988

The Power of Plants
Brendan Lehane
John Murray, 1977

Traditional Home and Herbal Remedies
Jan De Vries
Mainstream Publishing, 1986

HOMEOPATHY

The Challenge of Homeopathy
Margery Blackie
Unwin Hyman, 1981

The Complete Homeopathy Handbook
Miranda Castro
Pan Books, 1990

Emotional Healing with Homeopathy: A Self-help Manual
Peter Chappell
Element Books, 1994

The Family Guide to Homeopathy
Andrew Lockie
Hamish Hamilton, 1990

Homeopathic Drug Pictures
Margaret Tyler
Health Science Press, 1970

Homeopathy for Children
Henrietta Wells
Element Books, 1993

Homeopathy for Mother and Baby
Miranda Castro
Pan Books, 1995

Homeopathy: Medicine of the New Man
George Vithoulkas
Thorsons, 1985

The New Concise Guide to Homeopathy
Nigel and Susan Garion-Hutchings
Element Books, 1993

The Woman's Guide to Homeopathy
Andrew Lockie and Nicola Geddes
Hamish Hamilton, 1992

HYDROTHERAPY

The Complete Book of Water Therapy
Dian Dinsin Buchman
Keats, 1994

Hydrotherapy – Water and Nature Cure
C L Thomson
Kingston Publications, 1970

Water and Nature Cure
C Leslie Thomson
Kingston Clinic, Edinburgh, 1955

Water and Sexuality
Michel Odent
Arkana, 1990

Water Babies
Erik Sidenbladh
A and C Black, 1983

HYPNOTHERAPY

Principles of Hypnotherapy
Vera Peiffer
Thorsons, 1996

Self-Hypnosis
Elaine Sheehan
Element, 1995

NUTRITION

The Complete Book of Minerals for Health
J I Rodale
Rodale Books, 1976

The Complete Guide to Food Allergy and Environmental Illnesses
Dr Keith Mumby
Thorsons, 1993

The Complete Home Guide to All the Vitamins
Ruth Adams
Larchmont Books, 1972

The Doctor's Book of Vitamin Therapy: Megavitamins for Health
Harold Rosenberg and A N Feldzaman
Putnam's, 1974

The Doctors' Vitamin and Mineral Encyclopedia
Sheldon Saul Hendler, M.D., Ph.D.
Simon and Schuster, 1995

Food and Health
Elizabeth Morse, John Rivers, and Anne Heughan
Barrie and Jenkins, 1990

Food: Your Miracle Medicine
Jean Carper
Simon and Schuster, 1993

Healing Nutrients
Patrick Quillen
Penguin, 1989

Health Essentials: Vitamins Guide
Hasnain Walji
Element Books, 1992

In a Nutshell: Vitamins and Minerals
Karen Sullivan
Element Books, 1997

Nutritional Medicine
Stephen Davis and Alan Stewart
Pan Books, 1987

Raw Energy
Leslie and Susannah Kenton
Arrow Books, 1991

Superfoods
Michael Van Straten and Barbara Griggs
Dorling Kindersley, 1992

Thorsons Complete Guide to Vitamins and Minerals
Leonard Mervyn
Thorsons, 1995

The Vitamin Bible
Earl Mindell
Arrow Books, 1993

The Vitamin Guide: Using Vitamins for Optimum Health
Hasnain Walji
Element Books, 1992

Vitamins and Minerals: The Amino Revolution
Robert Erdmann and Meirion Jones
Century, 1987

Which Vitamins Do You Need?
Martin Ebon
Bantam Books, 1974

The Zinc Solution
Derek Bryce-Smith
and Liz Hodgkinson
Arrow Books, 1987

MASSAGE

The Bassett Atlas of Human Anatomy
Robert A Chase
Benjamin Cummings, 1989

Beard's Massage
Wood and Becker
3rd Edition, W.B. Saunders, 1964

The Complete Book of Massage
Clare Maxwell-Hudson
Dorling Kindersley, 1988

Manipulation and Mobilisation
Susan L Edmond
Mosby, 1993

Massage: A Practical Introduction
Stewart Mitchell
Element, 1992

Mosby's Fundamentals of Therapeutic Massage
Sandy Fritz
Mosby, 1995

The New Atlas of the Human Body
Vannini and Pogliano (translated R Jolly)
Chancellor Press, 1980

Tidy's Massage and Remedial Exercises 11th ed
John Wright and Son, 1968

Visualising Muscles
John Cody
Kansas University Press, 1990, USA

MEDITATION

The Meditator's Handbook
David Fontana
Element Books, 1992

How to Meditate
K McDonald
Wisdom, 1984

Teaching Meditation to Children
David Fontana and Ingrid Slack
Element Books, 1997

Teach Yourself Meditation
James Hewitt
Hodder and Stoughton, 1978

POLARITY THERAPY

The Polarity Process: Energy as a Healing Art
Franklyn Sills
Element Books, 1989

Polarity Therapy
A Siegel
Prism Press, 1987

QI GONG AND TAI QI

Art of Chi Kung: Making the Most of Your Vital Energy
Wong Kiew Kit
Element Books, 1997

Between Heaven and Earth
H Beinfield and E Korngold
Ballantine, New York, 1991

Chi Kung
J McRitchie
Element Books, Shaftesbury, 1993

The Complete Book of Tai Chi Ch'uan
Wong Kiew Kit
Element Books, 1996

The Elements of Tai Chi
Paul Crompton
Element Books, 1990

Embrace Tiger, Return to Mountain
Chungliang Al Huang
Celestial Arts, Berkeley, CA, 1973

Movements of Magic
B Klein
Newcastle, California, 1984

Tai Chi Ch'uan for Health and Self-Defense
T T Liang
Vintage, New York, 1977

Taiji
Chungliang Al Huang
Celestial Arts, Berkeley, CA, 1989

The Way of Energy
Lam Kam Chuen
Gaia Books, London, 1991

The Way of Harmony
H Reid
Gaia Books, London, 1988

REFLEXOLOGY

The Complete Illustrated Guide to Reflexology
Inge Dougans
Element Books, UK/US, 1996

The Reflexology and Colour Therapy Workbook
Pauline Wills
Element Books, 1992

The Reflexology Partnership
Adamson and Harris
Kyle Cathie, 1995

Reflexology – The Ancient Answer
Ann Gilanders
Jenny Lee Publishing, 1994

Reflexology: The Definitive Practitioner's Manual
Beryl Crane
Element Books, 1997

Zone Therapy Using Foot Massage
Astrid Goosman-Legger
C W Daniel, 1983

SHIATSU

The Book of Shiatsu
P Lundberg
Gaia Books, 1992

The Complete Illustrated Guide to Shiatsu
Elaine Leichti
Element Books, 1998

Shiatsu: Japanese Massage for Health and Fitness
Elaine Liechti
Element Books, 1992

Shiatsu: The Complete Guide
C Jarmey and G Mojay
Thorsons, 1991

The Shiatsu Workbook
N Dawes
Piatkus Books, 1991

TIBETAN MEDICINE

The Tibetan Art of Living
Christopher Hansard
Hodder and Stoughton, 2001

YOGA

The Complete Yoga Course
Howard Kent
Headline Press, 1993

Elements of Yoga
Godfrey Devereux
Element Books, 1994

Preparing for Birth with Yoga
Janet Balaskas
Element Books, 1994

The Yoga Book
Stephen Sturgess
Element Books, 1997

Useful Addresses

Investigations

Where possible, if the text recommends investigations or tests enquire of your local GP or health practitioner as to whether they can perform or organize them. Failing to do so, which may be the case, especially for the more pioneering or alternative techniques, please contact the following:

General

Dr Sharma
Integrated Health Consultancy
87 North Road, Parkstone, Poole,
Dorset, BH14 0LT, England.

E-mail enquiries to:
drsharma@101clinic.co.uk *or*
drrsharma@healersworld.com

All the complementary products mentioned in this book can be obtained from the above addresses, by letter or e-mail.

Most investigations can be obtained through the mail. Please enquire through the above address about which tests can be done at home and which can be sent to your physician.

Dr Sharma has a wide network of practitioners and may be able to direct you to somebody within your area. Such enquiries should be sent by post or e-mail to the above addresses.

The following laboratory will deal only with doctors and practitioners registered with them:

Biolab Medical Unit
The Stonehouse, 9 Weymouth Street,
London, W1W 6BB

Australia

Australian College of Alternative Medicine
11 Howard Avenue, Mount Waverley,
Victoria 3149

Australasian College of Natural Therapies
620 Harris Street, Ultimo,
NSW 2007
Tel: 02212 6699

Australian Traditional Medicine Society
Suite 3, First Floor,
120 Blaxland Road, Ryde,
NSW 2112
Tel: 612 808 2825
Fax: 612 809 7570

Canada

Canadian Holistic Medical Association
42 Redpath Avenue, Toronto,
Ontario M4S 2J6
Tel: 416 485 3071

Europe

The 101 Group Practitioners
87 North Road, Parkstone, Poole,
Dorset BH14 0LT, United Kingdom
(practices in London and elsewhere)

British Holistic Medical Association
59 Landsdowne Place, Hove,
East Sussex, BN3 1FL, United Kingdom
Tel: 01273 725951

The Centre for The Study of Complementary Medicine
51 Bedford Place, Southampton,
Hampshire SO15 2DT,
United Kingdom
Tel: 02380 334752
Fax: 02380 231835

The Hale Clinic
7 Park Crescent, London W1B 1PF,
United Kingdom
Tel: 020 7631 0156

The Institute for Complementary Medicine
PO Box 194, London SE16 7QZ,
United Kingdom
Tel: 020 7237 5165
Fax: 020 7237 5175

USA

Alliance/Foundation for Alternative Medicine
160 NW Widmer Place, Albany,
OR 97321
Tel: 503 926 4678

American Holistic Medical Association
4101 Lake Boone Trail, Suite 201,
Raleigh, NC 27607
Tel: 919 787 5181
Fax: 919 787 5146

Holistic Health Association
PO Box 17400, Anaheim
CA 92817 7400
Tel: 714 779 6152

(*see also* **Shiatsu**)

Australia

The Shiatsu Therapy Association of Australia
332 Carlisle St, Balaclava,
3182 Victoria
Tel: 0061 395 344780

Europe

ITHMA
PO Box 6555, London N8 9DF,
United Kingdom

Tony Rusli
82 Ashville Road, London E11 4DU,
United Kingdom
Tel: 020 8558 9676

Jon Sandifer
PO Box 69, Teddington, Middlesex
TW11 9SH, United Kingdom
Tel: 020 8977 8988

USA

Michael Blate
Falknor Books, PO Box 8060
Pembroke Pines, Florida 33023

ACUPUNCTURE

Australia

**Acupuncture Ethics and Standards
Organization**
PO Box 84, Merrylands, NSW
Tel: 0061 296 827882

Canada

Acupuncture Foundation of Canada
7321 Victoria Park Avenue,
Unit 18, Markham,
Ontario L3R 2Z3
Tel: 905 881 5540

Europe

British Acupuncture Council (BAC)
66 Jeddo Road, London W12 9HQ,
United Kingdom
Tel: 020 8735 0400

Richard Field/Andrew Mullen
87 North Road, Parkstone, Poole,
Dorset BH14 0LT, United Kingdom
(practice in London)

The Kailash Centre
7 Newcourt Street, London NW8,
United Kingdom
Tel: 020 7722 3939
Fax: 020 7586 1642

**London School of Acupuncture and
Traditional Chinese Medicine**
University of Westminster,
115 New Cavendish Street,
London W1W 6UW, United Kingdom
Tel: 020 7911 5000

New Zealand

NZRA
PO Box 9950, Wellington 1
Tel: 00648 016 400

South Africa

**Western Cape Su Jok Acupuncture
Institute**
3 Periwinkle Close,
Kommetjie 7975
Tel: 021 783 3460

USA

**American Association of Acupuncture
and Oriental Medicine**
1424 16th Street NW,
Suite 501
Washington DC 20036

ALEXANDER TECHNIQUE

Australia

**The Australian Society of Teachers
of the Alexander Technique**
19 Princess Street, Kew,
VIC 3101
Tel: 0398 531 356

Brazil

**Association Brasilieria da Tenica
Alexander**
Rua dos Miranhaas, 333 Pinheiros,
05434-040 Sao Paulo

Canada

**The Canadian Society of Teachers of
the Alexander Technique**
PO Box 47025, 19–555 West 12th Avenue,
Vancouver BC, V5Z 3X0

Europe

**Alexander Technique Training Centre
(Ireland)**
Richard Brennan ATI, STAT (cert.)
Kirkullen Lodge, Tooreeny, Moycullen,
Co. Galway, Eire
Tel: 00 353 91 555800

APTA
42 Terrasse de l'iris, La Defense 2,
92400 Coubevoire, France
Tel: 0033 1409 00623

**Danish Society of Teachers of the
Alexander Technique**
c/o Mr Marc Grue, Secretary,
Otto Rud's 38 Stsh,
DK-8200 Aarhus, Denmark

GLAT
Postfach 5312, 79020 Frieburg,
Germany
Tel: 0049 76138 3357

ISTAT
PO Box 715, Karkur 37106

**Netherlands Society of Teachers of the
Alexander Technique**
Postbus 15591, 1001 NB Amsterdam,
Netherlands
Tel: 0031 20623 8260

**The Society of Teachers of the
Alexander Technique**
129 Camden Mews, London N1 9AH,
United Kingdom
Tel: 020 7284 3338
Fax: 020 7482 5435

SVLAT
Postfach, CH 8032,
Zurich, Switzerland

South Africa

SASTAT
5 Leinster Road, Green Point 8001,
Cape Town

ALLERGIES

Europe

Individual Well-being
99 Kings Road, London SW3 4PA,
United Kingdom

ANTHROPOSOPHICAL MEDICINE

Europe

Anthroposophical Medical Trust
Park Attwood Clinic, Trimpley Lane,
Bewdley, Worcestershire DY12 1RE,
United Kingdom
Tel: 01299 861561
Fax: 01299 861375

Anthroposophical Society in Great Britain
Ruldolf Steiner House, 35 Park Road, London NW1 6XT, United Kingdom
Tel: 020 7723 4400
Fax: 020 7724 4364

Australia

International Federation of Aromatherapists
1/390 Burwood Road, Hawthorn, BIC 3122, Australia
Tel: 03 9530 0067

Europe

Aromatherapy Trades Council
PO Box 387, Ipswich, IP2 9AN, United Kingdom
Tel: 01473 603630

International Federation of Aromatherapists
182 Chiswick High Road, London W4 1PF, United Kingdom
Tel: 020 8742 2605
Fax: 020 8742 2606

International Federation of Professional Aromatherapists (IFPA)
82 Ashby Road, Hinckley, Leicestershire LE10 1AG, United Kingdom
Tel: 01455 637987
Fax: 01455 890956

South Africa

Association of Aromatherapists
PO Box 23924, Claremont 7735, South Africa
Tel: 021 531 297

USA

American Alliance of Aromatherapy
PO Box 750428, Petaluma, California 94975–0428

American Aromatherapy Association
PO Box 3679, South Pasadena, California 91031

The Aromatherapy Institute and Research
PO Box 1222, Fair Oaks, California 95628

National Association of Holistic Aromatherapy
PO Box 17622, Boulder, Colorado 80308–0622

Nature's Apothecary
6350 Gunpark Drive 500, Boulder, Colorado 80301
Tel: 001 303 664 1600

The Pacific Institute of Aromatherapy
PO Box 6842, San Raphael, California 94903
Tel: 001 415 479 9129
Fax: 001 415 479 9121

Europe

British Association of Art Therapists
Maryward House, 5 Tavistock Place, London WC1M 9SH, United Kingdom
Tel: 020 7383 3774

Lisa Elle
87 North Road, Parkstone, Poole, Dorset BH14 0LT, United Kingdom
(practice in London)

USA

American Art Therapy Association
1202 Allanson Road, Mundelein Illinois 60060

(see also **Reflexology***)*

Europe

British Acupuncture Council (BAC)
66 Jeddo Road, London W12 9HQ, United Kingdom
Tel: 020 8735 0400
Fax: 020 8735 0404

Europe

British Association for Autogenic Training and Therapy
Heath Cottage, Pitch Hill, Ewhurst, nr Cranleigh, Surrey GU6 7NP, United Kingdom

USA

Mind Body Health Sciences
393 Dixon Road, Boulder, Colorado 80302
Tel: 030 440 8460

Australia

Maharishi Ayurveda Health Centres
PO Box 81, Bundoora, Victoria 3083

Europe

Ayurvedic Company of Great Britain
81 Wimpole Street, London W1G 9RS, United Kingdom
Tel: 020 7224 6070
Fax: 020 7224 6080

Ayurvedic Living
PO Box 188, Exeter, Devon EX4 5AB, United Kingdom

Ayurvedic Medical Association Great Britain
The Hale Clinic, 7 Park Crescent, London W1B 1BF, United Kingdom
Tel: 020 7631 0156

Eastern Clinic
1079 Garratt Lane, Tooting, London SW17 0LN, United Kingdom
Tel: 020 8682 3876
Fax: 020 8333 7904

South Africa

The Himalayan Drugs Company
Tel: 020 7935 0028
(please call for the address)

Maharishi Ayurveda Health Centre
PO Box 5155, Halfway House 1685

South African Ayurvedic Medicine Association
85 Harvey Road, Morningside,
Durban 4001
Tel: 031 303 3245

USA

American Holistic Medical Association
4101 Lake Boone Trail, Suite 201,
Raleigh, North Carolina 27607

The Ayurveda Institute
11311 Menaul NE, Suite A,
Albuquerque, New Mexico 87112
Tel: 505 291 9698

The Ayurveda Institute
PO Box 282, Fairfield,
Iowa 52556
Tel: 310 454 5531

Dr Edward Bach Healing Society
644 Merrick Road, Lynbrook,
New York 11563
Tel: 516 593 2206

Ellon (Bach United States of America) Inc
PO Box 32, Woodmere,
New York 11598
Tel: 516 825 2229

International Federation for Ayurveda
Ayurvedic Medicine of New York,
Scott Gerson, MD,
13 West Ninth Street, New York,
NY 10011
Tel: 212 505 8971

Mapi, Inc
Garden of the Gods Business Park,
1115 Elkton Drive, Suite 401,
Colorado Spring, Colorado 80907

Andrew Weil MD
1975 West Hunter Road, Tucson,
Arizona 85737

BACH FLOWER REMEDIES

Australia

Martin & Pleasance
137 Swan Street, Richmond,
Victoria 3121
Tel: 61 39 427 7422

Europe

Dr Edward Bach Centre
Mount Vernon, Sotwell, Wallingford,
Oxon OX10 0PZ, United Kingdom
Tel: 01491 834678
Fax: 01491 825022

Morris Griffin
Trinders Cottage, Calcot, Colm St
Denys, Cheltenham, Gloucestershire
GL54 3JZ, United Kingdom
Fax: 01285 720 931

USA

Nelson Bach USA Limited
Wilmington Technology Park,
100 Research Drive, Wilmington,
Massachusetts 01887-4406
Tel: 978 988 3833
Fax: 978 988 0233

BATES METHOD FOR EYES

Europe

The Bates Association of Great Britain
46 Hollingbury Road, Brighton,
West Sussex BN1 7JA, United Kingdom
Tel: 0870 2417458

Karen Banks
70 Station Road, Finchley,
London N3 2SA, United Kingdom

BEHAVIOURAL THERAPY

(*see also* **Psychotherapy/Stress management**)

Europe

The Hale Clinic
7 Park Crescent, London W1B 1PF,
United Kingdom
Tel: 020 7631 0156
Fax: 020 7631 3377

BIOFEEDBACK

Europe

Aleph One Ltd
The Old Courthouse, Bottisham,
Cambridge CB5 9BA, United Kingdom
Tel: 01223 811 679
Fax: 01223 812 713

USA

Association for Applied Psychophysiology and Biofeedback
10200 West 44th Avenue, Apt 304,
Wheat Ridge,
Colorado 80033-8436
Tel: 303 422 8894
Fax: 303 422 8894

BUTEYKO THERAPY

Europe

The Hale Clinic
7 Park Crescent, London W1B 1PF,
United Kingdom
Tel: 020 7631 0156

CHINESE HERBALISM

Australia

Australian College of Alternative Medicine
11 Howard Avenue,
Mount Waverley,
Victoria 3149

Chinese and Herbal Centre
1st Floor, 2392–2394 Sussex Street,
Sydney, NSW 2000

Canada

Canadian Holistic Medical Association
42 Redpath Avenue, Toronto,
Ontario M4S 2J6
Tel: 416 485 3071

Europe

British Herbal Medicine Association
Wickham Road, Bournemouth,
Dorset BH7 6JZ, United Kingdom
Tel: 01202 433691
Fax: 01202 417079

The Camden Practice
55 Dartmouth Park Road,
London NW5 1SL, United Kingdom
Tel: 020 7482 1248

Kailash Centre
7 Newcourt Street, London NW8,
United Kingdom
Tel: 020 7722 3939
Fax: 020 7586 1642

The Register of Chinese Herbal Medicine
21 Warbeck Road, London W12 8NS,
United Kingdom
Tel: 020 7224 0803

New Zealand

Holistic Health Centre
CPO Box 2273, Auckland

South Africa

The Herb Society of South Africa
PO Box 37721, Overport

USA

American Holistic Medical Association
6728 Old McLean Village Drive,
McLean,
Virginia 22101

American Holistic Nurses Association
PO Box 2130, 2133 E Lakin Drive,
Suite 2, Flagstaff,
Arizona 86003–2130

CHINESE & ORIENTAL MEDICINE

Australia

Australian College of Oriental Medicine
24 Price Road, Lalorama
Victoria 3766

Canada

Ontario Herbalists Association
1565 Carling Avenue, Suite 400, Ottawa
Ontario K1Z 8R1

Europe

Kailash Centre
7 Newcourt Street, London NW8,
United Kingdom
Tel: 020 7722 3939

USA

American Herb Association
PO Box 1673, Nevada City,
California 95959

CHELATION THERAPY

Europe

Dr Rodney Adenyi-Jones
Flat H, 21 Devonshire Place,
London W1G 6HZ, United Kingdom
Tel: 020 7486 6354

The Arterial Disease Clinic
Prospect House, 32 Bolton Road,
Atherton, Manchester, Gt Manchester
M46 9JY, United Kingdom
Tel: 01942 886644
Fax: 01942 889955

CHIROPRACTIC

Asia

Chiropractic Association (Singapore)
Box 23, Tanglin Post Office,
Singapore
Tel: 65 293 9843/734 8584
Fax: 65 733 8380

Australia

Australian Council on Chiropractic and Osteopathic Education
941 Nepean Highway,
Mornington,
Victoria 3931

Chiropractors' Association of Australia
PO Box 241, Springwood,
NSW 2777
Tel: 61 47 515 644
Fax: 61 47 515 856

Canada

Canadian Chiropractic Association
1396 Eglington Avenue, West,
Toronto,
Ontario M6C 2E4
Tel: 416 488 0470

Europe

Anglo-European College of Chiropractic
13–15 Parkwood Road, Bournemouth,
Dorset BH5 2DF, United Kingdom
Tel: 01202 436275
Fax: 01202 436278

British Chiropractic Association
Blagrave House, 17 Blagrave Street,
Reading, Berkshire RG1 1QB,
United Kingdom
Tel: 01189 505 950
Fax: 01189 588 946

Natureworks
Dr Douglas Diehl, 16 Bolderton Street,
London W1K 6TN, United Kingdom
Tel: 020 7355 4036

Chelsea and Fulham Chiropractic Clinic
1 Parson's Green Lane, Fulham,
London SW6 4HP, United Kingdom
Tel: 020 7731 3737
Fax: 020 7371 8644

Chiropractic Association of Ireland
28 Fair Street, Drogheda,
County Louth, Eire
Tel: 00353 41 98305999

European Chiropractors' Union
The Waldegrave Clinic,
82 Waldegrave Road, Teddington,
Middlesex TW11 8NY,
United Kingdom
Tel: 020 8943 2424
Fax: 020 8977 6626

New Zealand

New Zealand Chiropractors' Association
PO Box 7144, Wellesley Street,
Auckland
Tel: 64 9 373 4343
Fax: 64 9 373 5973

USA

American Chiropractic Association
1701 Clarendon Boulevard,
Arlington, Virginia 22209
Tel: 703 276 8800
Fax: 703 243 2593

World Chiropractic Alliance
2950 North Dobson Road, Suite One,
Chandler, Arizona 85224-1802
Tel: 800 347 1011
Fax: 602 732 9313

CLINICAL ECOLOGY

Europe

The British Society for Allergy, Environmental and Nutritional Medicine
PO Box 7, Totton, Southampton, Hants
SO40 2ZA, United Kingdom
Tel: 02380 812124

COLONIC HYDROTHERAPY

Europe

Colonic International Association (CIA)
16 Englands Lane, London NW3 4TG,
United Kingdom
Tel/Fax: 020 7483 1595

COLOUR THERAPY

Europe

Aura-Soma
South Road, Tetford, Horncastle,
Lincolnshire LN9 6QL, United Kingdom
Tel: 01507 533441

Colour & Reflexology
9 Wyndale Avenue, Kingsbury,
London NW9 9PT, United Kingdom
Tel: 020 8204 7672
Fax: 020 8204 7672

The Hygeia College of Colour Therapy
Brook House, Hampton Hill
Avening, Nr Tetbury, Gloucestershire
GL8 8NS, United Kingdom
Tel: 01453 832150
Fax: 01453 835757

The Institute for Complementary Medicine
PO Box 194, London SE16 7QZ,
United Kingdom
Tel: 020 7237 5165

The International Association for Colour Therapy
137 Hendon Lane, Finchley,
London N3, United Kingdom

Know Yourself Through Colour
Maria Louise Lacy,
5 Church Walk, Worthing, West Sussex
BN11 2LF, United Kingdom
Tel: 01903 216311

COUNSELLING

(*see also* **Psychotherapy**)

Europe

British Association for Counselling
1 Regent Place, Rugby, Warwicks
CV21 2PJ, United Kingdom
Tel: 01788 550899/578328
Fax: 01788 562189

Scott Galloway
The Hale Clinic, 7 Park Crescent
London W1B 1PF, United Kingdom
Tel: 020 7631 0156

The Institute of Stress Management
57 Hall Lane, London NW4 4TJ,
United Kingdom

Lisa Ekke/Kitty Kennedy/Sean Arnold
87 North Road, Parkstone, Poole,
Dorset BH14 0LT, United Kingdom
(*practice in London*)

USA

American Counseling Association
5999 Stevenson Avenue, Alexandrea,
Virginia 22304-9800

CRANIOSACRAL THERAPY

Europe

Craniosacral Association
Monmark House, 27 Old Gloucester
Street, London WC1N 3XX,
United Kingdom
Tel: 01737 767100

The Castle Street Clinic
36 Castle Street, Guildford GU1 3UQ,
United Kingdom
Tel: 01483 300400
Fax: 01483 300411

The Upledger Institute UK
2 Marshall Place, Perth PH2 8AH,
United Kingdom
Tel: 01738 444 404
Fax: 01738 442 275

CRYSTAL AND GEM THERAPY

Europe

Affiliation of Crystal Healing Organizations (ACHO)
International College of Crystal Healing
46 Lower Green Road, Esher,
Surrey KT10 8HD, United Kingdom
Tel: 01227 472435
Fax: 01227 761297

School of Electro-Crystal Therapy
117 Long Drive, South Ruislip,
Middlesex HA4 0HL, United Kingdom
Tel/Fax: 020 8841 1716

School of White Crystal Healing
Paradise Valley, Llangynin,
St Clears, Carmarthen SA33 4JY
Tel/Fax: 01994 230028

DANCE THERAPY

Europe

Association for Dance Movement Therapy
c/o Arts Therapies Department,
Springfield Hospital, Glenburnie
Road, Tooting, London SW17 7DJ,
United Kingdom
Tel: 020 8672 9911

USA

American Dance Therapy Association
10632 Little Pateuxent Parkway, 2000
Century Plaza, Suite 108, Columbia,
MD 21044-3265
Tel: 410 997 4040
Fax: 410 997 4048

FELDENKRAIS METHOD

Europe

The Feldenkrais Guild UK
PO Box 370, London N10 3XA,
United Kingdom

FENG SHUI

Australia

Feng Shui Design Studio
PO Box 705, Glebe, Sydney , NSW 2037
Tel: 00612 315 8258

Europe

Feng Shui Association
31 Woburn Place, Brighton,
E Sussex BN1 9GA, United Kingdom
Tel/Fax: 01273 693844

The Healthy Home
PO Box 249, Keighsley, North Yorkshire
BD20 8YN, United Kingdom
Tel: 07000 336474 / 01423 712868
Fax: 01423 712869

USA

Earth Design
PO Box 530725, Miami Shores,
Florida 33153
Tel: 305 756 6426
Fax: 305 751 9995

Feng Shui Designs
PO Box 399, Nevada City,
CA 95959
Tel: 800 551 2482

Feng Shui Institute of America
PO Box 488, Wabasso,
Florida 32970
Tel: 407 589 9900
Fax: 407 589 1611

FLOTATION

Europe

Float Tank Association
PO Box 11024, London SW4 7ZF,
United Kingdom
Tel: 020 7627 4962

FLOWER ESSENCES

Australia

**Martin and Pleasance Wholesale
Pty Ltd**
PO Box 4, Collingwood,
Victoria, NSW 3066
Tel: 419 9733

Nonsuch Botanical Pty Limited
PO Box 68, Mt Evelyn,
Victoria 3796
Tel: 762 8577

Europe

Bach Flower Remedies
The Bach Centre, Mount Vernon,
Sotwell, Wallingford, Oxfordshire
OX10 9PZ, United Kingdom
Tel: 01491 834 678

Flower Essence Fellowship
Laura Farm Clinic, 17 Carlincott,
Peasedown St John,
Bath BA2 8AN, United Kingdom

Healing Herbs
PO Box 65, Hereford HR2 0UW,
United Kingdom
Tel: 01873 890 218
Fax: 01873 890 314

USA

Dr Edward Bach Healing Society
644 Merrick Road, Lynbrook,
New York 11563
Tel: 516 593 2206

**Ellon (Bach United States of
America), Inc**
PO Box 32, Woodmere,
New York 11598
Tel: 516 825 2229

GESTALT THERAPY

Europe

Gestalt Centre London
62 Paul Street, London EC2A 4NA,
United Kingdom
Tel: 020 7613 4480
Fax: 020 7613 4737

USA

**Gestalt Centre for Psychotherapy
and Training**
510 East 89th Street, New York 10401
Tel: 212 879 3669

**Gestalt Therapy Institute of
Los Angeles**
Faculty Training Office, Suite 301,
1460 Seventh Street, Santa Monica,
California 90401
Tel: 909 629 9935

HEALING

Europe

**British Alliance of Healing
Associations**
26 Highfield Avenue, Herne Bay,
Kent CT6 6LN, United Kingdom

David Cunningham
The Hale Clinic, 7 Park Crescent,
London W1B 1PF, United Kingdom
Tel: 020 7631 0156

HELLERWORK

Europe

Hellerwork Inc (Rose-Marie Amoroso)
1 Finsbury Avenue, Broadgate,
London EC2M 2PA, United Kingdom
Tel: 020 7638 2322

USA

The Body of Knowledge Association
3468 Mt Daiblo Bulavard, Sre B203,
Ladayetter, CA 945 49 3917
Tel: 510 499 9050

Hellerwork International
406 Berry Street, Mount Shasta,
California 96067
Tel: 530 926 2500
Fax: 530 926 6839

HERBALISM

Australia

**National Herbalists Association of
Australia**
Suite 305, BST House, 3 Small Street,
Broadway, NSW 2007
Tel: 02 211 6437

Canada

Canadian Natural Health Association
439 Wellington Street, Toronto,
Ontario M5V 2H7
Tel: 416 977 2642

Europe

The General Council and Register of Consultant Herbalists
18 Sussex Square, Brighton,
East Sussex BN2 5AA, United Kingdom

The Herb Society
77 Great Peter Street, London SW1,
United Kingdom

National Institute of Medical Herbalists
56 Longbrooke Street, Exeter EX4 8HA,
United Kingdom
Tel: 01392 426 022

School of Herbal Medicine/Phytotherapy
Bucksteep Manor, Bodle Street Green,
Near Hailsham, Sussex BN27 4RJ,
United Kingdom

South Africa

South African Naturopaths and Herbalists Association
PO Box 18663, Wynberg 7824

USA

American Herbalists Guild
PO Box 1683, Sequel,
California 95073
Tel: 408 484 2441

Angelica's Traditional Herbs and Food
147 First Avenue, New York,
NY 10003
Tel: 212 677 1549

HERBAL MEDICINE

Australia

Australian Traditional Medicine Society
120 Blaxland Road, Ryde,
NSW 2112
Tel: 808 2825

National Herbalists Association of Australia
14/249 Kingsgrove Road, Kingsgrove,
NSW 2208

Europe

Healing Herbs Limited
PO Box 65, Hereford HR2 0UW,
United Kingdom
Tel: 01873 890 218
Fax: 01873 890 314

National Institute of Medical Herbalists
59 Longbrook Street, Exeter,
Devon EX4 6AH, United Kingdom
Tel: 01392 426022

USA

American Botanical Council
PO Box 201660, Austin, TX 78720
Tel: 512 331 8868
Fax: 512 331 1924

American Herbalists Guild
PO Box 1683, Sequel,
CA 95073
Tel: 408 484 2441

American Herb Association
PO Box 1673, Nevada City,
CA 95959
Tel: 916 265 9552
Fax: 916 274 3140

Herb Research Foundation
1007 Pearl Street, Suite 200,
Boulder, CO 80303
Tel: 300 449 2265

HOMEOPATHY

Australia

Australian Federation of Homeopaths
238 Ballarat Road, Footscray,
Victoria 3011
Tel: 03 9318 3057

Australian Institute of Homeopathy
7 Hampden Road, Artemon,
Sydney, NSW 2064

Australian Institute of Homeopathy
21 Bulah Close, Berdwra Heights,
NSW 2082

The National Centre for Homeopathy
801 N Fairfax 306, Alexandria,
VA 22314
Tel: 703 548 7790

Canada

Canadian Society of Homeopathy
87 Meadowlands Drive West, Nepean,
Ontario K2G 2R9

Europe

British Homoeopathic Association
15 Clerkenwell Close, London
EC1R 0AA, United Kingdom
Tel/Fax: 020 7566 7800

The Hahnemann College of Homeopathy
Humane Education Centre, Avenue
Lodge, Bounds Green Road,
London N22 4EU, United Kingdom
Tel/Fax: 020 8843 9220

The 101 Group
87 North Road, Parkstone,
Poole, Dorset BH14 0LT,
United Kingdom (practice in London)

The Society of Homeopaths
2 Artisan Road, Northampton NN1 4HU,
United Kingdom
Tel: 01604 621400
Fax: 01604 622622

New Zealand

Institute of Classical Homoeopathy
24 West Haven Drive,
Tawa, Wellington

New Zealand Homeopathic Society
Box 2929, Auckland
Tel: 9 630 9458

USA

American Foundation for Homeopathy
1508 Glencoe Street,
Suite 44, Denver,
Colorado 80220–1338

American Institute of Homeopathy
1585 Glencoe, Denver, CO 80220
Tel: 303 370 9164

Homeopathic Academy of
Naturopathic Physicians
PO Box 69565, Portland, OR 97201
Tel: 503 795 0579

Homeopathic Educational Services
2124 Kitteridge Street,
Berkeley,
California 94704
Tel: 800 359 9051 / 510 649 0294

International Foundation for
Homeopathy
2366 Eastlake Avenue,
East Suit 301,
Seattle, WA 98102
Tel: 206 776 4147

National Center for Homeopathy
801 North Fairfax Street,
Alexandria,
Virginia 22314
Tel: 703 548 7790

HYDROTHERAPY

Europe

The British College of Naturopathy
and Osteopathy
Lief House, 3 Sumpter Close,
120–122 Finchley Road,
London NW3 5HR, United Kingdom
Tel: 020 7435 6464
Fax: 020 7431 3630

Tyringham Naturopathic Clinic
Newport Pagnell, Bucks MK16 9ER,
United Kingdom
Tel: 01908 551935

HYPNOTHERAPY

Australia

Australian Society of Hypnosis (ASH)
Austin Hospital, Heidelberg, Victoria 3084

Canada

Canadian Society of Hypnosis (CSH)
Labelle, 7027 Edgemont Drive,
Calgary, Alberta T3A 2H9

Europe

British Society of Experimental and
Clinical Hypnosis
Department of Clinical Oncology,
Derby Royal Infirmary, London Road,
Derby DE1 2QY, United Kingdom
Tel: 01332 347141 ext. 4150

British Society of Medical and Dental
Hypnosis
17 Keppel View Road, Kimberworth,
Rotherham, South Yorks S61 2AR,
United Kingdom
Tel/Fax: 01709 554558

The Institute of Stress Management
57 Hall Lane, London NW4 4TJ,
United Kingdom

KINESIOLOGY

Australia

Association of Victoria
PO Box 155, Ormond, Vic 3204
Tel: 03 9578 1229

Europe

Body Balance UK Ltd
Kay McCaroll, 12 Golders Rise,
Hendon, London NW4 2HR,
United Kingdom
Tel: 020 8202 9747
Fax: 020 8202 3890

ICAK Executive European
Thea Marshal, 54 East Street, Andover,
Hampshire SP10 1ES, United Kingdom
Tel: 01264 339512

International College of Applied
Kinesiology UK
Donecchka Clinic, Mill Straight,
Southwater, W Sussex RH13 9EY,
United Kingdom

International Kinesiology College
Shifting
PO Box 3347, CH-8031 Zurich,
Switzerland
Tel: 41 1 272 4515

Maya Kraus
The Castle Street Clinic, 36 Castle Street,
Guildford GU1 3UQ, United Kingdom
Tel: 01483 300400
Fax: 01483 300 411

Mr E Levin
42 Harley Street, London W1,
United Kingdom
Tel: 020 7935 6202

South Africa

Association of Specialized Kinesiology
14 Osborne Road, Claremont,
7700 South Africa
Tel: 012 61 8021

USA

International College of Applied
Kinesiology
PO Box 25276, Shawnee Mission,
Kansas 66255-5276
Tel: 913 648 2828

MAGNETIC THERAPY

Europe

British Biomagnetic Association
31 St Marychurch Road, Torquay,
Devon TQ1 3JF, United Kingdom

MARMA THERAPY

Europe

The Hale Clinic
7 Park Crescent, London W1B 1PF,
United Kingdom
Tel: 020 7631 0156

The 101 Group of Practitioners
67 North Road, Parkstone, Poole,
Dorset BH14 0LT, United Kingdom

MASSAGE

Australia

Association of Massage Therapists
18A Spit Road, Mosman,
NSW 1088, Australia

Society of Clinical Masseurs
PO Box 483, 9 Delhi Street,
Mitcham 3131, Victoria
Tel: 613 874 6973

Canada

**Association of Physiotherapists &
Massage Practitioners of BC**
Suite 103, 1089 West Broadway,
Vancouver, BC V6H 0V3

Europe

Academy of Aromatherapy & Massage
50 Cow Wynd, Falkirk,
Stirlingshire FK1 1PU, United Kingdom
Tel: 01324 612658

British Massage Therapy Council
Greenbank House, 65a Adelphi Street,
Preston, Lancs PR1 7BH,
United Kingdom
Tel: 01772 881063

London College of Massage
5 Newman Passage, London W1T 1EH,
United Kingdom
Tel: 020 7323 3574
Fax: 020 7637 7125

Massage Training Institute
24 Highbury Road, London N5 2DQ,
United Kingdom
Tel: 020 7226 5313

Justin Sharma/Alison Underhill
87 North Road, Parkstone, Poole,
Dorset BH14 0LT, United Kingdom
(practice in London)

USA

**Association of Bodyworkers and
Massage Professionals**
28677 Buffalow Park Road,
Evergreen,
Colorado 80439
Tel: 303 674 8478
Fax: 303 674 0859

**International Association of Infant
Massage**
PO Box 438, Elma,
New York 14059-0438
Tel: 1 716 652 9789
Fax: 1 716 652 1990

MEDITATION

Australia

Counselling and Meditation Service
20 Pitt Street, Parramatta,
NSW 2150
Tel: 02 891 1628
Fax: 02 891 5675

USA

**Himalayan International Institute of
Yoga Science and Philosophy of the USA**
RR1, Box 400, Honesdale, PA 18431
Tel: 717 253 5551
Fax: 717 253 9078

Europe

Himalayan Institute of Great Britain
70 Claremont Road, West Ealing,
London W13 0DG, United Kingdom
Tel: 020 8991 8090

**The International School of
Meditation**
87 North Road, Parkstone, Poole,
Dorset BH14 0LT, United Kingdom
(practice in London)

The Kailash Centre
7 Newcourt Street, London NW8,
United Kingdom
Tel: 020 7722 3939

MUSIC THERAPY

Europe

**Association of Professional Music
Therapists**
Chestnut Cottage, 38 Pierce Lane,
Fulbourn, Cambridge CB1 5DL,
United Kingdom

British Society for Music Therapy
25 Rosslyn Avenue, East Barnet,
Hertfordshire EN4 8DH,
United Kingdom
Tel/Fax: 020 8368 8879

USA

**American Association for Music
Therapy**
PO Box 80012, Valley Forge, PA 19484
Tel: 610 265 4006

**National Association for Music
Therapy**
8455 Colesville Road, Suite 930,
Silver Spring, MD 20920
Tel: 301 589 3300
Fax: 301 589 5175

NATUROPATHY

Australia

**Australia Naturopathy Practitioners
and Chiropractors Association**
1st Floor, 609 Camberwell Road,
Camberwell, Vic 3124

**Australian Natural Therapists
Association (ATNA)**
PO Box 308, Melrose Park,
South Australia 5039
Tel: 61 8 371 3222
Fax: 61 8 297 0003

**Federation of Natural and Traditional
Therapists (FNTT)**
238 Ballarat Road, Victoria 3011
Tel: 61 3 9318 3057

Europe

**British College of Naturopathy and
Osteopathy**
3 Sumpter Close, 120-22 Finchley Road,
London NW3 5HR, United Kingdom
Tel: 020 7435 6464
Fax: 020 7431 3630

Dr Harald Gaier
The 101 Group of Practitioners,
87 North Road, Parkstone, Poole,
Dorset BH14 0LT, United Kingdom
(practice in London)

General Council and Register of Naturopaths
Goswell House, 2 Goswell Road, Street,
Somerset BA16 0JG, United Kingdom
Tel: 01458 840072
Fax: 01458 840075

USA

American Association of Naturopathic Physicians
2366 Eastlake Avenue East, Suite 322,
Seattle, Washington 98102
Tel: 206 323 8510

American Naturopathic Association
1413 King Street, First Floor,
Washington DC 20005
Tel: 202 682 7352
Fax: 202 289 2027

NEURO-LINGUISTIC PROGRAMMING (NLP)

Australia

The Australian Institute of NLP
c/o Askawn Quality Solutions Pty Ltd,
PO Box 31, Kippa-Ring, Queensland 4021
Tel: 07 3204 0824
Fax: 07 3204 0825

Europe

Nancy Blake/Ross Myers
102 Park Avenue, Kingston-Upon-
Hull, East Yorkshire HU5 3ET,
United Kingdom

Lynne Crawford
The Hale Clinic,
7 Park Crescent, London W1B 1PF,
United Kingdom
Tel: 020 7631 0156

The Institute of Stress Management
57 Hall Lane, London NW4 4TJ,
United Kingdom

Dominique Radclyffe
87 North Road, Parkstone, Poole,
Dorset BH14 0LT, United Kingdom
(practice in London)

NEUROTHERAPY

Europe

The 101 Group of Practitioners
87 North Road, Parkstone, Poole,
Dorset BH14 0LT, United Kingdom
(practice in London)

NUTRITIONISTS/DIETETICS

Europe

Cotswold Allergy Clinic
Trinders Cottage, Calcot, Colm St
Denys, Cheltenham, Gloucestershire
GL54 3JZ, United Kingdom
Fax: 01285 720 931

Dominique Radclyffe
The Kailash Centre,
7 Newcourt Street, London NW8,
United Kingdom
Tel: 020 7722 3939

OSTEOPATHY

Australia

Australian Osteopathy Association
PO Box 699, Turramurra,
NSW 2074
Tel: 02 4494799

Chiropractors and Osteopaths' Registration
Board of Victoria, P O Box 59,
Carlton Street, Victoria 3053
Tel: 61 3 349 3000
Fax: 61 3 349 3003

NSW Chiropractors and Osteopathic Registration Board
PO Box K599, Haymarket, NSW 2000
Tel: 61 2 281 0884
Fax: 61 2 281 2030

Europe

The Camden Practice
West Hill House, 6 Swains Lane,
London N6 6QU, United Kingdom

General Osteopathic Council and Osteopathic Information Service
Premier House, 10 Greycoat Place,
London SW1P 1SB, United Kingdom
Tel: 020 7357 6655

Richard Field/Andrew Mullen
87 North Road, Parkstone, Poole,
Dorset BH14 0LT United Kingdom
(practice in London)

USA

American Academy of Osteopathy
3500 DePauw Boulevard, Suite 1080,
Indianopolis, Indiana 46268-139
Tel: 317 879 1881
Fax: 317 879 0563

American Association of Colleges of Osteopathic Medicine
6110 Executive, Boulevard Apt 405,
Rockville, Maryland 20852
Tel: 301 468 0990

American Osteopathic Association
142 East Ohio Street, Chicago,
Illinois 60611
Tel: 312 280 5800
Fax: 312 280 3860

POLARITY THERAPY

Europe

The Federation of Polarity Training
7 Nunney Close, Golden Valley,
Cheltenham, Gloucestershire
GL51 0TU, United Kingdom

The Castle Street Clinic
36 Castle Street, Guildford GU1 3UQ,
United Kingdom
Tel: 01483 300400
Fax: 01483 400 411

UK Polarity Therapy Association
Monomark House,
27 Old Gloucester Street, London
WC1N 3XX, United Kingdom
Tel: 0700 7052748

Zero Balancing Association UK
36 Richmond Road, Cambridge
CB4 3PU, United Kingdom
Tel/Fax: 01223 315480

USA

American Polarity Therapy Association
2888 Bluff Street\Suite 149, Boulder, Colorado 80301
Tel: 303 545 2080
Fax: 303 545 2161

Zero Balancing Association
PO Box 1727, Capitola, California 95010
Tel: 408 476 0665

PSYCHOTHERAPY

(*see also* **Counselling**)

Europe

British Association of Psychotherapists
37 Mapesbury Road, London NW2 4HJ, United Kingdom
Tel: 020 8452 9823
Fax: 020 8452 5182

European Association for Psychotherapy (EAP)
Rosenbursenstrasse, 8/3/7
a-1010 Vienna, Austria
Tel: 0043 1 512 7090
Fax: 0043 1 512 7091

UK Council for Psychotherapy
167–9 Great Portland Street, London W1N 5F, United Kingdom
Tel: 020 7436 3002
Fax: 020 7436 3013

USA

American Psychological Association
750 First Street NE, Washington, DC20002
Tel: 415 327 2066

Association for Humanistic Psychology (International)
45 Franklin Street, 315 San Francisco, CA 94102

International Transpersonal Association
20 Sunnyside Avenue, A-257 Mill Valley, CA 94941
Tel: 415 389 6912

QI GONG

Australia

Qi Gong Association of Australia
458 White Horse Road, Surrey Hills, Victoria 3127
Tel: 03 836 6961

Europe

The Institute of Stress Management
57 Hall Lane, London NW4 4TJ, United Kingdom

Tse Qigong Centre
PO Box 59, Altrincham, Cheshire WA15 8FS, United Kingdom
Tel: 0161 929 4485
Fax: 0161 929 4489

USA

Qi Gong Human Life Research Foundation
PO Box 5327, Cleveland, Ohio 44101
Tel: 216 475 4712

Qi Gong Institute
East West Academy of Healing Arts
450 Sutter Street, Suite 916, San Francisco, California 94108
Tel: 415 788 2227/323 1221

Qi Gong Resources Associates
1755 Homets Road, Pasadena, California 94122
Tel: 818 564 9751

RADIESTHESIA/RADIONICS

Europe

Confederation of Radionic and Radiesthesic Organisations
Maperton, Wincanton, Somerset BA9 8EH, United Kingdom

The Radionic Association
Baerlein House, Goose Green, Deddington, Banbury, Oxon OX15 0SZ, United Kingdom
Tel/Fax: 01869 338852

REFLEXOLOGY

Australia

Association of Reflexology
2 Stewart Avenue, Matraville, NSW 2036
Tel: 02 311 2322

Canada

Cecile Myslicki
70 Parkville Drive, Winnipeg, Manitobe R2M 2H5
Tel: 204 253 9375

Karen Nel
1951 Glenarie Avenue, North Vancouver V7P 1X9
Tel: 604 986 7121

Europe

Association of Reflexologists
27 Old Gloucester Street, London WC1N 3XX
Tel: 0870 5673320

Carol Bosiger
PO Box 93, Tadworth, Surrey KT20 7JL, United Kingdom
Tel/Fax: 01737 842961

Alberto Carnevale-Maffe
Via Procaccini 47, Milan, Italy
Tel/Fax: 39 2 311116

Ann-Chatrine Jonsson
Varmlandsvagen 438, 12348 Farsta, Sweden
Tel/Fax: 46 8 942 485

Karine van Niekerk
Frankenstraat 31A, 2582 SE Den Haag, Netherlands
Tel: 31 70 354 304

Andrea Schippers
Domkeweg 23, 37213 Witzenhausen, Germany
Tel: 49 5542 71463

Lena Walters
Vale Da Telha, Apartado 173, Aljezue 8670, Algarve, Portugal
Tel: 351 82 98566

South Africa

Inge Dougans
PO Box 68283, Bryanston,
Johannesburg 2021
Tel/Fax: 27 11 706 4206

USA

Jill Tonkovich
2222 Kilkare Parkway, Pt Pleasant,
New Jersey 08742
Tel: 908 892 7566

ROLFING

Australia

Rolf Institute
Pacific Branch Office, 28 Davies Street
Brunswick 3056, Victoria
Tel: 61 3 383 5045

Europe

The Rolfing Institute
PO Box 14793, London SW1V 2WB,
United Kingdom

Rolf Institute: European Branch Office
Herzogstrasse 40, D-800 Munich 40,
Germany
Tel: 49 8939 6802

USA

The Rolf Institute
205 Canyon Boulevard, Boulder,
Colorado 80302-4920
Tel: 303 449 5903
Fax: 303 449 5978

SHIATSU

Australia

**The Shiatsu Therapy Association of
Australia**
332 Carlisle Street, Balaclava, 3183 Victoria
Tel: 039530 0067

Europe

Paul Lambeth
Albert Cottage, Town Head, Alston,
Cumbria CA9 3SR, United Kingdom
Tel: 01434 381 088

The Shiatsu College of London
Kim Lovelace, 25 Parchment Street,
Chichester, W. Sussex PO19 3BX,
United Kingdom
Tel: 01243 778599
(courses run in London)

Shiatsu Society of Ireland
Greenville Lodge, Esker Road, Lucan,
Co. Dublin

The Shiatsu Society (UK)
Eastlands Court, St Peters Road, Rugby
CV21 3QP, United Kingdom
Tel: 01788 555051

Michael Woolly/Ismail Mazzara
87 North Road, Parkstone, Poole,
Dorset BH14 0LT, United Kingdom
(practice in London)

Japan

Japanese Shiatsu College
2-15-6 Koishikawa, Bunkyoku, Tokyo
Tel: 00 813 3813 7354

Iokai Centre
1-8-9 Higashiuena, Daito-Ku, Tokyo

SOUND THERAPY

Europe

The Hale Clinic
7 Park Crescent, London W1N 3HE,
United Kingdom
Tel: 020 7631 0156

Inner Sound
8 Elms Avenue, London N10 2JP,
United Kingdom

The Tomatis Centre UK Ltd
3 Wallands Crescent, Lewes,
E Sussex BN7 2QT, United Kingdom
Tel: 01273 474 877
Fax: 01273 487 500

TAI CHI CH'UAN

Europe

The Institute of Stress Management
57 Hall Lane, London NW4 4TJ

The North Pole School of Tai Chi
83 St Quintin Avenue, London W10 6PB
United Kingdom

Tai Chi Union for Great Britain
23 Oakwood Avenue, Mitcham,
Surrey CR4 3DQ, United Kingdom

The UK Tai Chi Association
PO Box 159, Bromley,
Kent BR1 3XX, United Kingdom

VITAMINS AND MINERALS

Australia

**Australian College of Nutritional and
Environmental Medicine**
13 Hilton Road, Beamaris,
Victoria 3193
Tel: 03 9589 6088

Canada

**Canadian College of Naturopathic
Medicine**
60 Berl Avenue, Etobicoke,
Ontario M8Y 3C7
Tel: 416 251 5261

National Institute of Nutrition
2565 Carling Avenue, Suite 400, Ottawa,
Ontario K1Z 8R1
Tel: 613 235 3355

Europe

**The Council for Nutrition Education
of Therapy (CNEAT)**
1 The Close, Halton, Aylesbury,
Buckinghamshire HP22 5NJ,
United Kingdom

Health Development Agency
Holborn Gate, 330 High Holborn,
London WC1V 7BA, United Kingdom
Tel: 020 7430 0850
Fax: 020 7061 3390

Institute of Optimum Nutrition
Blades Court, Dodar Road,
London SW15 2MU, United Kingdom
Tel: 020 8877 9993
Fax: 020 8877 9980

Nutritional Science Research Institute
Mulberry Tree Road, Brookthorpe,
Gloucester GL4 0UU, United Kingdom

The 101 Group Dispensary
87 North Road, Parkstone, Poole,
Dorset BH14 0LT
United Kingdom
(practice in London)

The Vegetarian Society
Parkdale, Dunham Road,
Altrincham, Cheshire WA14 4QG,
United Kingdom
Tel: 0161 928 0793

USA

American College of Advancement in Medicine
PO Box 3427, Laguna Hills,
California 92654

VIZUALIZATION
(see also **Psychotherapy** *and* **Counselling**)

Europe

Holistic Health and Healing Centre
10 Connaught Hill, Loughton,
Essex IG10 4DU, United Kingdom

The International School of Meditation
87 North Road, Parkstone, Poole,
Dorset BH14 0LT *(practice in London)*

USA

Academy for Guided Imagery
PO Box 2070, Mill Valley,
CA 94942
Tel: 800 726 2070

YOGA

Australia

BKS Iyengar Association of Australia
1 Rickman Avenue, Mosman, 2088 NSW
Tel: 2 9969 4052

International Yoga Teachers' Association
c/o 14/15 Huddart Avenue,
Normanhurst
NSW 2076

Canada

Sivananda Yoga Vedanta Centre
5178 St Lawrence, Boulevard,
Montreal, Quebec H2T 1R8

Sivananda Yoga Vedanta Centre
77 Harbord Street, Toronto,
Ontario M5S 1G4

Unity Yoga International
303 2495 West 2nd Avenue,
Vancouver, British Columbia VKG 1J5

Europe

British Wheel of Yoga
25 Jermyn Street, Sleaford, Lincs
NG34 7RU, United Kingdom
Tel: 01529 306851
Fax: 01529 303233

Institute of Iyengar Yoga
223A Randolf Avenue,
London W9 1NL,
United Kingdom
Tel/Fax: 020 7624 3080

Kailash Centre
7 Newcourt Street, London NW8,
United Kingdom
Tel: 020 7722 3939

Kitty Kennedy
87 North Road, Parkstone, Poole,
Dorset BH14 0LT *(practice in London)*

Patanjali Yoga Centre & Ashram
The Cottage, Marley Lane,
Battle, Sussex TN33 0RE,
United Kingdom
Tel/Fax: 01424 870 538

Sivananda Yoga Vendanta Centre
51 Felsham Road,
London SW15 1AZ,
United Kingdom
Tel: 020 8780 0160
Fax: 020 8780 0128

Yoga for Health Foundation
Ickwell Bury, Biggleswade,
Bedfordshire SG18 9EF
Tel: 01767 627271

USA

International Association of Yoga Therapists
109 Hillside Avenue,
Mill Valley,
California 94941
Tel: 415 383 4587
Fax: 415 381 0876

Sivananda Yoga Vendanta Centre
243 West 24th Street,
New York 10011

Unity in Yoga International
PO Box 281004, Lakewood,
Colorado 80228

Unity Yoga International
7918 Bolling Drive, Alexandria,
Virginia 22308

Yogaville
Buckingham, Virginia 23921

ZEN

Europe

The Buddhist Society
58 Eccleston Square,
London SW1V 1PH,
United Kingdom
Tel: 020 7834 5858
Fax: 020 7976 5238

INDEX